Gustavo Machicote Goth

# Canine and Feline DERMATOLOGY ATLAS

SECOND EDITION

Foreword by
**Candace Sousa**

edra
PUBLISHING

This book was originally published in Spanish under the title:
*Atlas de dermatología canina y felina. 2.ª edición*

ISBN Spanish edition: 978-84-18339-56-1

**Canine and Feline Dermatology Atlas. Second Edition**
**Gustavo Machicote Goth**


ISBN: 978-1-957260-31-0
eISBN: 978-1-957260-39-6

Book Publishing Manager: Ana Hernández Marín, Grupo Asís Biomedia SL, Zaragoza, Spain
Illustrator: Jacob Gragera Artal, Grupo Asís Biomedia SL, Zaragoza, Spain
Cover, Layout and Copyediting: Grupo Asís Biomedia SL, Zaragoza, Spain
Translation: Owen Howard
Project Manager: Teresa García Rubio, Grupo Asís Biomedia SL, Zaragoza, Spain



**Edra Publishing US LLC**
3309 Northlake Boulevard, Suite 203
Palm Beach Gardens, FL, 33403
EIN: 844113980
info@edrapublishing.com
www.edrapublishing.com

edra
PUBLISHING

Printed by Monterreina Comunicación, Pinto (Madrid), España, January 2023

# DEDICATION

Nine years after the publication of the first edition of this atlas, I believe that the original acknowledgements hold true. Family, friends, colleagues, and pets in the ideal environment make for a full life and accomplishment of one's projects. This has been even more evident in the context of the COVID-19 pandemic, during which we have been able to appreciate the true value of these relationships, whether in person or through virtual contact, a form of communication that seems so natural to us now.

I dedicate this book to my wife, Lina, and to my two daughters, María José and Carolina, to all my family and, of course, to my dogs and cats who keep me company during my hours of study and writing.

I also dedicate this book to all my veterinary colleagues, who have taught me so much during my long career, both those who have shared time with me in the clinic and the many colleagues on either side of the Atlantic who have shared the same passion: animal health. These animals motivate us every day and teach us behaviours that, although basic, are full of kindness and affection, and from which we can continually learn. When we provide them with medical care, we are caring not only for their health, but also for the emotions, affections, and needs of their owners.

**Gustavo Machicote Goth**

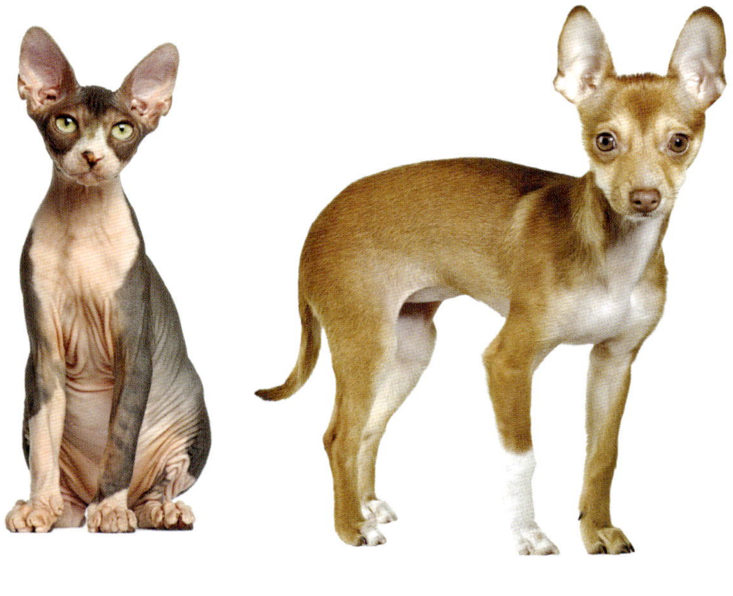

# THE AUTHOR

## GUSTAVO MACHICOTE GOTH

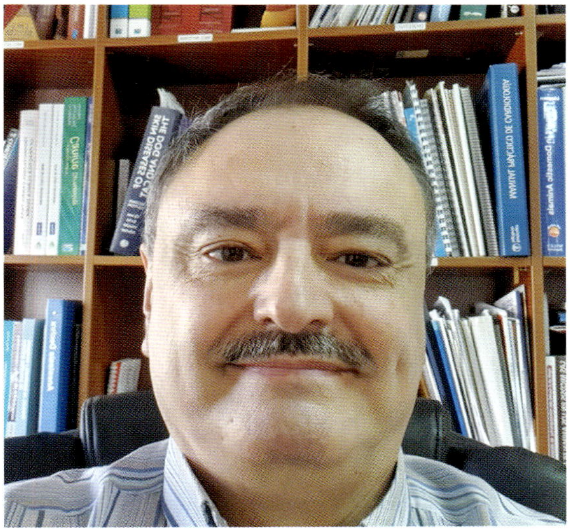

Gustavo Machicote Goth was awarded his degree in Veterinary Medicine from the University of Buenos Aires, Argentina. He is a veterinary practitioner at the Vilanova Veterinary Clinic and head of the Dermapet dermatology referral service in Santiago de Compostela and Vilanova de Arousa, Spain. He has acquired over 25 years of experience in dermatology, a specialty that he continues to practice exclusively.

He is a member of the scientific committee of the GEDA (the specialist dermatology group of the Spanish Association of Small Animal Specialists [AVEPA]), of which he was secretary from 2004 to 2008; a full member of the European Society of Veterinary Dermatology (ESVD); certified in dermatology by the European School for Advanced Veterinary Studies (ESAVS); and AVEPA-certified in dermatology. He has taught numerous training courses in dermatology in different countries in South and North America and in Europe.

He has published a range of articles on dermatology in both national and international journals. He is coauthor of several books and author of *Dermatología canina y felina* (Canine and Feline Dermatology), *Canine and Feline Dermatology Atlas*, *Servet Clinical Guides: Allergies* and *Guía Servet de Manejo Clínico: Prurito en perros y gatos* (Servet Clinical Guides: Pruritus in Dogs and Cats).

He works as a dermatology consultant for multiple veterinary consulting services.

He was awarded the Miguel Luera Award from AVEPA in both 2005 and 2017. He holds a Master's degree in Oncology from AEVA and the Miguel de Cervantes European University.

# FOREWORD

It is an honor to have been asked to write the foreword for the second edition of the *Canine and Feline Dermatology Atlas*, authored by Dr. Gustavo Machicote Goth. It makes my heart sing to know that there is another veterinarian who shares my passion for veterinary dermatology. I spent most my veterinary career practicing and teaching this specialty and recognize how important it is to both veterinarians and pet owners.

Dermatology constitutes a large percentage of the cases seen in a small animal clinic. One common thing practitioners say is that dermatology can be challenging. This is primarily because they are looking for the best way to manage, cure or control a condition without knowing exactly what they are treating. Success first involves obtaining an accurate diagnosis so that we can prescribe the best and safest therapies, and much of the diagnosis relies on the physical examination.

In this atlas, Gustavo has assembled a collection of hundreds of beautiful images of a wide variety of dermatologic conditions of dogs and cats and presents them in a logical and orderly way. He brings a wealth of clinical experience, and the fabulous pictures are what make this book so unique.

There are many good dermatology textbooks currently available, but few of them can be as clinically useful as this atlas. For each of the conditions described, clinical—and many times histopathologic—pictures are provided, along with a short discussion of their etiopathogenesis, diagnostic methods and treatment. This book can therefore help the veterinarian develop a list of differentials, decide on the diagnostic tests to be performed and select the most appropriate therapy.

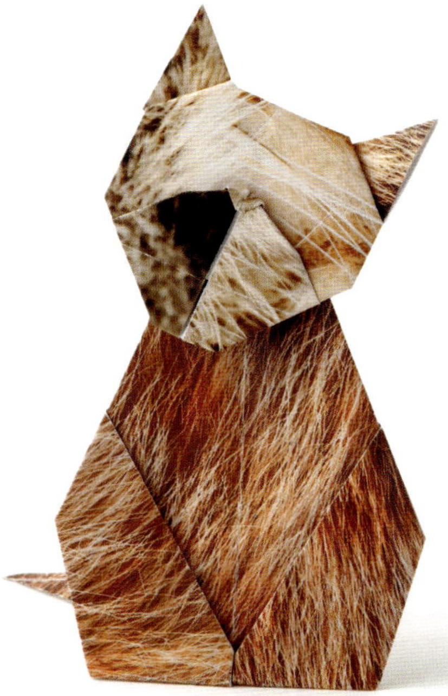

This book will be extremely useful for veterinary students, general practitioners, veterinary assistants and even dermatology specialists. The first chapter should be particularly helpful to veterinary students and recent graduates as it introduces dermatology, including lesion and pattern recognition

I invite you all to use and share this beautiful atlas, which will help us to further advance in treating dogs and cats with skin disease. I thank Gustavo for continuing to share his knowledge with all who love and treat animals.

**Candace Sousa**, DVM
DABVP (Emeritus), Canine & Feline
DACVD (Emeritus)

# PREFACE

The clear objective of this second edition is to update and improve the atlas' graphical content, with the addition of many new images, as well as the written content, which has been updated in accordance with the latest therapeutic and diagnostic advances. In addition, some clinical pictures not included in the first edition have been added.

The aim of this atlas has always been to help clinicians recognise the different dermatoses encountered in routine clinical practice. While dermatology is based on direct observation of the affected organ, which should theoretically facilitate diagnosis, it is not always easy to find pathognomonic images of a disease, and differential diagnoses should always be considered when establishing the most likely diagnosis

Part of the value of this atlas is that it associates the clinical picture, the presentation, with the likely corresponding dermatological pattern and diagnoses.

In this second edition the image gallery has been expanded, in many cases including corresponding cytology or microscopy images that can help establish diagnosis.

As the author, I will be more than happy if this atlas helps veterinary clinicians to orient diagnoses and resolve cases.

**Gustavo Machicote Goth**

# Table of contents



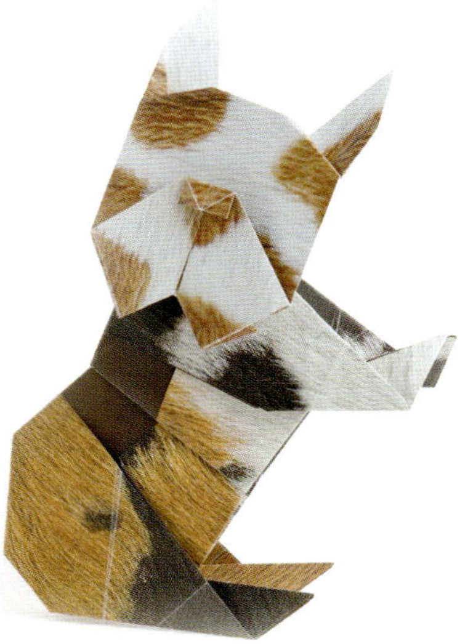

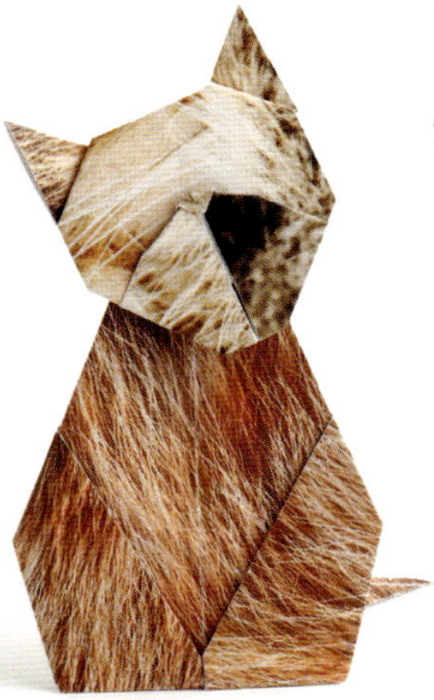

# 01

# Introduction to dermatological diagnosis

# Introduction

After years of experience in dermatological clinical practice, the most characteristic presentations of skin diseases become etched in one's memory. Phenotypic expression describes the ways in which these clinical pictures manifest, and is the consequence of biomolecular mechanisms called endotypes.

A disease can manifest with different phenotypic expressions depending on the characteristics of the affected individual (e.g. breed, age).

Dermatological diagnosis is based mainly on the ability to recognise lesions and knowledge of why they occur (i.e. aetiology and pathogenesis).

Therefore, visual examination of the presentation is often essential and in most cases, together with a thorough clinical history, allows us to draw up a list of differential or more probable diagnoses compatible with the disease. How comprehensive this list is will depend in part on the veterinary clinician's proficiency (visual memory and questioning the owner).

In dermatology, it is very important to be able to recognise primary and secondary lesions, which, depending on their presence either alone or in combination, describe the macroscopic clinical picture of the disease. In this introductory chapter we will review these primary and secondary lesions (see below).

| Primary lesions | Secondary lesions |
|---|---|
| • Macule | • Scale |
| • Papule | • Crust |
| • Plaque | • Scar |
| • Pustule | • Erosion |
| • Vesicle | • Epidermal collarette |
| • Bulla | • Ulcer |
| • Nodule | • Comedone |
| • Tumour | • Fissure |
| • Cyst | • Excoriation |
| • Wheal | • Lichenification |
| | • Hyper/hypopigmentation |
| | • Callus (hyperkeratosis) |

These lesions can occur in combination, creating clinical patterns that, together with a particular distribution on the animal's body and specific clinical signs, produce the clinical picture of a given dermatological disease.

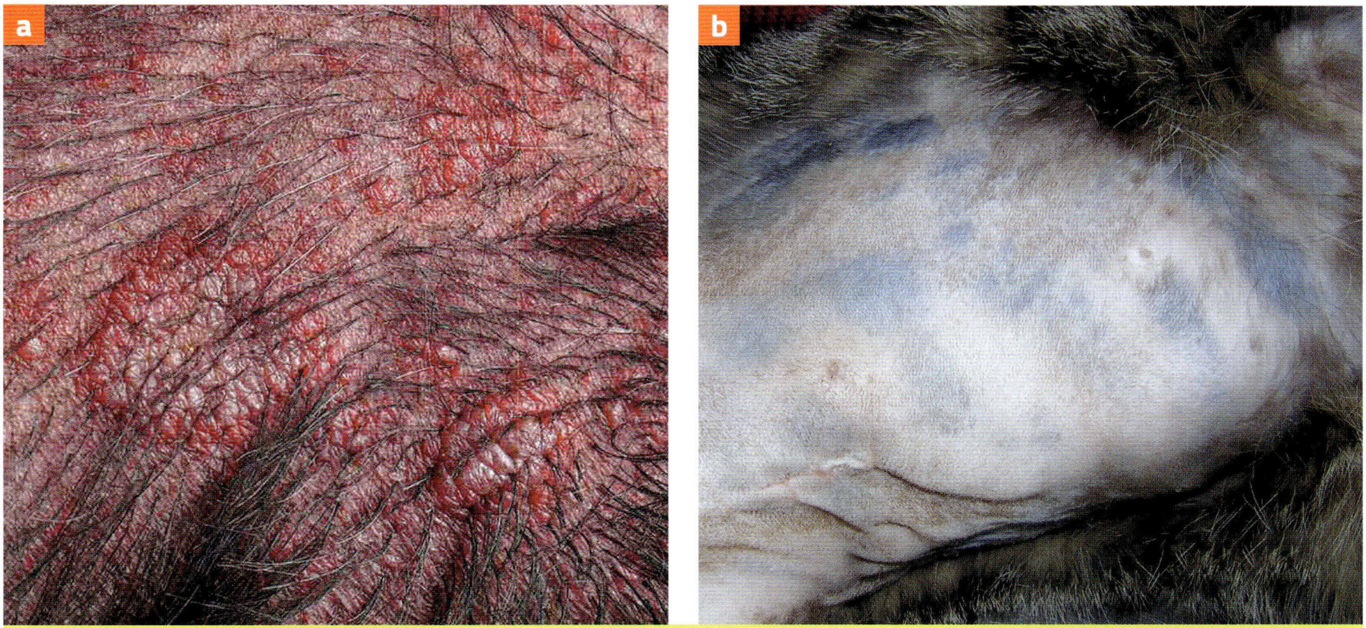

01 Erythematous macules (a); macules in the deep dermis caused by melanin incontinence (b).

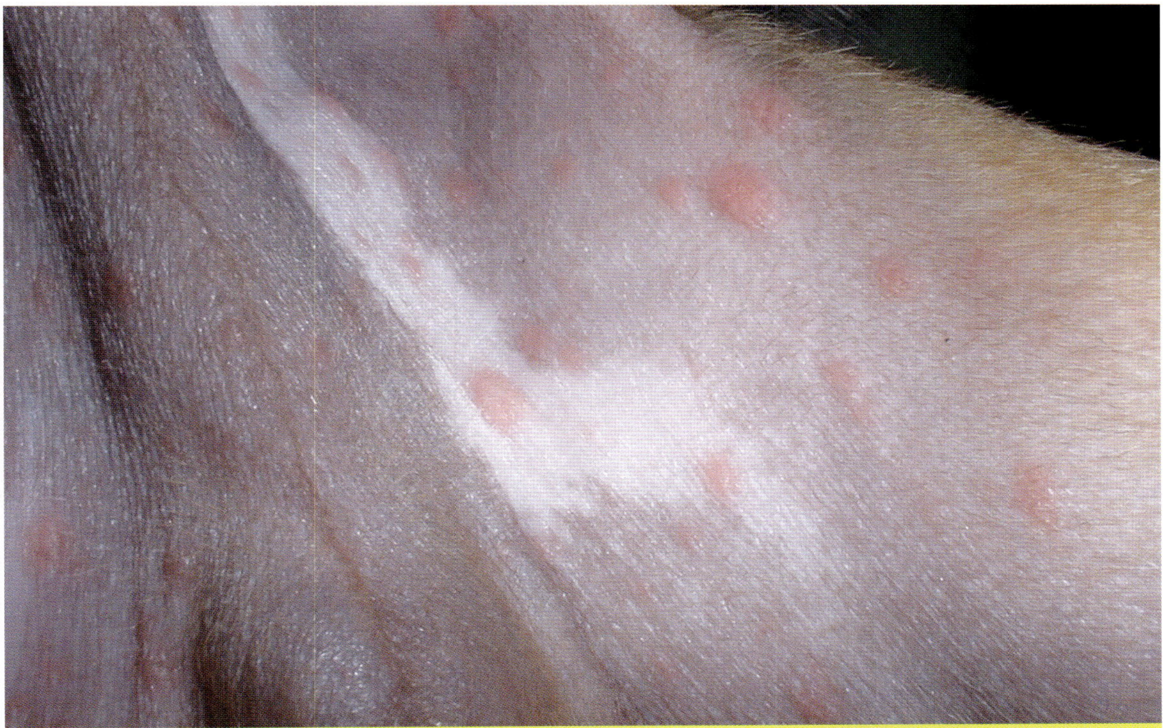

02 Papules in an allergic reaction.

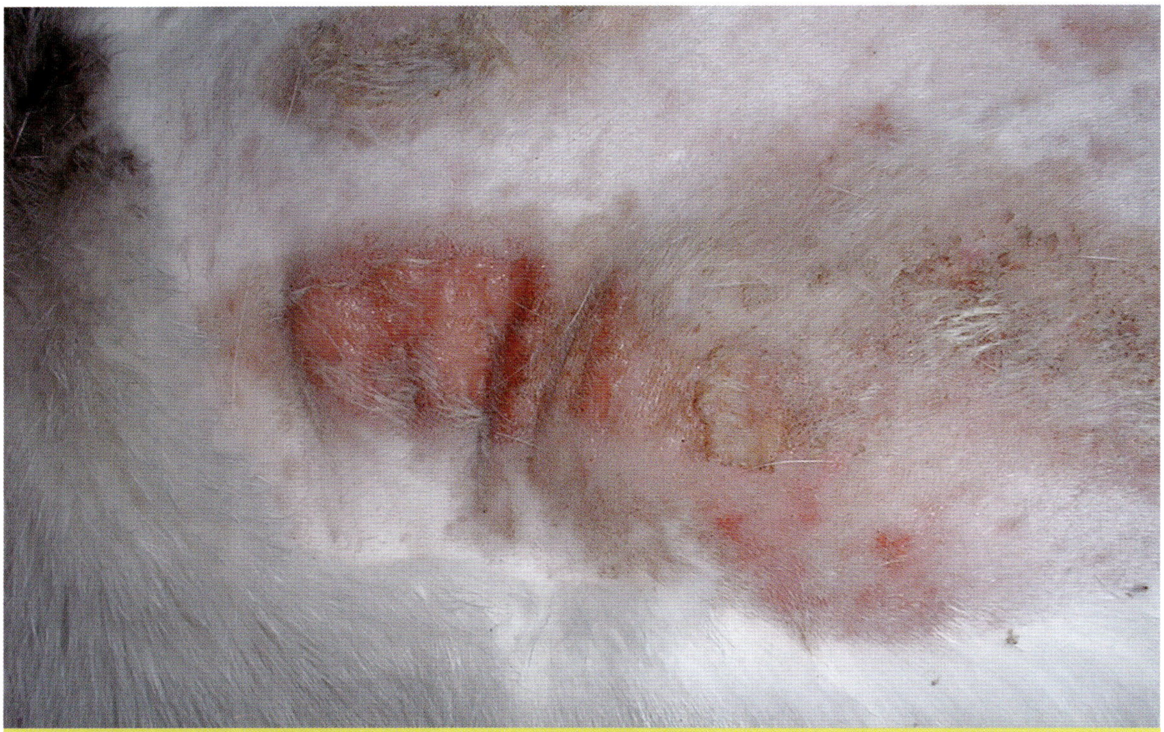

03 Eosinophilic plaque.

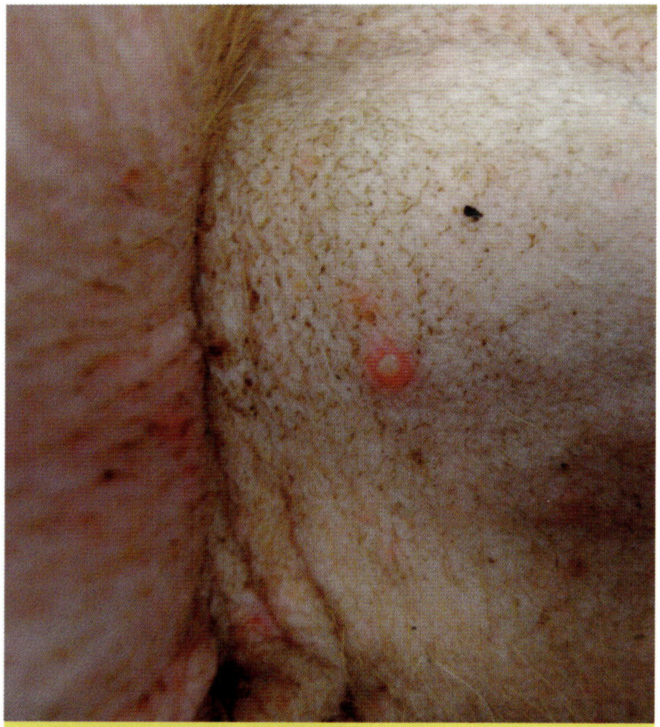

04 Pustule in a case of pyoderma.

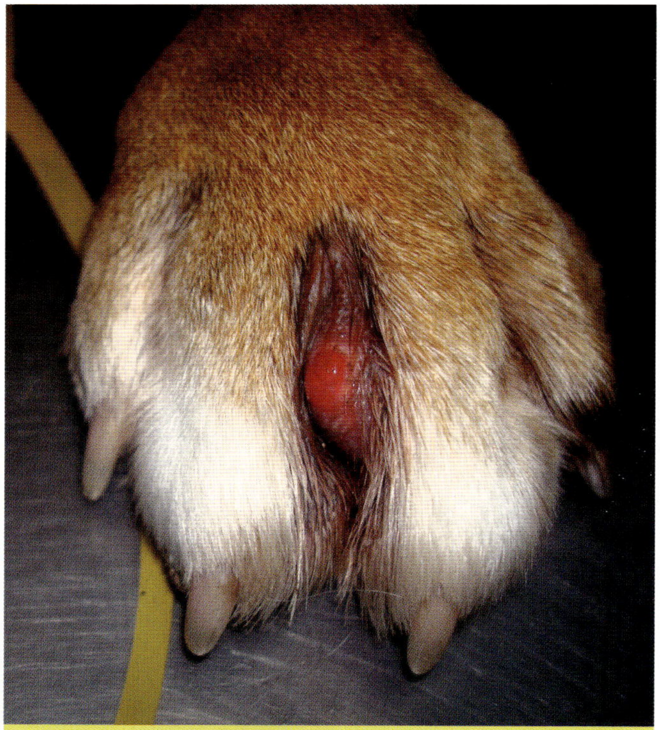

05 Vesicle caused by an interdigital cyst.

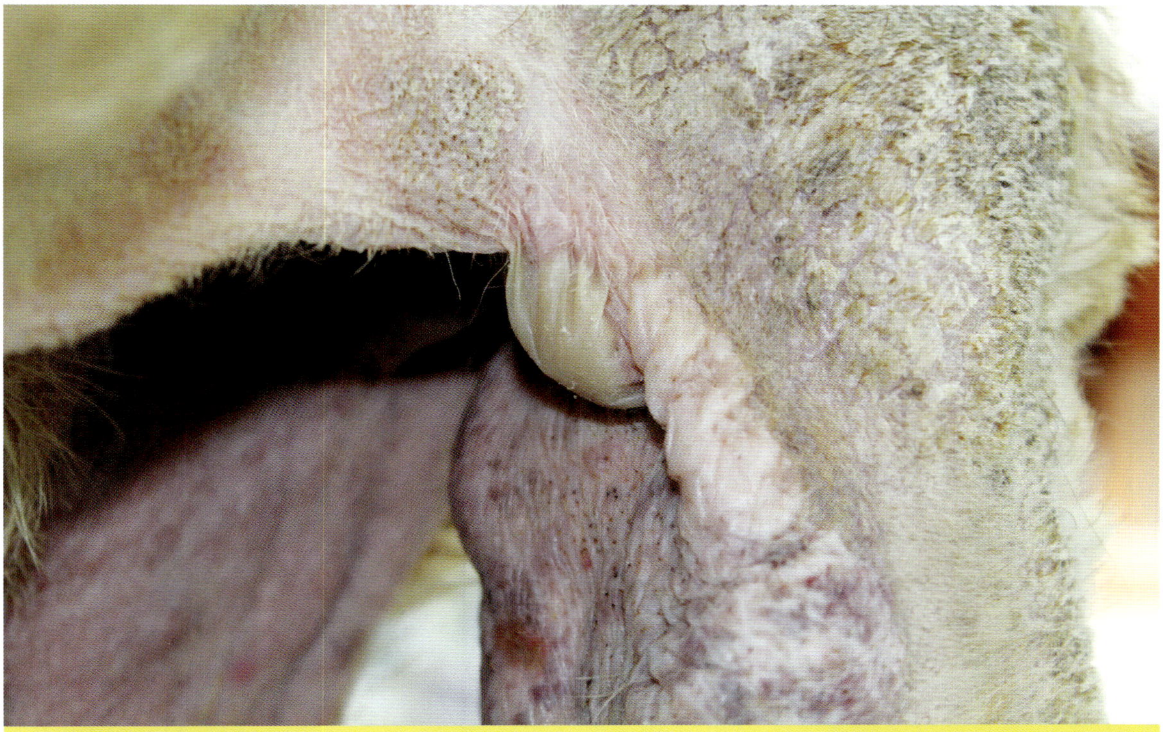

06 Purulent bulla due to autoimmune dermatosis.

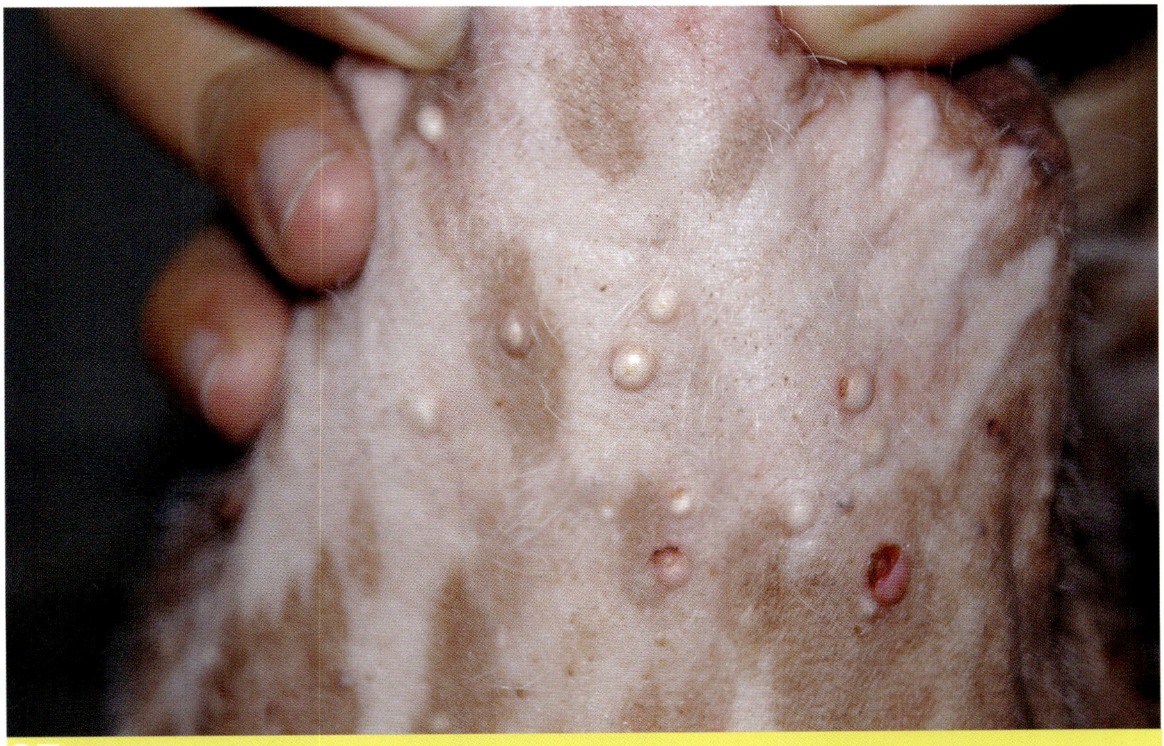

07 Hamartoma nodules.

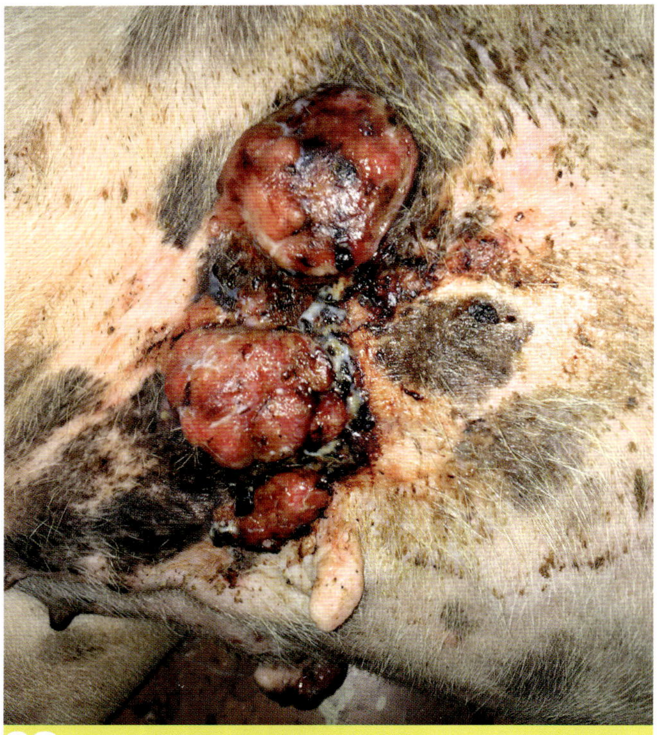

08 Squamous cell carcinoma.

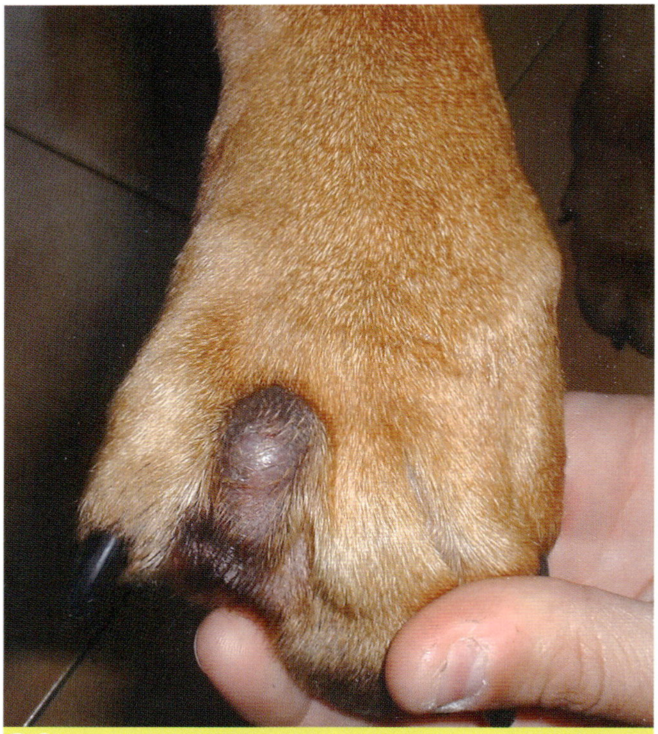

09 Interdigital cyst.

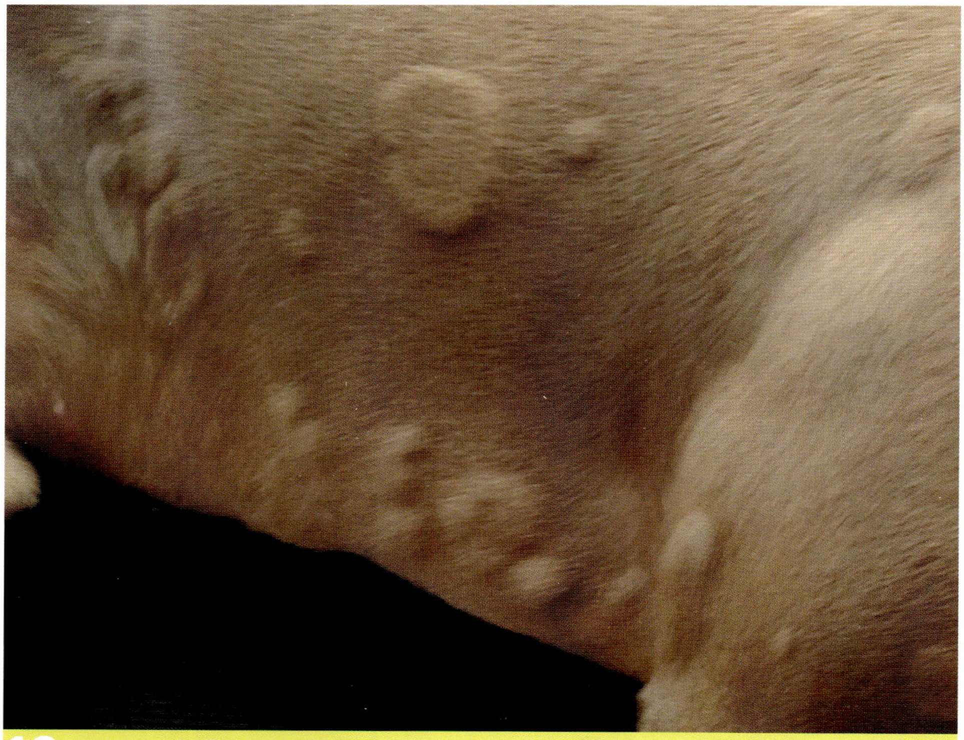

10 Wheals in a case of urticaria.

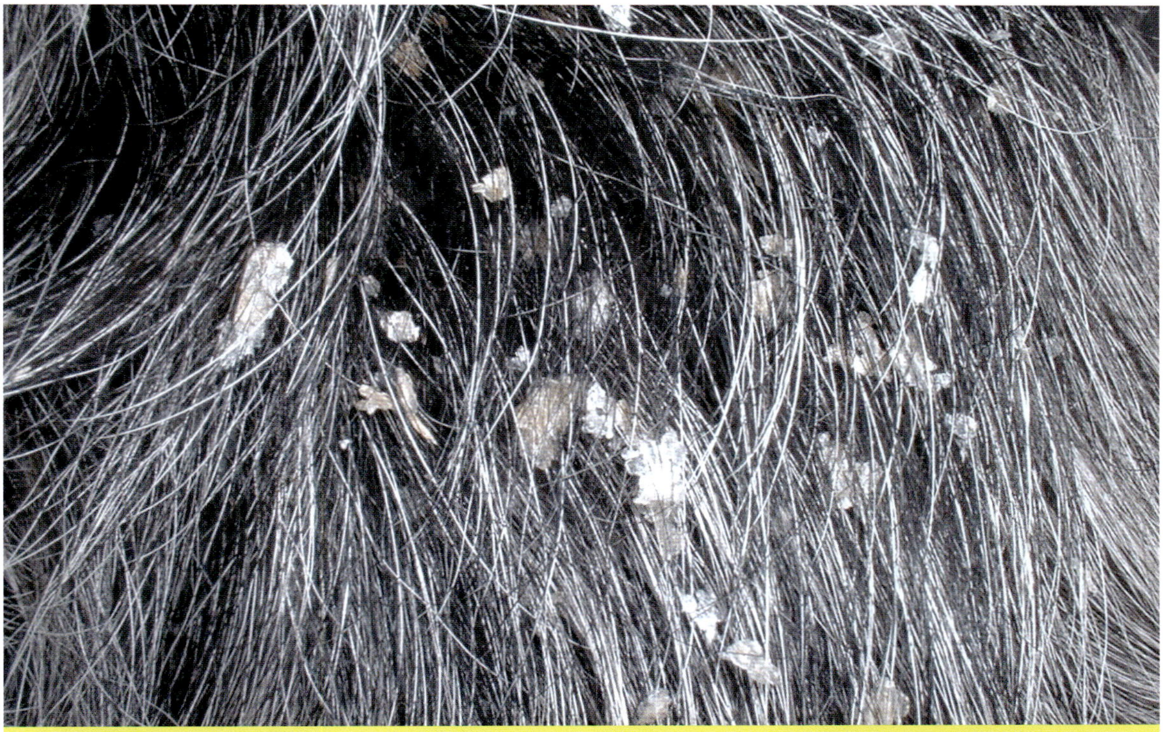

11 Scales in a seborrhoeic disorder.

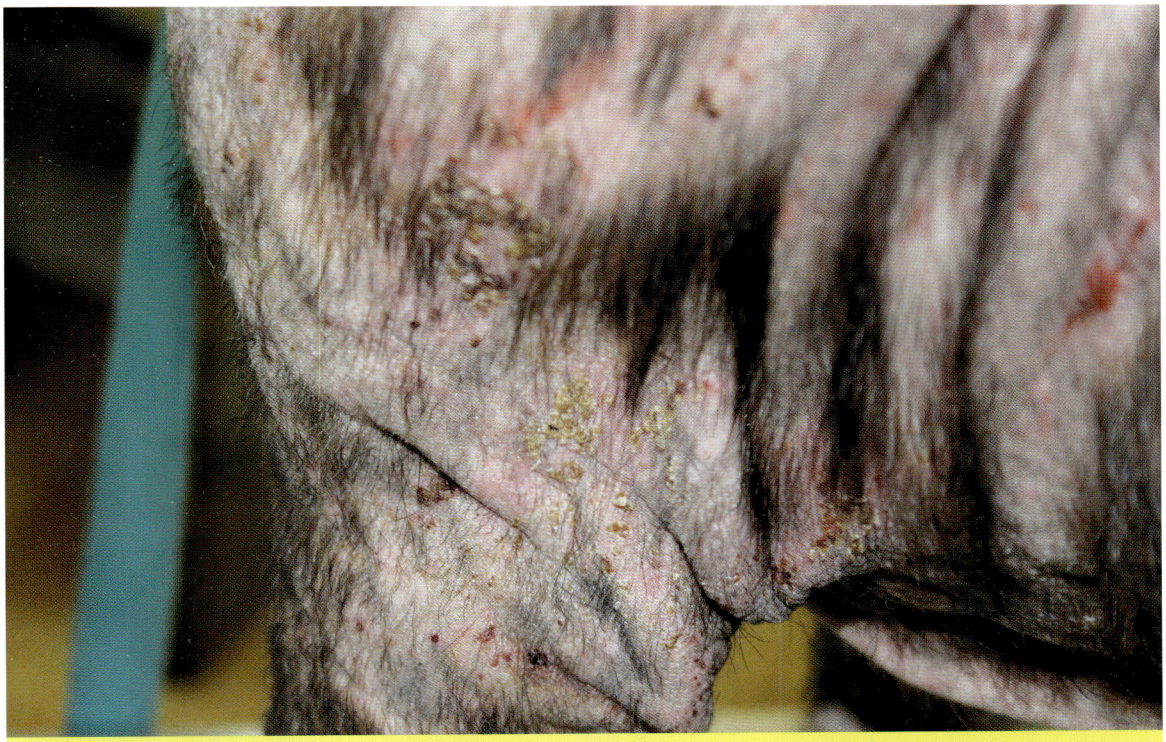

12 Crusts in a dog with scabies.

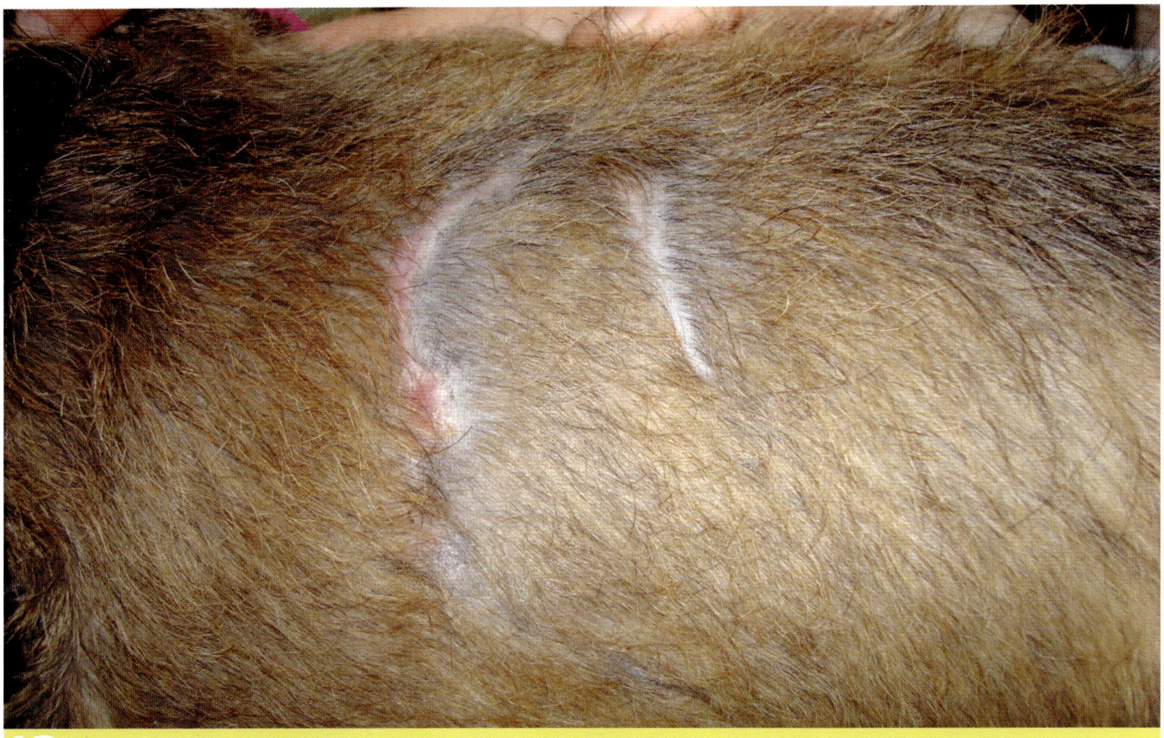

13 Scar.

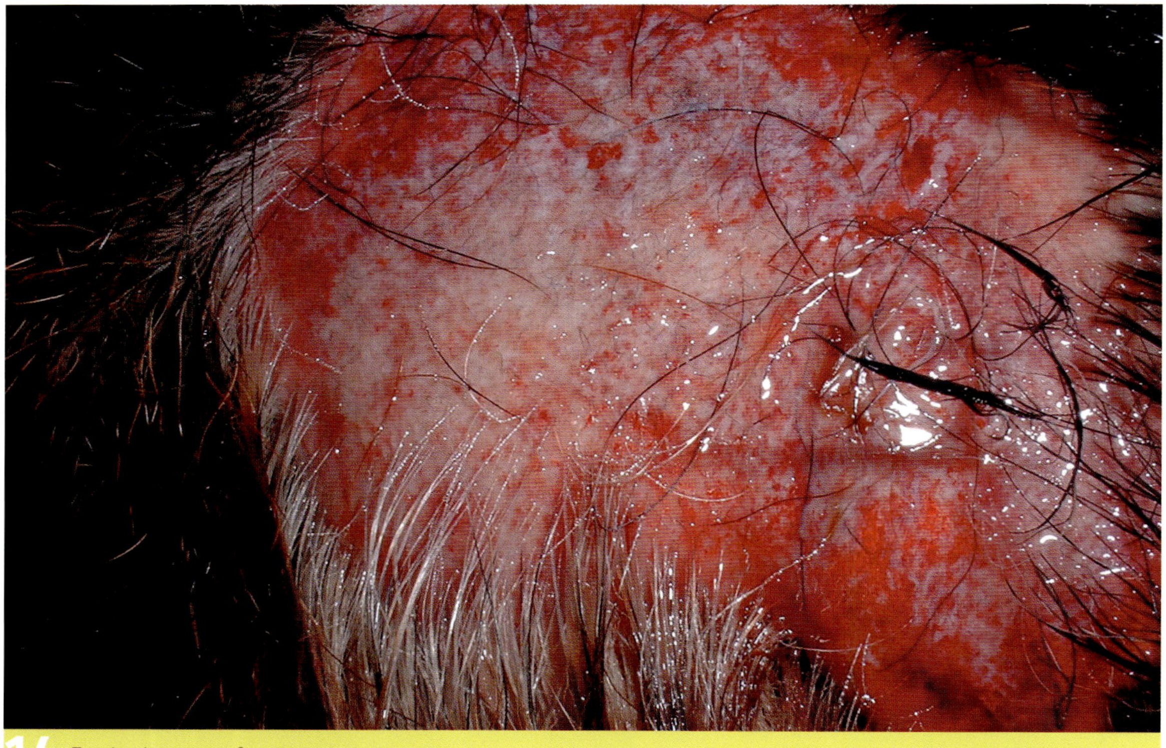

14 Erosion in a case of pyotraumatic dermatitis.

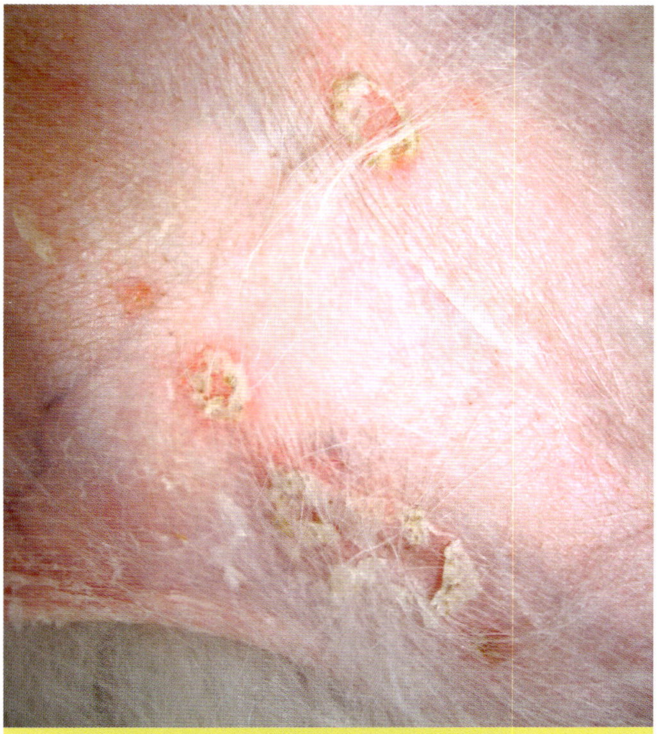

15 Epidermal collaretes in a *Staphylococcus* infection.

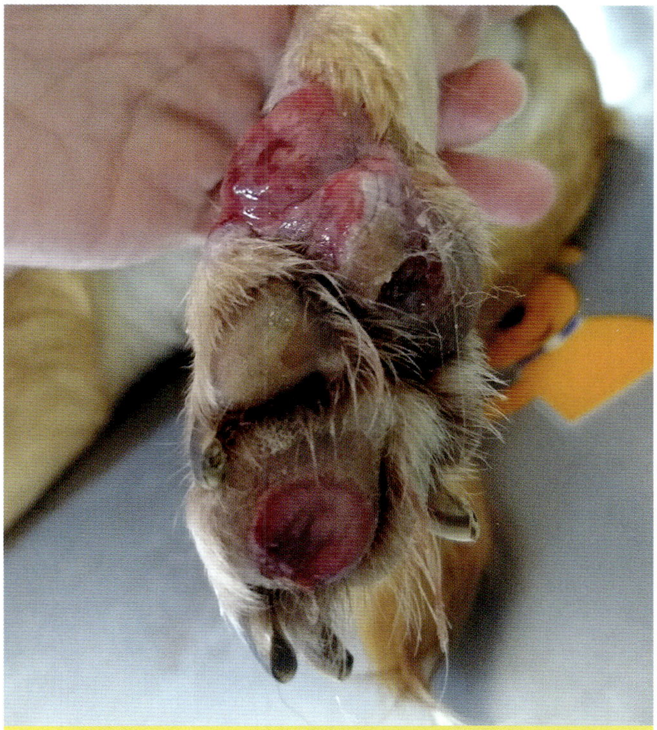

16 Ulcers in a dog with protothecosis.

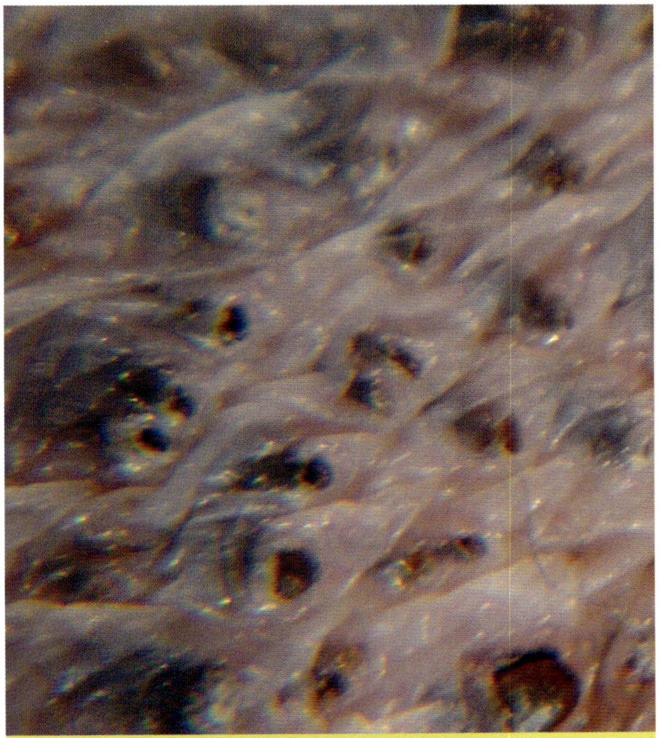

17 Comedones in a dog with Cushing's syndrome.

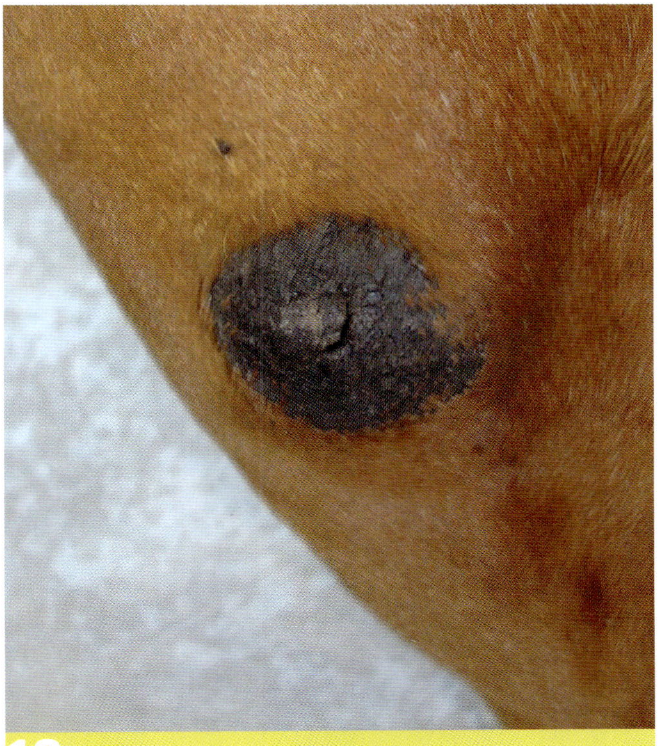

18 Fissure in a callus.

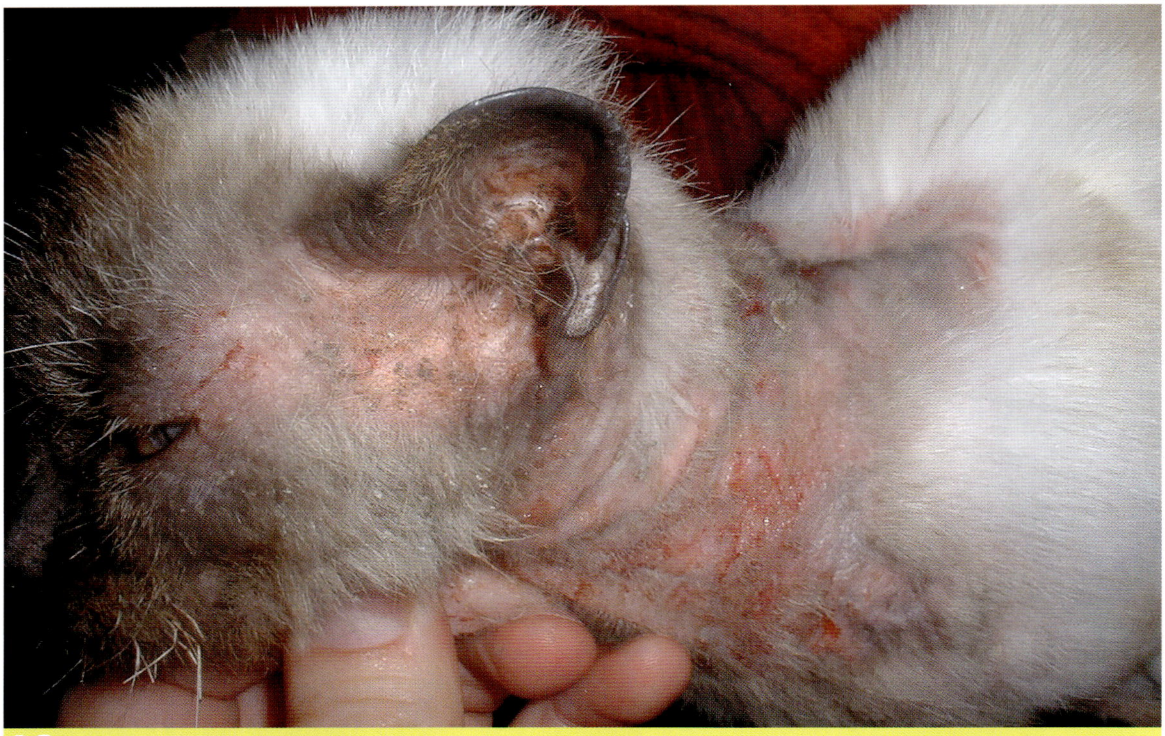

19 Excoriation on the face of a cat.

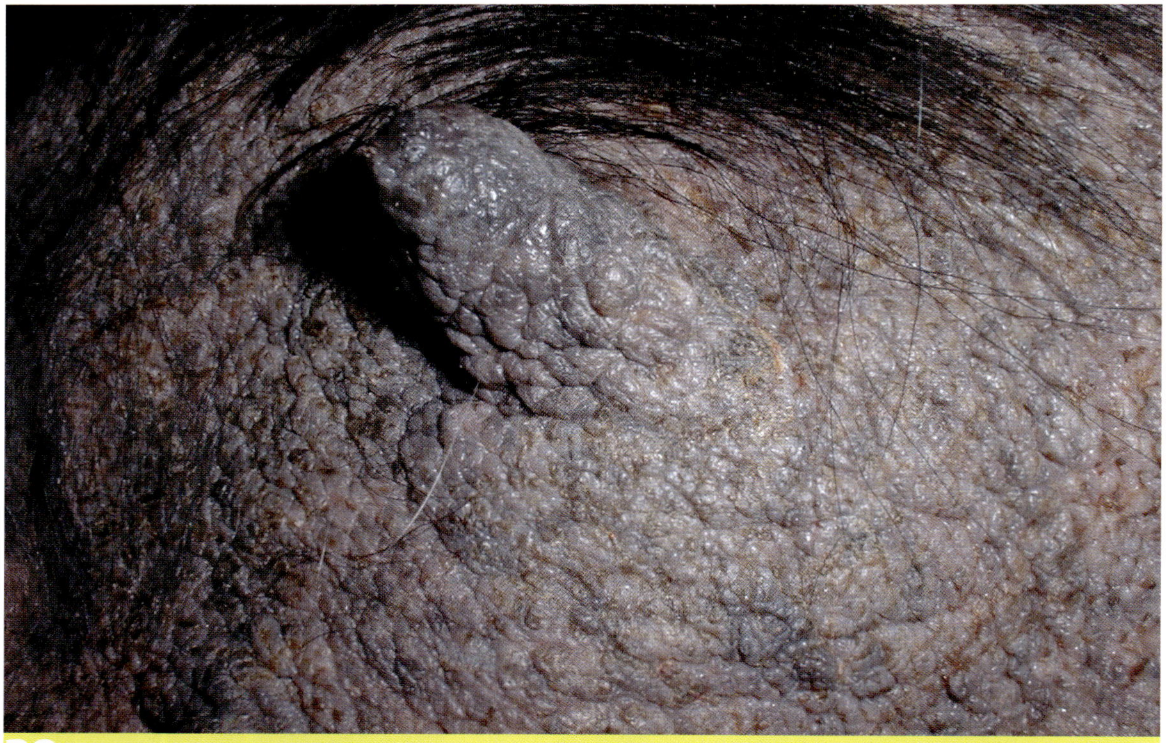

20 Lichenification due to chronic inflammation.

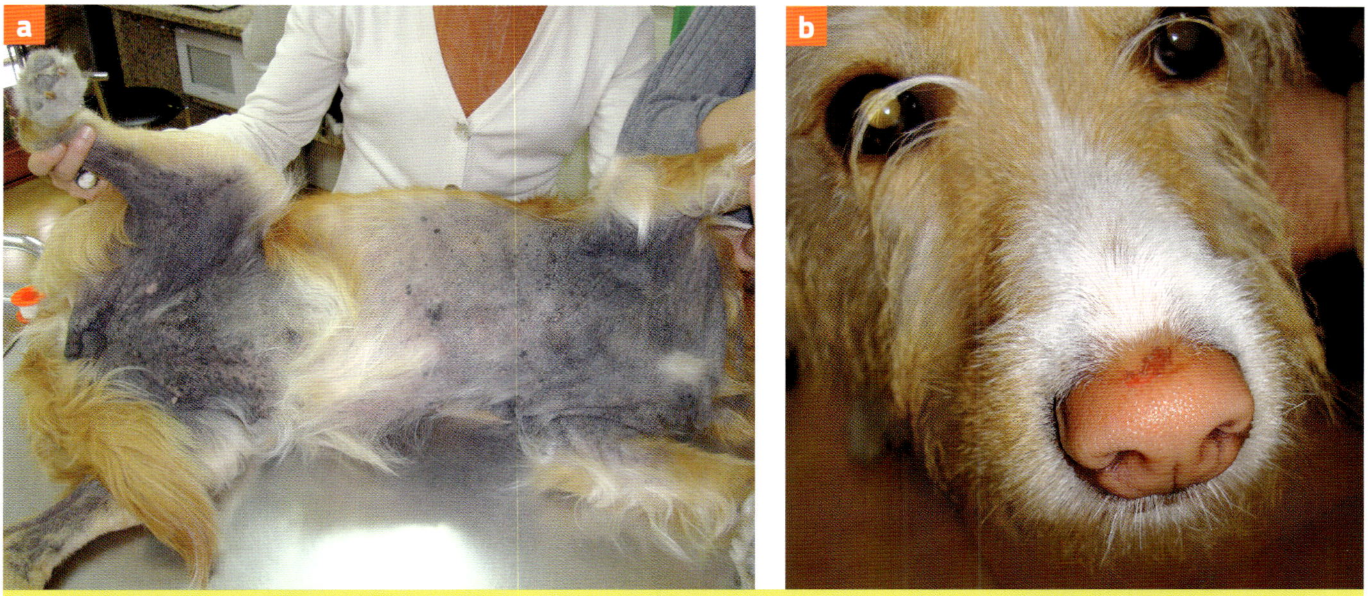

21 Hyperpigmentation in a case of hypersensitivity (a); hypopigmentation in a dog with snow nose (b).

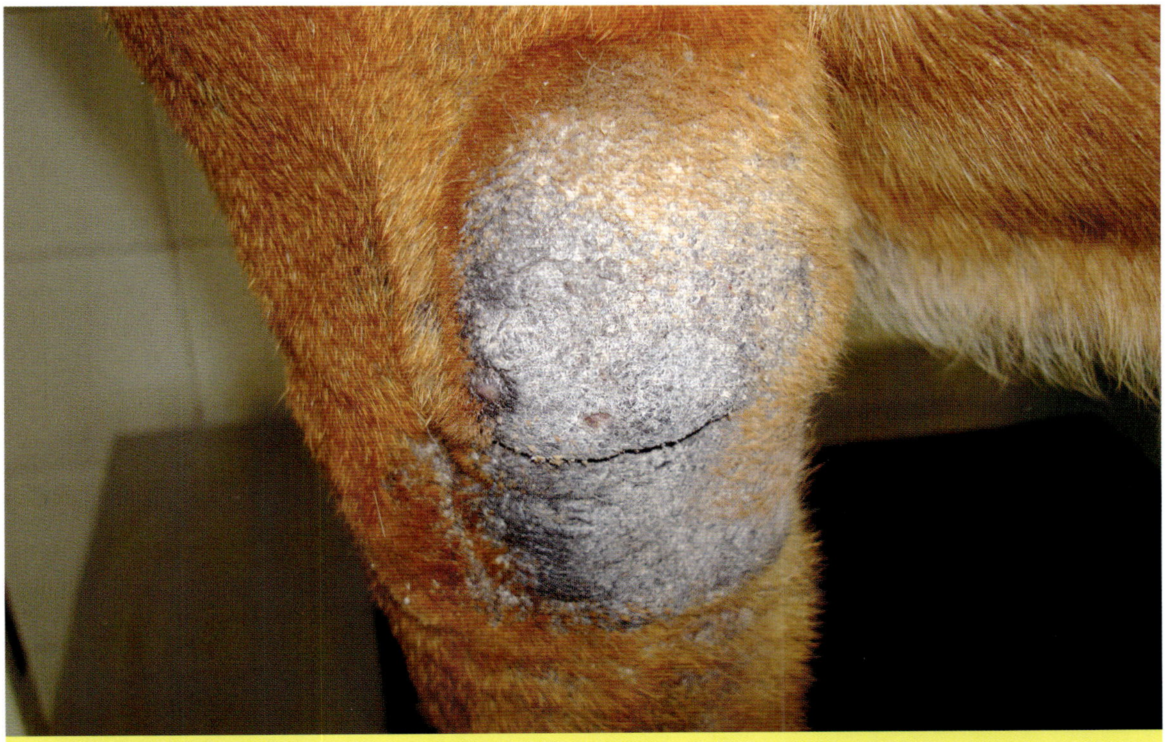

22 Callus at a pressure point.

# Clinical patterns

It is important not to assume that a given clinical picture is pathognomonic. This rarely occurs in dermatology, in which a correct diagnosis is typically established by following the corresponding protocol and performing the necessary diagnostic tests.

The classical clinical patterns of most skin diseases can be categorised as follows:

| Clinical patterns of skin diseases |
|---|
| • Focal, multifocal, regional, generalised, diffuse, or symmetric alopecia. |
| • Erosive–ulcerative (self-inflicted or due to evolution of primary lesions). |
| • Exfoliative, scaling, seborrhoeic, or combined. |
| • Papule/pustule/crusting, due to normal evolution of primary lesions. |
| • Nodular, due to developmental, inflammatory, or neoplastic alterations. |
| • Pigmentary changes, due to stimulation or suppression of melanocytes. |

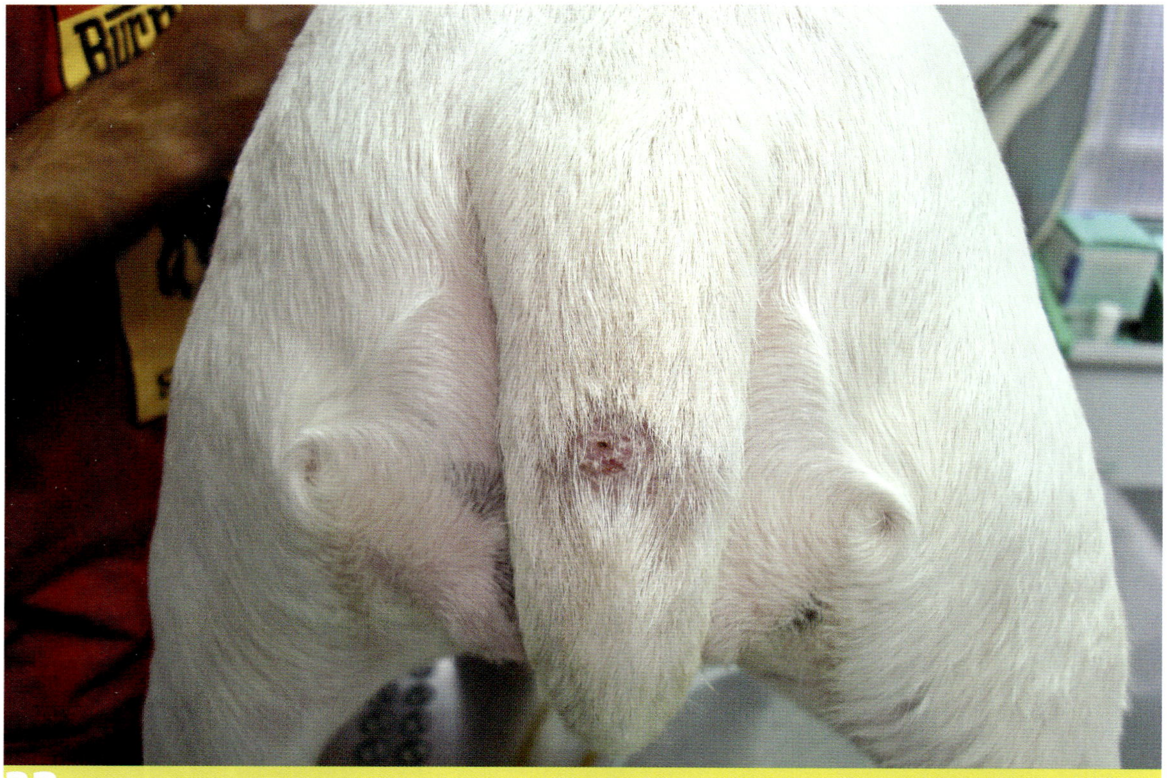

23 Focal alopecia. Dog with a seborrhoeic plaque on the dorsal aspect of the tail.

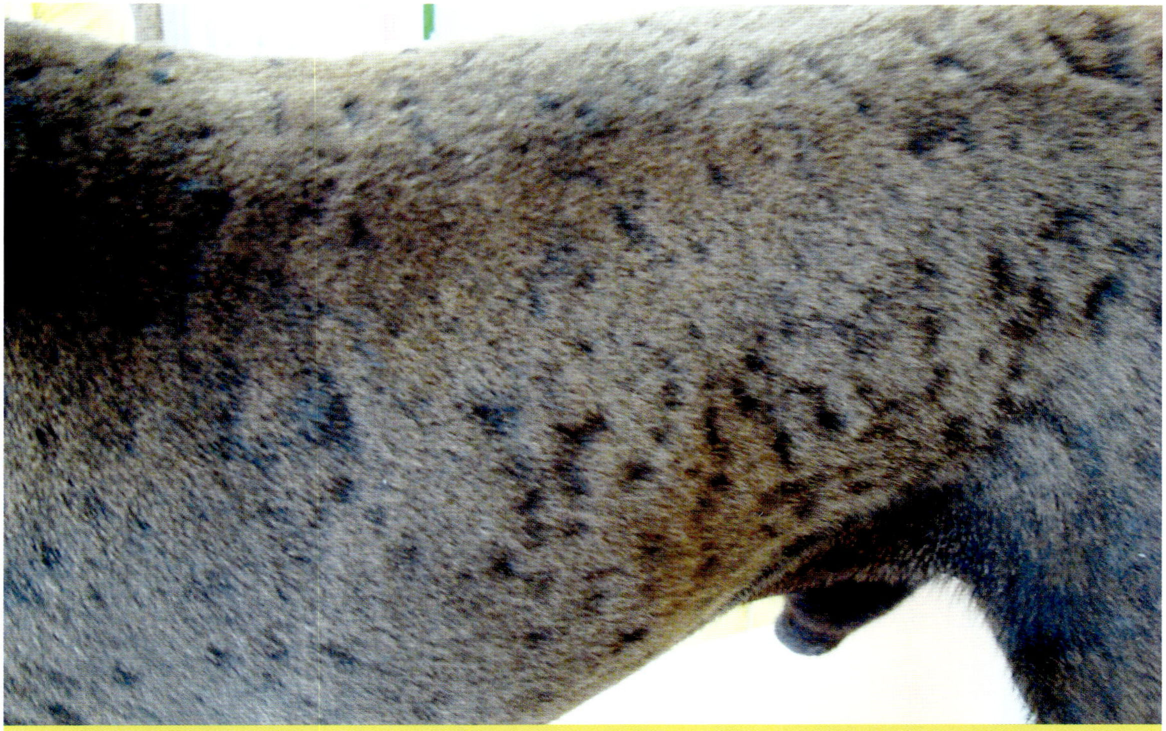

24 Multifocal alopecia. Shar Pei with a moth-eaten appearance.

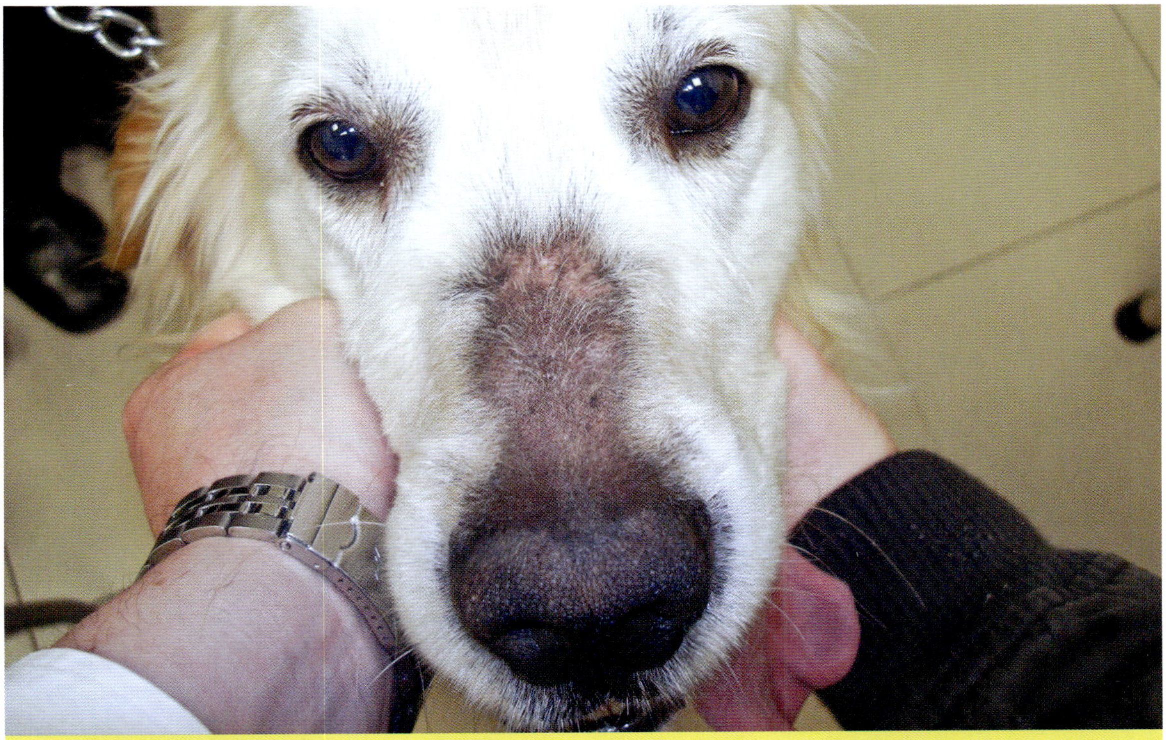

25 Local alopecia on the nasal bridge. Cyclic alopecia.

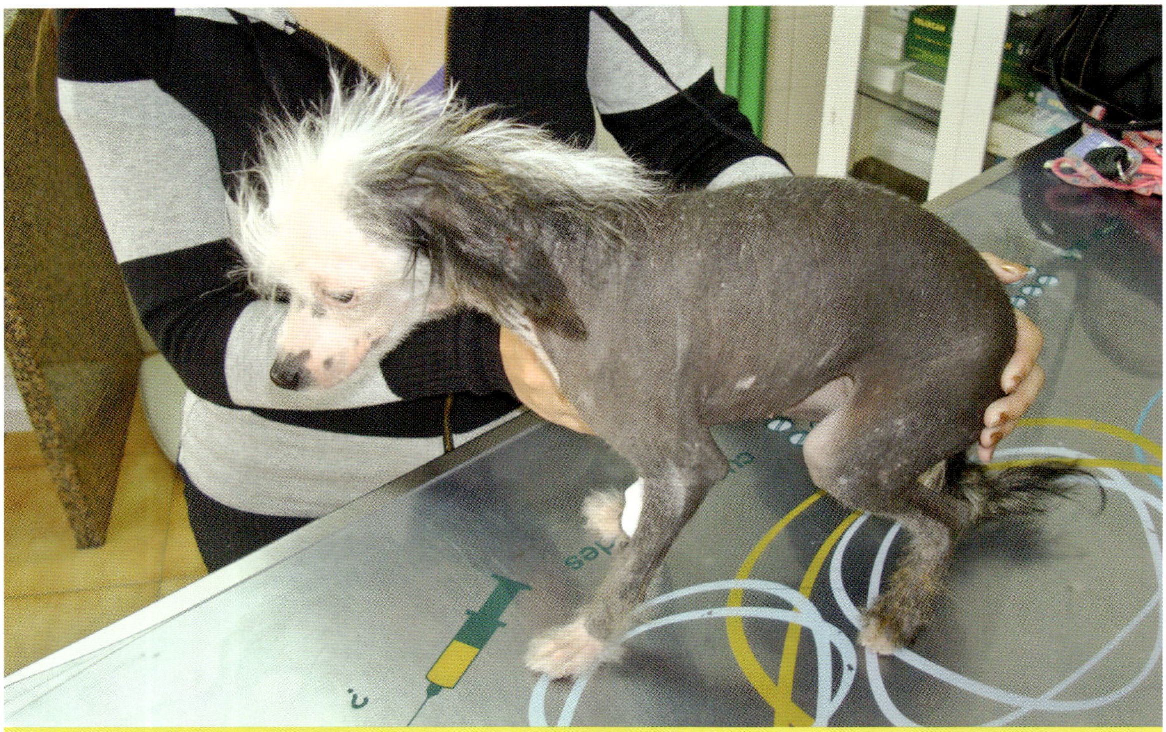

26 Generalised alopecia. Chinese Crested Dog.

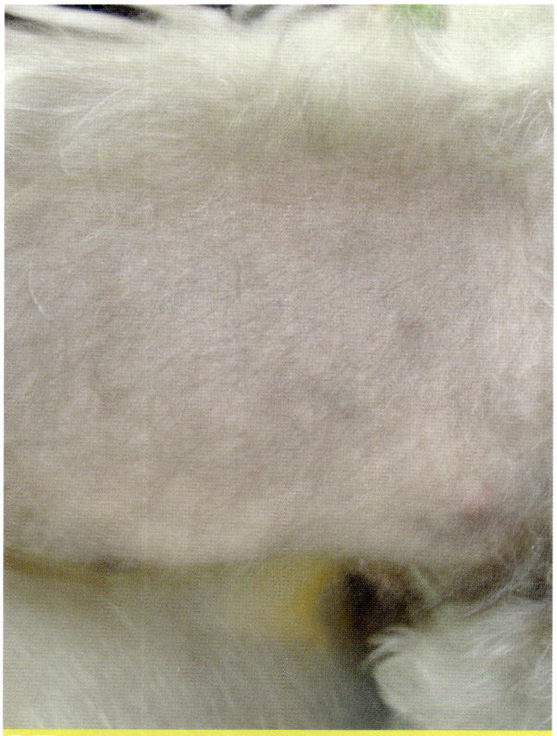

27 Diffuse alopecia. Dog with Cushing's syndrome.

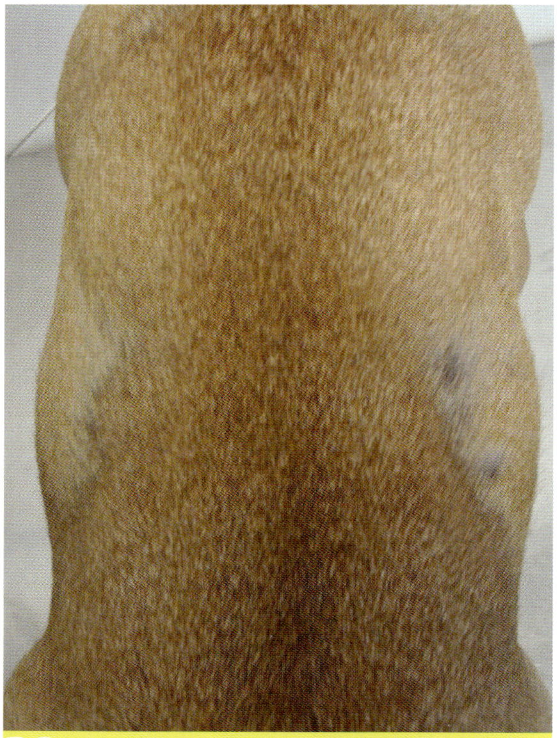

28 Symmetric alopecia. Pug with cyclic flank alopecia.

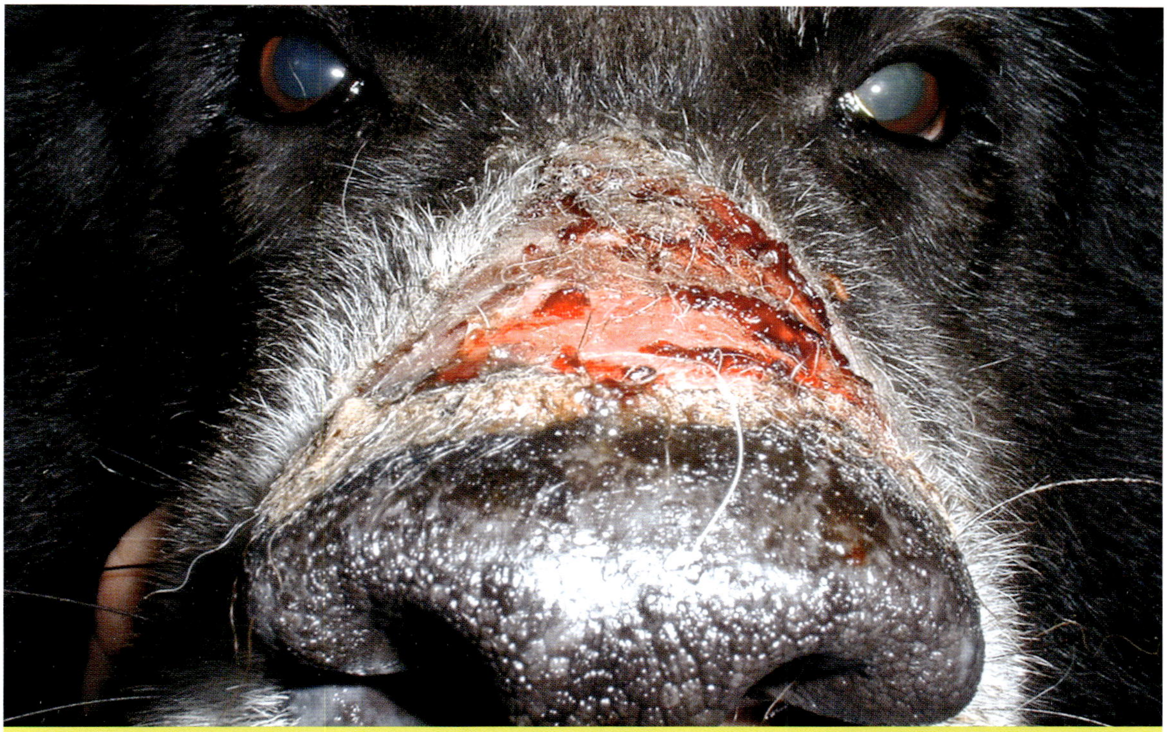

29 Erosive–ulcerative pattern. Dog with discoid lupus erythematosus.

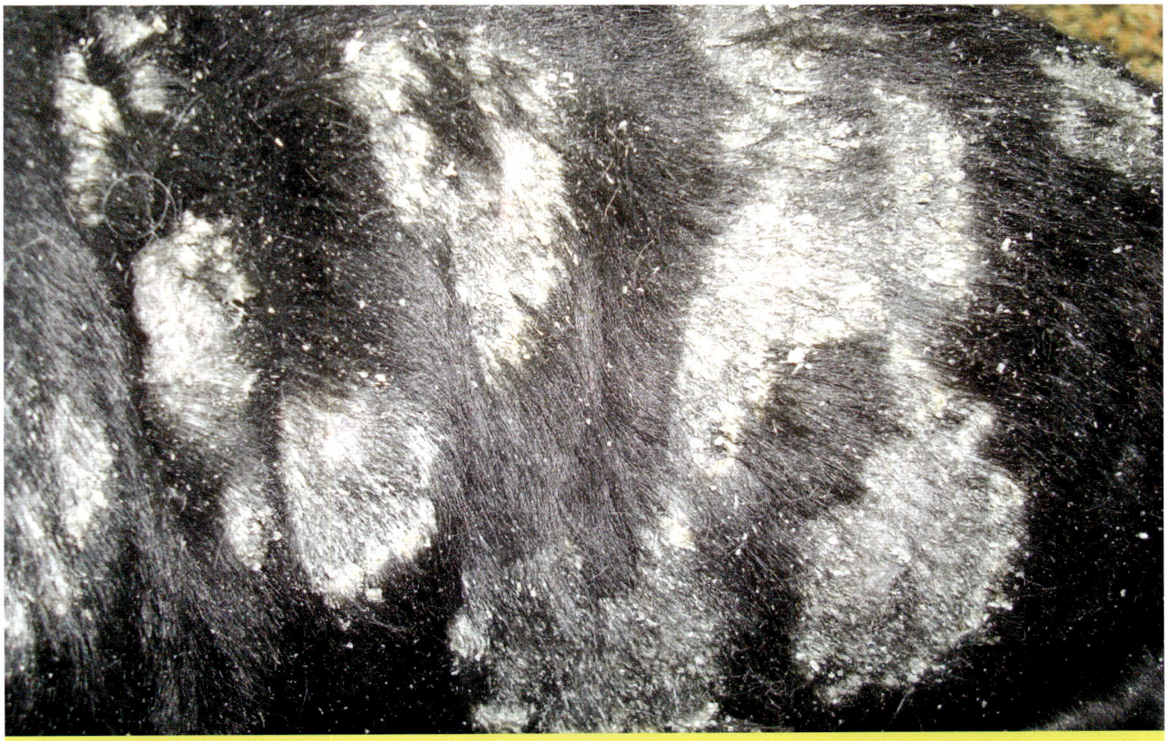

30 Scaling seborrhoea. Cocker Spaniel with vitamin A-responsive seborrhoea.

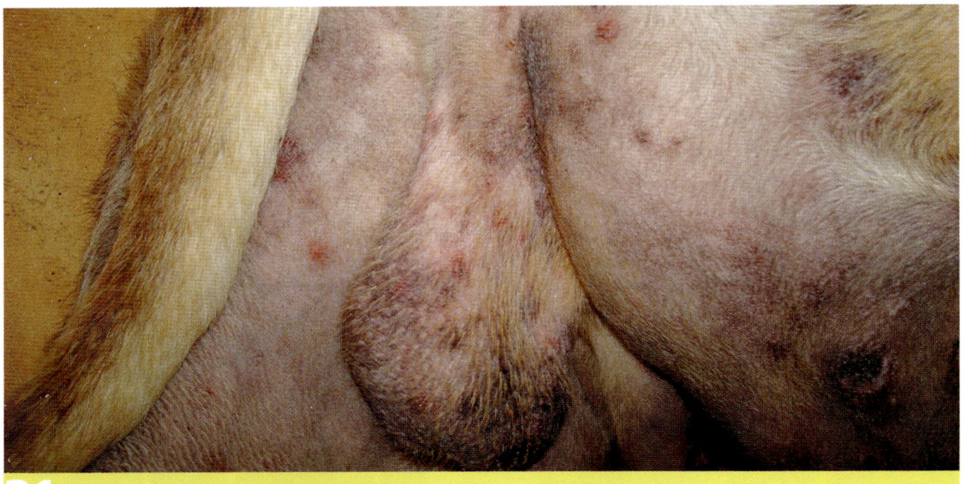

31 Papules/pustules/crusting. Dog with pyoderma.

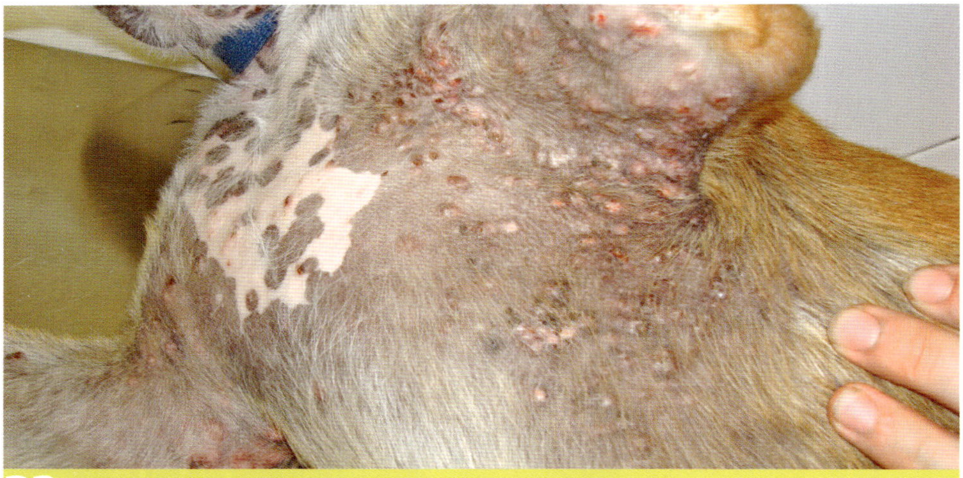

32 Nodular pattern. Dog with nodular demodicosis.

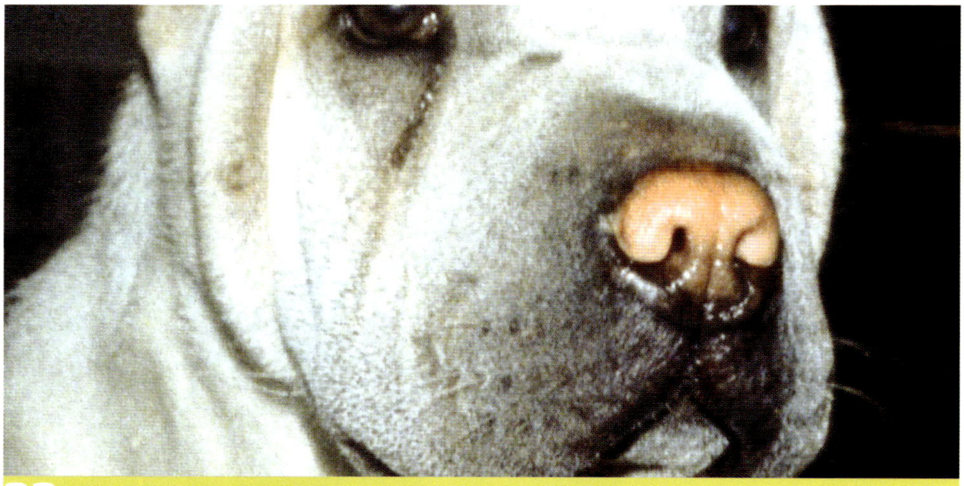

33 Pigmentary changes. Dog with initial vitiligo on the muzzle and upper lip.

# Histopathological patterns

The aforementioned clinical patterns are caused by microscopic changes at the cellular level and by the lesions produced by the actions of these cells and their cytokines.

Compared with the histological patterns of normal skin, these patterns reveal alterations in cell location and morphology. The resulting lesions can be classified as follows:

- **Perivascular dermatitis:** this is a very frequent pattern, but also very nonspecific. It is caused mainly by allergies or parasites. It is characterised by the migration of inflammatory cells around the blood vessels.

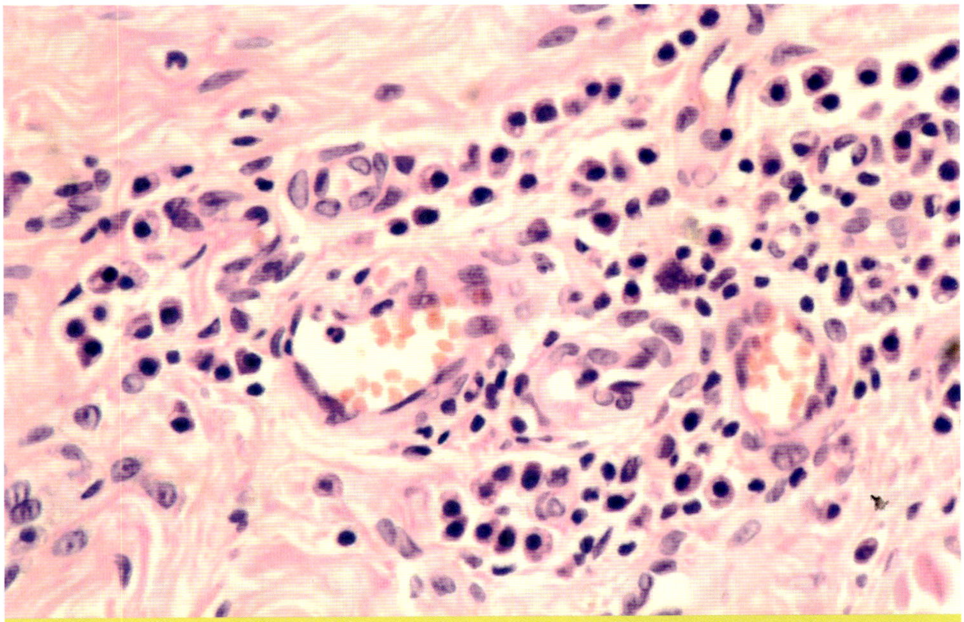

34 Perivascular dermatitis. Image courtesy of José Luis González Arribas.

- **Interface dermatitis:** inflammatory cells are observed at the dermoepidermal junction. This can be accompanied by alterations in basal keratinocytes, which undergo hydropic degeneration and/or apoptosis. Interface dermatitis can be inflammatory cell–poor, as occurs in dermatomyositis, ischaemic dermatopathies, erythema multiforme, toxic epidermal necrolysis, and thymoma-associated exfoliative dermatitis.

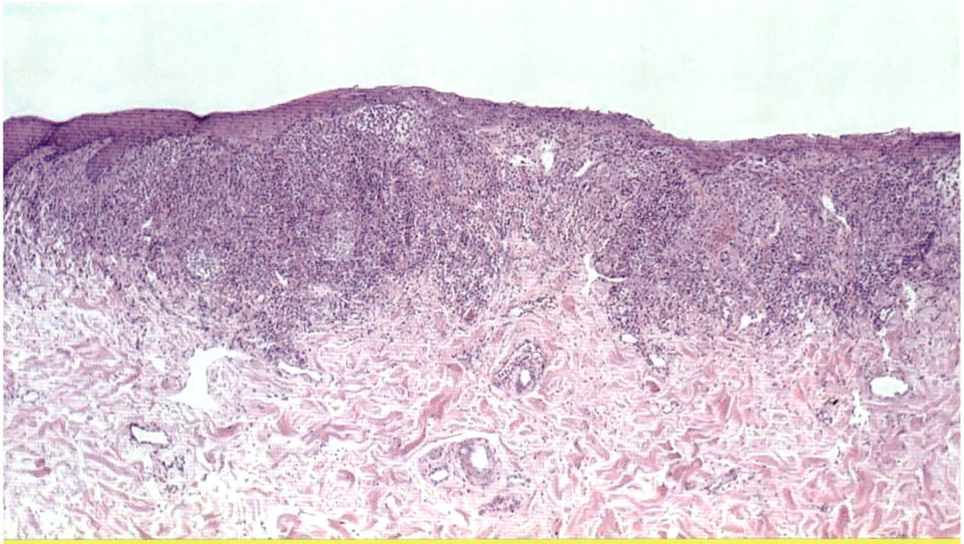

35 Interface dermatitis. Image courtesy of José Luis González Arribas.

- **Nodular and/or diffuse dermatitis:** inflammatory cells infiltrate the dermis, forming nodules or acquiring a diffuse distribution. This pattern is observed in some infectious diseases such as actinomycosis, nocardiosis, and leishmaniasis, as well as sterile granuloma and pyogranuloma, reactive histiocytosis, juvenile cellulitis, xanthoma, and foreign body reaction. It can also be observed in diseases in which eosinophils, neutrophils, or plasma cells predominate, including eosinophilic furunculosis, herpesvirus dermatitis, eosinophilic granuloma complex, and plasmacytic pododermatitis.

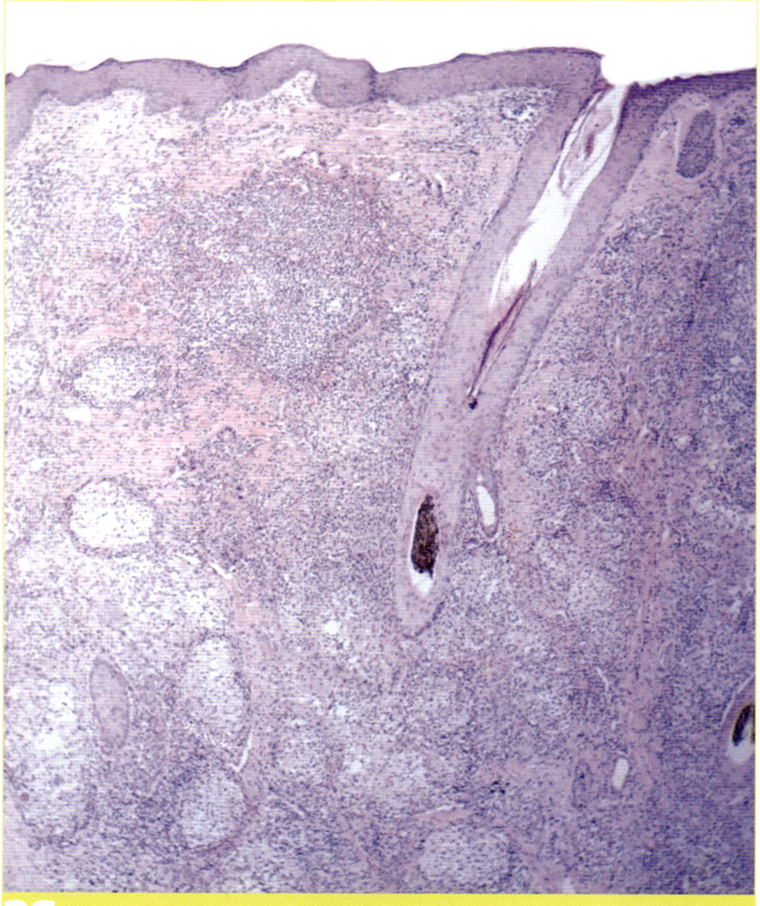

36 Nodular and diffuse dermatitis. Image courtesy of José Luis González Arribas.

- **Vesicular dermatitis and intraepidermal pustular dermatitis:** these are characterised by the formation of vesicles and pustules, respectively, which can result from bacterial infections or allergies that cause spongiosis (oedema between epidermal cells), herpesvirus infections that cause intracellular oedema, or autoimmune diseases that cause acantholysis.

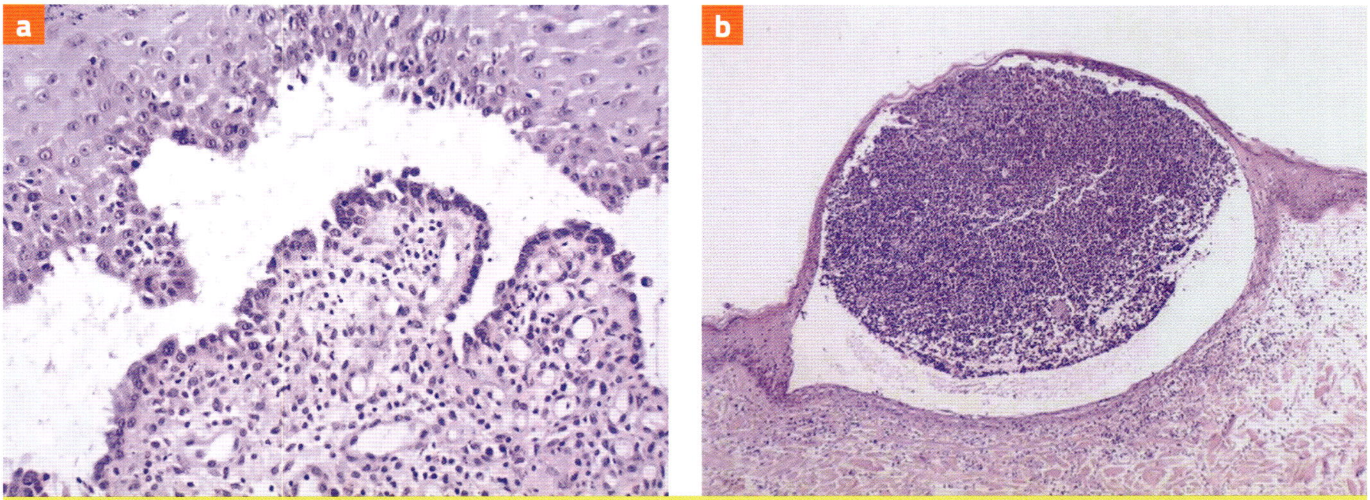


37 Intraepidermal vesicular pustular dermatitis; separation due to acantholysis (a) and intact pustule (b). Images provided by José Luis González Arribas.

- **Subepidermal vesicular and/or pustular dermatitis:** separation of the dermoepidermal junction occurs. Cellular content is usually low. The main diseases in which this pattern is observed are epidermolysis bullosa and bullous pemphigoid.

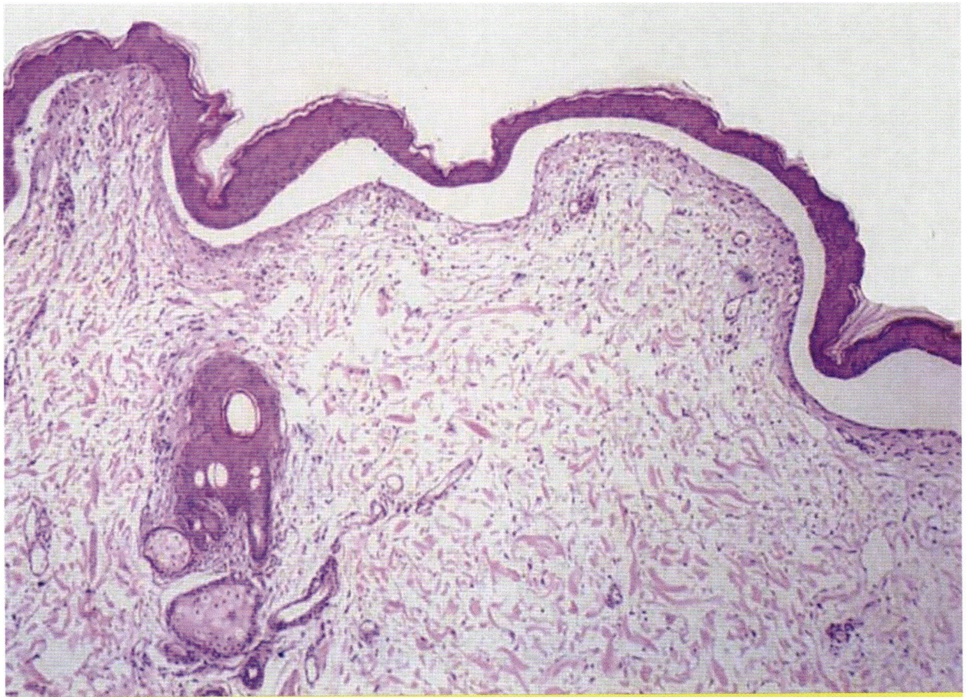

38 Subepidermal vesicular pustular dermatitis. Image courtesy of José Luis González Arribas.

- **Perifolliculitis, folliculitis, and furunculosis:** occur in diseases that affect the range of structures associated with the hair follicle. Inflammatory cells accumulate outside the follicle wall in perifolliculitis; in the wall of the follicle itself in mural folliculitis; and in the lumen of the follicle in luminal folliculitis (dermatophytosis, demodicosis, etc.). Perifolliculitis can occur in the initial stages of follicular inflammation, in which cells migrate towards the wall or accumulate outside it, indicating a general follicular problem. The mural pattern can manifest at the junction with the dermis (ischaemic dermatopathies, demodicosis, lupus, etc.) in the form of intramural pustules (pemphigus foliaceus) with intramural infiltrate, or as a necrotising form (herpesvirus infections, mosquito bite hypersensitivity). The level at which inflammation occurs can be characteristic of specific conditions. For example, alopecia areata is characterised by the presence of bulbitis.

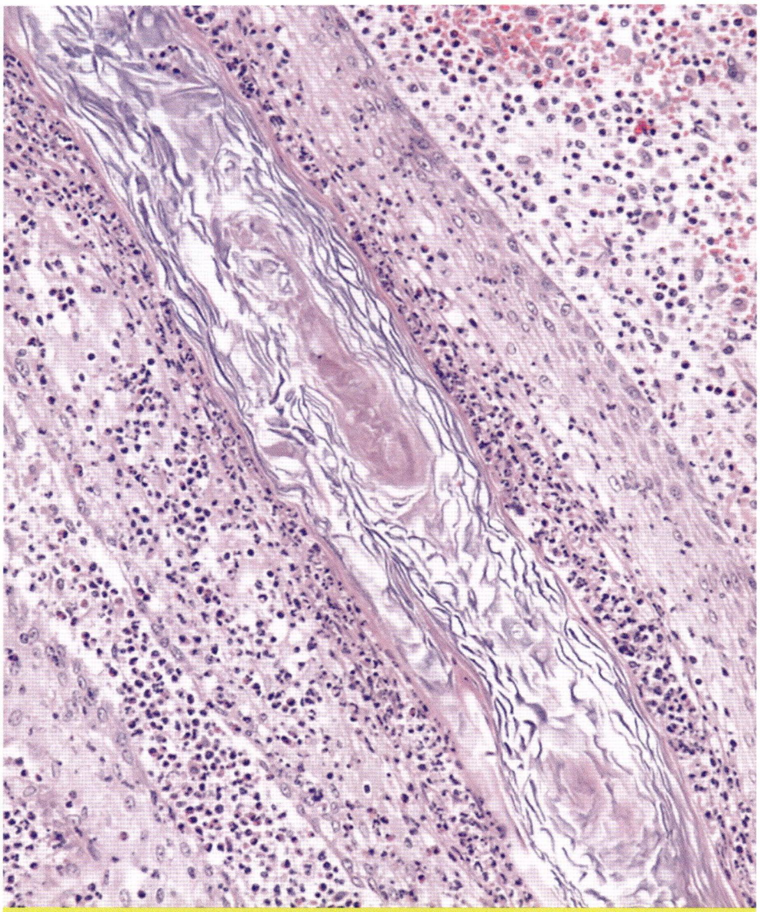

39 Perifolliculitis. Image courtesy of José Luis González Arribas.

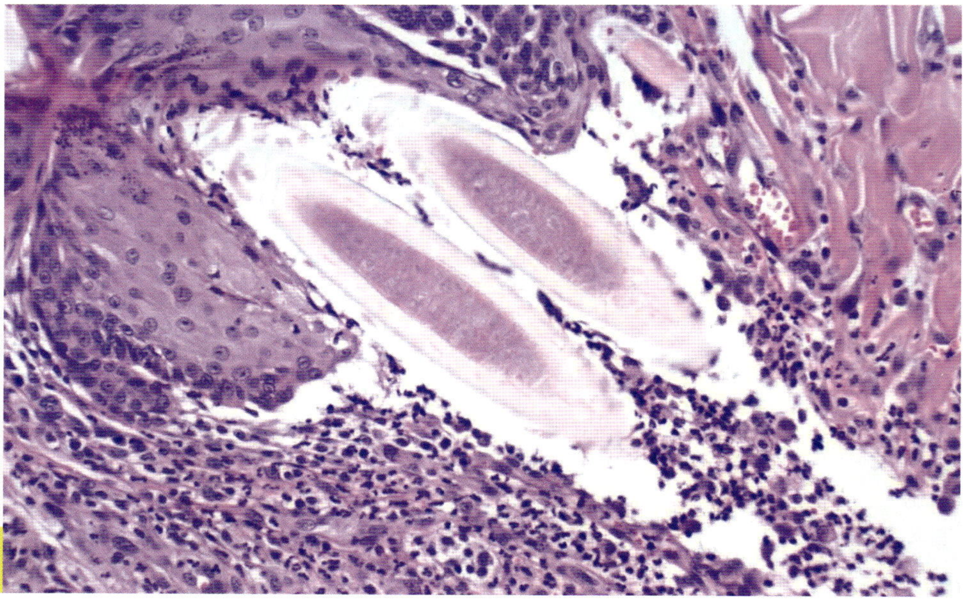

40 Furunculosis. Image courtesy of José Luis González Arribas.

- **Vasculitis:** inflammatory cells infiltrate the blood vessel walls. This can occur in septic vasculitis, urticaria and angioedema, thrombovascular necrosis of the ear, cell-poor immune vasculitis, etc.

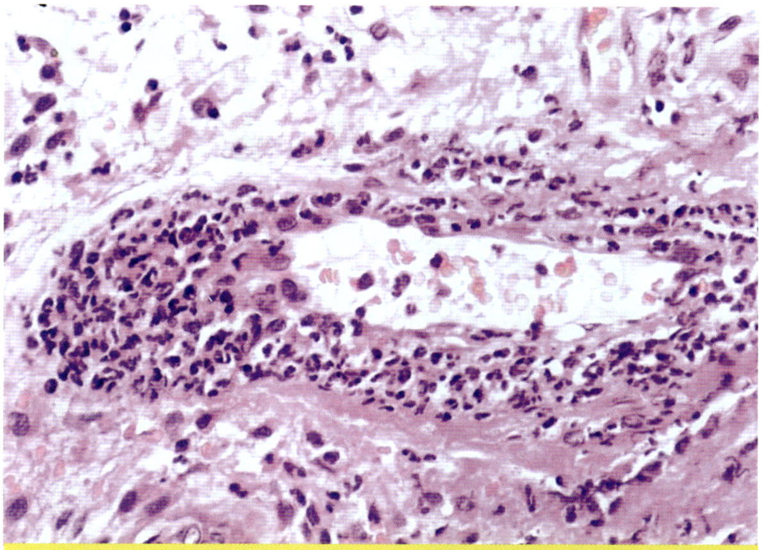

41 Vasculitis. Image courtesy of José Luis González Arribas.

- **Panniculitis:** as its name suggests, this is an inflammatory process of the adipose tissue. It can have an infectious origin (mycobacteria, viruses, bacteria, and fungi). It can also result from non-infectious causes such as a foreign body, injectable products, trauma, and pancreatic disease.

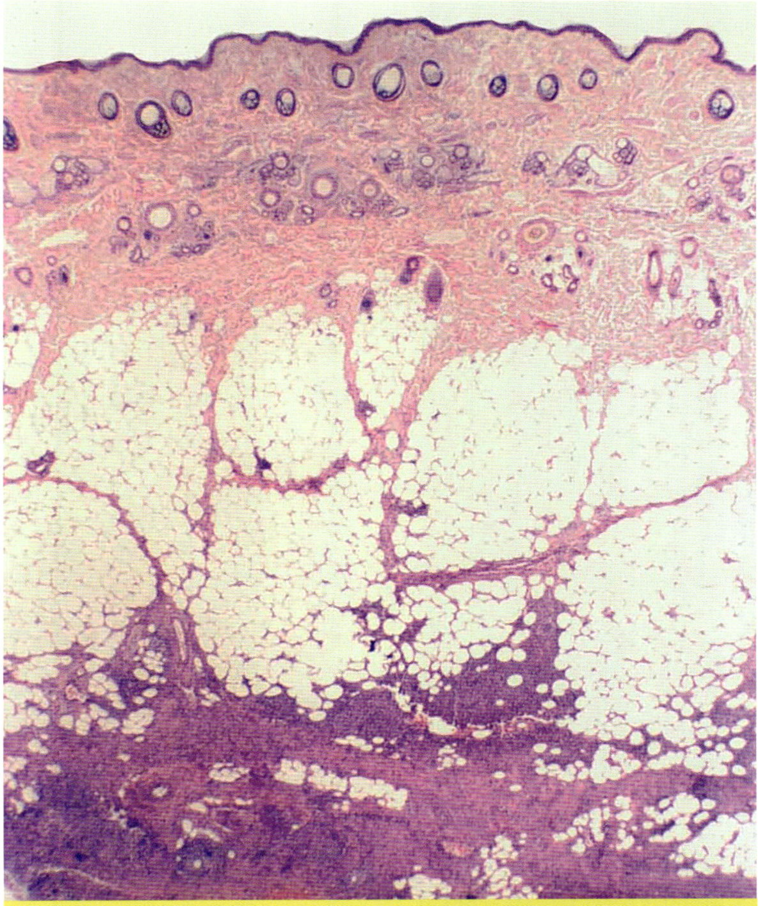

42 Panniculitis. Image courtesy of José Luis González Arribas.

- **Noninflammatory diseases of the adnexa:** this pattern includes alterations in the follicular cycle, as occurs in Cushing's syndrome and hypothyroidism, and follicular atrophy, which occurs in traction alopecia, post-injection reaction, and pattern alopecia. Other adnexal alterations occur in follicular dysplasia and sebaceous adenitis.

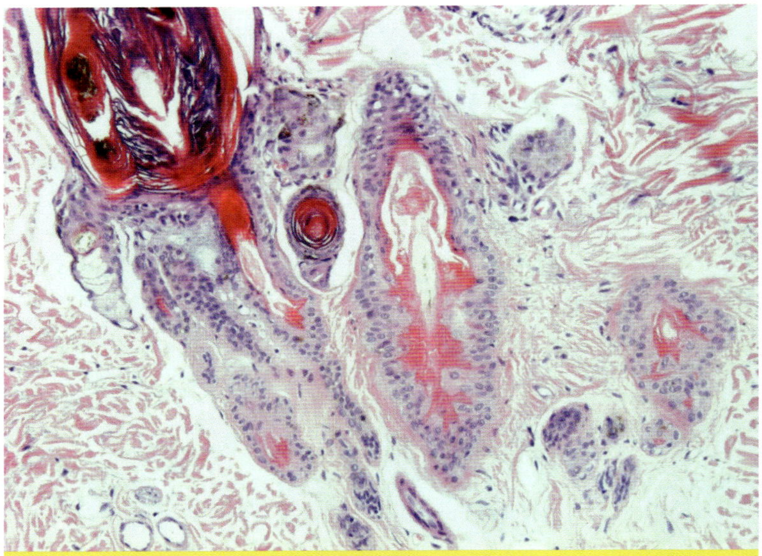

43 Noninflammatory diseases of the adnexa. Image courtesy of José Luis González Arribas.

- **Dermal alterations:** this pattern includes nonspecific inflammatory diseases of the dermis (e.g. degeneration or dysplasia, mineral deposition, dermal fibrosis). The diseases in which this pattern occurs include calcinosis cutis, cutaneous amyloidosis, elastosis, and solar fibrosis.

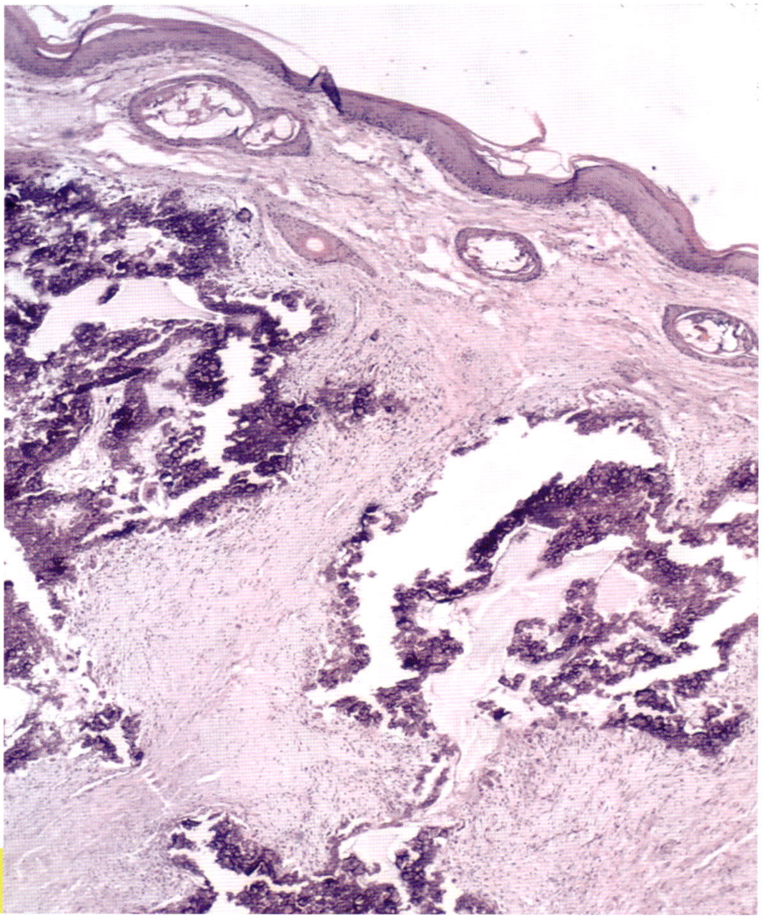

44 Dermal alterations. Image courtesy of José Luis González Arribas.

## Age of presentation

During the diagnostic process, it is useful to bear in mind that certain skin diseases tend to present at a particular age, as shown in the following table.

| Age at onset | Disease |
|---|---|
| Less than 6 months | Demodicosis |
| | Dermatophytosis |
| | Juvenile cellulitis |
| | Dermatomyositis |
| | Impetigo |
| | Pituitary dwarfism |
| | Histiocytoma |
| | Zinc-responsive dermatosis |
| | Congenital skin diseases |
| | Food hypersensitivity |
| 1 week to 3 years | Atopic dermatitis |
| | Primary seborrhoea |
| | Histiocytoma |
| | Zinc-responsive dermatosis |
| 6 years and older | Cushing's syndrome or hypothyroidism |
| | Cutaneous neoplasia, paraneoplasia, and pseudoneoplasia |
| | Cutaneous manifestations of systemic diseases |
| | Food allergen-induced atopic dermatitis |

Adapted from Peter B., Hill. *Small Animal Dermatology*. Elsevier Science Ltd., 2002.

## Lesion distribution

Lesions in general can be distributed as follows:

- Regional or focal
- Multiregional or multifocal
- Generalised or universal
- Symmetric
- Nonsymmetric

The following table shows lesions grouped by the most frequently affected body regions in the main skin diseases.

It is important to note that there are obviously many exceptions in which skin diseases can affect other, less commonly involved areas.

## Body regions most frequently affected in the main skin diseases.

| Disease | | Most frequently affected region | | | | | | | | | | | | |
|---|---|---|---|---|---|---|---|---|---|---|---|---|---|---|
| General | Specific | FACE | | | | TRUNK | | | | PERINEAL REGION | | | LIMBS | |
| | | Ears | Periocular region and forehead | Perioral region and muzzle | Nasal bridge | Dorsal/flanks | Abdomen | Axillae | Groin | Tail | Perivulvar and periprepucial regions | Perianal region | Feet-nails | Forelimbs and hindlimbs |
| Bacterial skin diseases | Intertrigo | | ■ | ■ | ■ | ■ | | | | ■ | ■ | | | |
| | Impetigo | | | | | | ■ | ■ | ■ | | | | | |
| | Bacterial overgrowth | | | | | ■ | ■ | ■ | ■ | | | | | |
| | Pyotraumatic dermatitis | | ■ | ■ | | ■ | | | | ■ | | ■ | | |
| | Superficial bacterial folliculitis | | | | | ■ | ■ | ■ | ■ | | | | | |
| | Pyotraumatic folliculitis/ furunculosis | | ■ | ■ | | ■ | | | | | | ■ | | |
| | Mucocutaneous pyoderma | | | ■ | | | | | | | ■ | ■ | | |
| | Deep pyoderma of the nasal bridge | | | | ■ | | | | | | | | | |
| | Deep pyoderma of the chin | | | ■ | | | | | | | | | | |
| | German Shepherd deep pyoderma | | ■ | ■ | ■ | ■ | ■ | ■ | ■ | | ■ | ■ | ■ | ■ |
| | Bacterial pododermatitis | | | | | | | | | | | | ■ | |
| | Callus pyoderma | | | | | | | | | | | | | ■ |
| | Furunculosis cellulitis | | ■ | ■ | ■ | ■ | ■ | ■ | ■ | | ■ | ■ | ■ | ■ |
| | Skin abscesses | | ■ | ■ | ■ | ■ | ■ | ■ | ■ | ■ | ■ | ■ | | ■ |
| | Pyoderma due to atypical bacteria | | ■ | ■ | ■ | ■ | ■ | ■ | ■ | | ■ | ■ | ■ | ■ |
| Fungal skin diseases | Dermatophytosis | ■ | ■ | ■ | ■ | ■ | ■ | ■ | ■ | ■ | ■ | ■ | ■ | ■ |
| | *Malassezia* dermatitis | ■ | | ■ | | | | ■ | ■ | | ■ | ■ | ■ | |
| | Uncommon mycoses | | | | ■ | | | | | | | | ■ | ■ |
| Parasitic skin diseases▾ | Cheyletiellosis | | | | | ■ | ■ | ■ | ■ | ■ | ■ | ■ | | |
| | Ticks | ■ | ■ | ■ | | ■ | ■ | | | | ■ | ■ | ■ | |
| | Pediculosis | ■ | ■ | ■ | ■ | ■ | ■ | ■ | ■ | ■ | ■ | ■ | ■ | ■ |
| | Myiasis | | ■ | ■ | | | ■ | ■ | ■ | ■ | ■ | ■ | ■ | |
| | Canine demodicosis | | ■ | ■ | ■ | ■ | ■ | ■ | ■ | ■ | ■ | ■ | ■ | ■ |
| | Feline demodicosis | | ■ | ■ | ■ | ■ | ■ | ■ | ■ | | | | ■ | ■ |
| | Scabies | ■ | ■ | | | | ■ | | | | | | | ■ |
| | *Notoedres* | ■ | ■ | ■ | ■ | | | | | | ■ | ■ | ■ | |
| | *Otodectes* | ■ | ■ | | | | | | | | | | | |

Continued ▸

| Disease | | Most frequently affected region | | | | | | | | | | | | |
|---|---|---|---|---|---|---|---|---|---|---|---|---|---|---|
| General | Specific | FACE | | | | TRUNK | | | | PERINEAL REGION | | | LIMBS | |
| | | Ears | Periocular region and forehead | Perioral region and muzzle | Nasal bridge | Dorsal/flanks | Abdomen | Axillae | Groin | Tail | Perivulvar and periprepucial regions | Perianal region | Feet-nails | Forelimbs and hindlimbs |
| Parasitic skin diseases ▲ | *Neotrombicula* | ■ | | | | | | | | | | | ■ | |
| | *Straelensia cynotis* | | ■ | | | ■ | | | | ■ | | | | |
| Viral skin diseases caused by protozoa and algae | Canine distemper virus | | ■ | ■ | ■ | | | | | | | | ■ | |
| | Feline herpes | | ■ | ■ | ■ | | | | | | | | | |
| | Leishmaniasis | ■ | ■ | ■ | ■ | | | | | | | | ■ | ■ |
| | Protothecosis | | ■ | ■ | | | | | | | ■ | ■ | ■ | |
| Allergic skin diseases | Urticaria and angioedema | ■ | ■ | ■ | | ■ | ■ | ■ | ■ | | ■ | ■ | ■ | ■ |
| | Atopy/food allergy | ■ | ■ | ■ | | | ■ | ■ | ■ | | ■ | ■ | ■ | ■ |
| | Contact hypersensitivity | ■ | | ■ | | | ■ | ■ | ■ | | ■ | ■ | ■ | |
| | Flea allergy dermatitis | | | | | ■ | ■ | | ■ | ■ | ■ | ■ | | |
| | Insect bite (cat) | ■ | | | ■ | | | | | | | | ■ | |
| | Facial eosinophilic furunculosis | | ■ | ■ | ■ | | | | | | | | | |
| | Drug reaction | | | | | ■ | ■ | ■ | ■ | | ■ | ■ | | ■ |
| Feline allergies | Miliary dermatitis | | ■ | | | ■ | | | | ■ | | | | |
| | Symmetric alopecia | | | | | ■ | ■ | ■ | ■ | | ■ | ■ | | |
| | Eosinophilic granuloma complex | | | ■ | | | ■ | ■ | ■ | | | | | ■ |
| | Dermatoses of the face and neck | ■ | ■ | ■ | ■ | | | | | | | | | |
| Dermatoses of endocrine and metabolic origin | Hypothyroidism | ■ | ■ | ■ | ■ | ■ | ■ | ■ | ■ | ■ | ■ | ■ | | ■ |
| | Cushing's syndrome | | | | | ■ | ■ | ■ | ■ | ■ | ■ | ■ | | ■ |
| | Pituitary dwarfism | | | | | ■ | ■ | ■ | ■ | ■ | ■ | ■ | | ■ |
| | Acromegaly | ■ | ■ | ■ | ■ | ■ | ■ | ■ | ■ | ■ | ■ | ■ | ■ | ■ |
| | Sex hormone dermatoses, females | | | | | ■ | ■ | ■ | ■ | ■ | ■ | ■ | | |
| | Sex hormone dermatoses, males | | | | | ■ | ■ | ■ | ■ | ■ | ■ | ■ | | |
| | Alopecia X | | | | | ■ | ■ | | | ■ | ■ | ■ | | ■ |
| | Shar Pei mucinosis | ■ | ■ | ■ | ■ | ■ | ■ | ■ | ■ | ■ | ■ | ■ | ■ | ■ |
| | Hepatocutaneous syndrome | | | ■ | | | ■ | | | | | | ■ | ■ |
| | Calcinosis circumscripta | ■ | ■ | ■ | ■ | | | | | | | | ■ | ■ |

Continued ▶

| Disease | | Most frequently affected region | | | | | | | | | | | | |
|---|---|---|---|---|---|---|---|---|---|---|---|---|---|---|
| **General** | **Specific** | FACE | | | | TRUNK | | | | PERINEAL REGION | | | LIMBS | |
| | | Ears | Periocular region and forehead | Perioral region and muzzle | Nasal bridge | Dorsal/flanks | Abdomen | Axillae | Groin | Tail | Perivulvar and periprepucial regions | Perianal region | Feet-nails | Forelimbs and hindlimbs |
| Autoimmune or immune-mediated skin diseases | Juvenile cellulitis | ■ | ■ | ■ | | | | | | | ■ | | | |
| | Pemphigus complex | ■ | ■ | ■ | ■ | ■ | ■ | ■ | ■ | | ■ | ■ | ■ | ■ |
| | Subepidermal bullous diseases | | ■ | ■ | | | ■ | | | | ■ | ■ | ■ | |
| | Cutaneous lupus | | ■ | ■ | | | ■ | | | | ■ | ■ | ■ | |
| | Lupoid onychodystrophy | | | | | | | | | | | | ■ | |
| | Sterile nodular panniculitis | | | | | ■ | ■ | | | | | | | |
| | Cold agglutinin disease | ■ | | | | | | | | | | | ■ | |
| | Sebaceous adenitis | ■ | ■ | ■ | | ■ | ■ | ■ | ■ | ■ | ■ | ■ | | ■ |
| | Vasculitis dermatomyositis | ■ | ■ | ■ | ■ | | | | | ■ | | | ■ | ■ |
| | Uveodermatologic syndrome | | ■ | ■ | ■ | | | | | | | | | |
| | Perianal fistulas | | | | | | | | | ■ | ■ | ■ | | |
| | Metatarsal fistulas | | | | | | | | | | | | ■ | |
| Dermatoses due to keratoseborrhoeic and pigmentary alterations | Generalised seborrhoea | ■ | ■ | ■ | ■ | ■ | ■ | ■ | ■ | ■ | ■ | ■ | ■ | ■ |
| | Ear margin seborrhoea | ■ | | | | | | | | | | | | |
| | Anal sac impaction | | | | | | | | | | | ■ | | |
| | Supracaudal gland hyperplasia (stud tail) | | | | | | | | | ■ | | | | |
| | Lichenoid dermatosis | ■ | ■ | ■ | ■ | ■ | ■ | ■ | ■ | ■ | ■ | ■ | ■ | ■ |
| | Zinc-responsive dermatosis | | ■ | ■ | | | | | | | | | ■ | ■ |
| | Facial dermatosis of Persian and Himalayan cats | ■ | ■ | ■ | ■ | | | | | | | | | |
| | Vitiligo | | ■ | ■ | ■ | ■ | ■ | ■ | ■ | ■ | ■ | ■ | ■ | ■ |
| | Lentigo | | ■ | ■ | ■ | | ■ | | | | | | | |
| | Split paw pad disease | | | | | | | | | | | | ■ | |

Continued ▸

| Disease | | Most frequently affected region | | | | | | | | | | | | |
|---|---|---|---|---|---|---|---|---|---|---|---|---|---|---|
| **General** | **Specific** | FACE | | | | TRUNK | | | | PERINEAL REGION | | | LIMBS | |
| | | Ears | Periocular region and forehead | Perioral region and muzzle | Nasal bridge | Dorsal/flanks | Abdomen | Axillae | Groin | Tail | Perivulvar and periprepucial regions | Perianal region | Feet-nails | Forelimbs and hindlimbs |
| Most frequent tumours | Lipoma | | | | | ■ | ■ | ■ | ■ | | | | | ■ |
| | Mast cell tumour | ■ | ■ | ■ | ■ | ■ | ■ | ■ | ■ | ■ | ■ | ■ | ■ | ■ |
| | Histiocytoma | ■ | ■ | ■ | ■ | | | | | | | | | ■ |
| | Reactive histiocytosis | ■ | ■ | ■ | ■ | ■ | ■ | ■ | ■ | ■ | ■ | ■ | ■ | ■ |
| | Epitheliotrophic lymphoma | | ■ | ■ | | ■ | ■ | ■ | ■ | | | | ■ | |
| | Feline paraneoplastic alopecia | | | | | | ■ | ■ | ■ | | | | ■ | ■ |
| | Hepatoid cell adenoma/carcinoma | | | | | | | | ■ | ■ | ■ | ■ | | |
| | Papilloma | ■ | ■ | ■ | ■ | ■ | ■ | ■ | ■ | ■ | ■ | ■ | ■ | ■ |
| | Basalioma | | ■ | ■ | ■ | | | | | | | | | ■ |
| | Soft tissue sarcoma | ■ | ■ | ■ | ■ | ■ | ■ | ■ | ■ | ■ | ■ | ■ | ■ | ■ |
| | Squamous cell carcinoma | ■ | ■ | ■ | ■ | ■ | ■ | ■ | ■ | ■ | ■ | ■ | ■ | ■ |
| | Actinic keratoses | ■ | ■ | ■ | ■ | | ■ | ■ | ■ | | | | | |
| | Plasma cell pododermatitis | | | | | | | | | | | | ■ | |
| Noninflammatory and nonendocrine forms of alopecia | Breed-related | | ■ | ■ | ■ | ■ | ■ | ■ | ■ | ■ | ■ | ■ | | ■ |
| | Follicular dysplasia | | | | | ■ | ■ | ■ | ■ | | | ■ | | ■ |
| | Pattern alopecia | ■ | ■ | | | | | ■ | ■ | | | ■ | | ■ |
| | Cyclic alopecia of the flanks and nasal bridge | | | | ■ | ■ | | | | | | | | |
| | Anagen and telogen effluvium | | | | | ■ | ■ | ■ | ■ | ■ | ■ | ■ | | ■ |
| | Post-clipping alopecia | | | | | ■ | ■ | ■ | ■ | ■ | | | | |
| | Traction alopecia | | ■ | | | | | | | | | | | |
| | Post-injection alopecia | | | | | ■ | | | | | | | | |
| | Alopecia areata | | ■ | ■ | ■ | ■ | ■ | ■ | ■ | ■ | ■ | ■ | ■ | ■ |
| | Pseudopelade | | ■ | ■ | ■ | ■ | ■ | ■ | ■ | ■ | ■ | ■ | ■ | ■ |
| | Feline psychogenic alopecia | | | | | ■ | ■ | ■ | ■ | | | | | |

# 02 Bacterial dermatoses

# Introduction

Pyoderma is a form of dermatitis that is caused by bacteria and is much more common in dogs. Depending on the depth of skin involvement, it can be classified as surface, superficial, or deep pyoderma.

The conditions described in this chapter are:

- Intertrigo
- Impetigo
- Bacterial overgrowth
- Pyotraumatic dermatitis
- Pyotraumatic folliculitis–furunculosis
- Superficial bacterial folliculitis
- Pyoderma of the mucocutaneous junctions
- Deep pyoderma of the nasal bridge
- Infectious blepharitis
- Pyoderma of the chin
- Bacterial pododermatitis
- German Shepherd deep pyoderma
- Callus pyoderma
- Furunculosis–cellulitis complex
- Subcutaneous abscesses
- Botryomycosis
- Superficial and deep pyoderma in cats
- Pyoderma due to atypical bacteria
- Acral lick dermatitis

A common feature of all these conditions is that they are almost always secondary to other conditions and may require antibiotic treatment for 3–8 weeks, depending on the depth of the pyoderma. Topical therapy should not be underestimated: antiseptic shampoos and antibiotic ointments, sprays, or lotions can help considerably. Topical treatment is always a good therapeutic strategy if it reduces or replaces the use of systemic antibiotics. This helps avoid alterations in the microbiome and possible selection of antibiotic-resistant bacterial strains. Fluorescent light energy (FLE) is an alternative option to reduce the duration of antibiotic treatment or stimulate the resolution of various skin disorders.

In general, empirical use of beta-lactam antibiotics such as cephalosporins or amoxicillin + clavulanic acid is advisable. Recurrent, refractory, or deep pyodermas should be treated with antibiotics selected based on the results of an antibiotic sensitivity test.

# Intertrigo

## Lesion aetiology/pathogenesis and clinical picture

This surface pyoderma with skin fold dermatitis is caused by friction and the accumulation of secretions and excretions (saliva, tears, faeces, urine, sweat, or sebaceous content). It is usually characterised by an erythematous, exudative, and erosive presentation, and more frequently affects brachycephalic breeds.

The most commonly affected areas are the facial, vaginal, interdigital, and caudal folds. Commonly affected sites include body folds in Shar Peis, the folds of the nasal bridge in brachycephalic breeds, labial folds in dogs with elongated lips, and the tail in French Bulldogs, obese dogs, and female dogs with hypoplastic genitalia.

Biofilm formation is common in this type of pyoderma, as well as in otitis and in any infection affecting areas in which cleaning and tissue renewal is difficult.

Deeper variants of intertrigo can be exacerbated by biofilm formation. In these cases treatment is difficult.

## Diagnostic method

Swab or imprint cytology can confirm the presence of bacterial agents and/or yeast with abundant inflammatory cells. The clinical presentation is usually unambiguous.

## Main differential diagnoses

- Dermatitis due to *Malassezia* or *Candida*
- Contact dermatitis
- Mucocutaneous pyoderma

## Treatment

Treatment usually seeks to restore the balance of the cutaneous ecosystem, either through surgical correction of the skin fold or by preventing accumulation of debris and consequent infection. Astringent topical antibiotic products can be used or, in more severe cases, systemic antibiotic treatment. First-generation cephalosporins are the antibiotics of choice.

Topical combinations of astringents (e.g. acetic and boric acid), antiseptics (e.g. chlorhexidine), and topical antibiotics (e.g. fusidic acid and mupirocin) are usually effective. Mupirocin should only be used where strictly necessary.

In cases of biofilm formation thorough cleaning and the use of products containing N-acetylcysteine are very important.

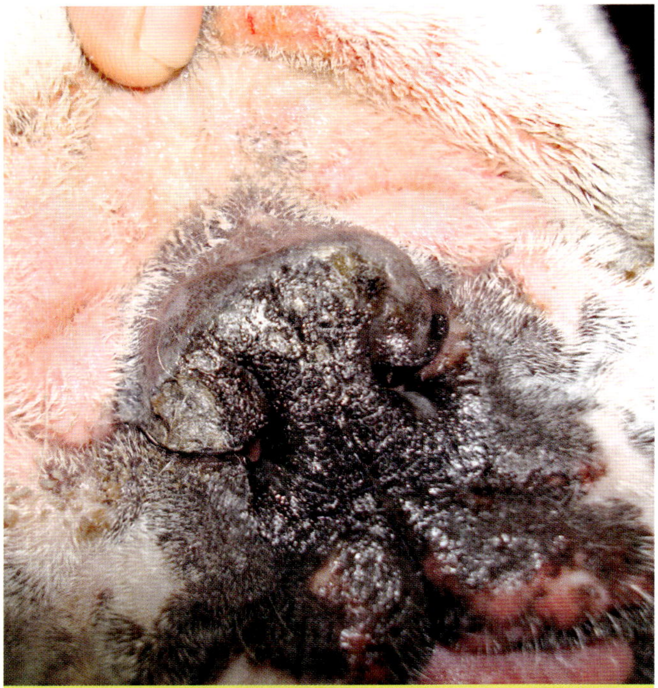

01 Intertrigo of the frontal facial fold in an English Bulldog. Note the abundant exudate and the depth of involvement.

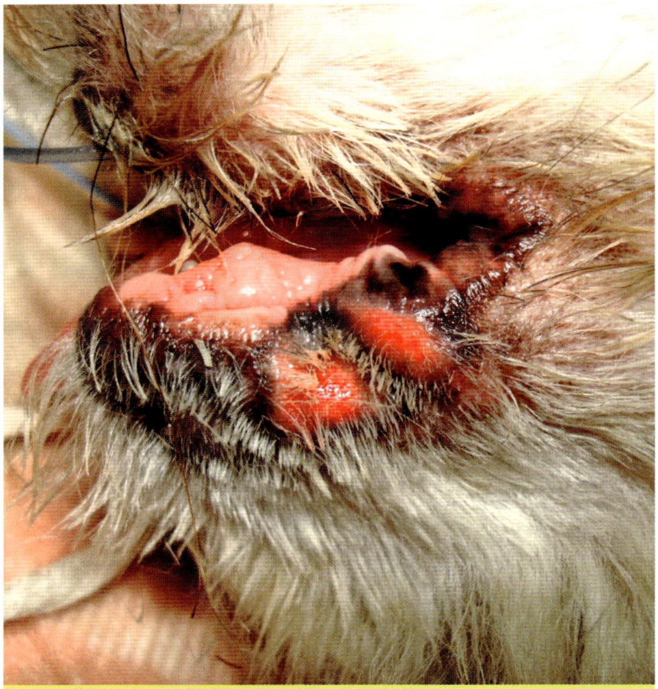

02 Intertrigo of the lip fold in a mixed-breed dog. The juxtaposition of the lips, together with saliva, can trigger the infection, which is characterised by a foul odour.

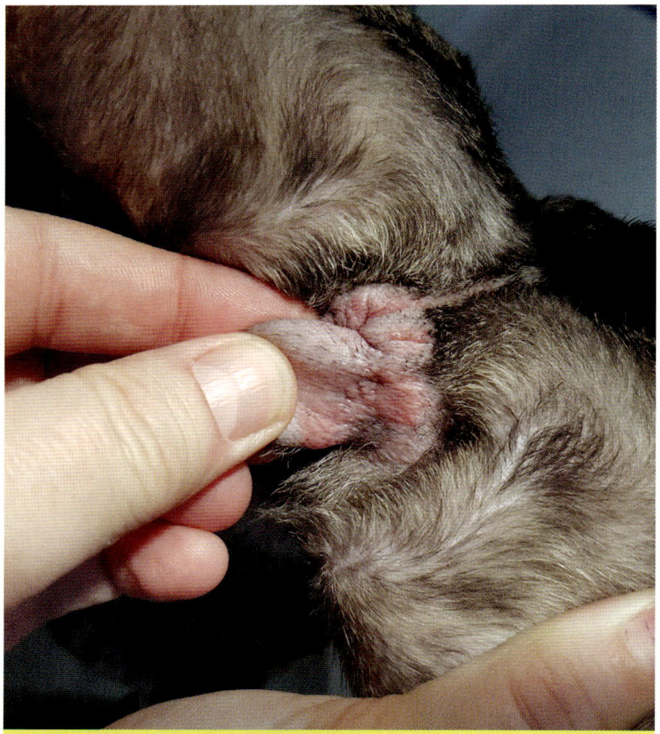

03 Perivulvar intertrigo. Hypoplastic vulva, causing excessive licking.

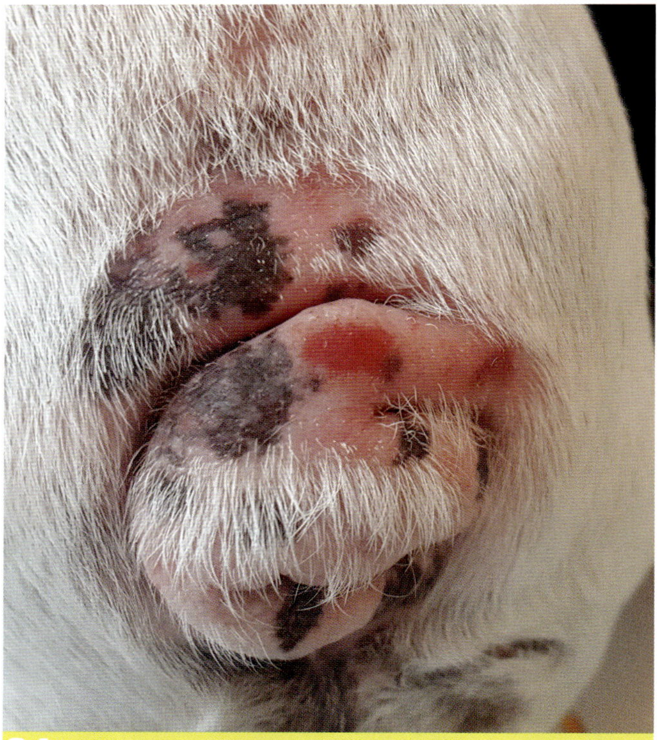

04 Tail fold intertrigo. French Bulldog with a deep skin fold.

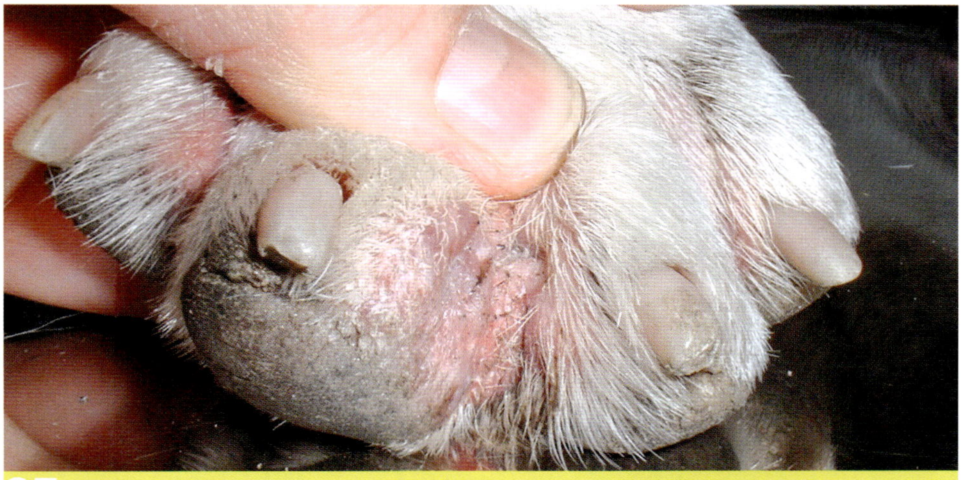

05 Interdigital intertrigo.

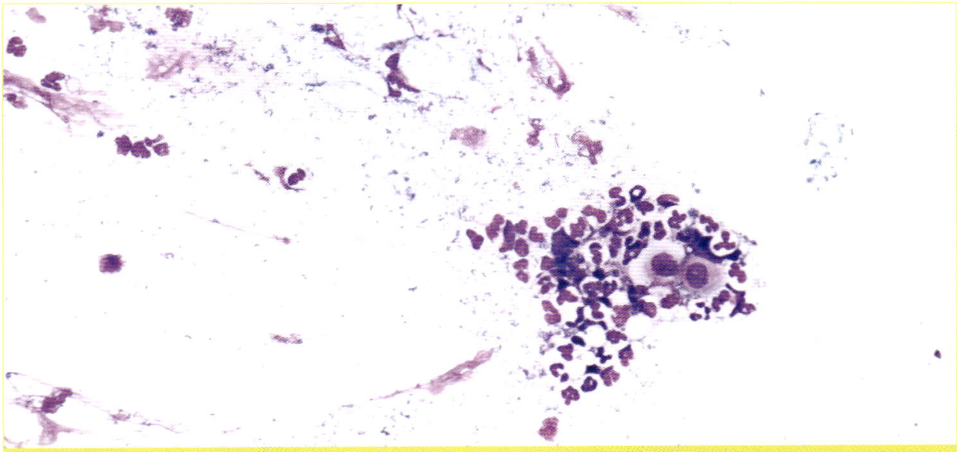

06 Intertrigo cytology. Note the bacterial formations and degenerated neutrophils, as well as some macrophages, in a sample taken from the exudate.

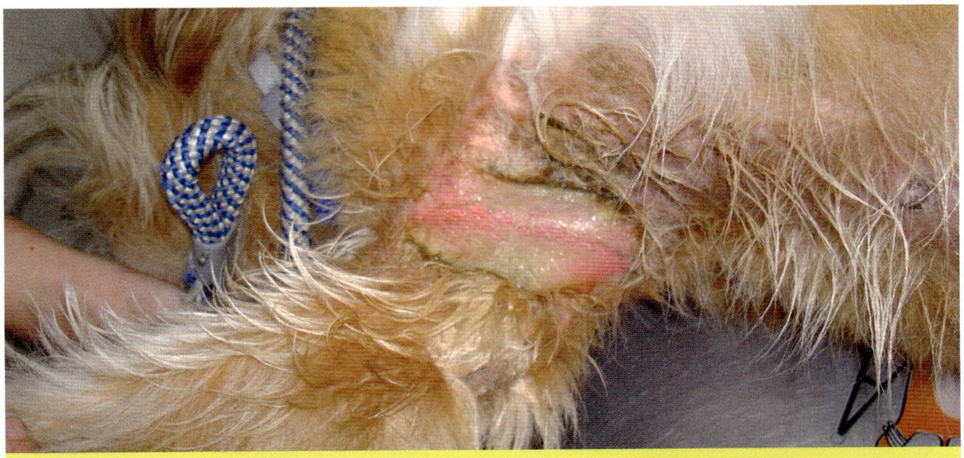

07 Deep intertrigo in the axillary area promoted by permanent dampness and obesity in a swimming dog. Note the biofilm formation.

# Impetigo

## Lesion aetiology/pathogenesis and clinical picture

This form of superficial pyoderma affects the ventroabdominal, axillary, and inguinal areas in young dogs, resulting in the formation of extrafollicular pustules.

It is usually associated with prepubertal immunosuppression and mainly affects dogs raised in poor conditions.

## Diagnostic method

The clinical appearance is characteristic, and diagnosis can be confirmed by ultrafine needle aspiration cytology of the pustules.

## Main differential diagnoses

- Other forms of pustular pyoderma
- Demodicosis
- Autoimmune pustular dermatosis

## Treatment

Improvement of the animal's environment is usually sufficient, together with the application of topical antiseptics. Correct internal deworming usually resolves the problem.

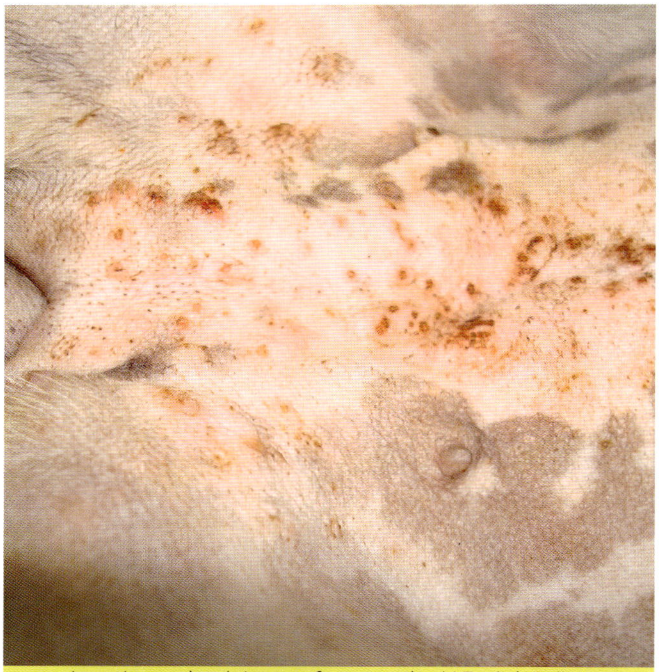

08 Impetigo on the abdomen of a 4-month-old English Bulldog puppy.

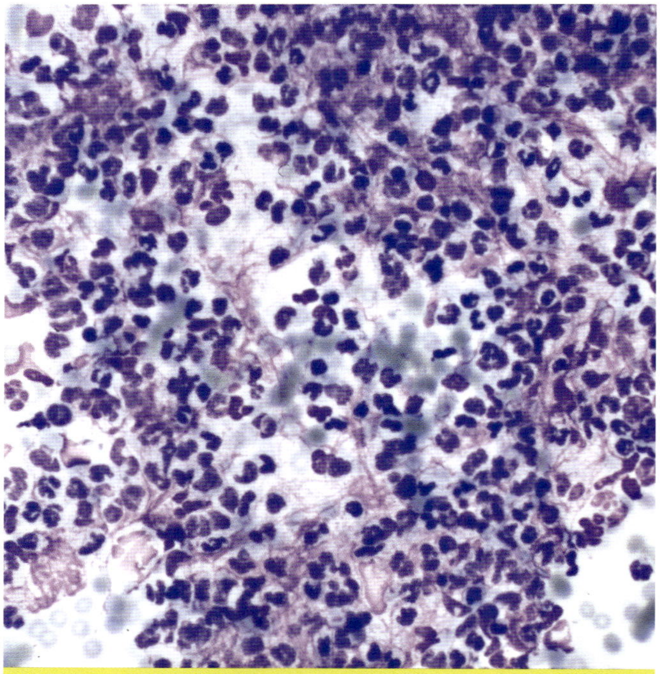

09 Typical pyogenic inflammation of an impetigo pustule.

# Bacterial overgrowth

## Lesion aetiology/pathogenesis and clinical picture

This is a form of surface pyoderma that typically affects dogs with allergic conditions, and is characterised by a scaling and seborrhoeic pattern, with diffuse alopecia in certain cases and hyperpigmentation and lichenification in advanced cases. Bacterial overgrowth usually has a significant impact on the severity of pruritus.

Excessive sebaceous production due to bacterial irritation of the sebaceous glands accounts for the seborrhoea and the rancid smell (caused by oxidation of sebaceous content).

## Diagnostic method

Adhesive tape cytology is usually the best diagnostic tool. Samples can be stained with rapid panoptic stain, which usually reveals keratinocytes, typically surrounded by cocci. Methylene blue or simply the blue component of panoptic stain can also be used to stain the sample.

## Main differential diagnoses

- *Malassezia* overgrowth
- Seborrhoea of other aetiology

## Treatment

Shampoo therapy with antiseptics and keratomodulators or moisturisers and, in some cases, antibiotic treatment, are the most commonly indicated therapies. Attempts should be made to control the underlying disease, which is usually allergic in nature.

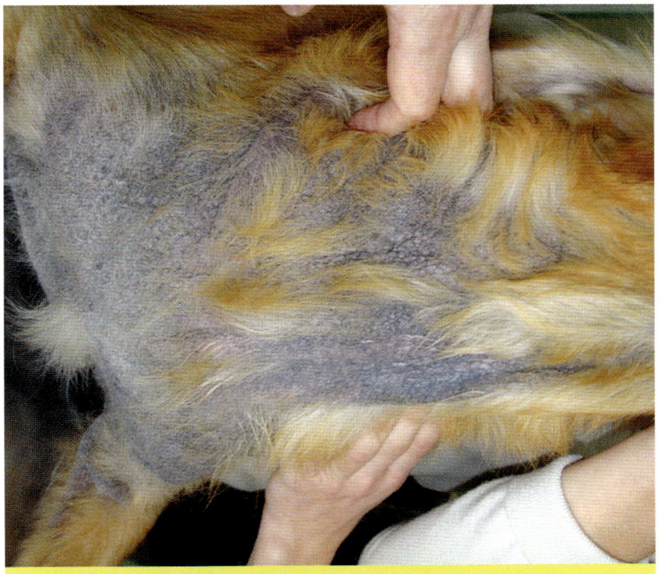

10 Bacterial overgrowth on the ventral part of the neck of an atopic Golden Retriever.

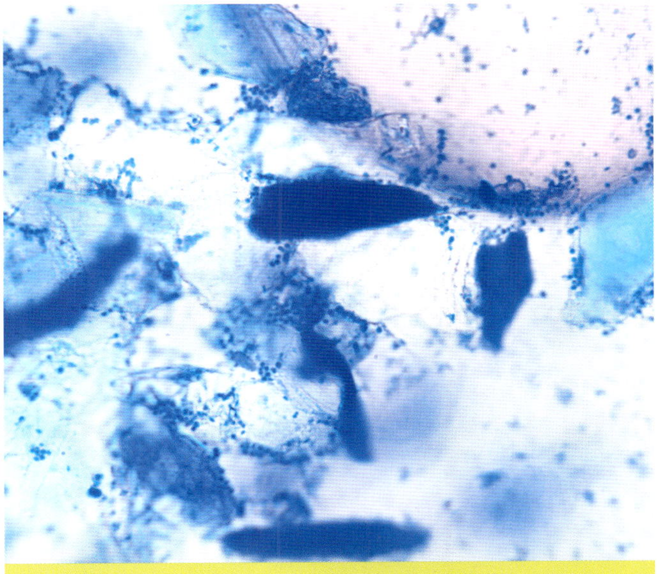

11 Cytology of bacterial overgrowth showing keratinocytes surrounded by cocci.

# Pyotraumatic dermatitis

## Lesion aetiology/pathogenesis and clinical picture

This form of surface pyoderma is caused by a self-induced lesion, with hyperacute onset. It is usually associated with conditions causing pain or pruritus in dogs. Certain breeds, including the German Shepherd, Golden Retriever, Labrador Retriever, Rottweiler, Newfoundland, Saint Bernard, and Bernese Mountain Dog appear to be predisposed. This type of pyoderma is also known as hot spot or wet eczema.

## Diagnostic method

The clinical picture is unmistakable, and is characterised by exudative and painful alopecia of abrupt onset. The caudal area, neck, and cheeks are the areas most often affected. It can be useful to investigate whether the site of the lesion corresponds to a region affected by possible pain or pruritus. For example, a lesion beneath the ear may be due to pruritus or pain affecting the ear. The same applies to pyotraumatic dermatitis of the rump, which may be due to orthopaedic problems in the hips or lumbar region, or conditions that affect the anus or adjacent anal sacs.

## Main differential diagnoses

- Pyotraumatic furunculosis
- Traumatic wound

## Treatment

Depending on the severity, treatment consists of topical or systemic antibiotics, corticosteroids, or oclacitinib, together with thorough cleaning of the area. It is very important to try to determine the cause of the self-induced injury. Avoidance of excess moisture may be necessary in recurrent cases, and proactive treatments (e.g. lokivetmab) may be required in patients with allergies. Proper flea control is essential, and NSAIDs should be administered if pain is present.

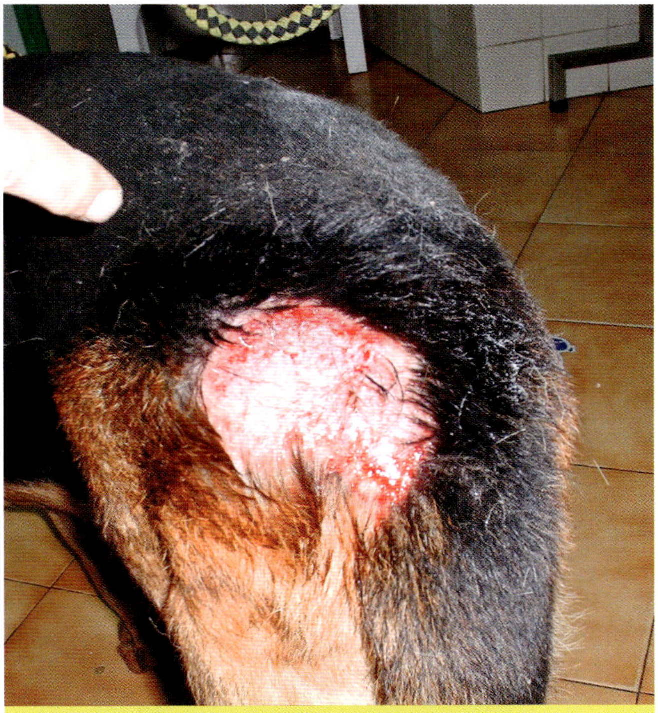

12 Pyotraumatic dermatitis on the rump of a German Shepherd.

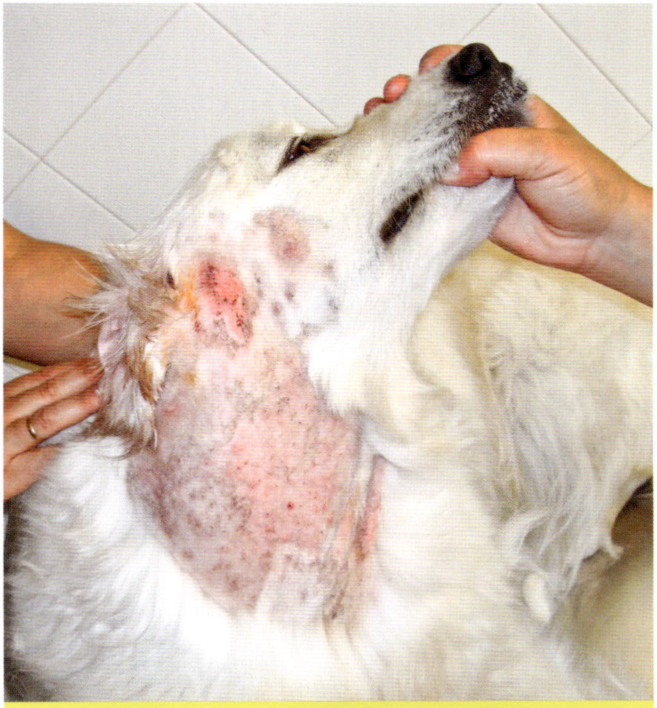

13 Subauricular pyotraumatic dermatitis with adjacent folliculitis in a Golden Retriever.

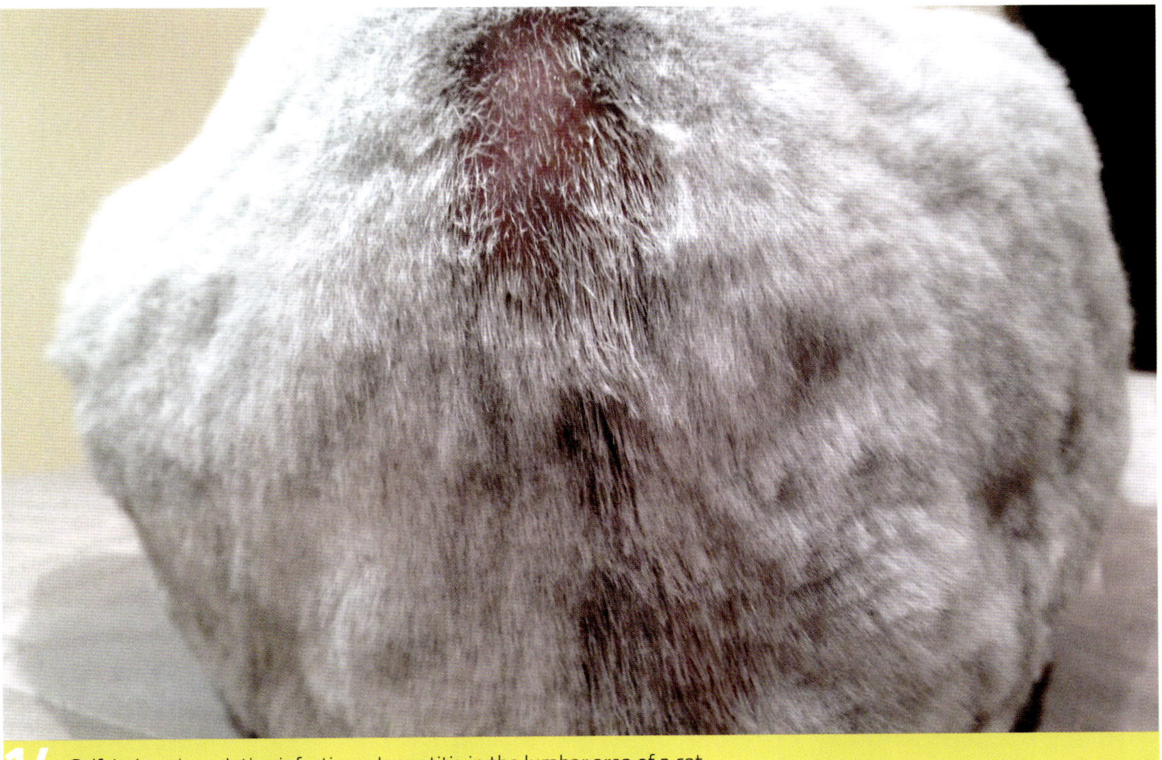

14 Self-induced exudative infectious dermatitis in the lumbar area of a cat.

# Pyotraumatic folliculitis-furunculosis

## Lesion aetiology/pathogenesis and clinical picture

This is a form of deep pyoderma resulting from a self-induced lesion, with hyperacute onset, that is usually associated with conditions causing pain or pruritus in dogs. The aetiology and pathogenesis are similar to those of pyotraumatic dermatitis, but the depth of skin involvement is much greater.

## Diagnostic method

This condition presents with furunculosis and sudden, exudative, and painful alopecia. It more commonly affects large breeds, particularly the subauricular area. The classic erosion caused by pyotraumatic dermatitis gives way to a deeper, sometimes ulcerative lesion, with hair in the centre emerging from areas of furunculosis.

## Main differential diagnoses

- Pyotraumatic dermatitis
- Traumatic wound

## Treatment

Treatment consists of systemic administration of antibiotics together with thorough cleaning of the affected area, which usually requires sedation of the animal. It is very important to try to identify the cause of the self-induced injury. The affected region should be examined. For example, if the subauricular area is affected, the ears and mouth should be examined, and if the lesion is in the rump area the examination should include the posterior locomotor apparatus and the anal region, as well as inspection for the presence of fleas.

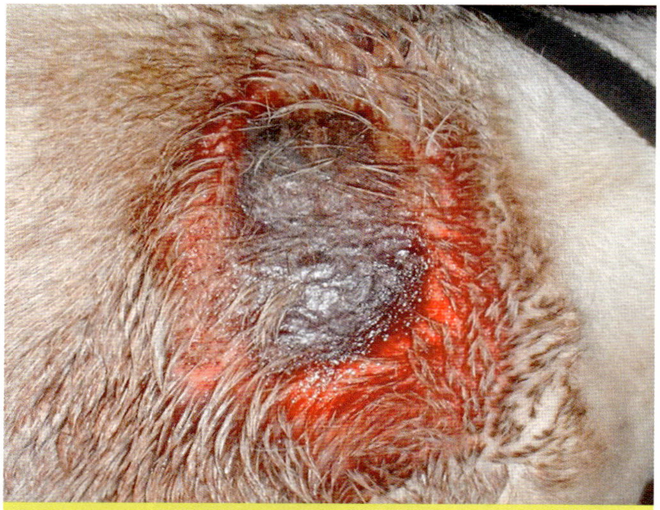

15 Pyotraumatic folliculitis furunculosis in the scapular area of an English Bulldog.

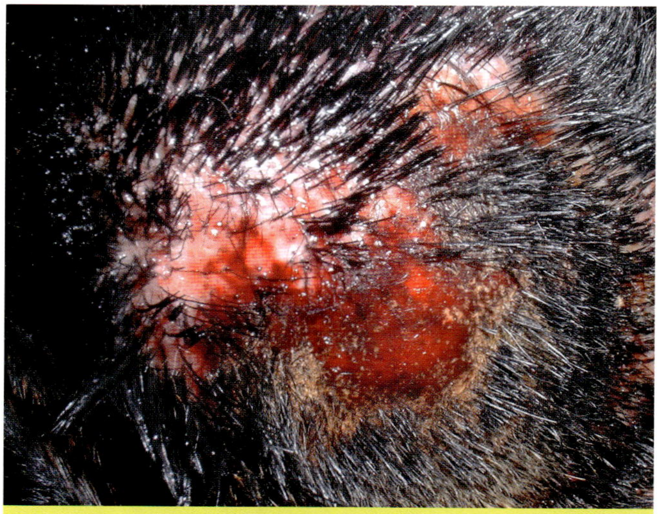

16 Close-up image of pyotraumatic furunculosis. Note the hairs emerging from the deeply inflamed central region of the lesion.

# Superficial bacterial folliculitis

## Lesion aetiology/pathogenesis and clinical picture

This is a superficial infection involving the hair follicle and the adjacent epidermis. It can be focal or multifocal, and is very common in short-haired dog breeds with allergic or endocrine diseases, resulting in a hair coat with a characteristic moth-eaten appearance. In some cases, the follicular condition can progress to furunculosis.

Although very rare in cats, it can occur secondary to miliary dermatitis.

## Diagnostic method

For the differential diagnosis it is essential to distinguish between the three main causes of folliculitis: bacterial, fungal, and parasitic. This can be achieved using adhesive tape cytology, skin scrapings, and dermatophyte test medium (DTM).

Autoimmune reactions, such as pemphigus, are a less common cause of folliculitis. In this case, the folliculitis is much more marked and does not usually respond well to antibiotic therapy.

## Main differential diagnoses

- Dermatophytosis
- Demodicosis
- Pemphigus foliaceus

## Treatment

Treatment usually consists of resolving or controlling the underlying cause, together with antiseptic shampoo and antibiotic therapy. Antibiotic sensitivity tests should be considered in problematic or recurrent cases, bearing in mind that certain strains are resistant to methicillin.

In allergic dogs, alterations in the skin microbiome can result in deficient control of the normal microbiota, leading to recurrence of the clinical picture.

Probiotic and prebiotic supplements can be beneficial. Other immunomodulators, including beta-glucans, nucleotides, and domperidone, can also be used.

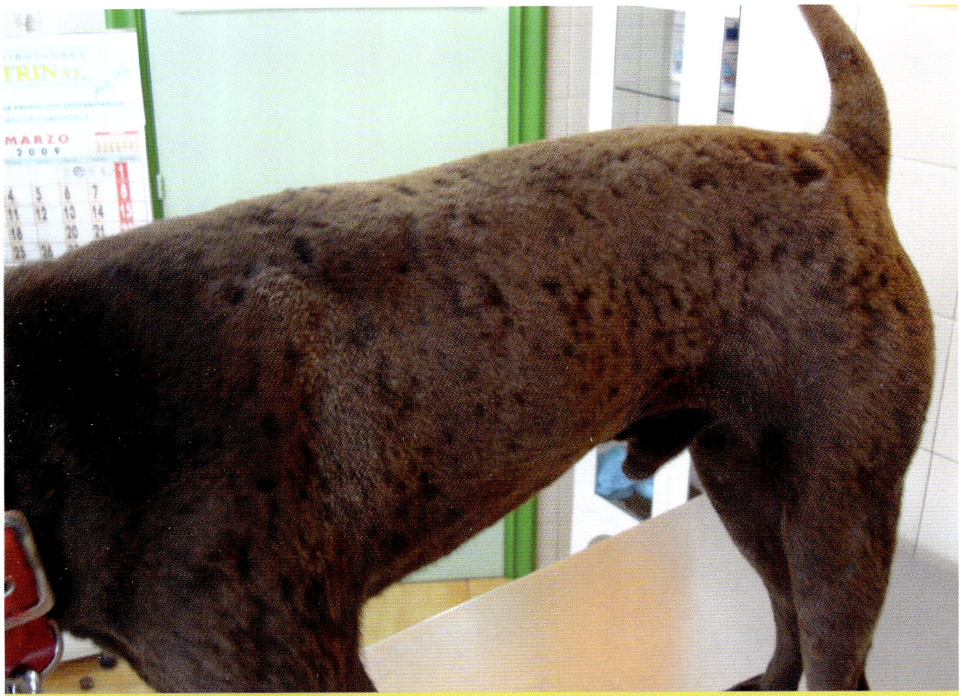


**17** Superficial folliculitis in a Shar Pei with a typical moth-eaten appearance.

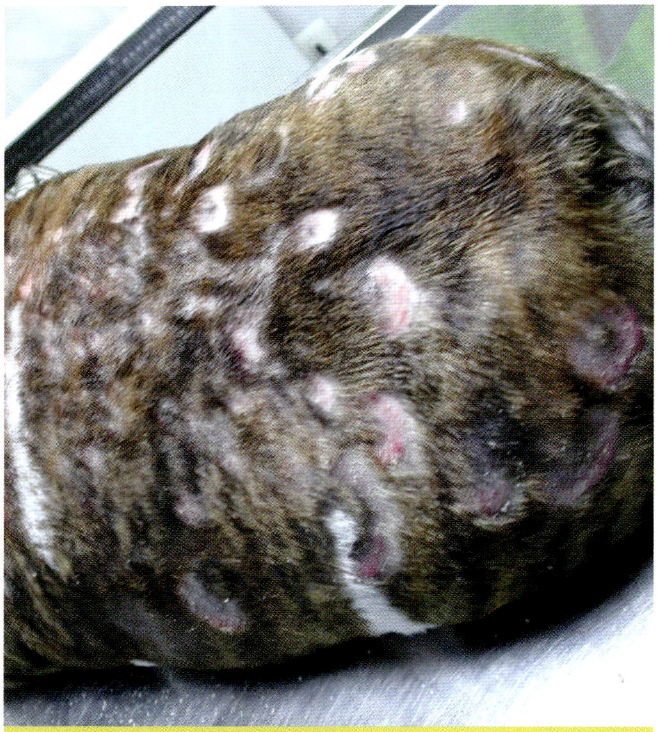

**18** Folliculitis and, in some lesions, severe disseminated furunculosis in a Bulldog. Image provided by the Somaza Pérez Veterinary Clinic (Spain).

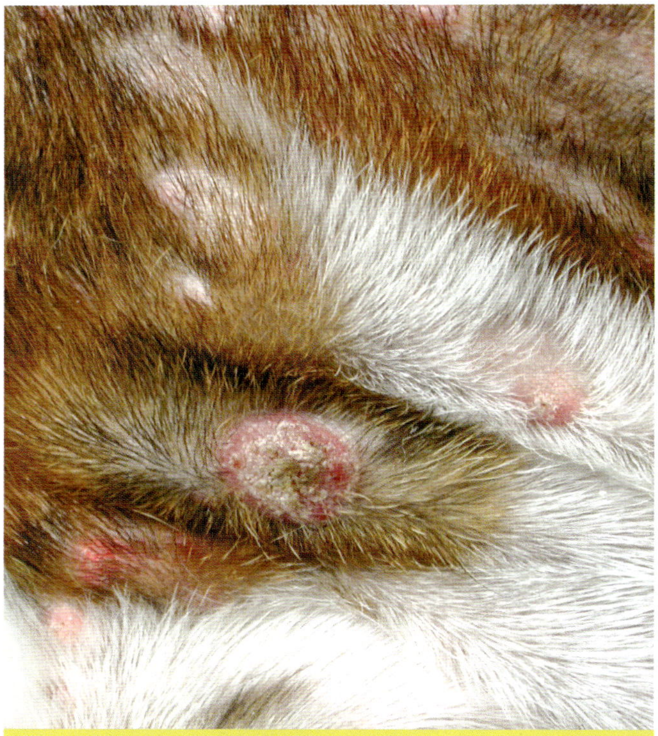

**19** Close-up image of the patient in Figure 18 in which the plaques can be seen.

# Pyoderma of the mucocutaneous junctions

## Lesion aetiology/pathogenesis and clinical picture

This superficial infection mainly affects the mucocutaneous junctions of the lips, although involvement of other mucocutaneous junctions is also described. It usually presents with an exudative–erosive picture, sometimes with ulceration, crusting, and depigmentation. It can result from various irritative causes, and mainly affects German Shepherds and their crosses.

## Diagnostic method

The differential diagnosis should include autoimmune diseases, intertrigo, candidiasis, and other diseases that affect the same body regions with a similar pattern. Antibiotic therapy is often required to confirm the diagnosis.

## Main differential diagnoses

- Contact dermatitis
- Intertrigo
- Cutaneous lupus erythematosus
- Tumours

## Treatment

Treatment usually consists of antibiotic therapy for 3 or 4 weeks and topical application of disinfectants, together with thorough cleaning of the affected area.

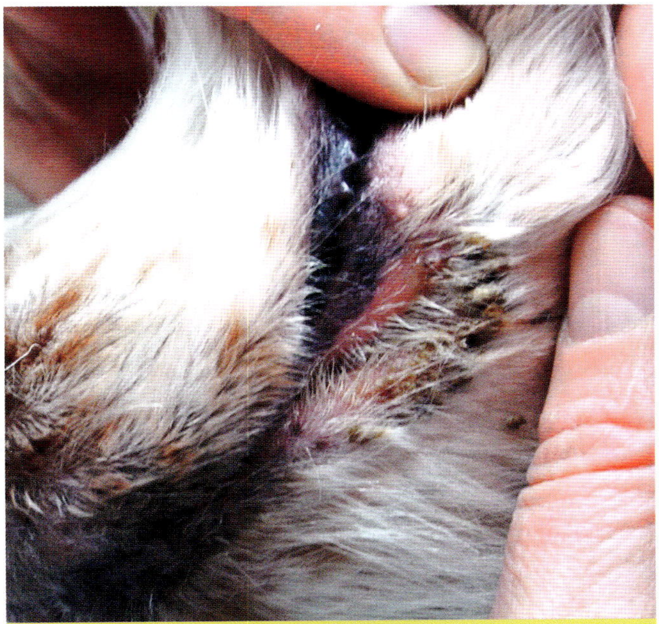

20 Mucocutaneous pyoderma of the lip in a mixed-breed dog.

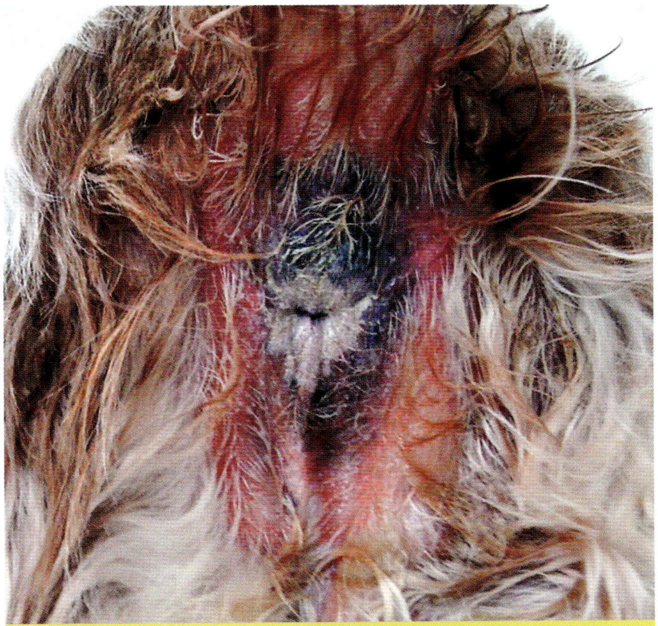

21 Perianal mucocutaneous pyoderma.

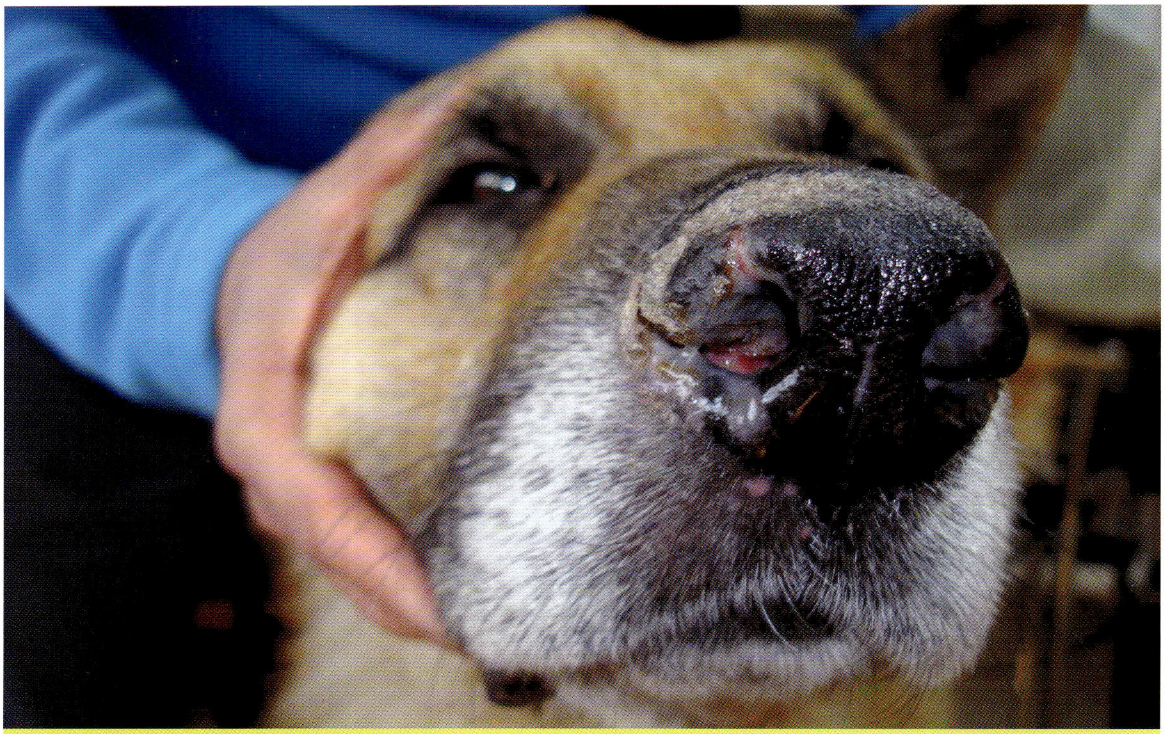

22 Nasal mucocutaneous pyoderma in a German Shepherd.

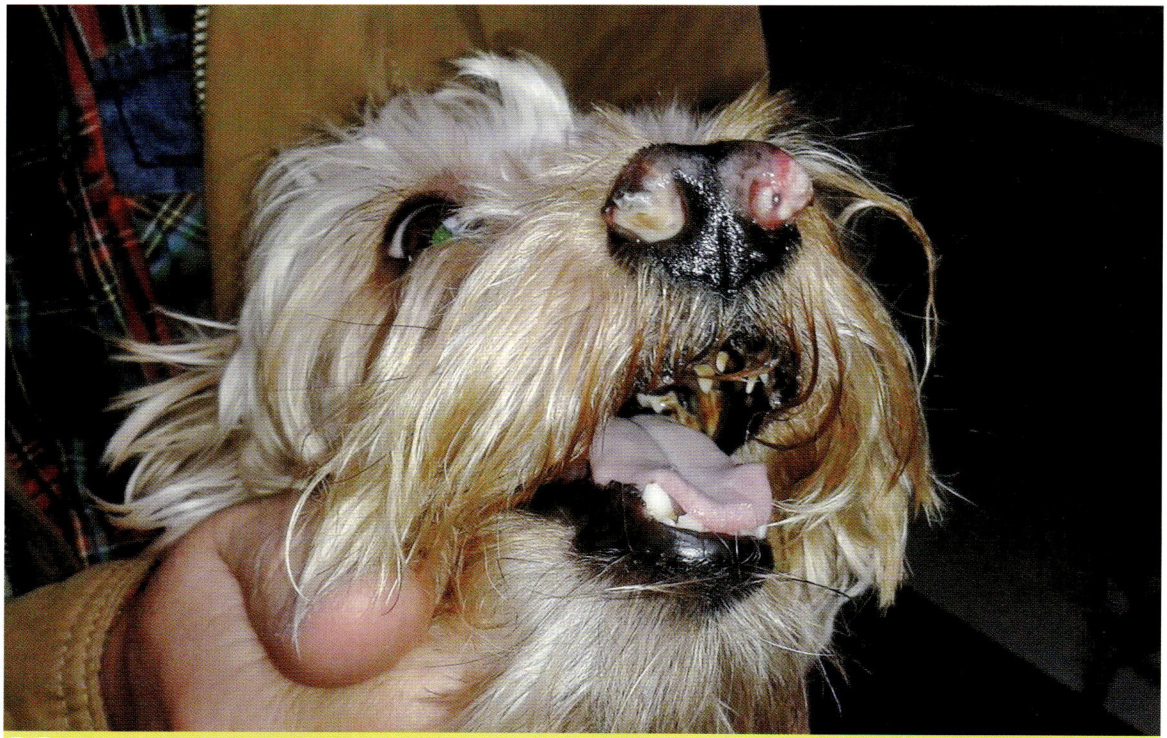

23 Mucocutaneous pyoderma of the muzzle. Note the ulcerative effect of the bacteria.

# Deep pyoderma of the nasal bridge

## Lesion aetiology/pathogenesis and clinical picture

This is a deep process that generally affects dogs, is often painful, and presents with erosions and crusts on the nasal bridge. It tends to be more common in breeds prone to cellulitis, such as the Bull Terrier. This breed usually rests the nasal bridge against the floor or wall while sleeping, which can promote follicular rupture.

In hunting dogs, this condition can be the result of trauma, actinic dermatosis, and certain autoimmune diseases.

## Diagnostic method

It is essential to include dermatophytosis in the differential diagnosis and to rule out other triggering diseases, such as pemphigus complex and discoid lupus erythematosus. Cytology is very important to determine the bacterial type (coccus or bacillus) and to detect the presence of acantholytic cells or exfoliating corneocytes, which must also be distinguished from one another. Eosinophilic furunculosis caused by Hymenoptera stings can cause a similar clinical picture, although in such cases abundant eosinophils will be visible on cytology.

In autoimmune diseases, the muzzle is usually affected.

## Main differential diagnoses

- Dermatophytosis
- Autoimmune disease
- Eosinophilic furunculosis

## Treatment

Like all forms of deep pyoderma, treatment for more than 1 month may be required, together with cleaning of the area. Efforts should be made to identify the primary cause of the problem.

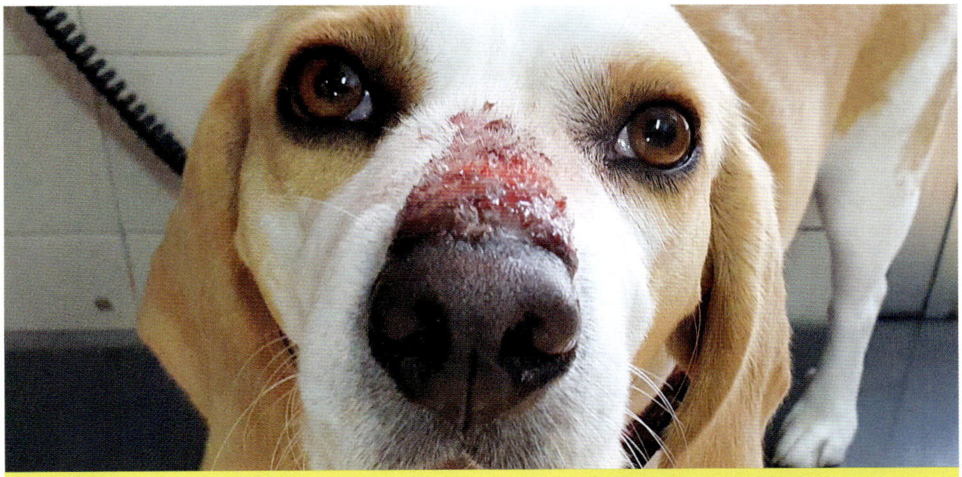

24 Pyoderma of the nasal bridge. Note that the muzzle is unaffected.

# Infectious blepharitis

## Lesion aetiology/pathogenesis and clinical picture

Itching of the eyelids, which is common in allergies, can trigger inflammation of the eyelash follicles and, in some cases, their adnexa, as occurs in meibomitis. This condition exacerbates the itching and leads to a vicious cycle, which is further aggravated by infection.

## Diagnostic method

Diagnosis is confirmed based on the clinical appearance, cytology of the exudate (obtained by lesion compression), and the response to topical antibiotics and antipruritic agents.

## Main differential diagnoses

- Chronic cutaneous lupus erythematosus
- Pemphigus
- Nodular leishmaniasis

## Treatment

In some cases, treatment with ophthalmic gels containing antibiotics and corticosteroids may suffice. In more severe cases the use of oclacitinib and antibiotics may be necessary and, if the problem recurs, proactive treatment with ophthalmic forms of tacrolimus ointment or cyclosporine can be instituted.

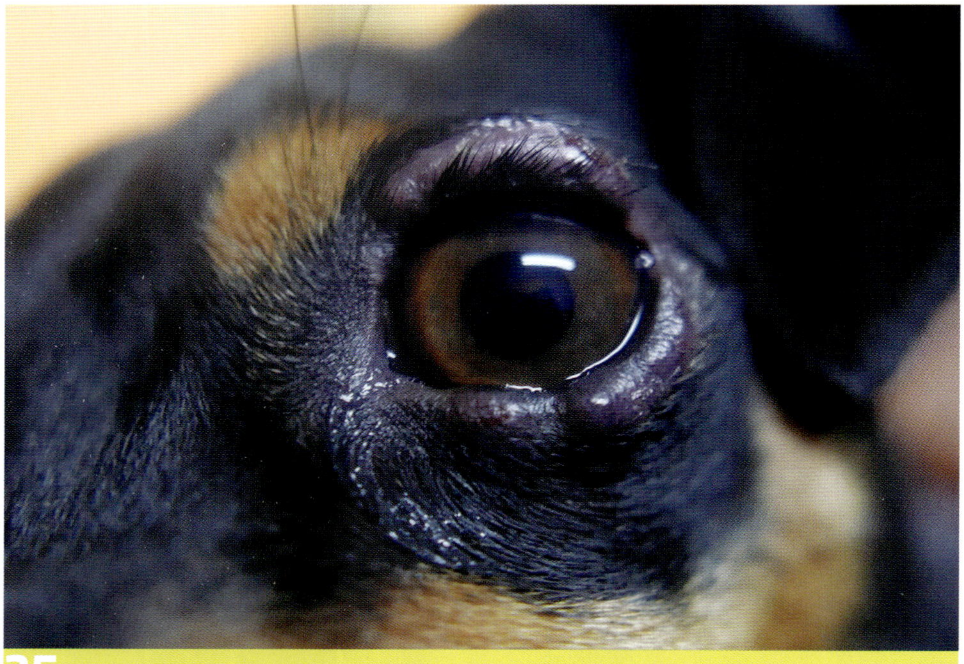

25 Blepharitis with meibomitis in an atopic Pinscher.

# Chin pyoderma

## Lesion aetiology/pathogenesis and clinical picture

This is a deep infection that generally affects dogs and cats, and is triggered by keratinisation disorders such as acne, or by other causes (often traumatic, fungal, or parasitic). It is characterised by furunculosis and, in many cases, the presence of comedones and abundant exudation. In some cases the condition can begin as intertrigo in the skin folds.

In this part of the body in cats, a keratinisation disorder can be the primary cause, affecting the area in the absence of any bacterial activity. In dogs, this condition is often caused by trauma and frequently occurs in animals that feed voraciously. The presentation can extend to affect the upper lip.

## Diagnostic method

Diagnosis is confirmed based on the clinical picture, after ruling out parasitic or fungal causes. Exudate cytology is an important complementary method to determine the type of bacteria involved.

## Main differential diagnoses

- Acne due to keratoseborrhoeic disorder
- Demodicosis
- Juvenile cellulitis
- Contact dermatitis
- Skin fold dermatitis of the chin

## Treatment

Treatment consists of antibacterial therapy and control of the underlying cause. Treatment with the exfoliating agent benzoyl peroxide and topical antiseptics can be effective.

In dogs, the use of anti-voracity feeders can be helpful to avoid rapid ingestion.

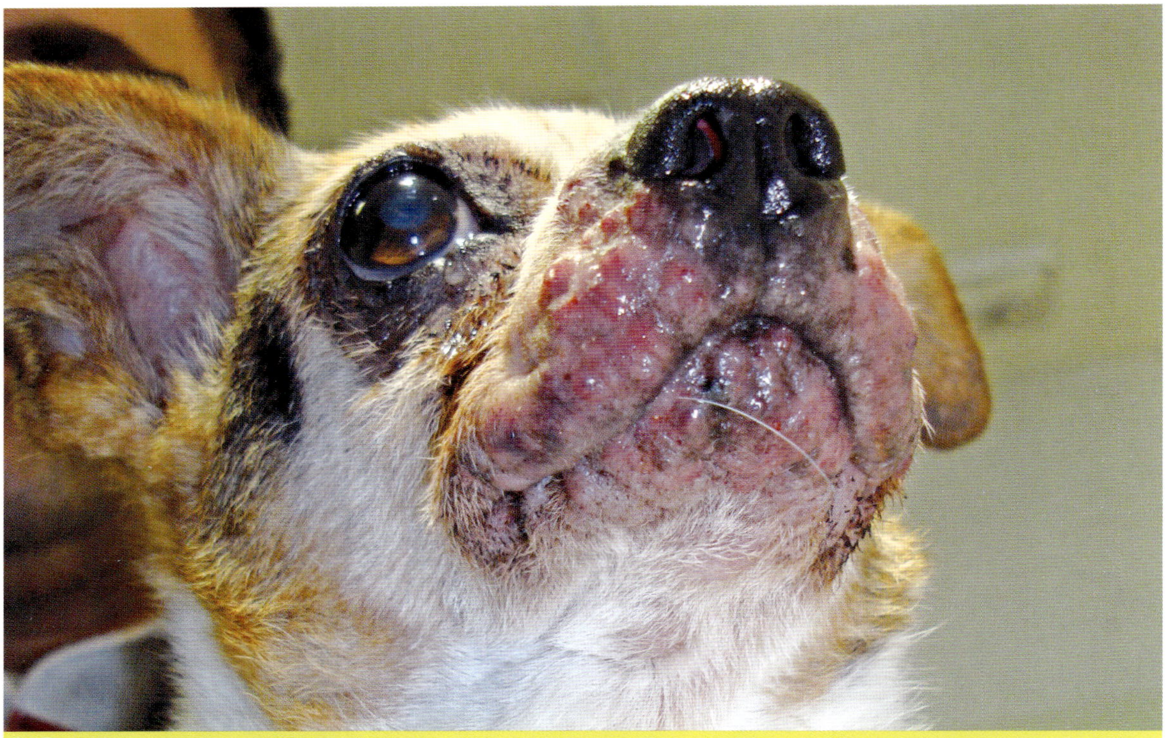

26 Dog with bacterial furunculosis on the chin and upper lip.

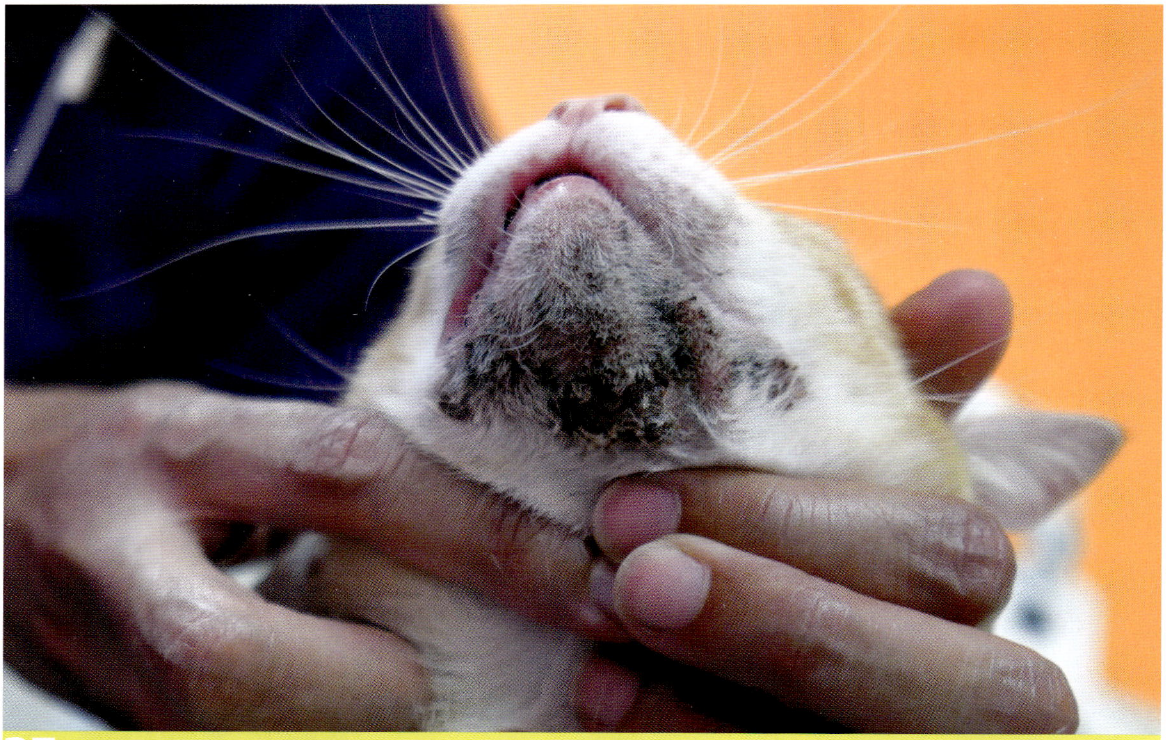

27 Feline acne with bacterial infection.

# Bacterial pododermatitis

## Lesion aetiology/pathogenesis and clinical picture

This usually deep pyoderma affects dogs and cats and is difficult to treat. It can result from primary allergic, parasitic, or traumatic causes. Due to involvement of the nail fold, the claws may be affected. In some cases licking of the digits is the trigger and can lead to pyoderma of the chin due to self-infection. German Shepherds appear to be predisposed.

In some dogs, interdigital furunculosis can lead to the formation of initially sterile granulomas that then become infected and form fistulas towards the dorsal surface.

## Diagnostic method

The differential diagnosis is achieved mainly based on cytology, which can reveal the bacterial type and the presence of *Malassezia* or parasites such as *Demodex*.

## Main differential diagnoses

- Demodicosis
- Sterile pyogranuloma
- Interdigital candidiasis or *Malassezia* infection
- Foreign body reaction (e.g. to grass awns)
- Feline pemphigus complex

## Treatment

Like all forms of deep pyoderma, treatment for more than 1 month may be required, together with cleaning of the area. Efforts should be made to identify the primary cause of the problem. It is very important to keep the area dry.

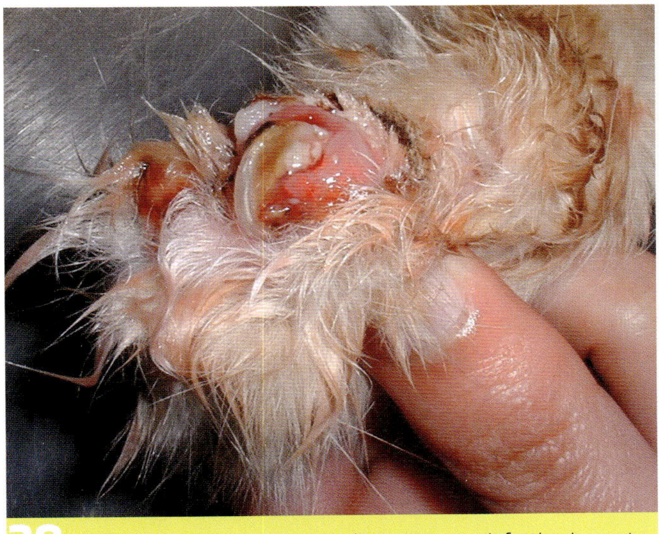

28 Onychodystrophy with paronychia and severe infection in a cat.

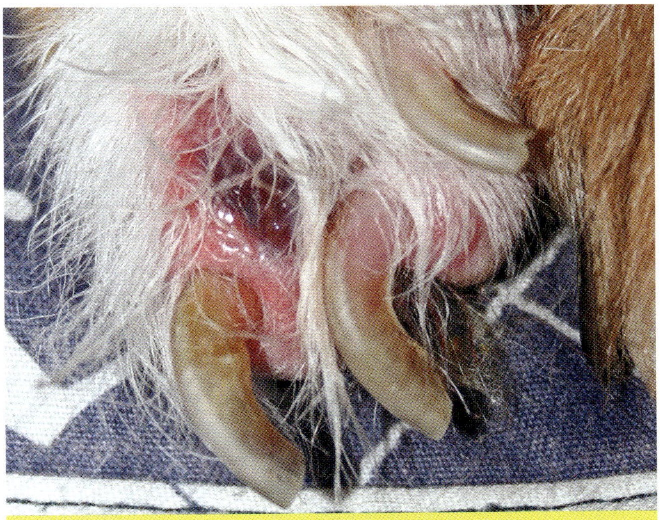

29 Pododermatitis in an atopic dog. Note the interdigital ulcer.

# German Shepherd deep pyoderma

## Lesion aetiology/pathogenesis and clinical picture

This highly characteristic disease may be associated with immunodeficiency in this breed. This is usually a very deep, painful infection, with abundant furunculosis and involvement of almost the entire body. It typically begins at 3–4 years of age.

Primary causes such as allergies, flea bites, demodicosis, hypothyroidism, ehrlichiosis, leishmaniasis, and babesiosis should always be ruled out. The presence of flies can significantly exacerbate the condition.

## Diagnostic method

Clinical manifestations are usually evident, although it is very important to rule out allergies, demodicosis, and deficient husbandry (e.g. very damp habitat, poor hygiene, flies). Some individuals of this breed tend to suffer recurrent infectious diseases due to their apparent immunodeficiency, although the aforementioned causes should be ruled out first.

## Main differential diagnoses

- Demodicosis
- Pyoderma due to allergy
- Pemphigus complex

## Treatment

As for all forms of deep pyoderma, treatment for more than 1 month may be required, together with cleaning of the area. Efforts should be made to identify the primary cause of the problem. It is very important to keep the body dry and free from parasites. A hair cut in spring or summer may be advisable in predisposed animals. Correct feeding with quality commercial food can be very important. It is advisable to avoid homemade food, which can attract flies, and to ensure a clean habitat by correctly cleaning faeces. In predisposed animals it is important to avoid aggressive brushing and walks through very wild areas. The use of some immunomodulators, such as nucleotides, domperidone, or prebiotics and probiotics, may be beneficial. Autologous bacterial lysate as a form of immunotherapy has also shown a high degree of efficacy.

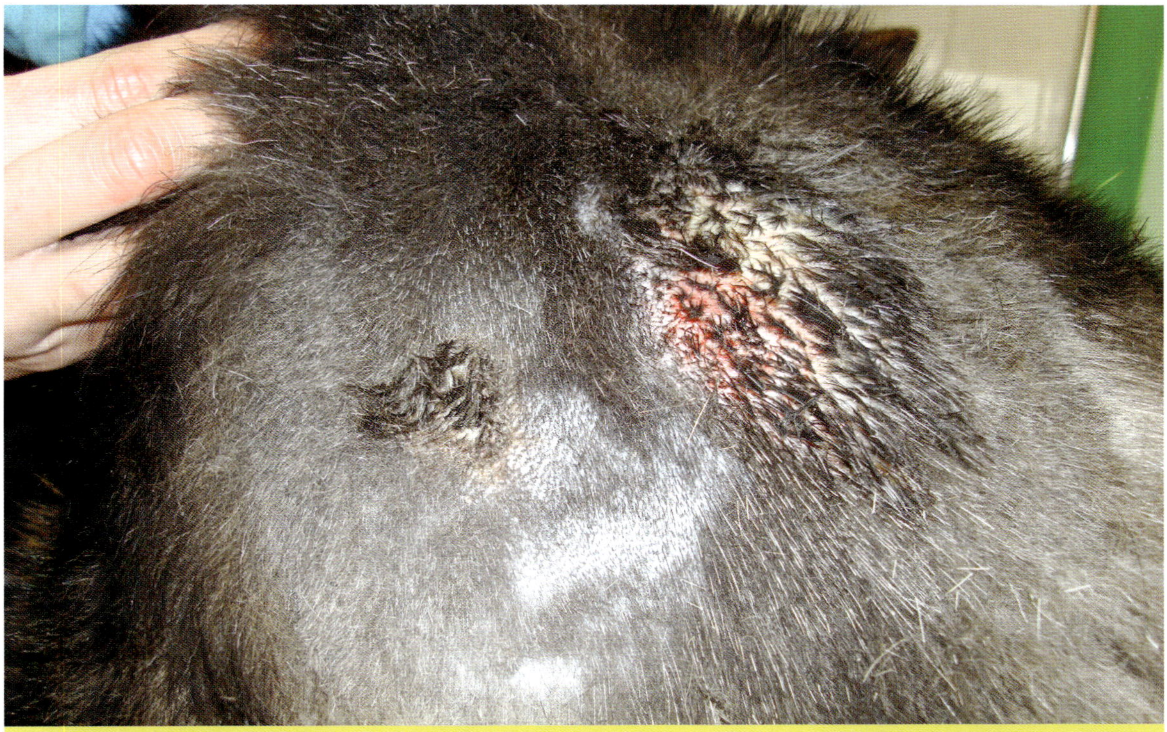

30 German Shepherd deep pyoderma. Initial condition.

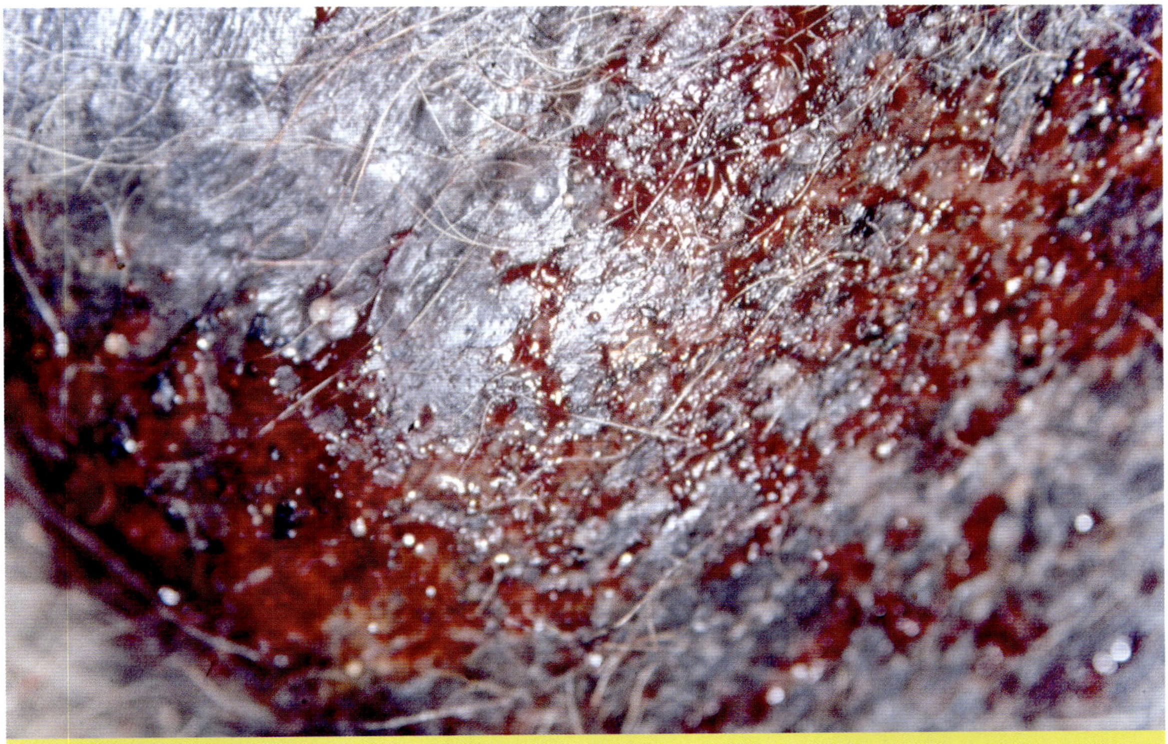

31 German Shepherd deep pyoderma. Detail showing exudation of pus and blood.

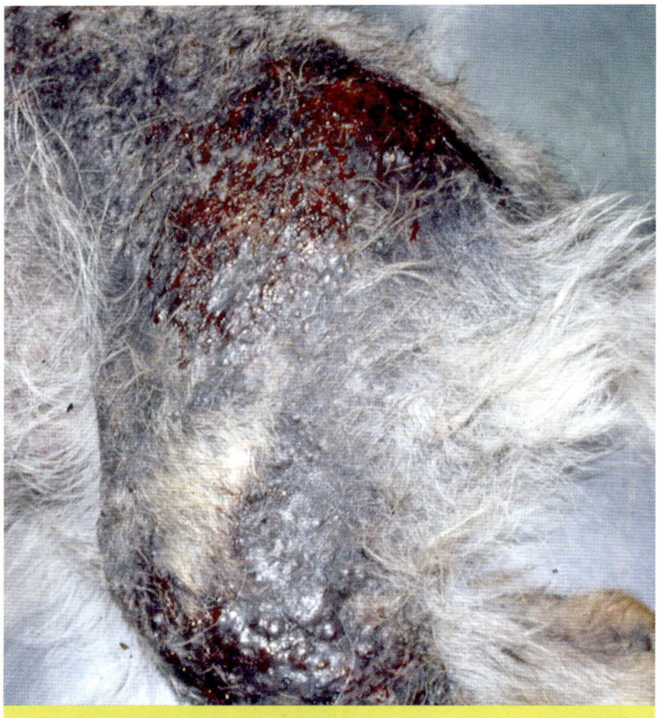

32 Severe generalised involvement in a case of German Shepherd deep pyoderma.

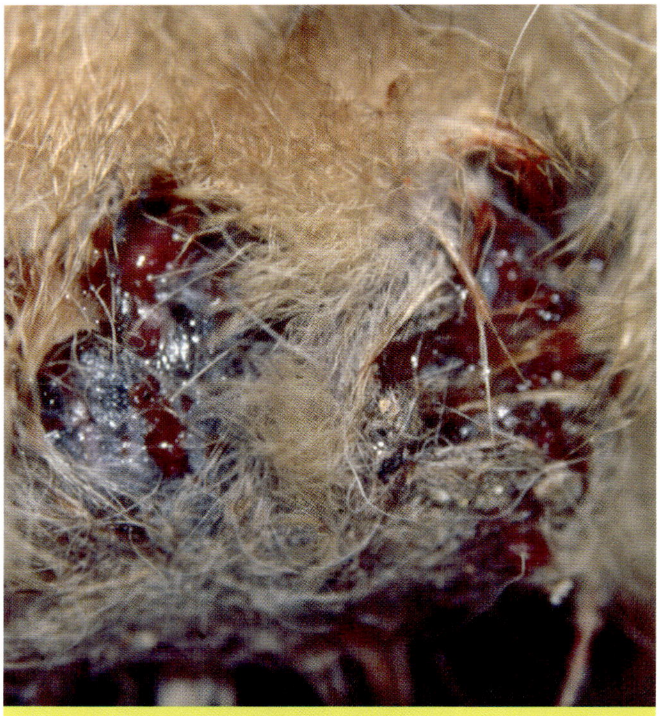

33 German Shepherd deep pyoderma. The typical fistulising lesion can be observed.

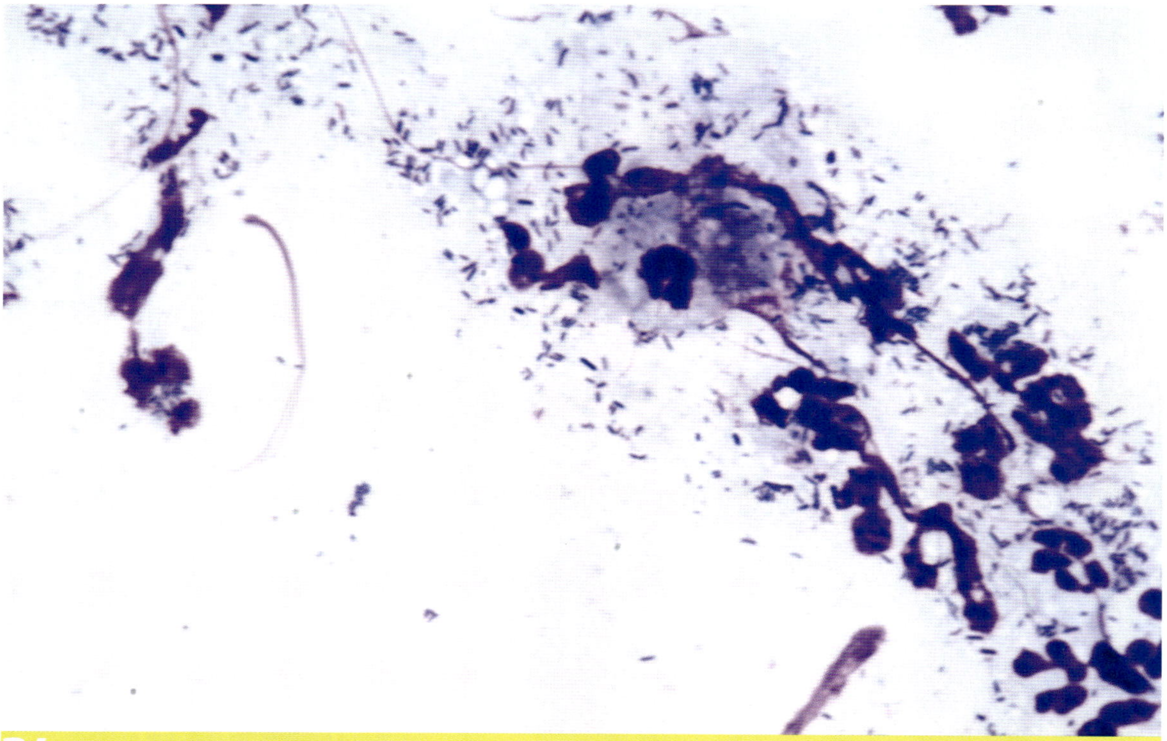

34 Cytology of the exudate showing degenerated bacilli and neutrophils.

# Callus pyoderma

## Lesion aetiology/pathogenesis and clinical picture

Also known as pressure point pyoderma, this is a deep infection that frequently presents with the formation of furuncles, and usually affects areas of skin covering bony prominences in dogs. A hyperkeratotic plaque usually forms, and later becomes infected and suppurates in response to self-trauma or formation of a fissure. It can affect the elbows, hocks, knees, sternum, or lateral carpus.

## Diagnostic method

Compression of the lesion releases fluid that can range from serohaemorrhagic to purulent. Cytology confirms infection due to the presence of cocci and/or bacilli, and reveals the presence of neutrophils. The presence of eosinophils and macrophages usually indicates a foreign body effect, resulting in the formation of trichogranulomas or keratogranulomas.

## Main differential diagnoses

- Infected wounds
- Hepatocutaneous syndrome
- Sarcoptic mange after a period of progression

## Treatment

Treatment consists of changing the animal's bed for one with padded material. This should be combined with moisturising creams and antibiotic therapy, which is usually required for several weeks until total remission of the condition is achieved. It is a recurring problem that can pose a challenge for the veterinary clinician in certain cases.

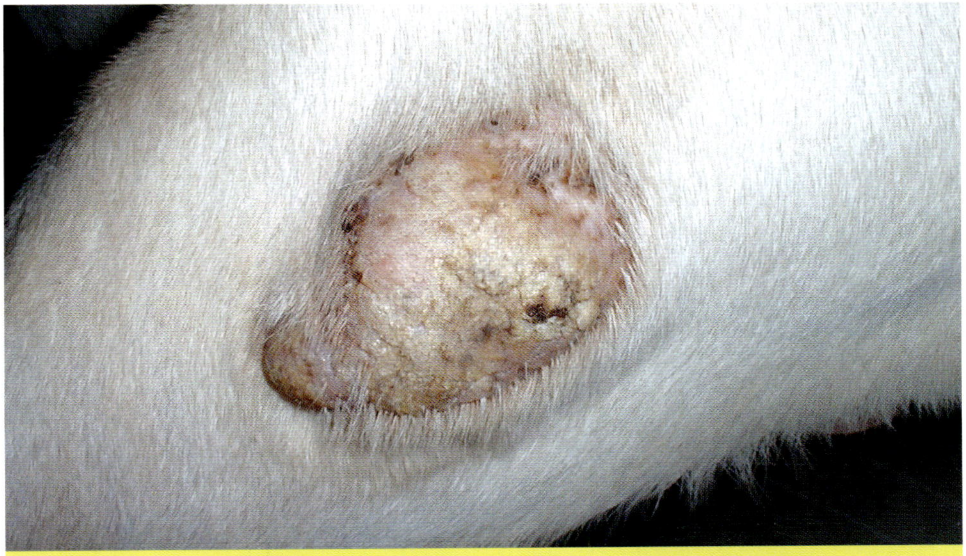

35 Calluses on skin covering bony prominences. Note the fissures, which tend to become infected.

# Furunculosis-cellulitis complex

## Lesion aetiology/pathogenesis and clinical picture

This is a highly problematic and recurrent dermatosis that is more prevalent in certain breeds such as the Bull Terrier and Staffordshire Bull Terrier. It is a deep pyoderma that can affect various areas of the body, including the head. It is much more common in short-haired dogs.

It consists of a vicious cycle that begins with licking and trauma, followed by follicular rupture, secondary infection, and pain, leading to further licking and infection. These conditions may be aggravated by sunlight, which can promote the formation of actinic comedones. The whole process is based on the formation of trichogranulomas and keratogranulomas.

## Diagnostic method

Diagnosis can be confirmed based on the clinical appearance, history, and cytology. This condition can affect predisposed dogs with an underlying allergy, although in many cases the underlying cause cannot be established.

## Main differential diagnoses

- Demodicosis
- Interdigital pyogranulomas
- Sterile panniculitis
- Actinic keratosis

## Treatment

It is very important to control these clinical signs with antibiotic therapy and shampoo (primarily benzoyl peroxide). Once the condition is controlled, relapses should be avoided by maintaining shampoo therapy and avoiding direct sunlight, which can have a negative effect on actin, and any trauma that can cause small wounds. Administration of cyclosporine as a maintenance immunomodulatory therapy after inducing remission with corticosteroids is effective in many cases.

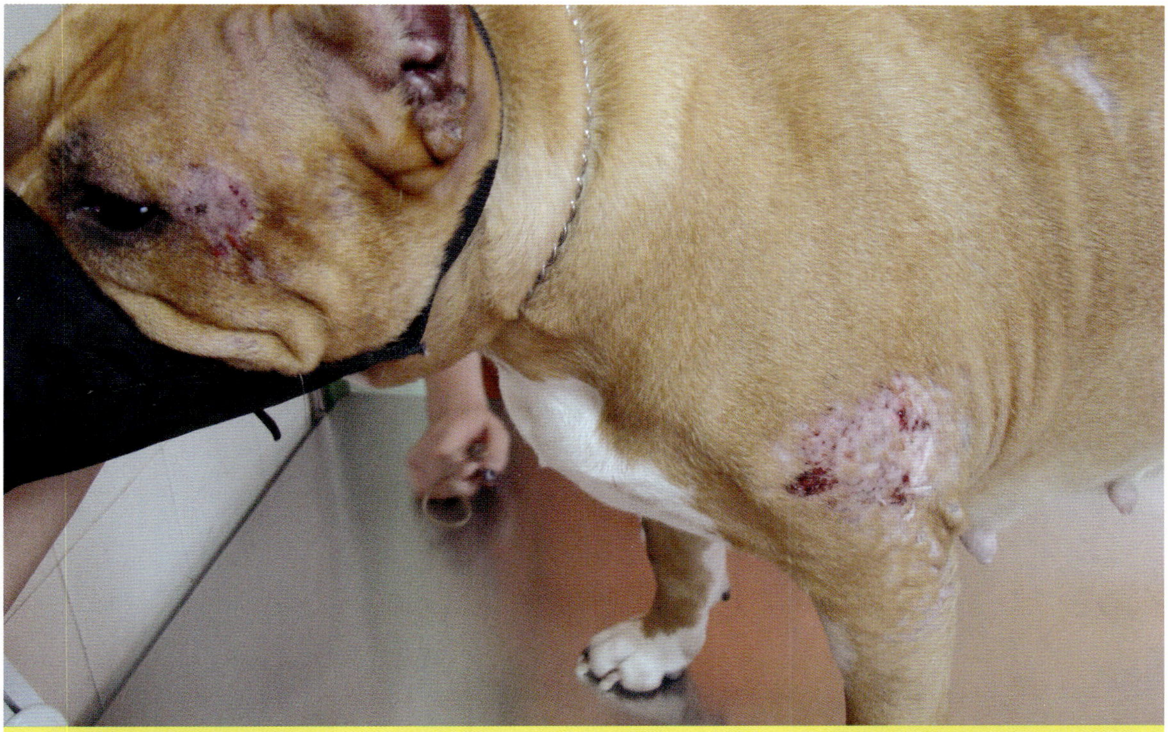

36 Furunculosis-cellulitis complex in a Pitbull.

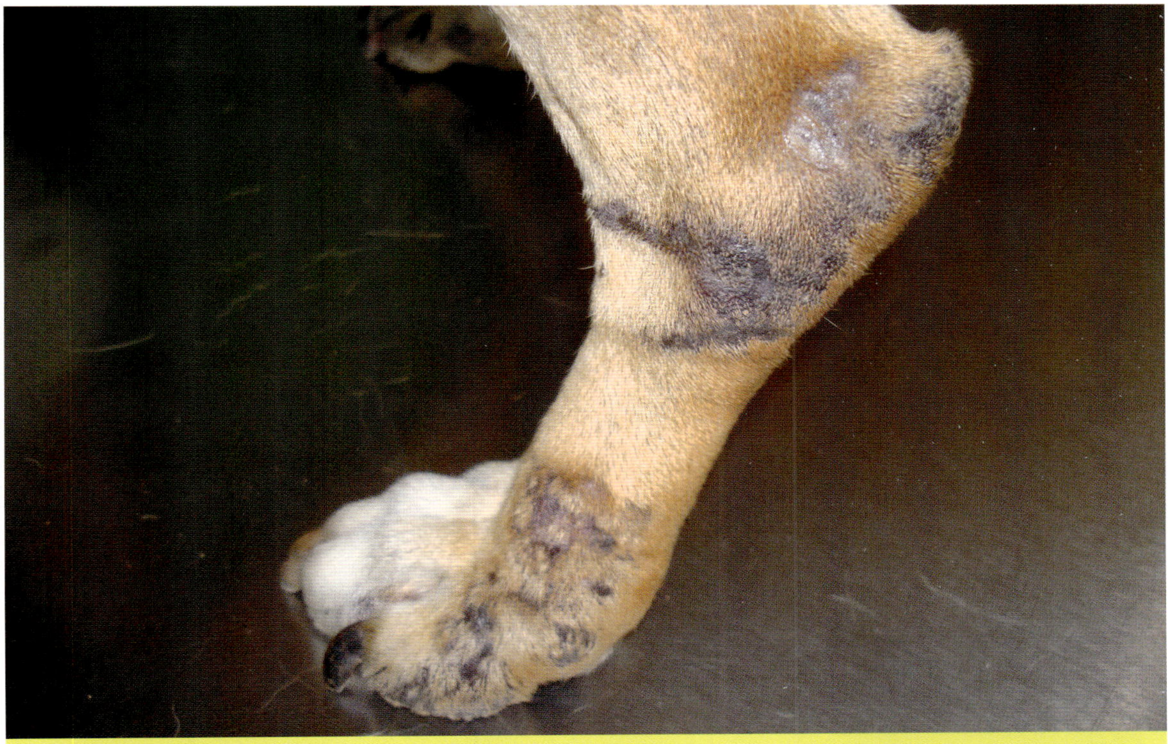

37 Pitbull from the previous image: note the papulopustular and fistulising presentation with serohaemorrhagic discharge.

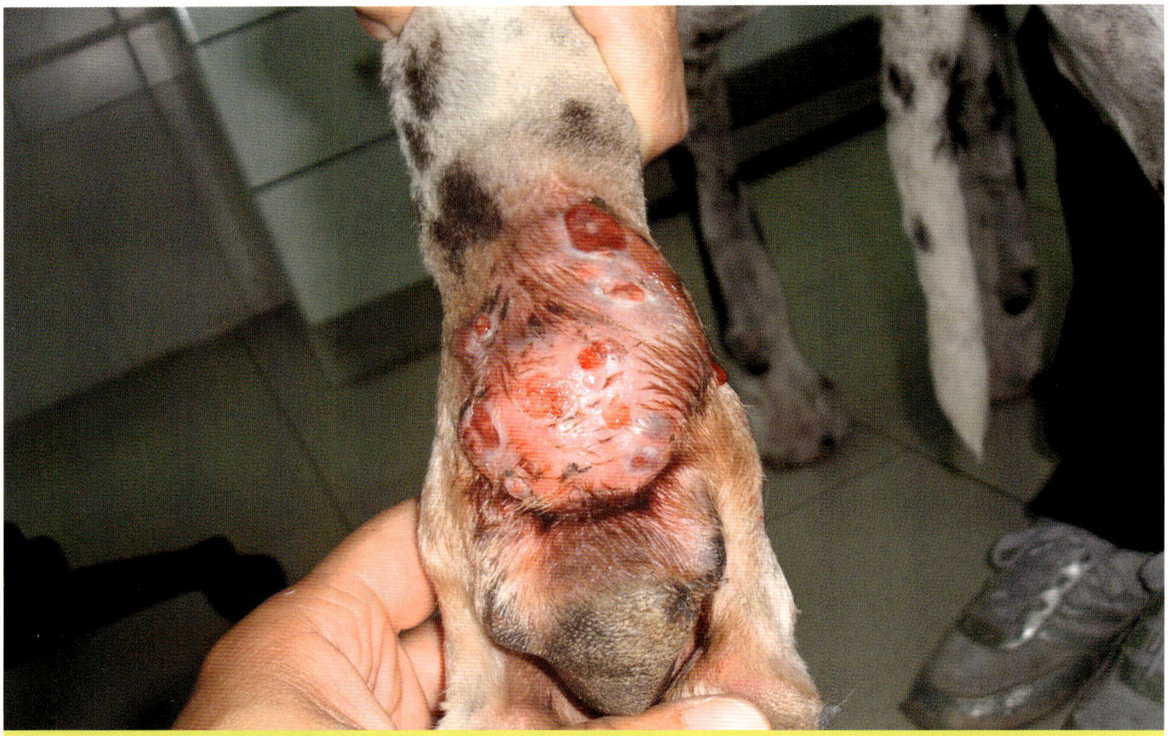

38 Cellulitis and digital furunculosis in a Great Dane.

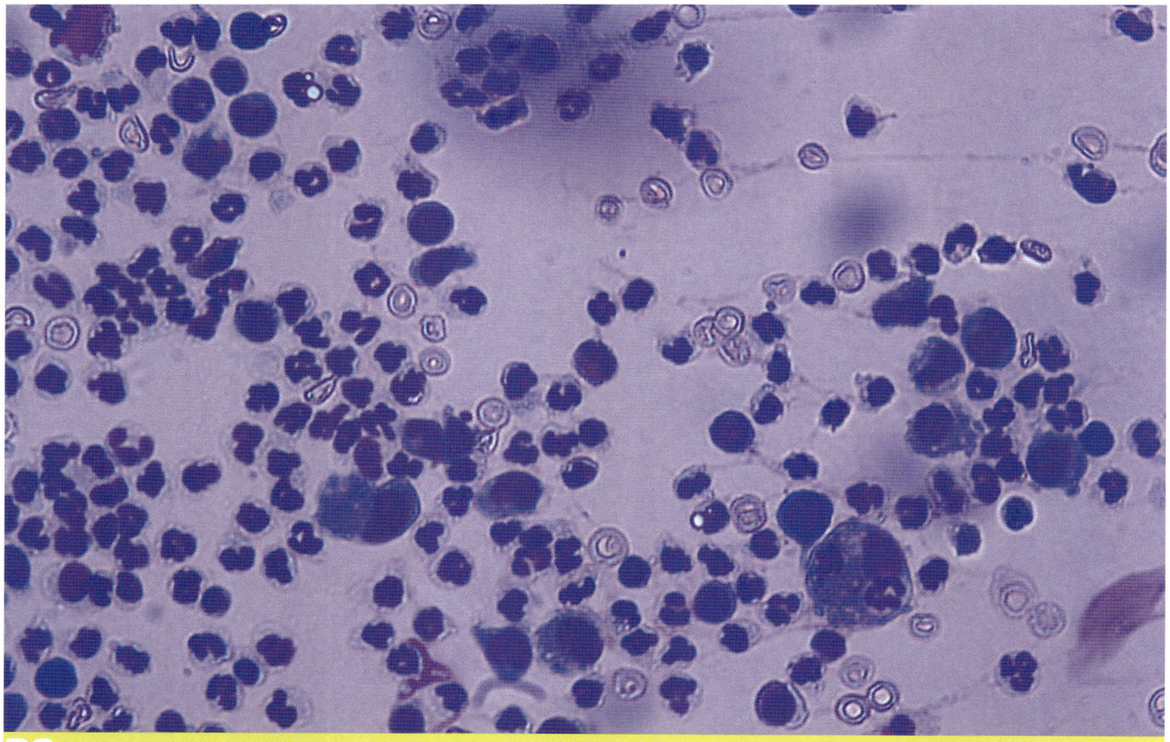

39 Cytology of furunculosis lesions showing neutrophils and eosinophils, some of which are being phagocytosed by macrophages.

# Subcutaneous abscesses

## Lesion aetiology/pathogenesis and clinical picture

These are cavities (often encapsulated) formed by the accumulation of pus in the dermis or hypodermis. This condition tends to be more frequent in cats with outdoor access due to their exposure to bites and scratches.

It can be caused by exogenous or systemic infection in immunosuppressed cats and dogs.

## Diagnostic method

Diagnosis is relatively straightforward, except when the fluid inside is under high pressure and the contents cannot be extracted to perform cytology. In cats, the characteristic thick pus also complicates fine needle aspiration. The most commonly affected areas are the perigenital area, head, and neck.

## Main differential diagnoses

- Tumour
- Hernia (inguinal area)
- Haematoma
- Fungal mycetoma
- Granuloma due to filamentous bacteria or mycobacteria

## Treatment

Surgical drainage and removal of the item causing the abscess are usually necessary. Together with antibiotic treatment, this approach is usually effective.

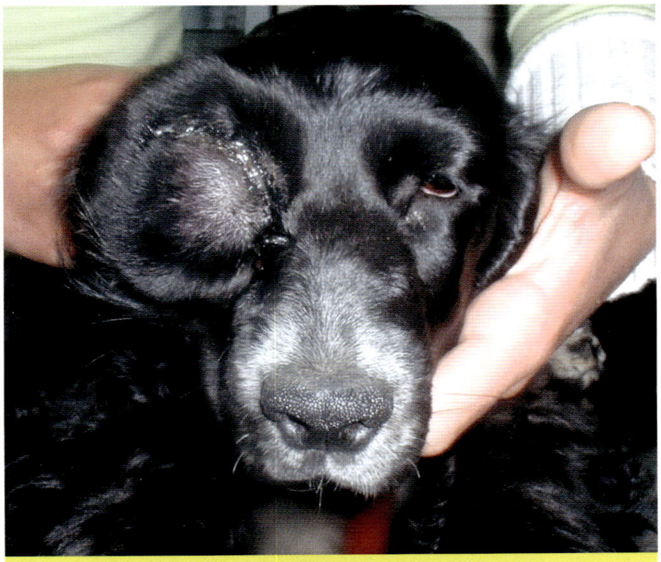

40 Cocker Spaniel with an abscess on the side of the face.

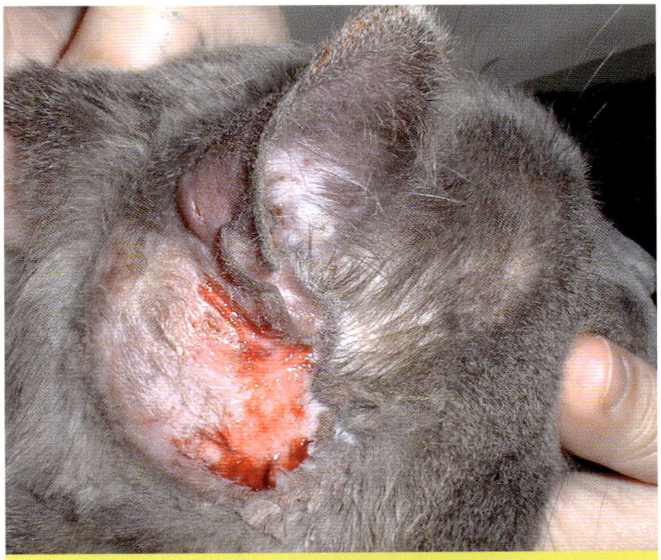

41 Cat with an ulcerated abscess caused by a fight.

# Botryomycosis

## Lesion aetiology/pathogenesis and clinical picture

This is a rare type of bacterial infection, caused mainly by staphylococci but in some cases by streptococci, in which the bacteria cluster together in small purulent clumps called pseudomycetomas.

This entity can affect the skin and mucous membranes exclusively, or can present with visceral involvement.

It can affect both dogs and cats. Predisposing factors include trauma, foreign bodies, and deficient defence mechanisms, although apparently healthy animals can also be affected.

## Diagnostic method

Cytology is insufficient for a definitive diagnosis.

Botryomycosis is a chronic suppurative granulomatous infection. Cytology reveals characteristic basophilic granules containing the causative microorganisms.

## Differential diagnoses

- Various fistulising, bacterial, or fungal infections
- Panniculitis
- Sterile pyogranuloma
- Tumours

## Treatment

The causative bacteria are usually resistant to antibiotics, despite being sensitive to many in the antibiotic sensitivity test.

Resolution in these cases, which can be especially challenging or refractory, may require prolonged antibiotic therapy or surgery.

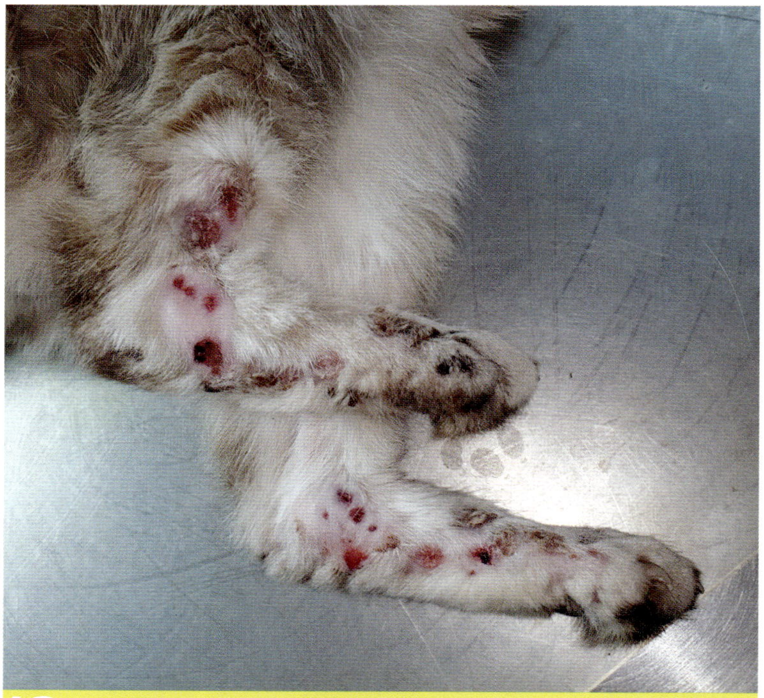

42 Hindlimb of a cat with botryomycosis caused by *Staphylococcus* spp.

# Superficial and deep pyodermas in cats

## Lesion aetiology/pathogenesis and clinical picture

In cats, skin infections tend to be caused by trauma, and are less likely to be self-induced by scratching or licking than in dogs.

However, some of the reactive processes that affect cats, such as miliary dermatitis and the eosinophilic complex, can be complicated by infection caused by licking or scratching.

Abscesses tend to be more common in cats than in dogs.

## Diagnostic method

The clinical presentation tends to be quite clear. Cytology does not help establish treatment.

## Main differential diagnoses

- Dermatophytosis
- Sterile reaction patterns
- Pemphigus complex
- Tumours

## Treatment

Depending on the patient, treatment may consist of topical therapy or, in the most stubborn cases, long-acting injectable antibiotics such as cefovecin.

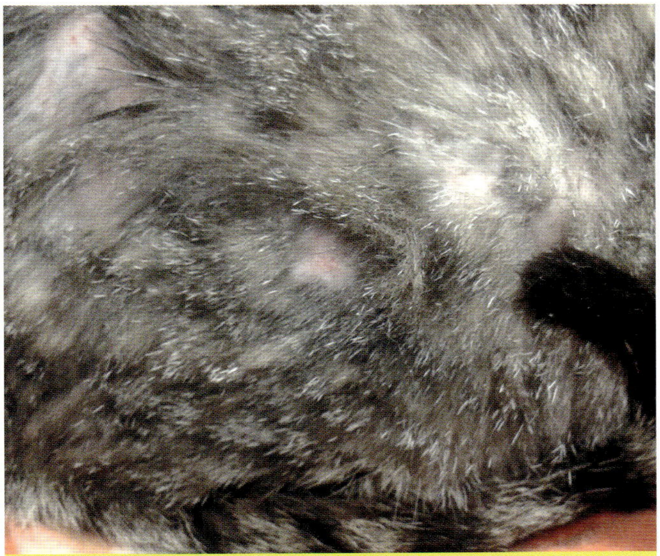

43 Bacterial overgrowth in a cat with miliary dermatitis.

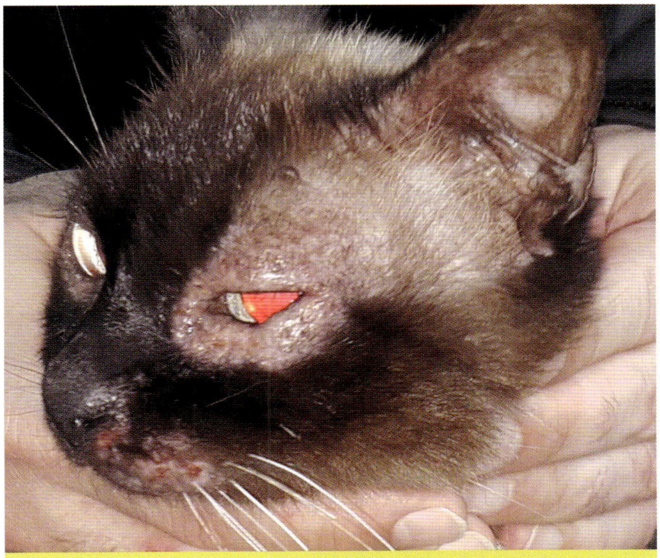

44 Infection of the periocular area and the lip caused by scratching.

# Pyoderma due to atypical bacteria

## Lesion aetiology/pathogenesis and clinical picture

Dogs and cats can develop nodules, abscesses, or granulomatous reactions caused by atypical opportunistic bacteria such as mycobacteria, *Nocardia*, and actinomycetes. Wounds in immunosuppressed animals offer conditions that favour the development of these lesions.

The abdomen is more frequently affected in cats, whereas in dogs different parts of the body can be affected.

## Diagnostic method

Lesions consist of occasionally fluctuant nodules that fistulise and exude thick, seropurulent content. Cytology and biopsy are usually essential. In many cases, special stains for acid-fast bacteria, specific cultures, or PCR testing are required.

## Main differential diagnoses

- Different types of infectious agents
- Deep mycoses
- Panniculitis
- Foreign body abscesses
- Tumours

## Treatment

Surgical removal of the affected area may be necessary, combined with specific antibiotic therapy.

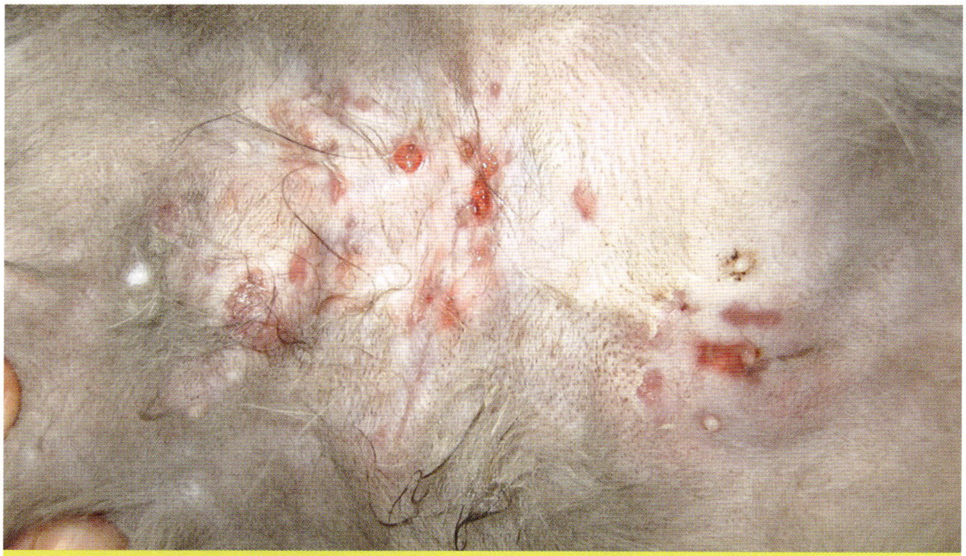

45 Mycobacterial infection in a cat. Image courtesy of Didier Carlotti (RIP).

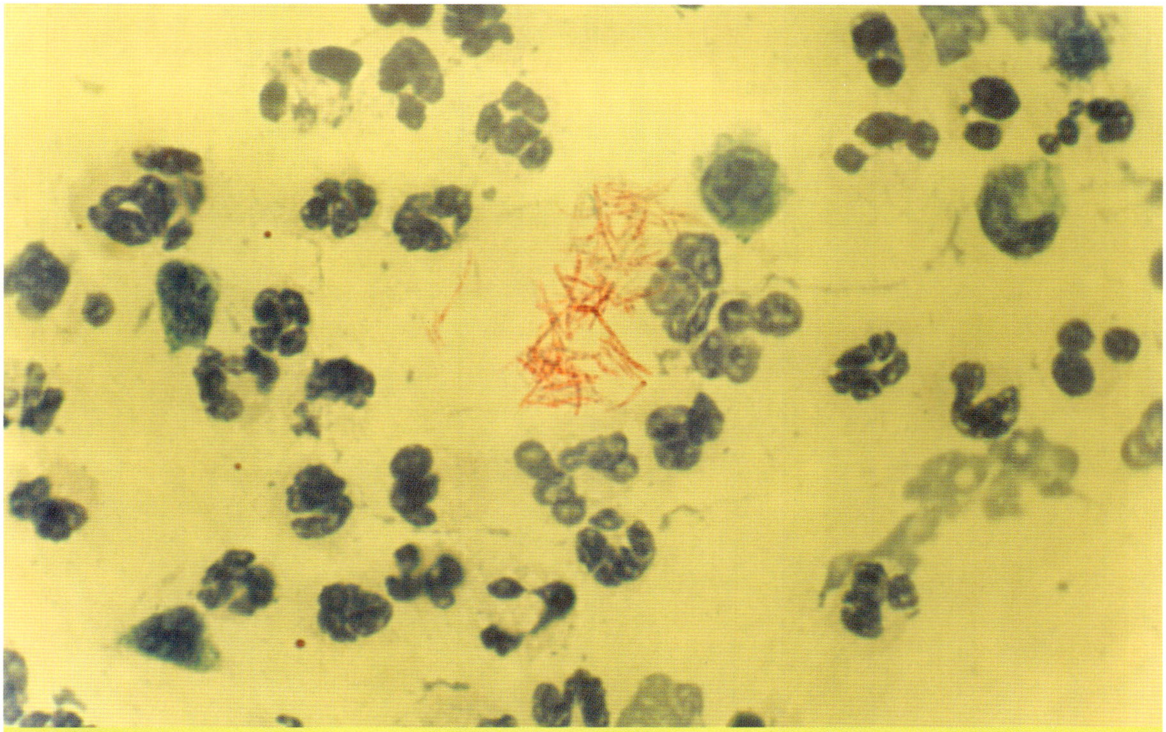

46 Cytology showing mycobacteria stained with Ziehl-Neelsen stain. Image courtesy of Didier Carlotti (RIP).

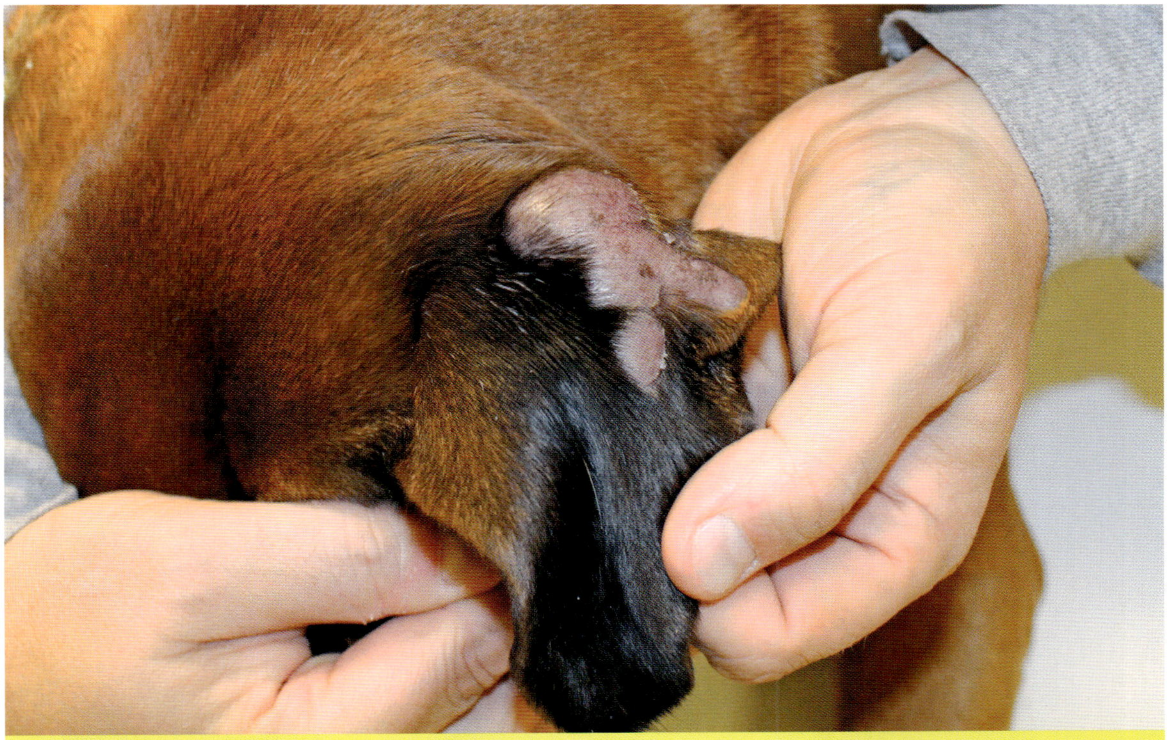

47 Leproid granuloma on the ears of a Boxer.

# Acral lick dermatitis

## Lesion aetiology/pathogenesis and clinical picture

This is a self-induced lesion caused by licking. It presents as an erythematous and exudative plaque of alopecia. It occurs mainly in large or giant breed dogs. It is important to determine the origin. It can be due to referred pain, allergy-induced obsessive licking, slow-healing wounds, or behavioural problems exacerbated by licking-induced endorphin release. Deep pyoderma and localised furunculosis develop due to the intensity of the licking and ultimately cause the lesion to become chronic.

## Diagnostic method

Diagnosis is based on the anamnesis, radiography to assess bone status, and the response to NSAIDs or antibiotics.

## Main differential diagnoses

- Demodicosis
- Dermatophytosis
- Histiocytoma or other tumours

## Treatment

Administration of long-term antibiotic therapy, NSAIDs, or corticosteroids, and, in many cases, fluoxetine (a psychomodulatory serotonin reuptake inhibitor). In certain situations amantadine, naltrexone, and gabapentin may be useful. Application of capsaicin cream around the lesion can reduce licking due to its caustic effect and its inhibition of substance P release.

Control of the vicious cycle of licking–infection–obsession requires highly resistant bandages. Otherwise, the dog will easily tear through them. Fluorescent light energy (FLE), which is used to treat other deep pyodermas, can also be used to treat this process, which is characterised by pyoderma with furunculosis.

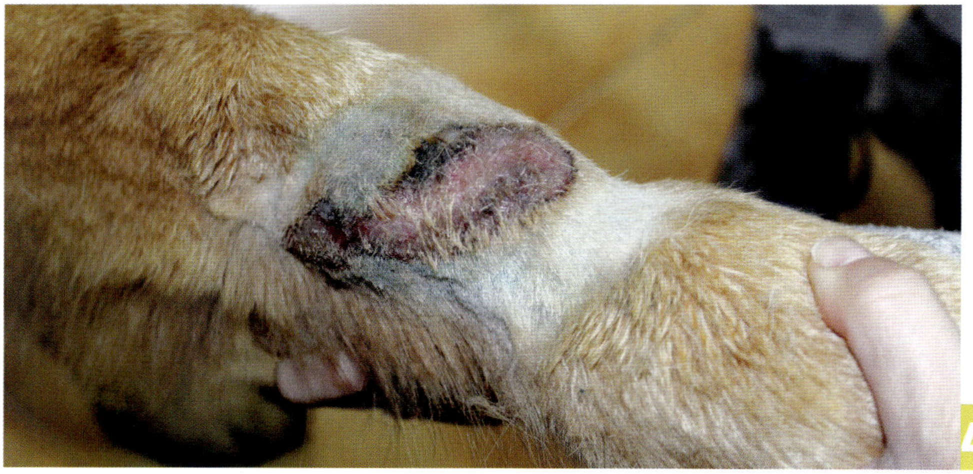

**48** Acral lick dermatitis on the carpus of a German Shepherd.

# 03 Fungal dermatoses

# Introduction

The following conditions are covered in this chapter:

- Canine dermatophytosis
- Feline dermatophytosis
- Systemic mycoses
- *Malassezia* infections
- Candidiasis

Points to consider:

- Dermatophytoses are usually highly overdiagnosed.
- *Malassezia* infections are, especially in dogs, complications that occur secondary to primary causes (mainly allergies and endocrine or keratinisation disorders) and exacerbate the pruritus and seborrhoea.
- Diagnosis of dermatophytoses by culture, performed in the clinic using DTM (dermatophyte test medium), is still a somewhat inexact method as its results can be misinterpreted.
- The prevalence of systemic mycoses varies greatly depending on the geographic location, although these diseases are generally rare.
- PCR tests are usually very sensitive but, for this very reason, can often produce false positives (e.g. animals that are already cured or that simply carry dermatophytes asymptomatically at the moment of testing).

# Canine dermatophytosis

## Lesion aetiology/pathogenesis and clinical picture

Infection caused by dermatophytes, mainly *Microsporum canis*, but also *Microsporum gypseum* and *Trichophyton mentagrophytes*. The incidence of infections caused by other dermatophytes is much lower. The zoonotic nature of this condition must be taken into account.

The clinical presentation, although highly variable, can be summarised as follows:

- Alopecic ring
- Folliculitis–furunculosis
- Seborrhoea
- Kerion (ring furunculosis)
- Onychomycosis
- Erythema–collarettes and scaling
- Pseudomycetoma (very rare in dogs)

Predisposed breeds include the Yorkshire Terrier and Jack Russell Terrier. Young or immunosuppressed animals are predominantly affected, as well as hunting dogs, which can have close contact with animals with *Trichophyton*. The infection is usually self-limiting.

## Diagnostic method

The clinical appearance is rarely sufficient for a definitive diagnosis, except in cases of ring-shaped scaling with a compatible clinical history. Analysis using Wood's lamp, DTM culture, microscopic observation of hairs, PCR tests and, in some cases, biopsy are usually necessary.

The lesions caused by these fungi consist of scaling alopecia with crusted borders, creating a pattern that can resemble the water's edge on the beach.

When taking the clinical history it is important to note whether the owner has been affected. This information can help orient the diagnosis.

## Main differential diagnoses

- Pyodermas
- Histiocytoma (in the case of a kerion)
- Acral lick dermatitis
- Folliculitis caused by bacteria or *Demodex*
- Pyoderma of the nasal bridge (mainly in cases of facial *Trichophyton*)
- Autoimmune disease
- Alopecia areata and pseudopelade
- Keratinisation defects

## Treatment

The use of topical and systemic antifungal medication is the most general recommendation. Treatment can be discontinued if the culture is negative.

Treatment usually consists of topical systemic azole derivatives combined with antiseptics such as chlorhexidine. Terbinafine is another molecule with demonstrated efficacy.

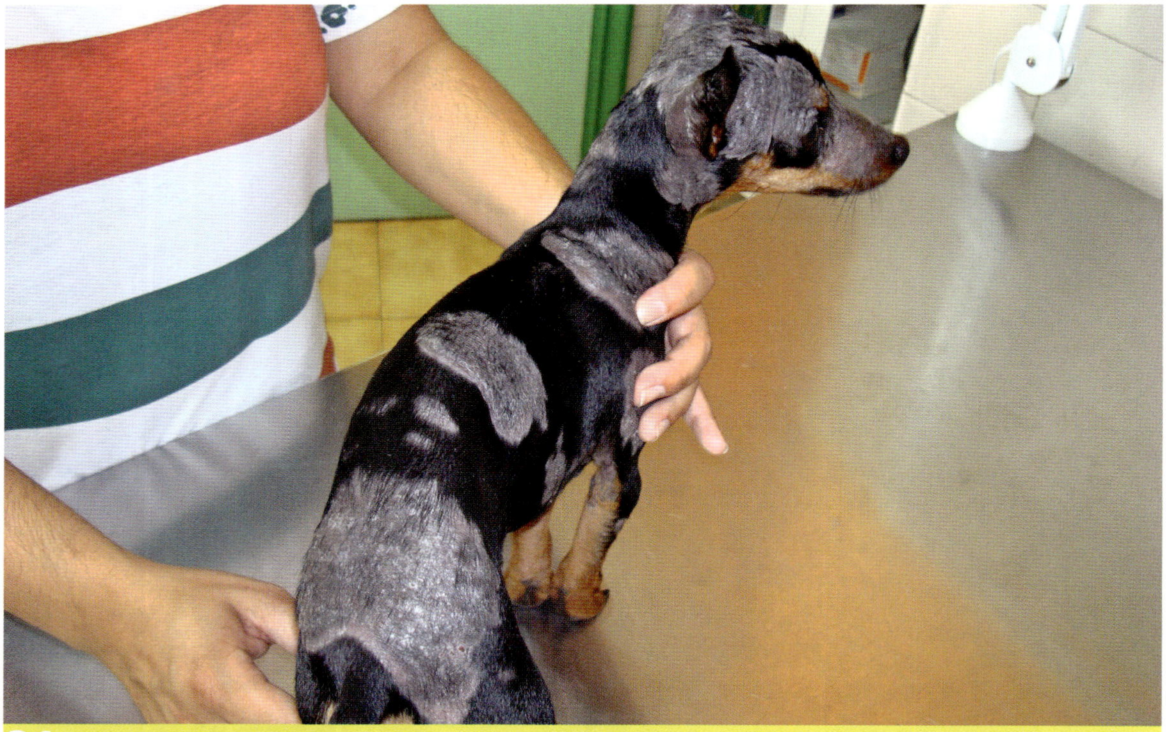

01 Generalised dermatophytosis in a Miniature Pinscher.

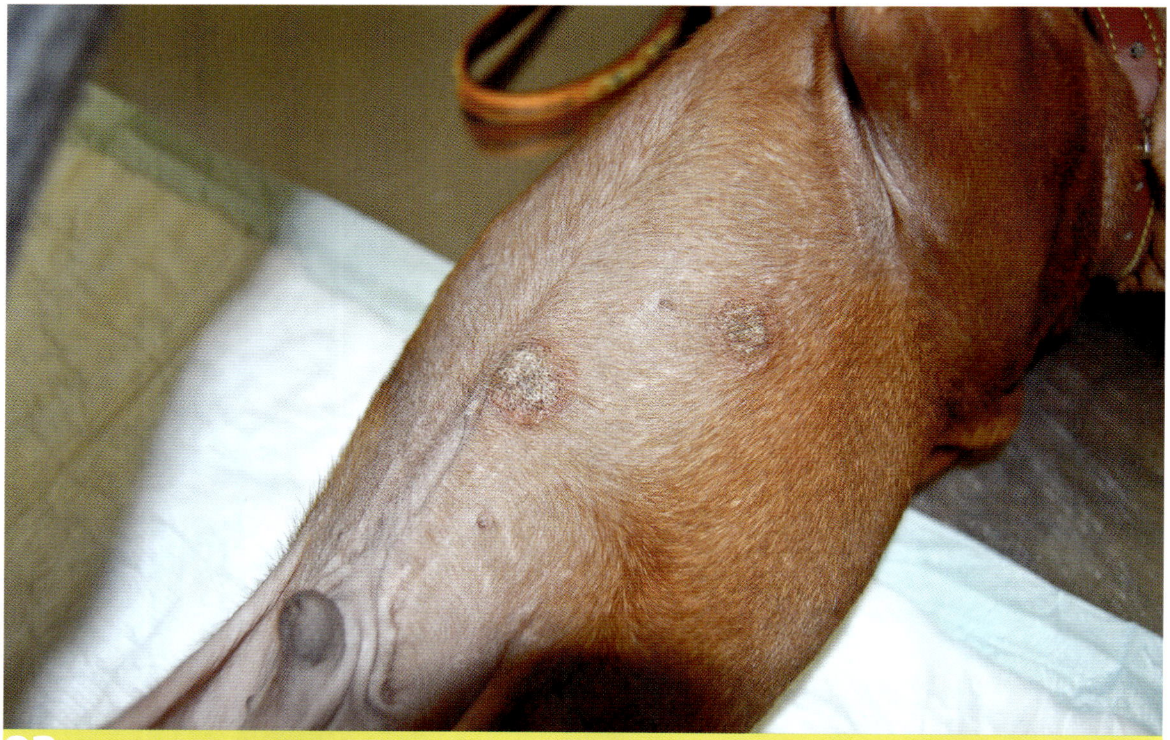

02 Classic ring pattern on the abdomen of a puppy.

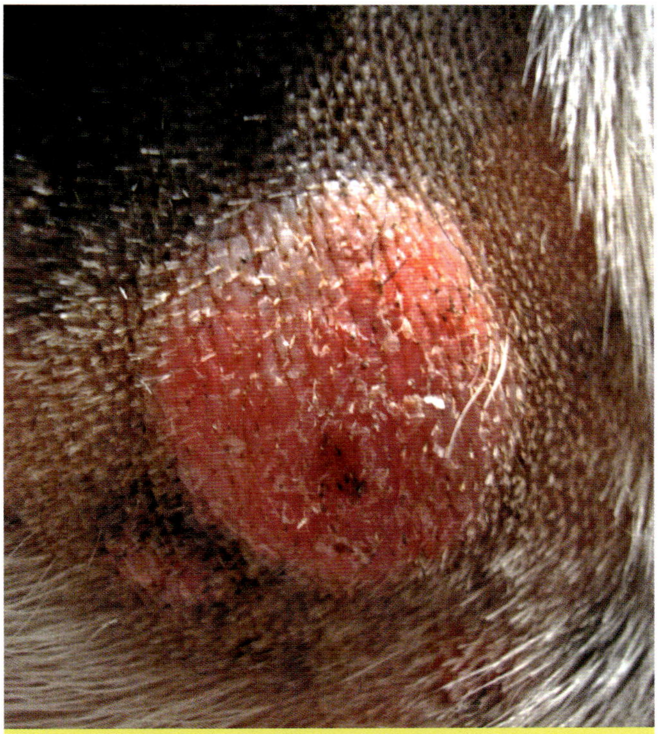

03 Typical appearance of a dermatophyte kerion.

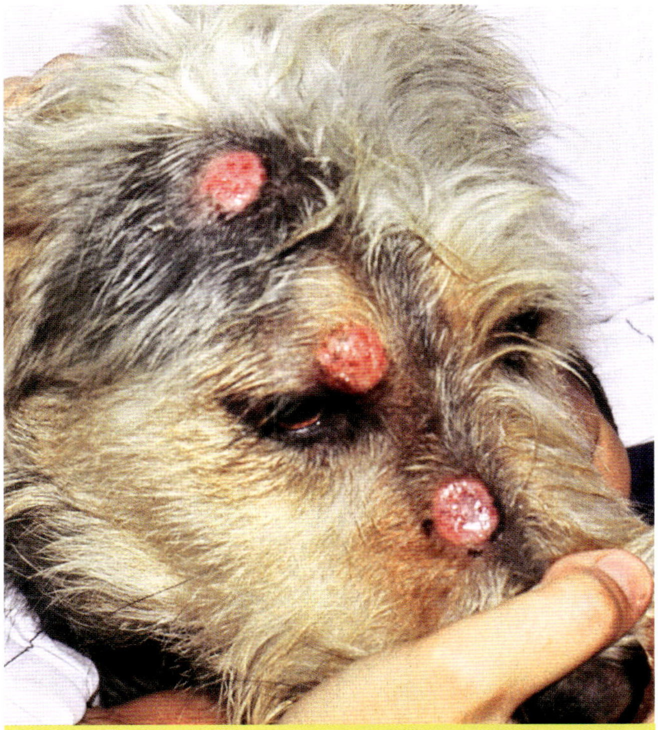

04 Dog with multiple kerions.

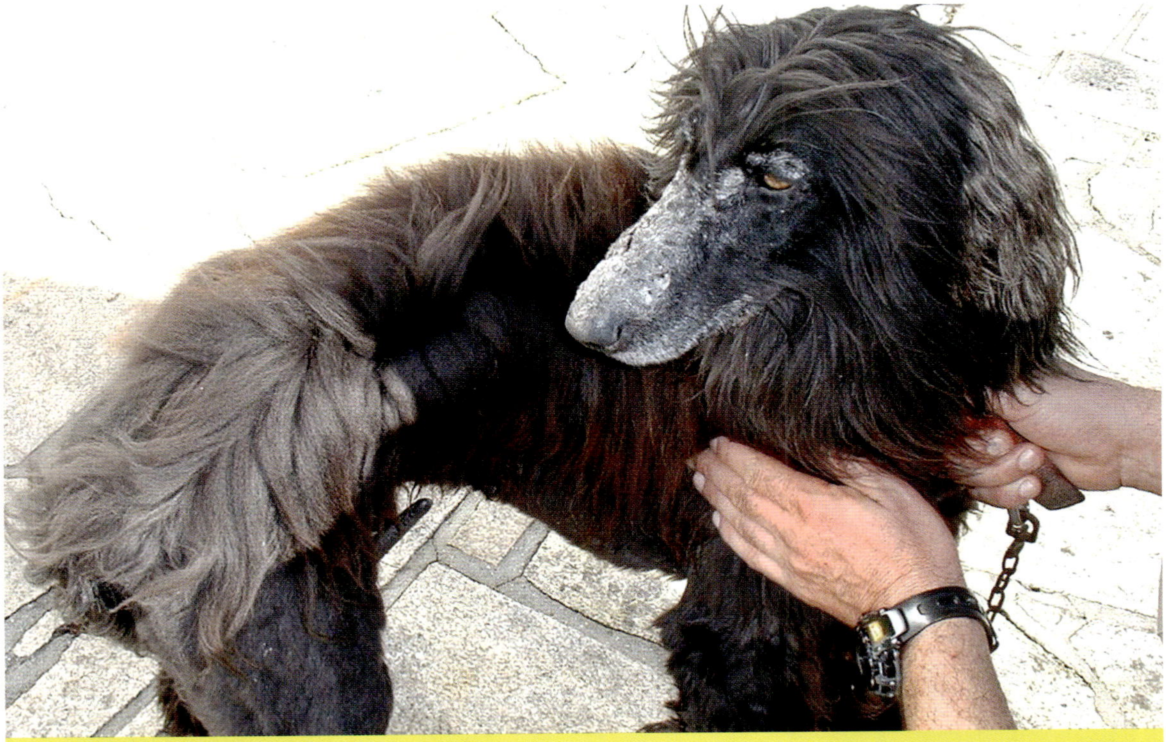

05 *Trichophyton*: involvement of the nasal bridge.

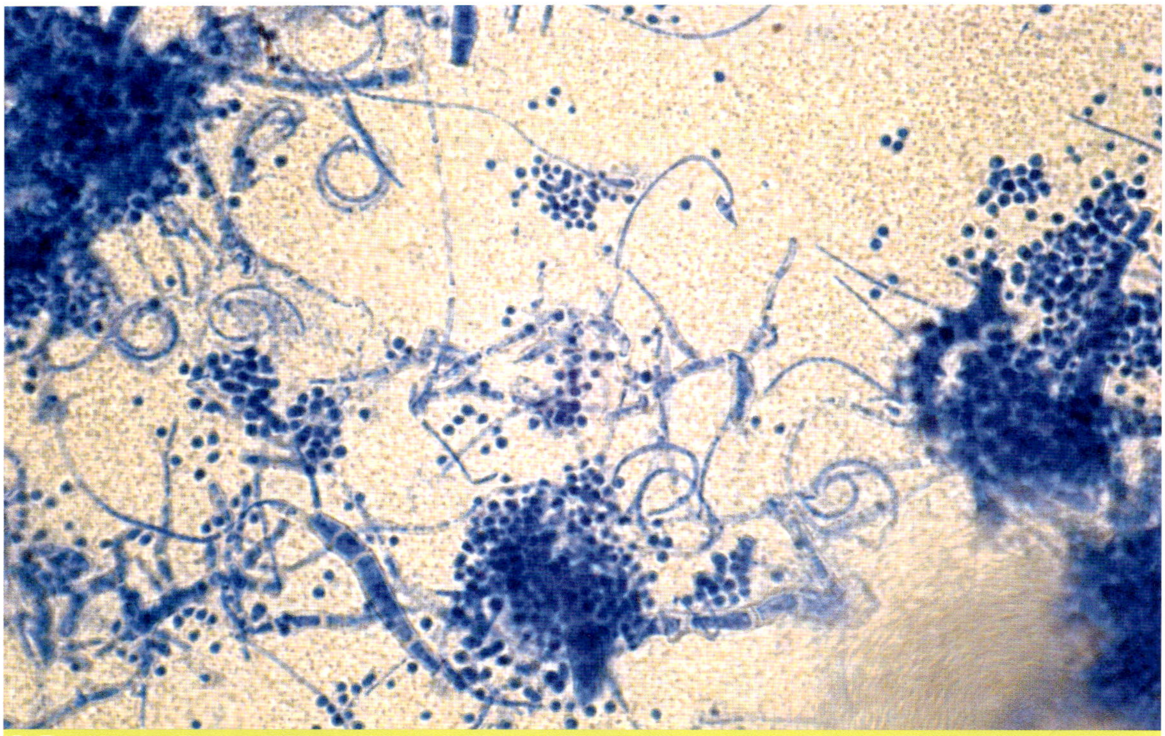

06 Twisted hyphae and macroconidia of *Trichophyton mentagrophytes*.

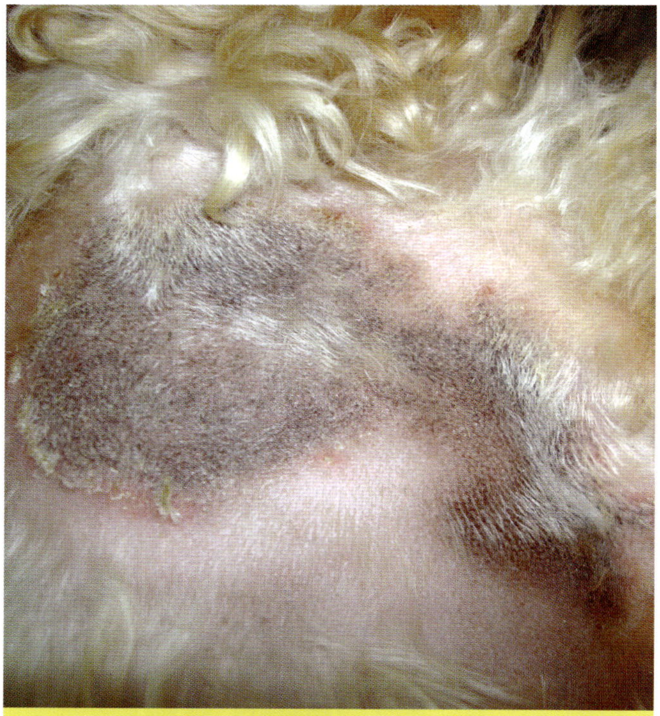

07 Dermatophyte lesion with characteristic borders in a Yorkshire Terrier.

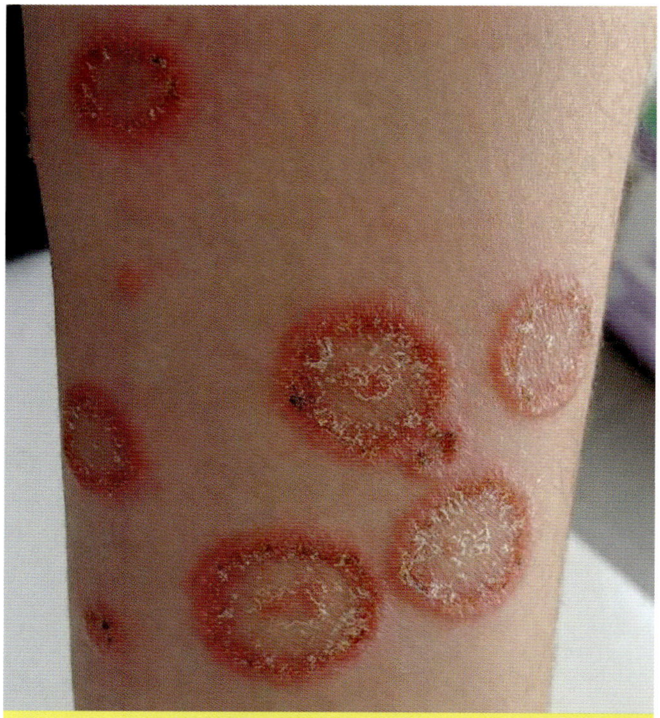

08 Classical lesions on a person's arm. Image provided by the Ciudad de Lugo Veterinary Hospital (Spain).

# Feline dermatophytosis

## Lesion aetiology/pathogenesis and clinical picture

This is the most common infectious dermatosis in cats, and is caused mainly by *M. canis*. The clinical picture can be highly variable, ranging from practically subclinical (microlesions) to a typical feline reaction pattern (e.g. miliary dermatitis). It can also present as focal or multifocal alopecia, otitis, or even a type of granuloma known as pseudomycetoma. Aspects to bear in mind include the zoonotic nature of this condition and the difficulty eradicating it in long-haired breeds.

## Diagnostic method

DTM culture is very important both for diagnosis and treatment monitoring. Wood's lamp and a trichogram may be useful. The presence of spores when observing the hair under a microscope can be diagnostically useful, although this is uncommon.

When using the Wood's lamp the light should be focused on the portion of the hair closest to the skin: analysis of the tip of the hair can produce a positive result even in animals that have recovered and are undergoing hair regrowth.

PCR testing can be useful not only for diagnosis, but also to monitor healing, provided the sample is taken from the same location at which a positive result was obtained.

## Main differential diagnoses

- Miliary dermatitis of other aetiology
- Demodicosis
- Ceruminous otitis
- Abscesses

## Treatment

Currently, itraconazole is the medication of choice and should be administered taking into account the culture results, the zoonotic nature of this disease, and the risk of spread to other cats in contact with the affected animal. Topical application of products such as enilconazole or chlorhexidine with miconazole is very important to treat the disease and prevent transmission.

Terbinafine is another potential treatment option.

Treatment must also be applied to the animal's environment and any fomites. Control of excessive moisture and use of antifungal agents for the environment, including bleach, are a key part of the treatment.

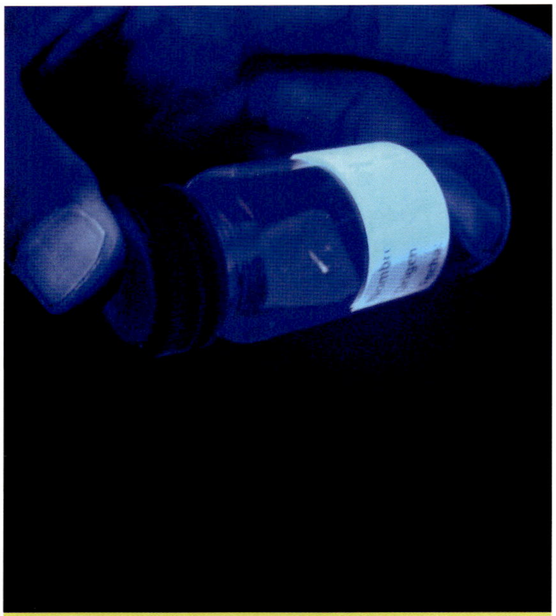

09 Examination of a hair under a Wood's lamp, revealing a positive result. The hair will subsequently undergo dermatophyte culture.

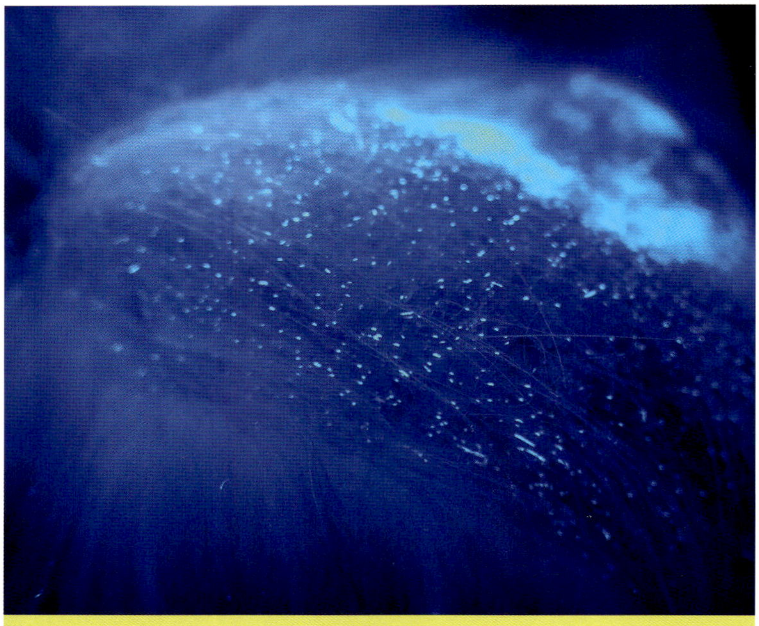

10 Positive Wood's lamp examination in a cat with dermatophytosis.

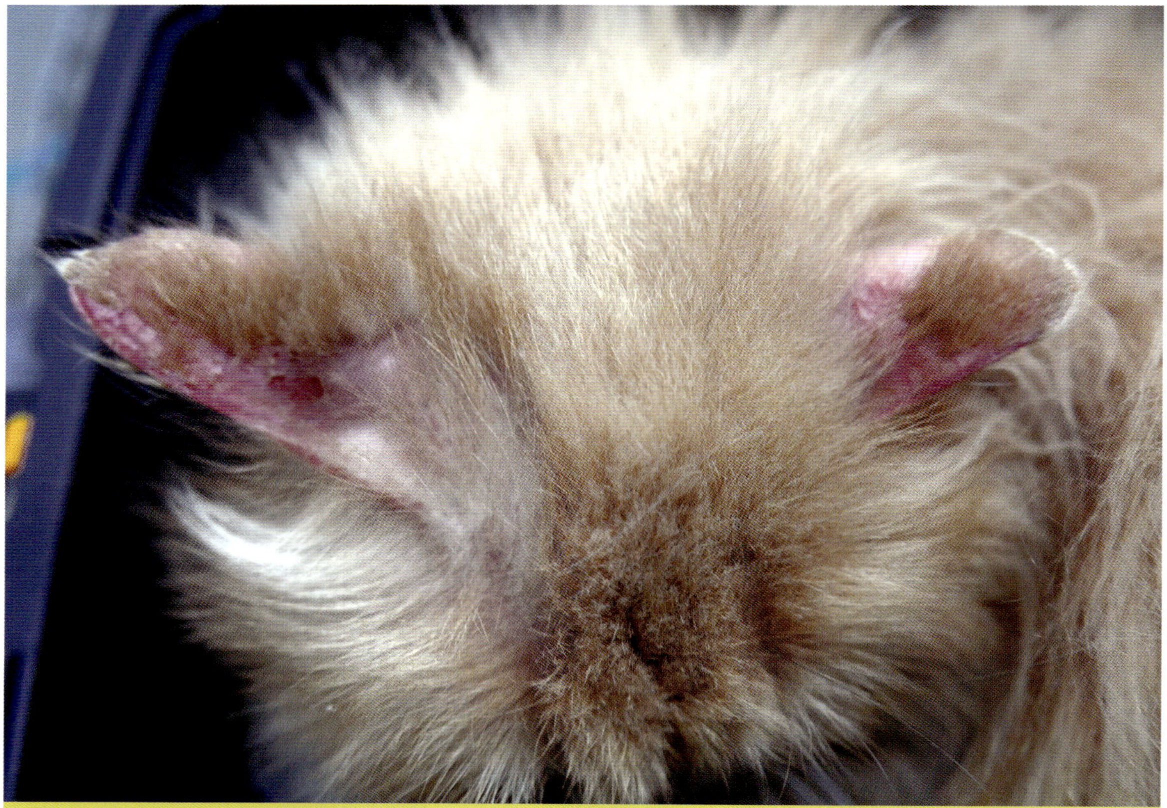

11 Feline dermatophytosis. Involvement of the ears in a Persian cat.

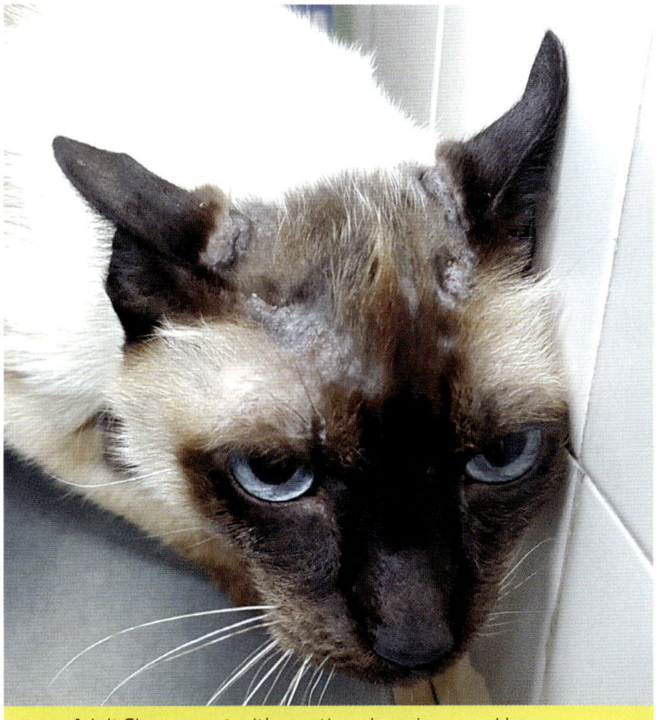

12 Adult Siamese cat with crusting alopecia caused by dermatophytes.

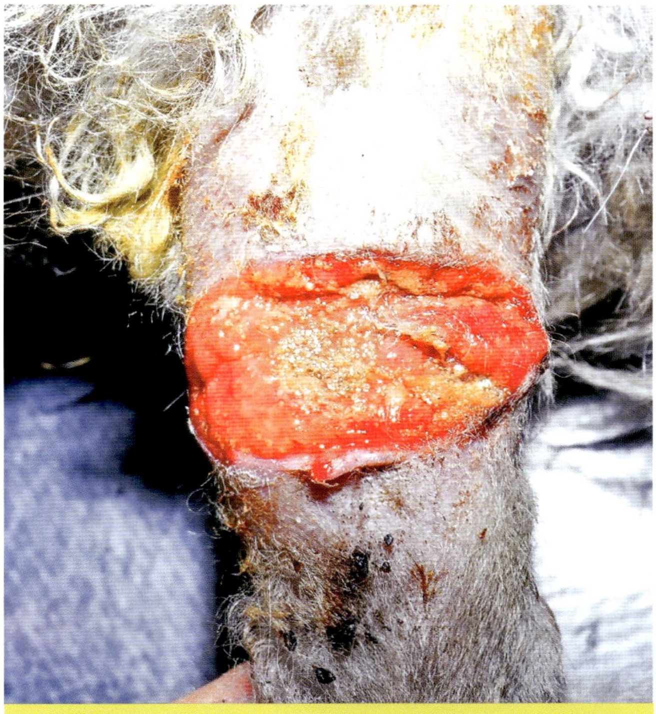

13 Mycetoma in a Persian cat. Image courtesy of D. Carlotti (RIP) and D. Pin.

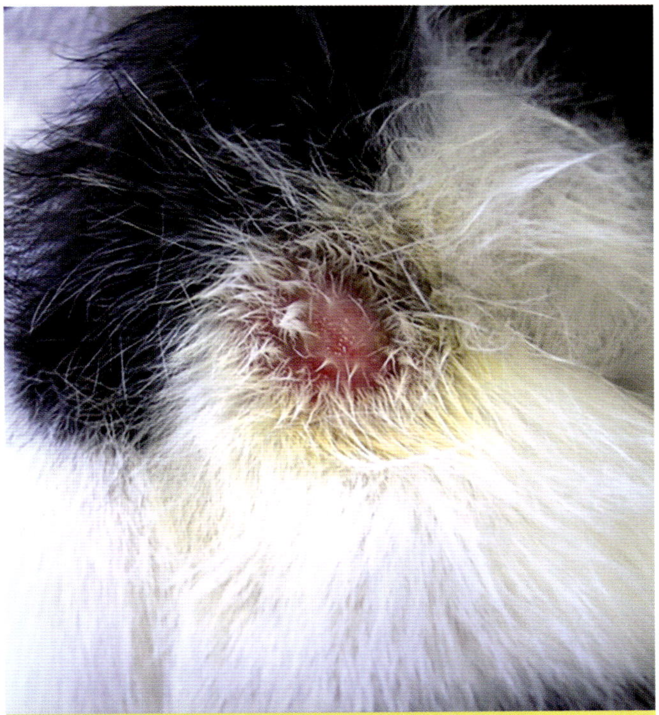

14 Cat with a dermatophyte kerion. This is a very uncommon lesion. Image courtesy of Annabel Dalmau.

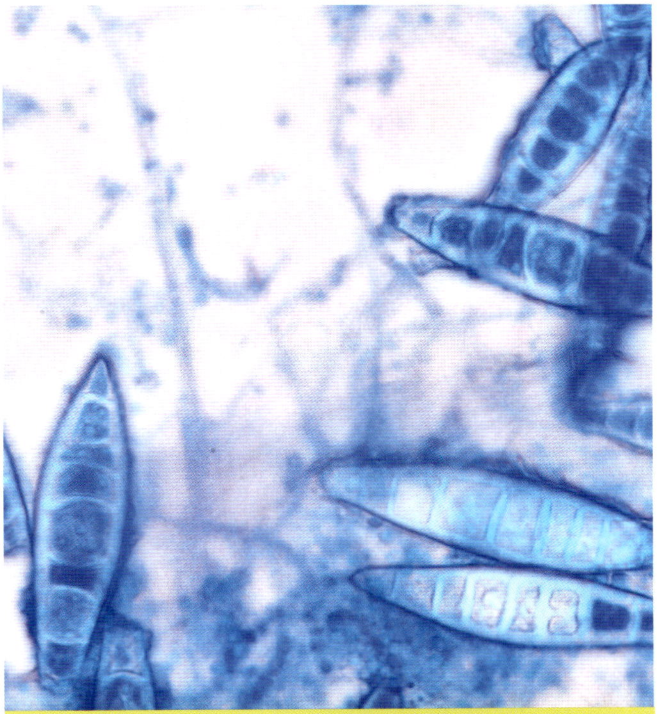

15 Macroconidia of *Microsporum canis* stained with methylene blue. Sample obtained from a colony cultured in DTM.

# Systemic mycoses

## Lesion aetiology/pathogenesis and clinical picture

These are mycoses caused by saprophytic fungi present in the soil and vegetation. They can affect various organs and spread via the bloodstream to the skin of dogs and cats.

These infections are caused by *Blastomyces dermatitidis*, *Coccidioides*, *Cryptococcus*, and *Histoplasma*.

They are characterised clinically by granuloma lesions and general illness.

## Diagnostic method

The clinical presentation, the clinical history, including any information linking the animal with endemic areas, and histology and cytology results are essential for diagnosis.

## Main differential diagnoses

- Granulomas or pyogranulomas of other aetiology
- Tumours

## Treatment

Azole derivatives (itraconazole, fluconazole, and ketoconazole) are often used, although in some refractory cases administration of amphotericin B may be necessary.

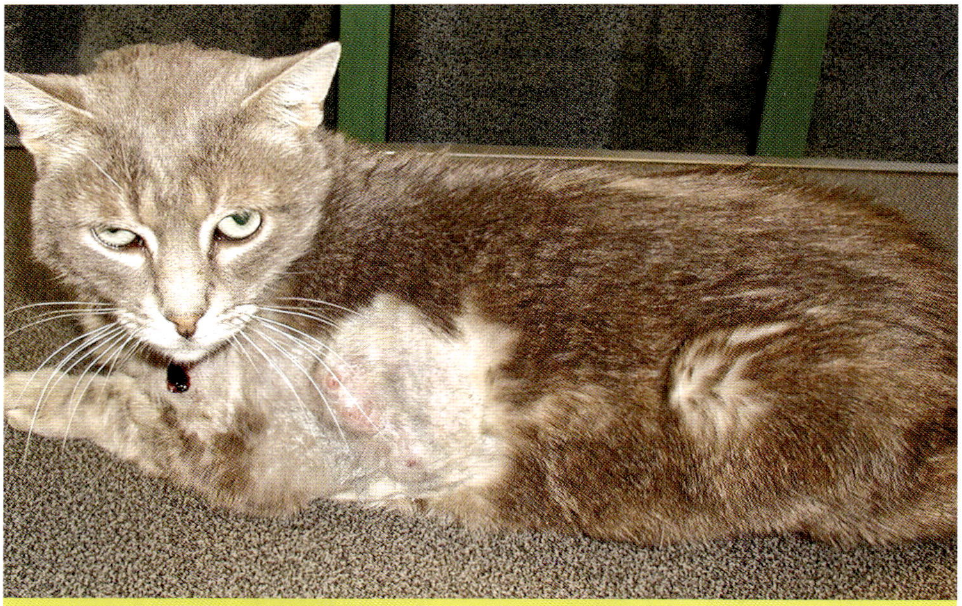

16 Skin lesion on the flank of a cat caused by *Cryptococcus neoformans*. Image courtesy of Didier Carlotti (RIP).

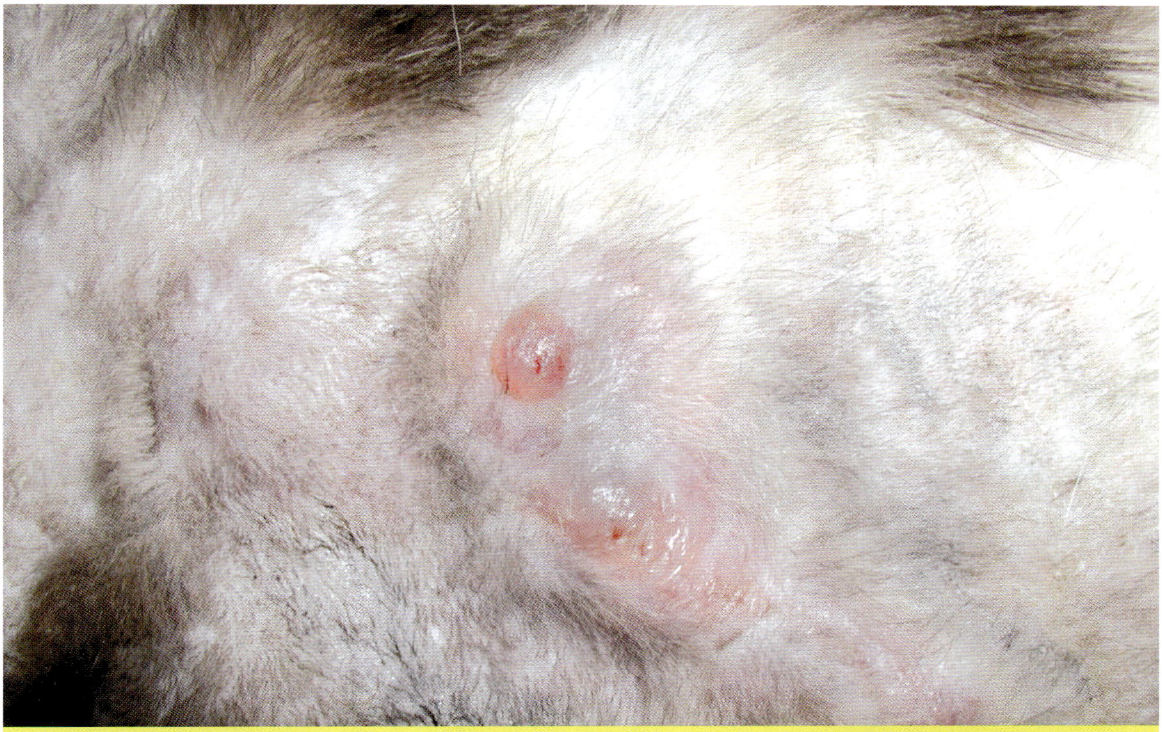

17 Close-up of the skin lesion from the cat in the previous image. Image courtesy of Didier Carlotti (RIP).

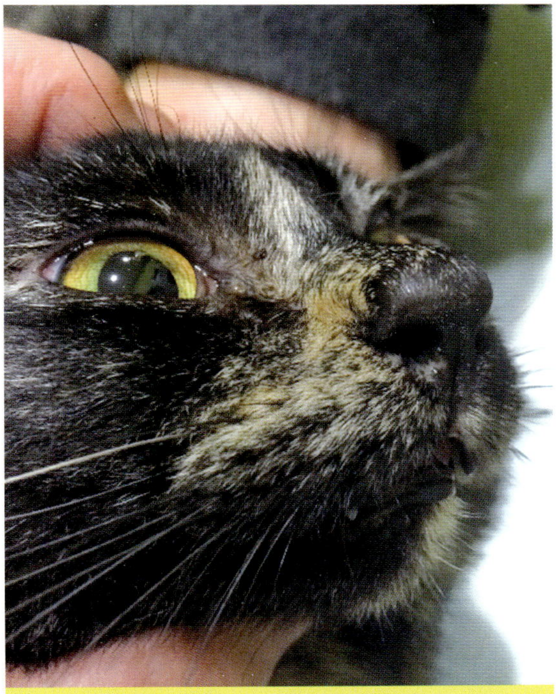

18 Classic subcutaneous inflammation of the nose in a cat with cryptococcosis.

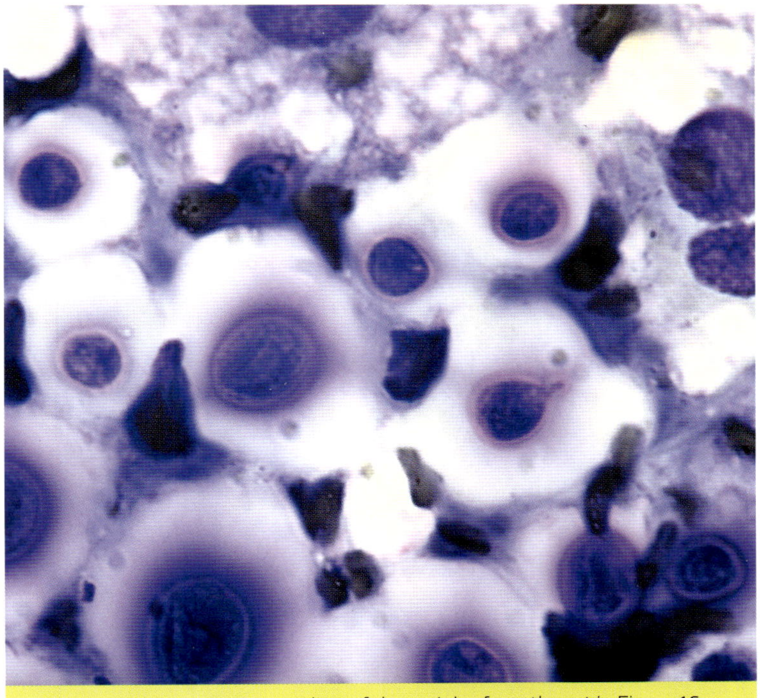

19 Fine needle aspiration cytology of the nodules from the cat in Figure 16. Fungi are visualised as spherical elements surrounded by a thick capsule (Diff-Quik, 1000×). Image courtesy of Didier Carlotti (RIP).

# *Malassezia* infections

## Lesion aetiology/pathogenesis and clinical picture

*Malassezia* spp. are commensal yeasts that form part of the microbiota of the skin and mucous membranes of dogs and cats. Predisposing factors that can trigger their proliferation include allergies and endocrine or keratinisation disorders in dogs, and tumours, endocrine diseases, and allergies in cats. Certain dog breeds, including the West Highland White Terrier and Blood Hound, are predisposed to *Malassezia* overgrowth.

This predominantly occurs in moist and greasy areas of the body, and generally gives rise to erythema and epidermal hyperplasia with excess production of seborrhoeic content. Chronic lesions tend result in hyperpigmentation and lichenification. In the ears, proliferation of *Malassezia* can lead to the formation of ceruminous otitis with erythema and, in many cases, hyperplasia of the external auditory canal.

These yeasts can also form biofilms, making them more difficult to eliminate.

## Diagnostic method

Cytology, using either a swab or adhesive tape, is usually the diagnostic method of choice.

The characteristic seborrhoeic clinical picture and rancid odour are unmistakable. There may be no direct relationship between the number of *Malassezia* observed and the severity of the clinical picture. The response to treatment is usually the best means of confirming the diagnosis.

## Main differential diagnoses

- Keratinisation defects
- Bacterial overgrowth
- Ectoparasites

## Treatment

Treatment of the primary cause is essential. Topical medication based on chlorhexidine and azole substances is usually effective. The combination of acetic acid and boric acid can also be effective.

Deep cleaning and the use of N-acetylcysteine are the methods indicated to eliminate biofilms.

Another option is systemic treatment with azole derivatives such as itraconazole or ketoconazole. Terbinafine, administered either topically or systemically, can also be highly effective.

Pulse therapy (e.g. 2 days per week) may be necessary in patients with recurrences.

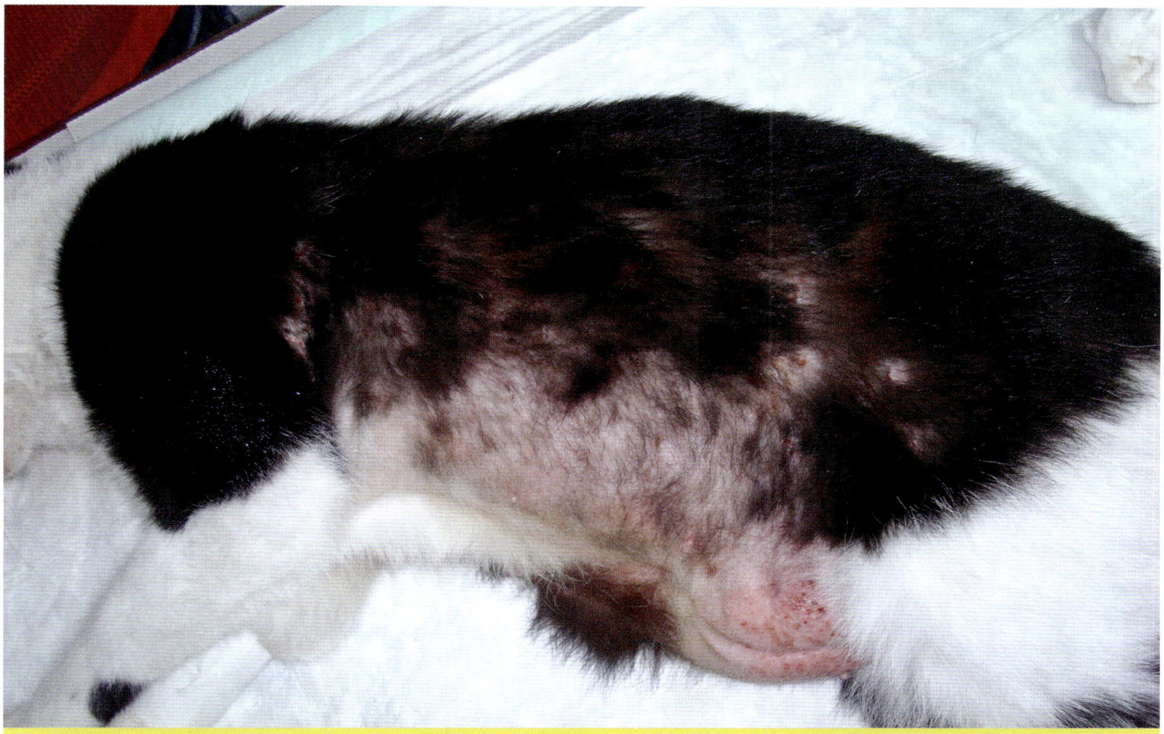

20 *Malassezia* overgrowth in an allergic cat.

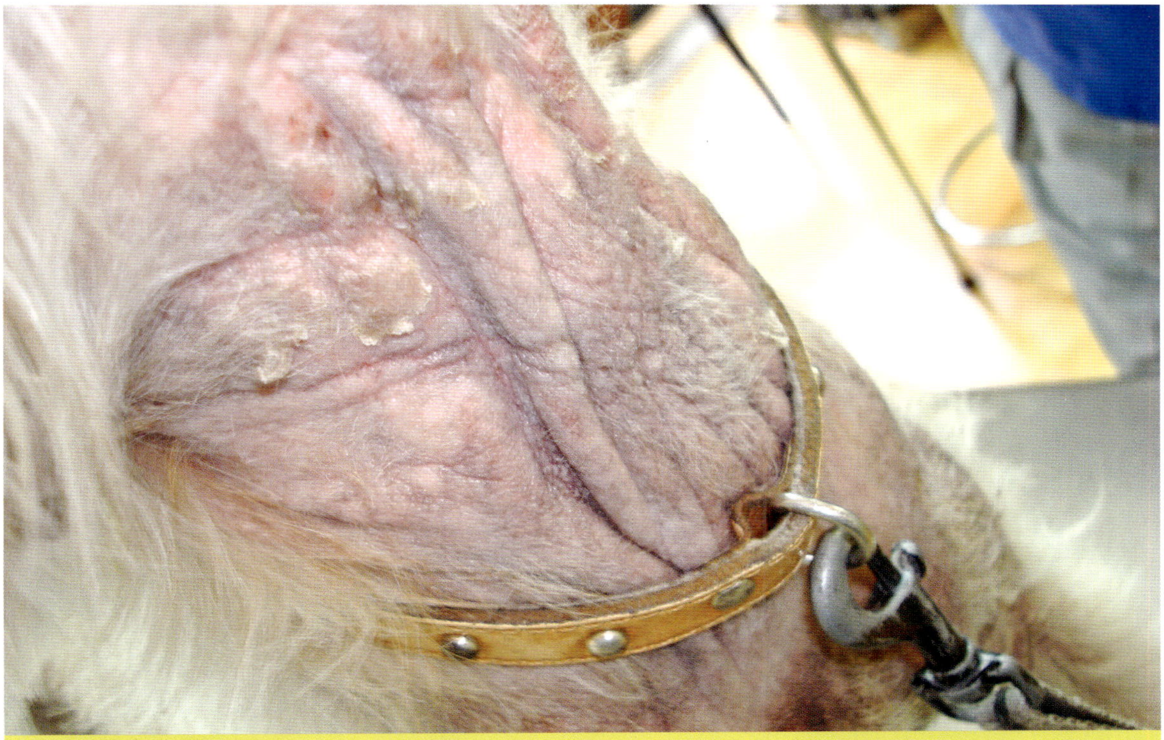

21 Classic presentation of *Malassezia* dermatitis.

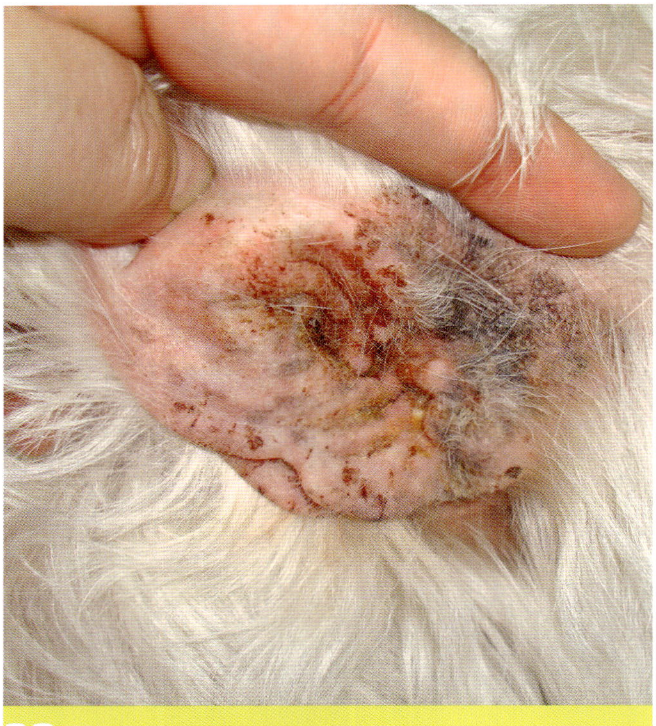

22 *Malassezia* otitis in a West Highland White Terrier.

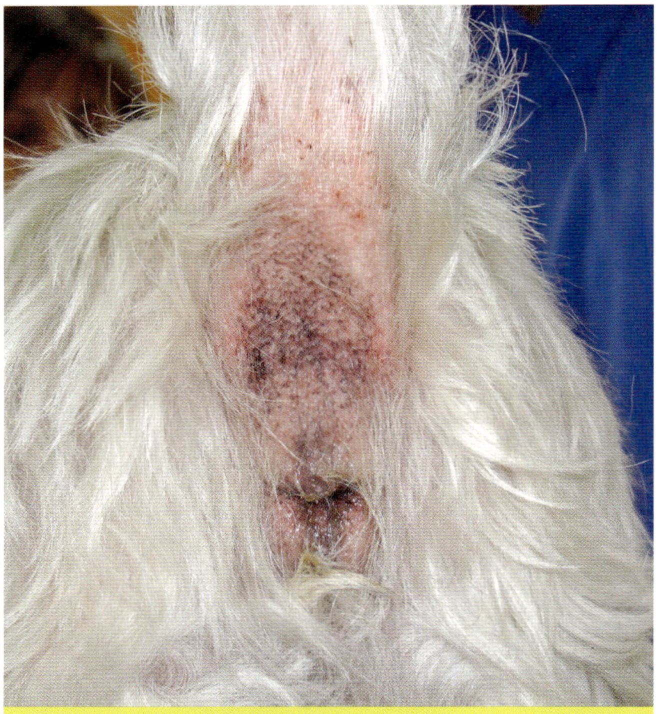

23 *Malassezia* overgrowth in the perineal region of a West Highland White Terrier.

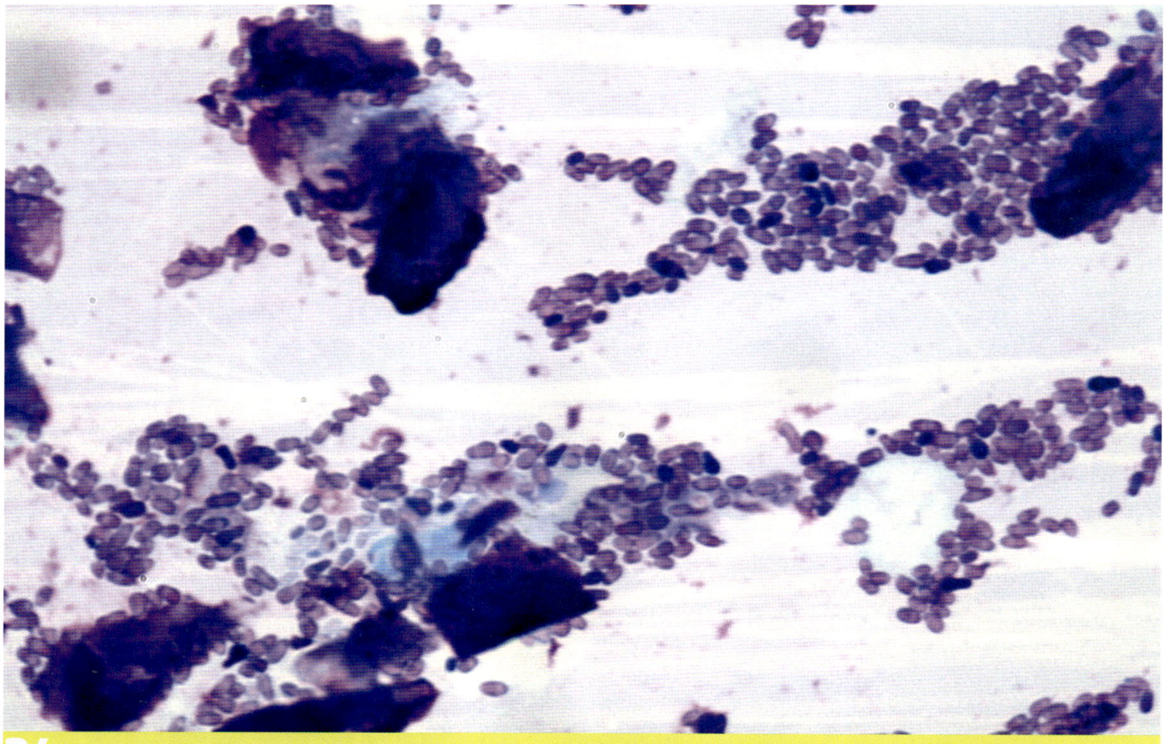

24 Grouped *Malassezia* in an animal with otitis of allergic origin. Image compatible with biofilm formation.

# Candidiasis

## Lesion aetiology/pathogenesis and clinical picture

This dermatitis is caused by *Candida* spp. yeasts and affects animals with immune compromise or those that have undergone excessive treatment with antibiotics, corticosteroids, or cytostatics. It can also be associated with certain endocrine diseases. It usually affects the mucous membranes, mucocutaneous junctions, and skin folds, resulting in moist and sometimes erosive erythematous dermatosis.

## Diagnostic method

This is a rare form of yeast overgrowth that can be diagnosed by direct smear. The clinical history, clinical presentation, and the presence of pain in the affected area are usually sufficient to establish diagnosis. The mucous membranes may have a characteristic whitish appearance. This condition should be distinguished from *Malassezia* overgrowth. In many cases, culture is necessary.

Microscopy of the yeast reveals characteristic budding at one pole, and not in the centre, as is observed in *Malassezia*.

## Main differential diagnoses

- *Malassezia* or bacterial dermatitis, mainly in intertrigo
- Stomatitis of other aetiology

## Treatment

Control of the primary cause, including discontinuation of triggering treatments, and topical application of antifungals such as nystatin or azoles are usually effective. In some cases, systemic itraconazole treatment is necessary to accelerate cure.

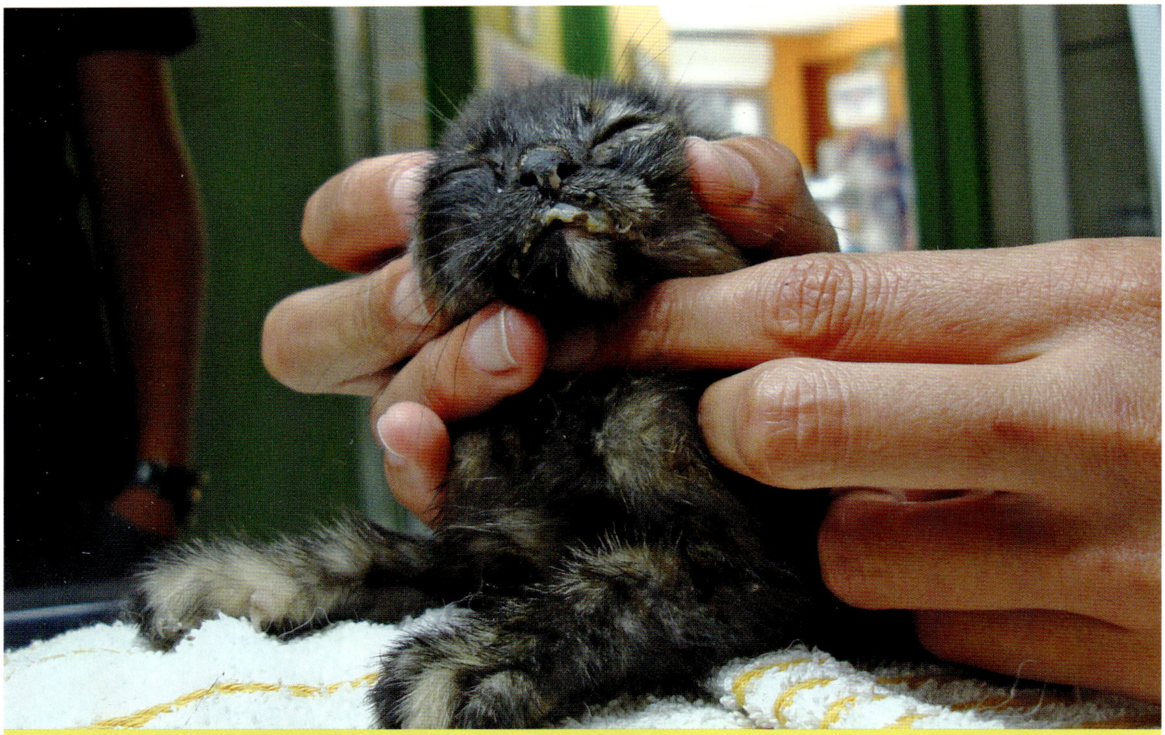

25 Typical appearance of oral candidiasis in a kitten.

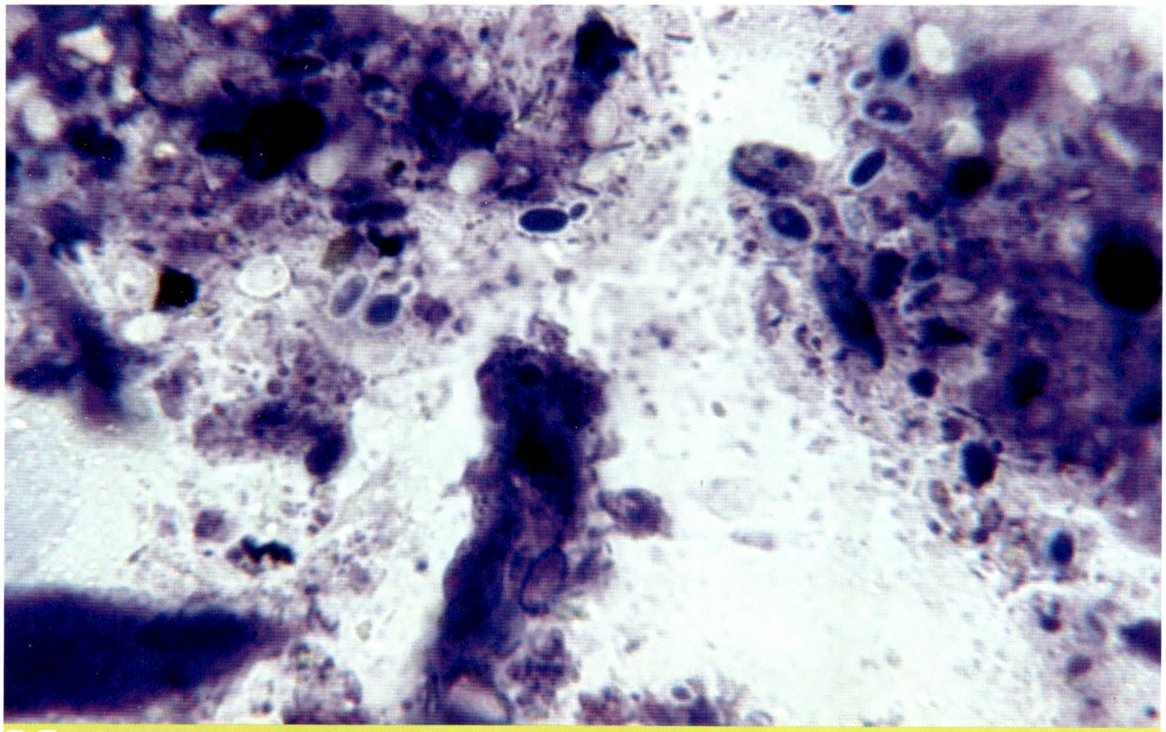

26 *Candida* spp. detected by cytology in the animal from the previous image. Note the asymmetric budding.

# 04 Parasitic dermatoses

# Introduction

The main parasitic dermatoses covered in this book are:

- Cheyletiellosis
- Tick infestation
- Pediculosis
- Pulicosis
- Myiasis
- Canine demodicosis or red mange
- Feline demodicosis
- Canine scabies or sarcoptic mange
- Feline notoedric mange or feline mange
- Otitis due to *Otodectes cynotis*
- Trombiculiasis:
  - *Neotrombicula autumnalis*
  - *Straelensia cynotis*

Cutaneous parasitic diseases in dogs and cats can be caused by mites, insects, or nematodes. This chapter deals with the main dermatoses caused by mites, insects, and fly larvae (myiasis).

# Cheyletiellosis

## Lesion aetiology/pathogenesis and clinical picture

This parasitic disease affects humans, cats, rabbits, and dogs, and is caused by all developmental stages of the mite *Cheyletiella*, which is an obligate parasite. This disease characteristically affects recently purchased puppies of uncertain origin.

The most common presentation consists of scaling, with abundant small white scales on the back. Pruritus is variable, and in cats can be masked by this species' constant grooming.

## Diagnostic method

Affected animals present with characteristic dry exfoliation on the back. Observation with a magnifying glass reveals whitish scales and mobile mites. An adhesive tape tests is usually the best diagnostic method, as it enables direct observation of mites. Nits, attached to hairs by small fibrils, may be observed.

## Main differential diagnoses

- Other keratinisation disorders
- Pediculosis
- Sarcoptic mange

- Flea dermatitis
- Feline miliary dermatitis of other aetiology
- Cats that do not groom themselves (e.g. due to osteoarthritis or obesity)

## Treatment

Treatment with antiparasitic pipettes, tablets, collars, or sprays is usually effective. The surrounding environment should also be treated.

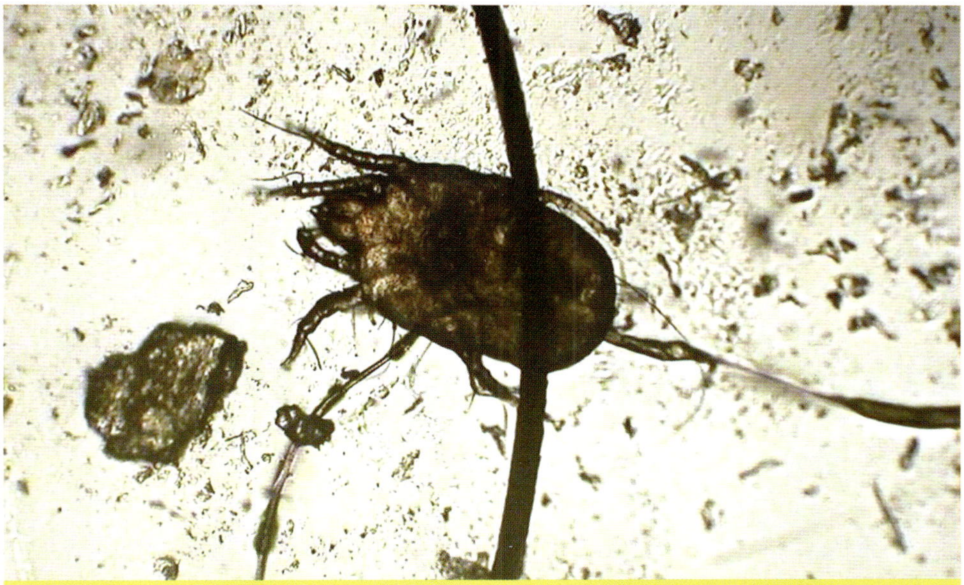

01 *Cheyletiella* observed using adhesive tape.

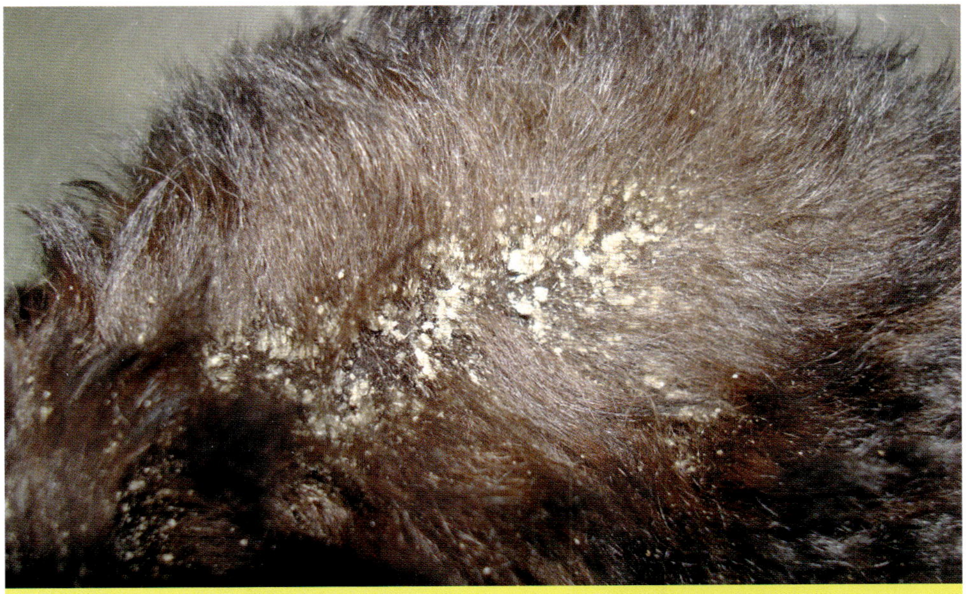

02 Dry exfoliation in a case of cheyletiellosis.

# Tick infestation

## Lesion aetiology/pathogenesis and clinical picture

Ticks are blood-sucking parasites that attach to the skin using a sucking mouthpart. They do this in several areas, but predominantly attach in areas that the animal cannot easily reach, such as the eyelids, back, or ears. They tend to cause a foreign body reaction in the host, especially when they are torn off, leaving the sucking apparatus embedded in the skin. They also transmit diseases such as ehrlichiosis, babesiosis, anaplasmosis, hepatozoonosis, Rocky Mountain spotted fever, and Lyme disease, which can cause neurological disorders, anaemia, jaundice, and clotting disorders, resulting in consequent petechiae and ecchymosis.

## Diagnostic method

These parasites do not pose any major diagnostic challenge, except in the very early stages, during which they can be confused with warts due to their small size. They can leave small nodules at their attachment site that self-resolve over a variable period of time.

## Main differential diagnoses

Nodules of various origins (differential diagnosis with encysted remnants of the sucking apparatus).

## Treatment

A variety of spray, pipette, and collar miticides can be used, and are quite effective. Isoxazolines constitute another important therapeutic breakthrough.

It is very important to treat the environment and avoid removing ticks, unless this is done with tweezers by grasping their sucking mouthpart.

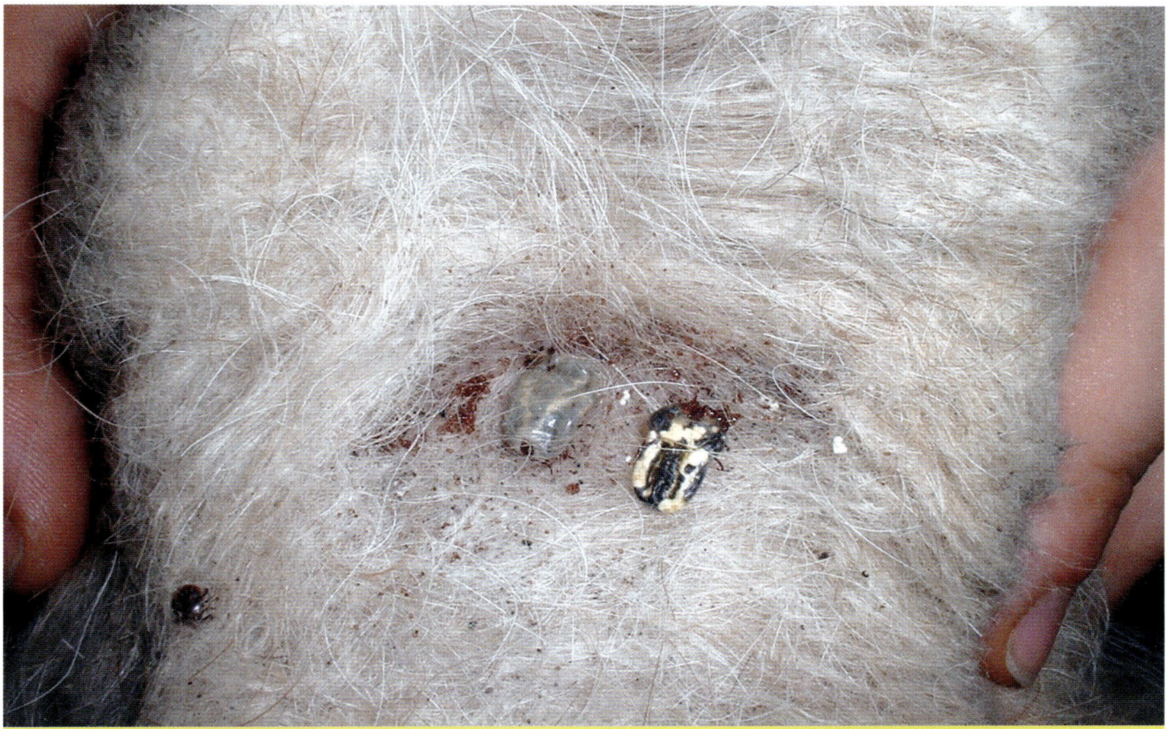

03 Ticks feeding on the back of a dog and another before insertion of the sucking apparatus.

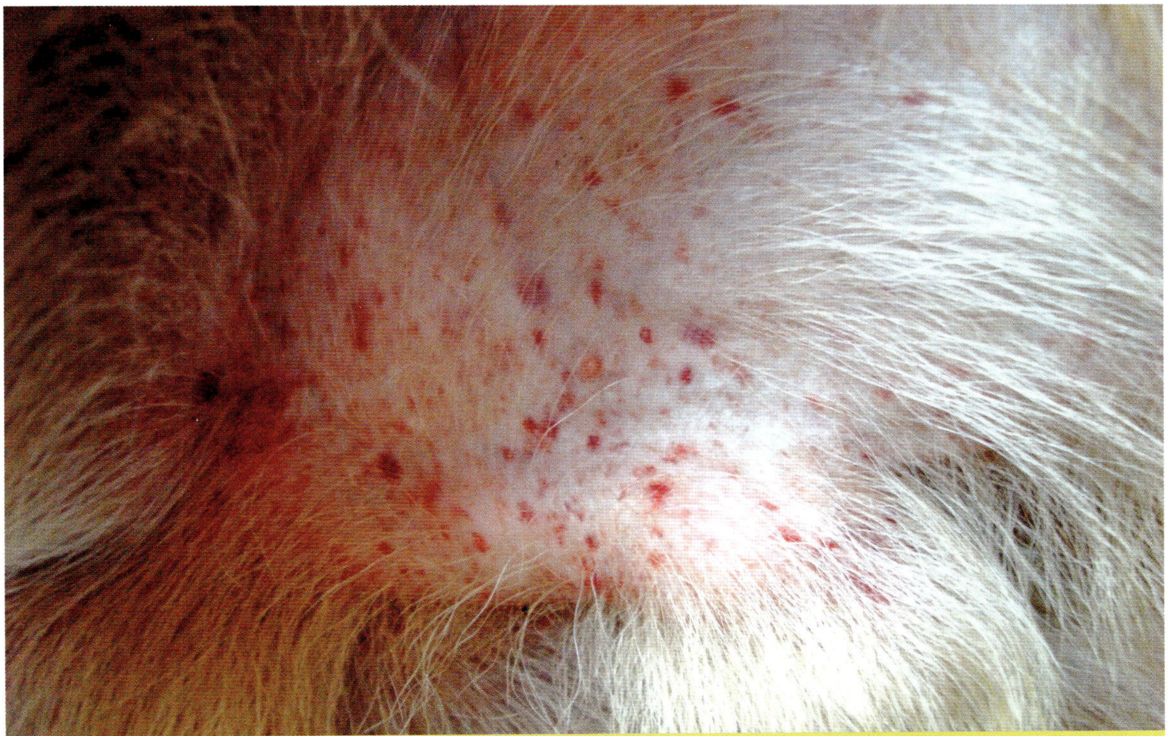

04 Petechiae on the skin of the abdomen due to tick-borne ehrlichiosis.

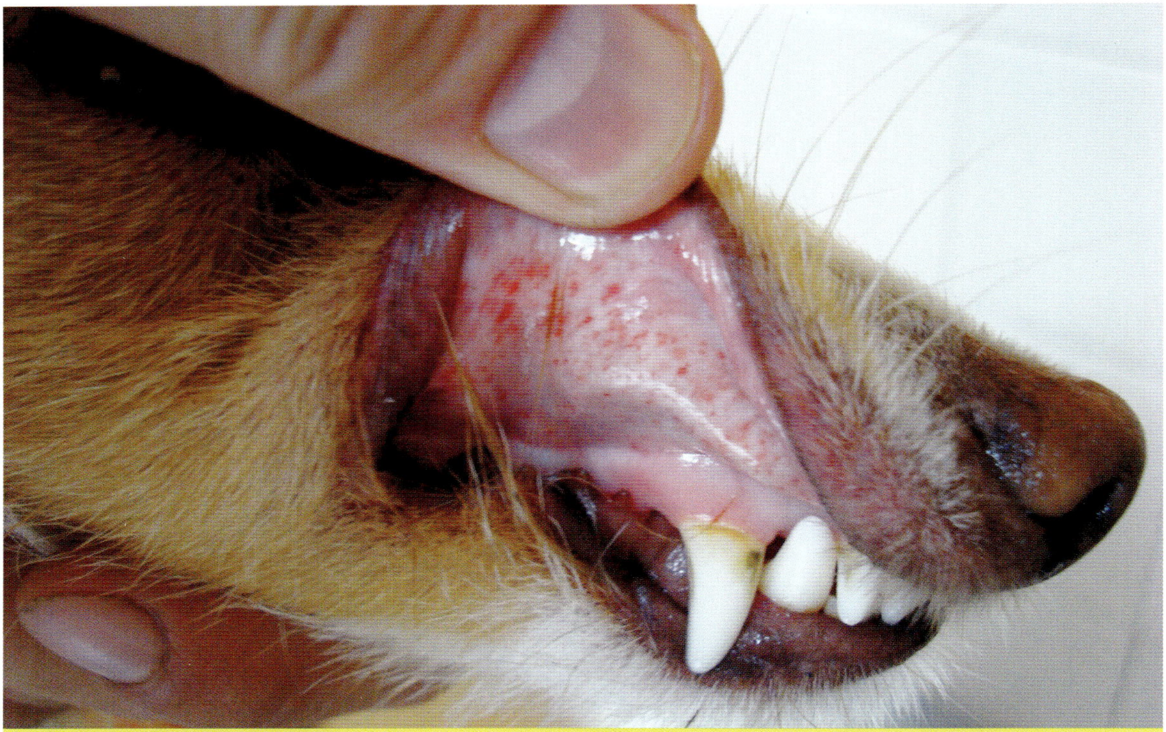

05 Petechiae in the oral mucosa due to tick-borne ehrlichiosis.

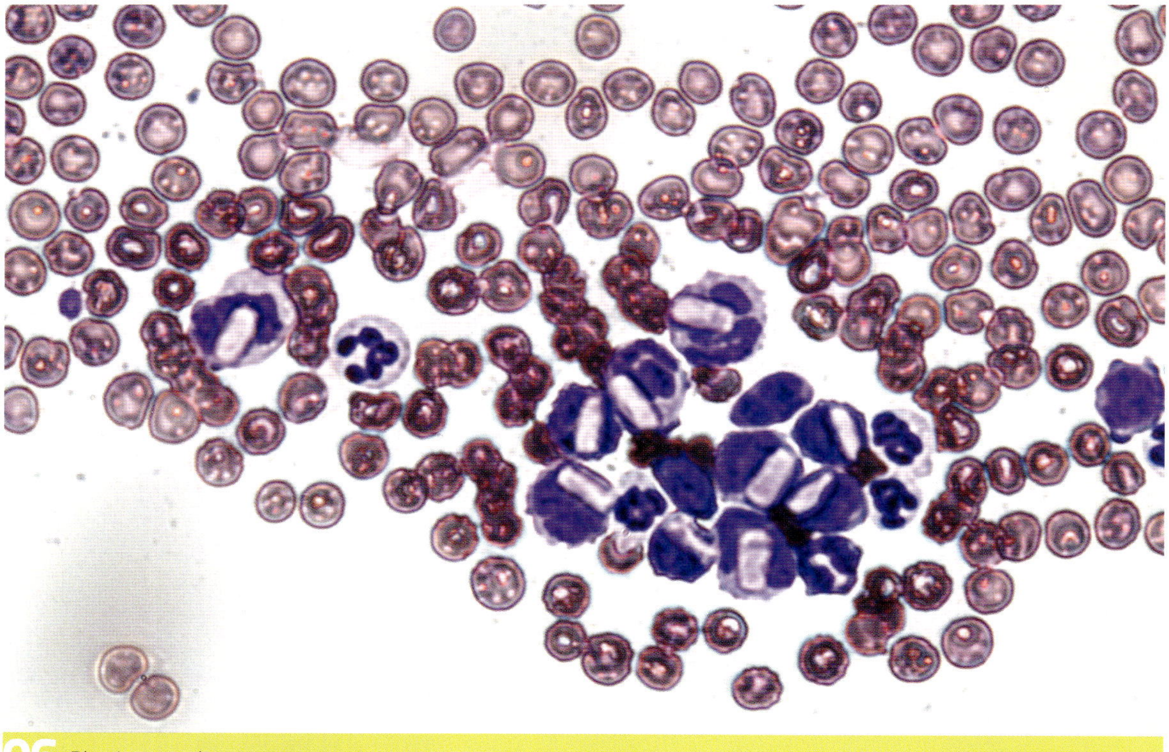

06 Blood smear showing *Hepatozoon canis*.

# Pediculosis

## Lesion aetiology/pathogenesis and clinical picture

This is a parasitosis of both dogs and cats caused by species-specific lice that do not affect humans. These insects cause pruritus of variable severity, mainly on the head, neck, and trunk. Clinical signs include excoriations, dry and brittle hair, and poor hair coat condition. Lice and their nits can be observed with the naked eye attached to hairs.

## Diagnostic method

Diagnosis is easily established based on the presence of the parasites, which are easy to identify, together with poor hair coat condition and pruritus.

## Main differential diagnoses

- Cheyletiellosis
- Flea dermatitis
- Allergies in general
- Grooming disorders in cats

## Treatment

Highly effective treatments in the form of tablets, pipettes, or sprays are available, and usually result in resolution without problems. It is important not to overlook treatment of fomites.

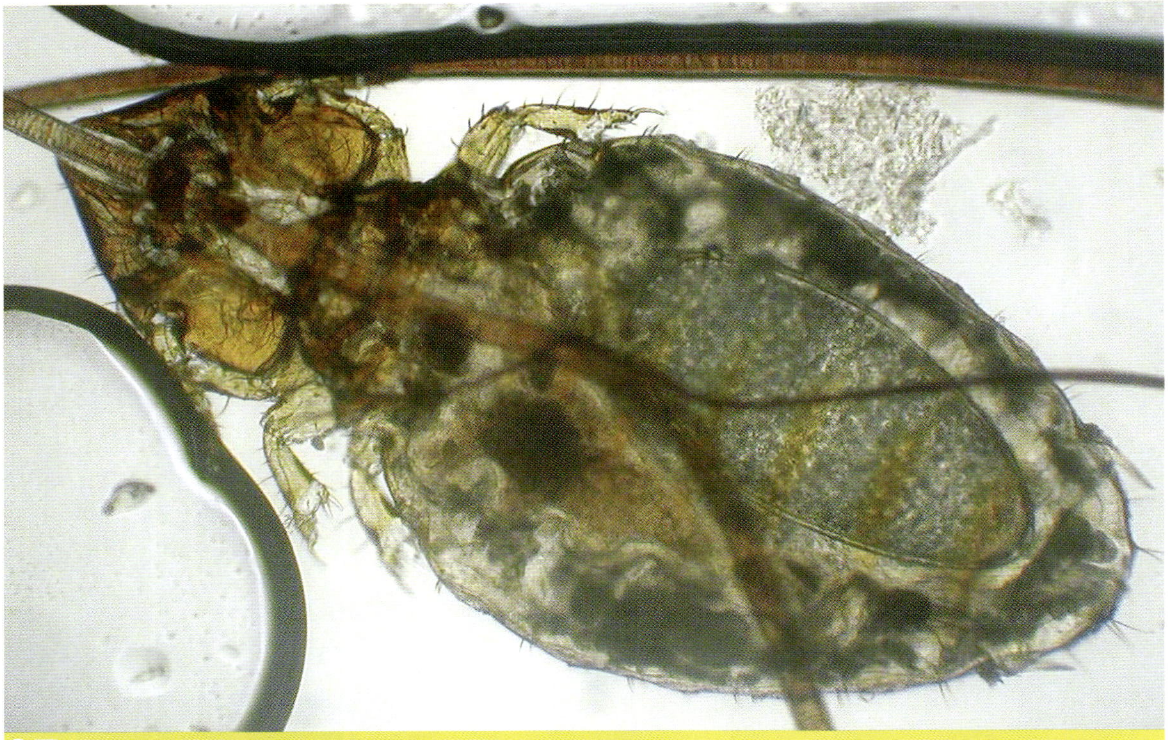

07 Louse with a nit inside.

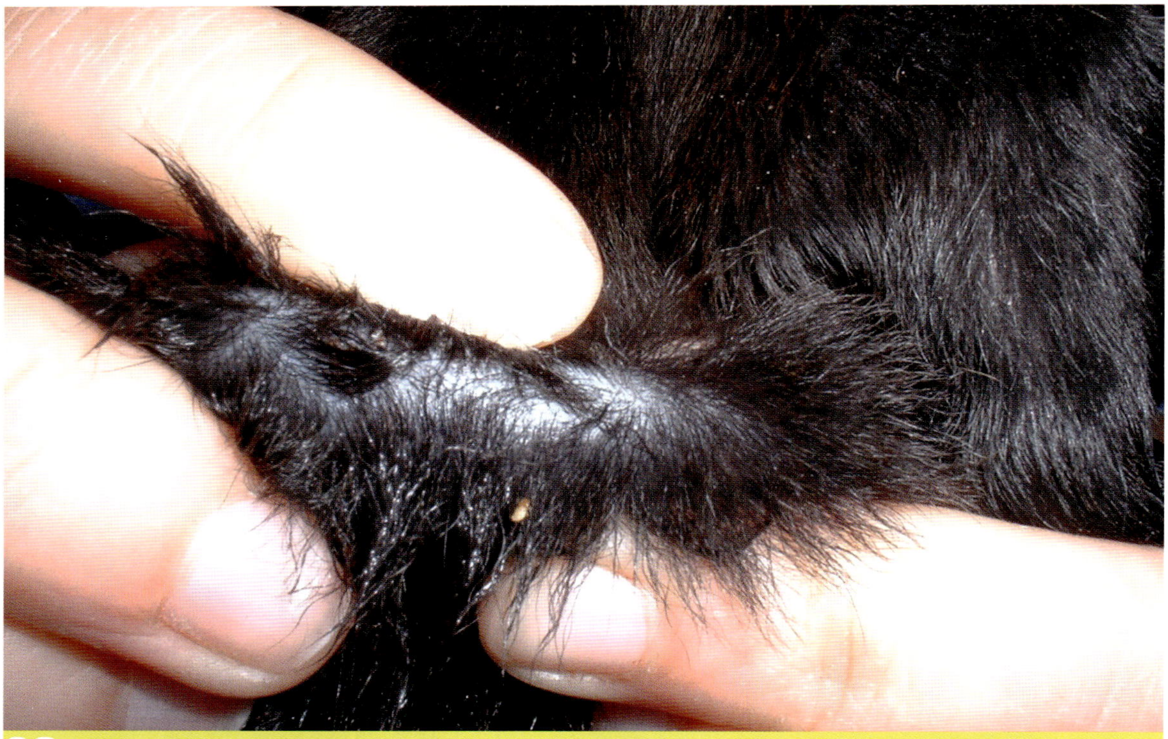

08 Close-up of lice between the hairs of a dog.

# Pulicosis

## Lesion aetiology/pathogenesis and clinical picture

Flea infestation, both in dogs and cats, must be differentiated from allergic dermatitis caused by this same insect.

In cases in which the host is not hypersensitive, skin conditions are usually milder and have distinct characteristics.

The presence of fleas can result in areas of trichorrhexis caused by biting. In dogs, this occurs mainly on limbs, while in cats the dorsal area is typically affected.

## Diagnostic method

Confirmation of the presence of the parasite or its droppings is the key to diagnosis. In cats, which groom continuously, fleas can be difficult to perceive, although broken hairs and even the accumulation of hairs on the teeth may be evident.

## Main differential diagnoses

- Other parasitic diseases
- Other causes of itching

## Treatment

Different insecticides in the form of collars, pipettes, sprays, or tablets can be effective. However, few can prevent the bite of at least some fleas, which triggers a clinical picture of variable intensity. It is very important to control the presence of ticks in the environment and avoid walks in areas where these insects reside.

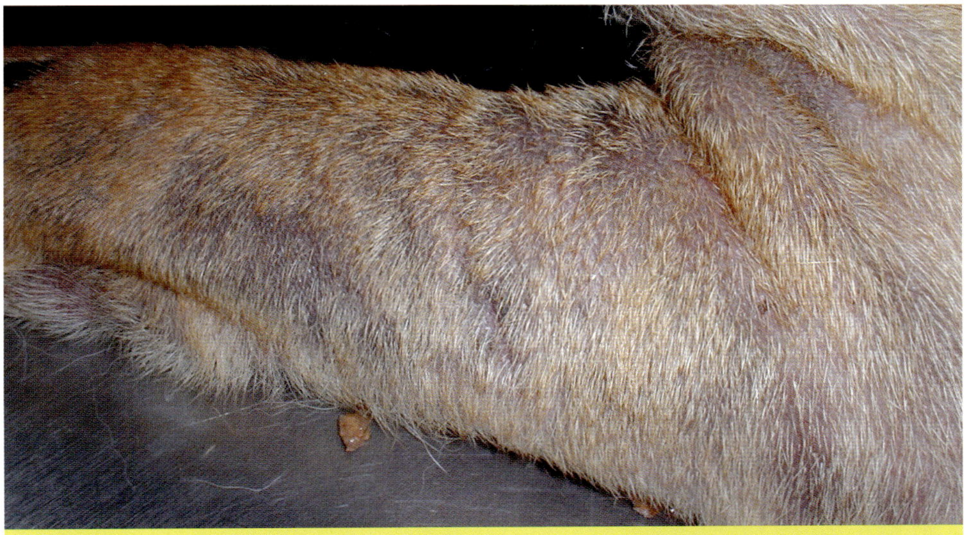

09 Note the broken hairs on the forelimb of a dog with fleas.

# Myiasis

## Lesion aetiology/pathogenesis and clinical picture

Lesions caused by fly larvae ranging from superficial to deep and severe. Depending on the species, flies deposit their eggs in moist areas of the skin or in the dead tissue in wounds. The resulting lesions are characterised by bleeding and the formation of large cavities.

## Diagnostic method

The clinical appearance is characteristic, although in some cases it is essential to clean the wound, clip the surrounding hair, and dissect the lesion to reveal the presence of larvae. Observation of larvae is confirmatory.

## Main differential diagnoses

Spike-type foreign bodies (in case of deep wounds).

## Treatment

Thorough cleaning of the wound, removal of the larvae, and application of antiseptic and antiparasitic agents is essential. Systemic macrocyclic lactones and isoxazolines are usually very effective. Appropriate insecticides can be applied locally.

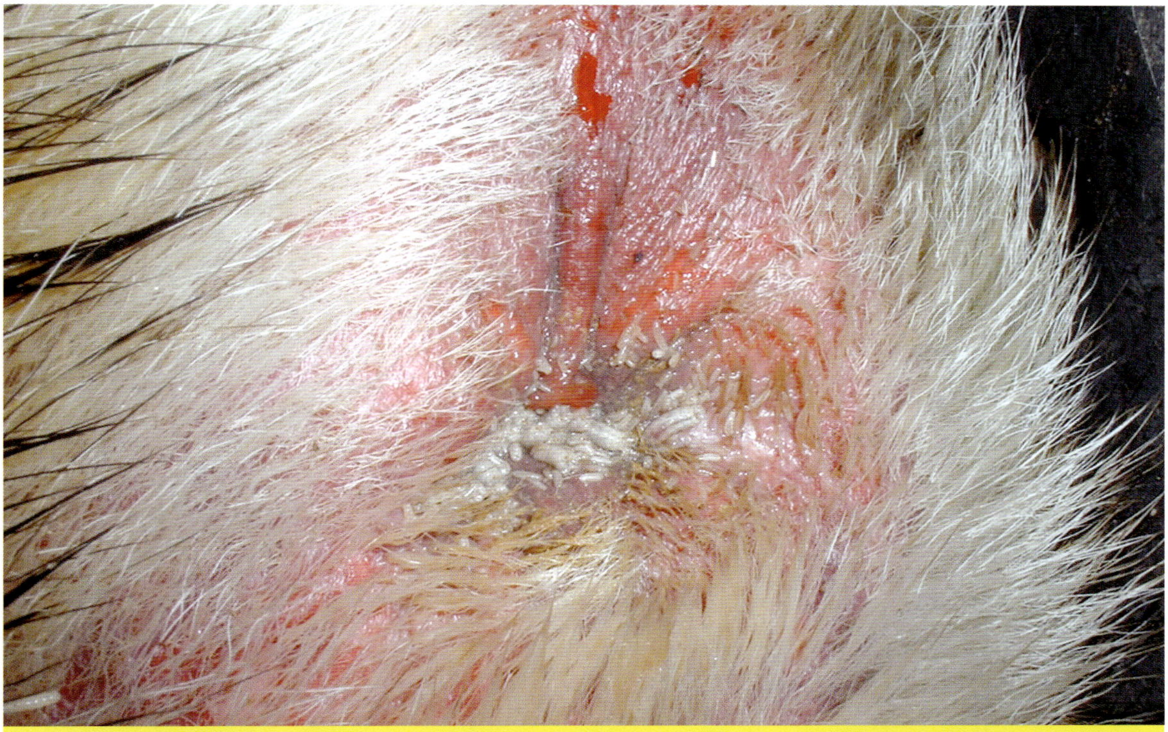

10 Myiasis in the anal area. Note the abundant larvae.

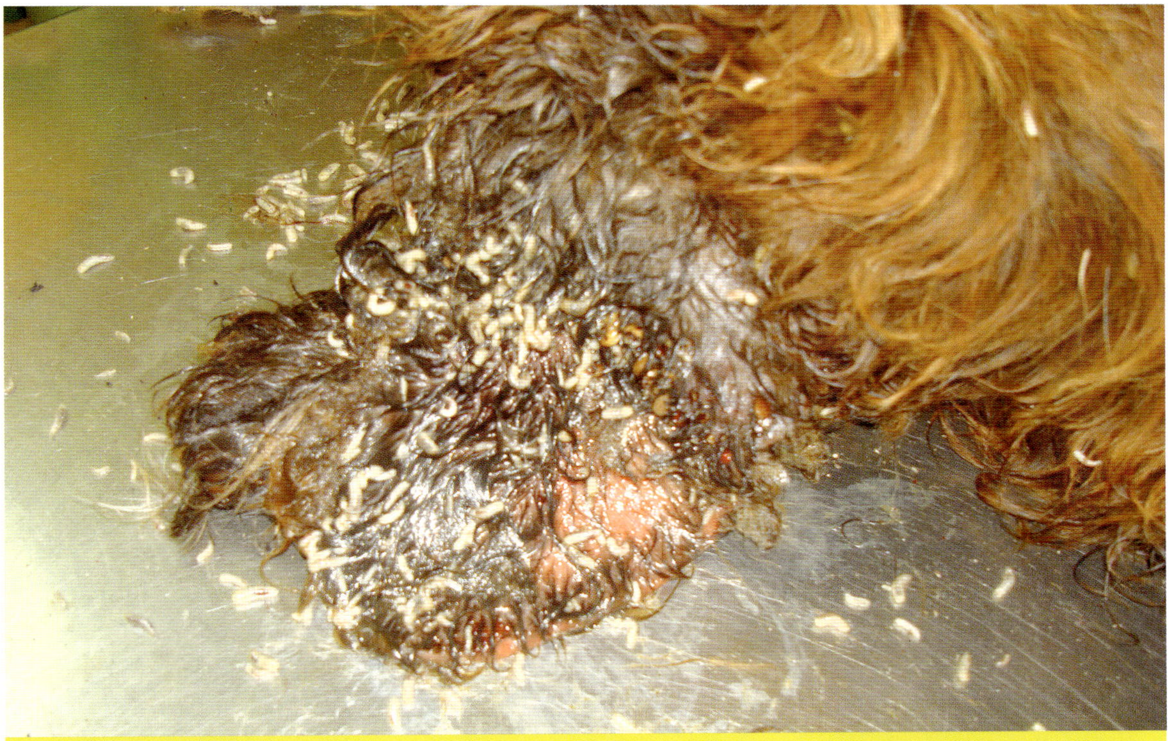

11 Myiasis in the ear of a dog.

# Canine demodicosis or red mange

## Lesion aetiology/pathogenesis and clinical picture

Skin condition caused by *Demodex* spp. in genetically predisposed and/or immunocompromised individuals. The clinical presentation can range from simple patches of alopecia to furunculosis, scaling, plaques, or even serious ulcers, with risk to life due to septicaemia. Depending on the affected areas, it can be classified as localised or generalised. In cases in which the affected animal is less than 2 years of age, it is usually considered a juvenile form. Adult demodicosis is more commonly due to immune deficiency caused by endocrine disorders, drugs, or neoplasia.

## Diagnostic method

The parasite can be located at the bottom of the hair follicle or in the sebaceous glands (*Demodex canis* or *Demodex injai*), or on the surface of the skin (short-bodied *Demodex*). Therefore, the methods of choice for diagnosis are deep scraping, trichography and, in some cases, superficial scraping or adhesive tape.

*Demodex cyonis,* a new species that is slightly thicker than the aforementioned species, has been associated with seborrhoeic and pruritic presentations in dogs.

## Main differential diagnoses

- Deep pyoderma
- Bacterial or dermatophyte folliculitis
- Dermatophyte kerion
- Histiocytomas
- Acral lick dermatitis

## Treatment

Localised forms of demodicosis are not usually treated, but follow-up is very important. Most generalised forms tend to respond to treatment with systemic macrocyclic lactones or isoxazolines. Antibiotic therapy is very important to control concomitant infections. The great efficacy of current treatments such as isoxazolines is transforming this disease into a sporadic finding.

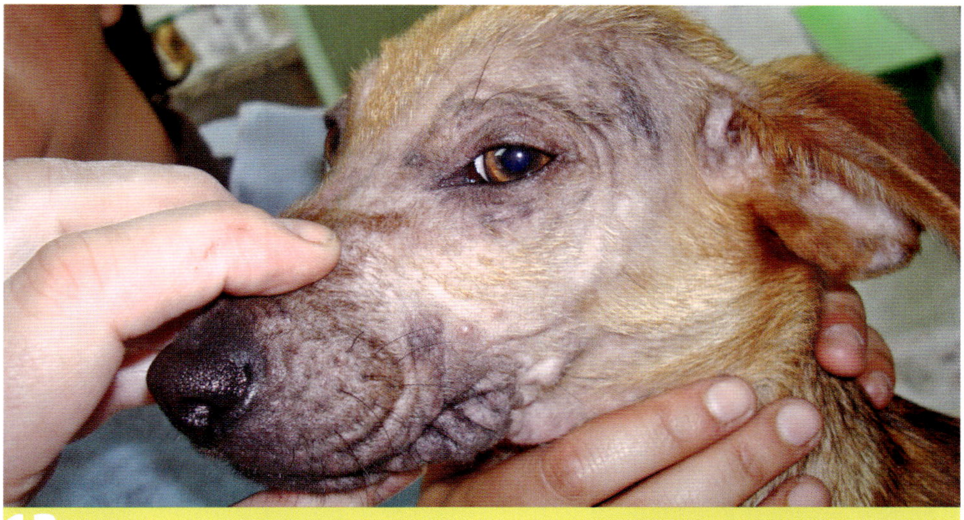

12 Facial involvement in a puppy with demodicosis.

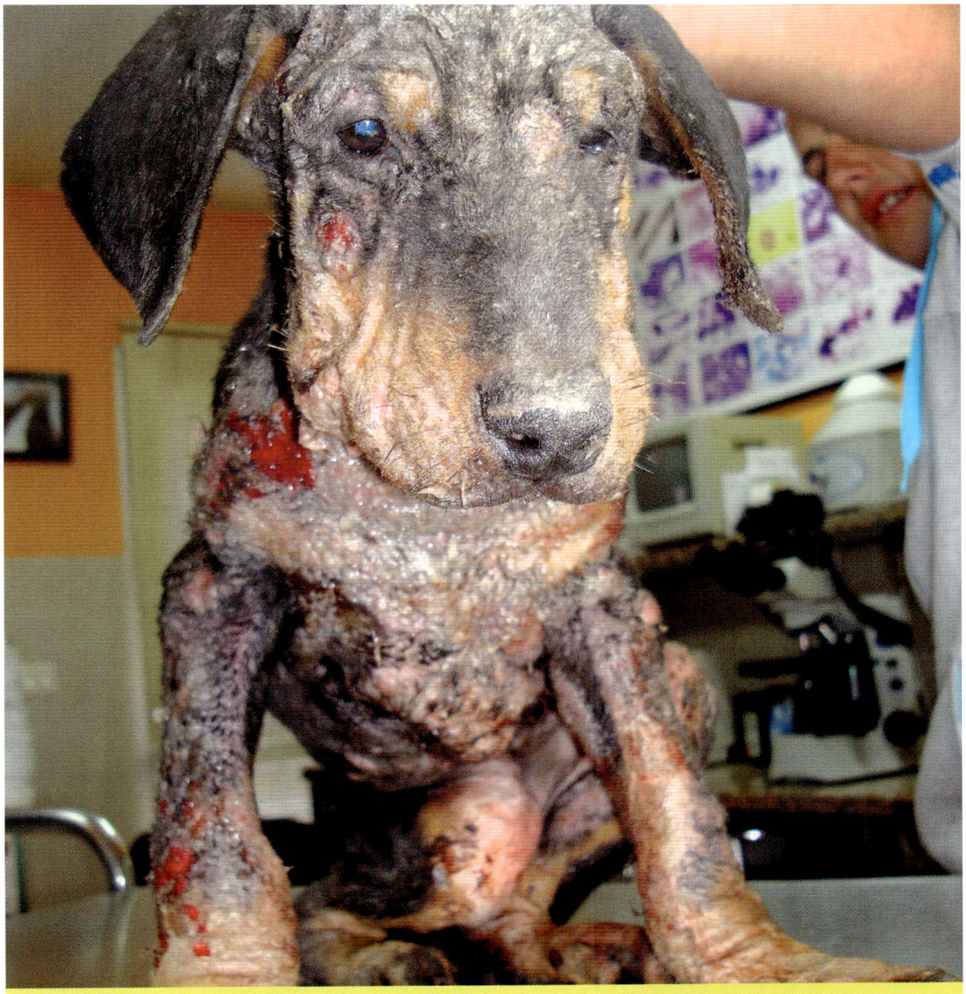

13 Severe demodicosis in a puppy with septicaemia.

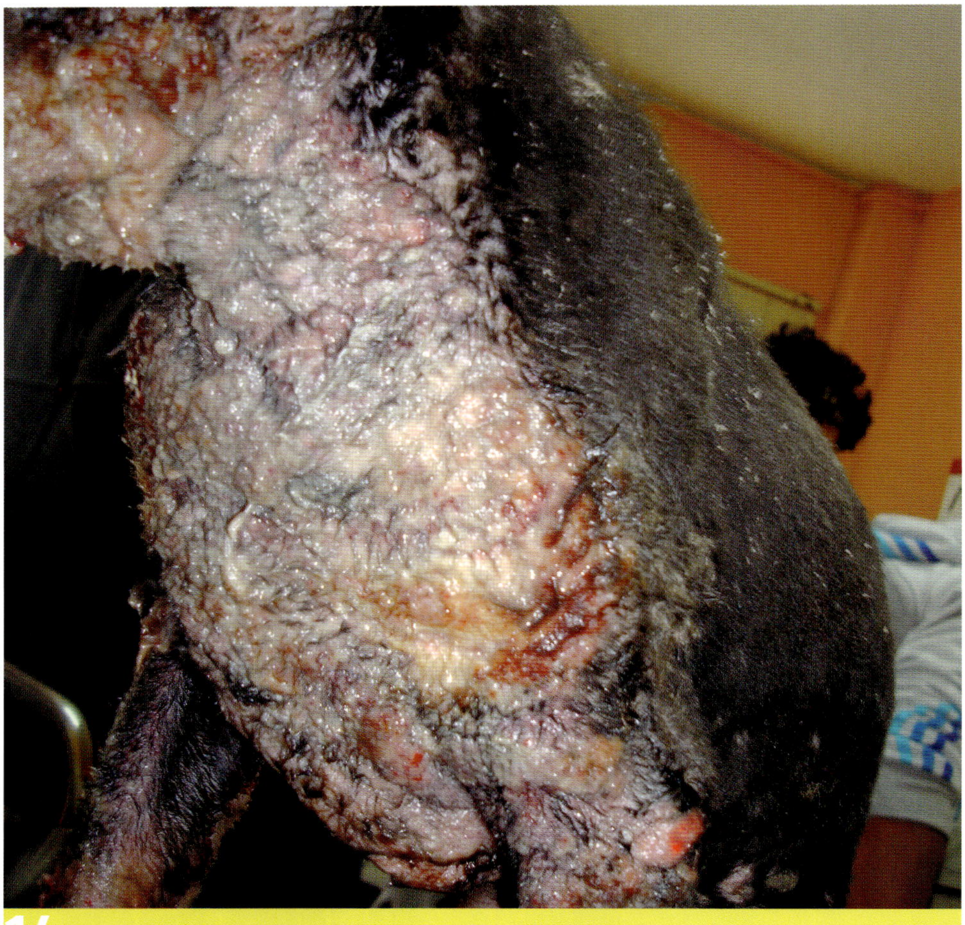

**14** Severe demodicosis in a puppy with septicaemia. Close-up of the skin.

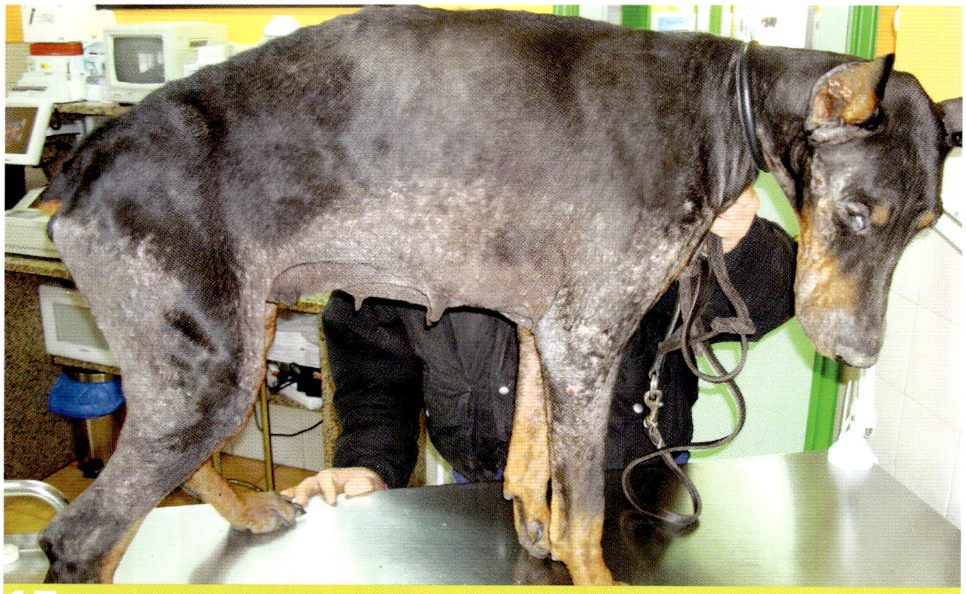

**15** Generalised adult demodicosis.

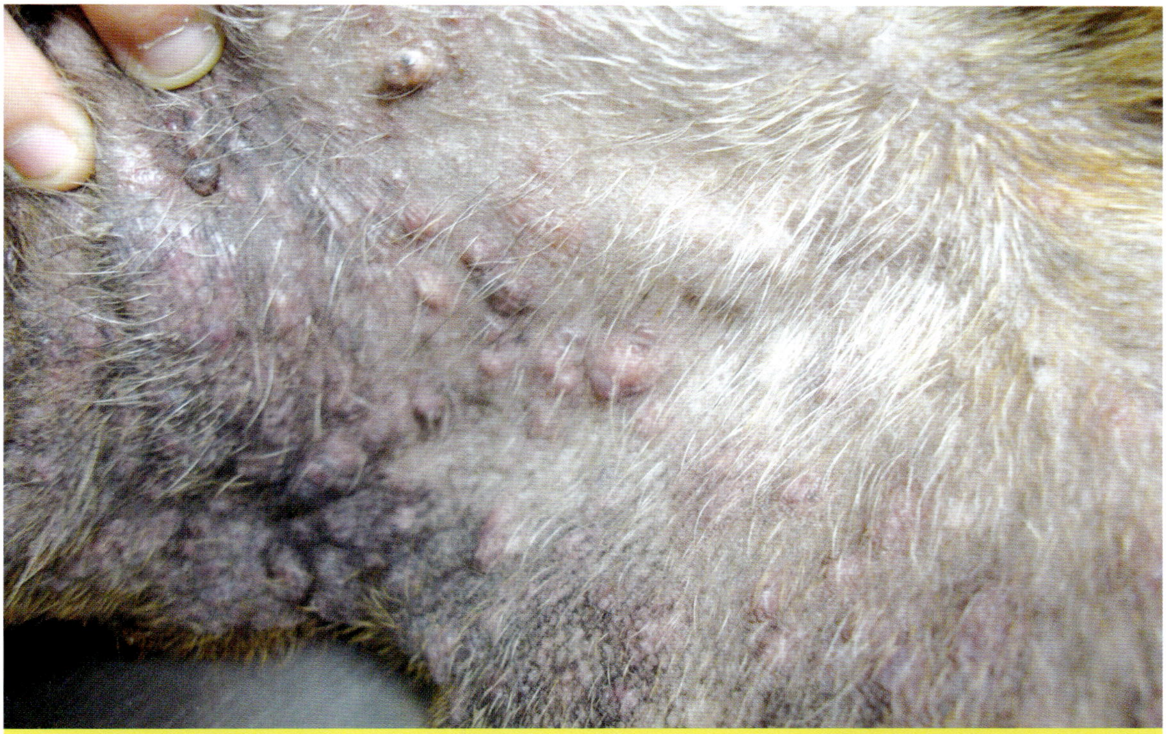

16 Nodular demodicosis in an adult Boxer.

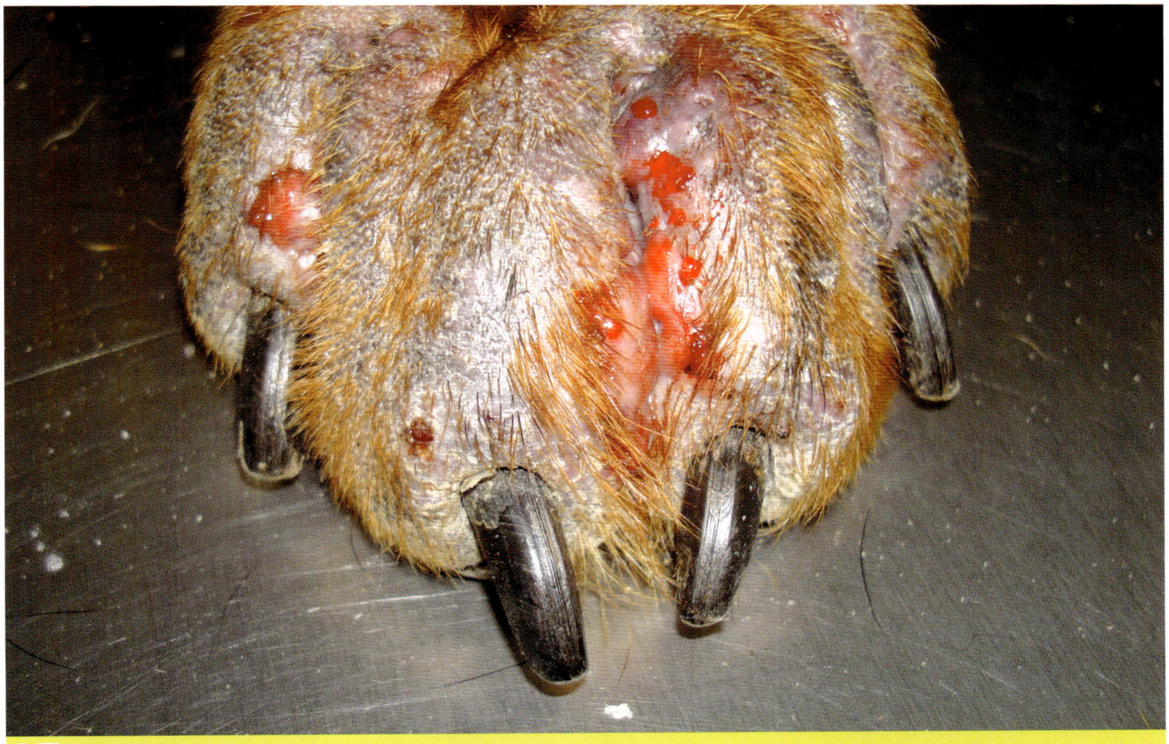

17 Severe pododemodicosis.

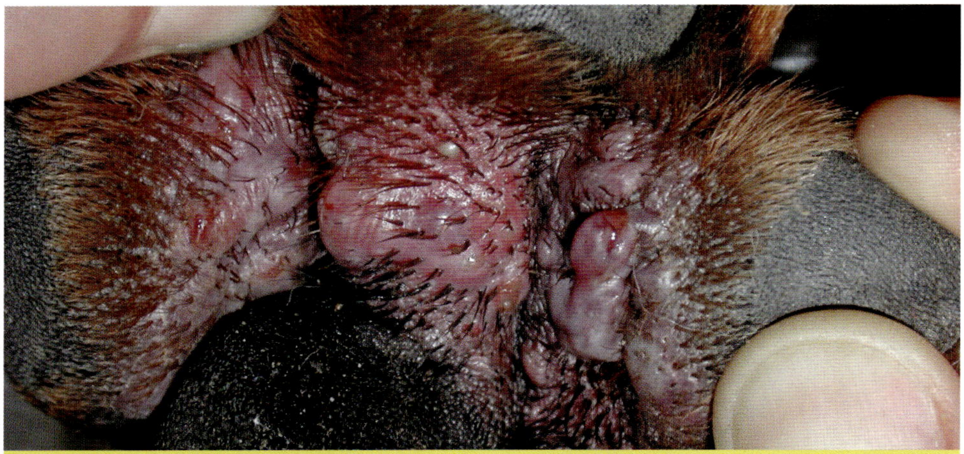

**18** Pododemodicosis, palmar view. Note the furuncles and pustules. Image provided by the Somaza Pérez Veterinary Clinic (Spain).

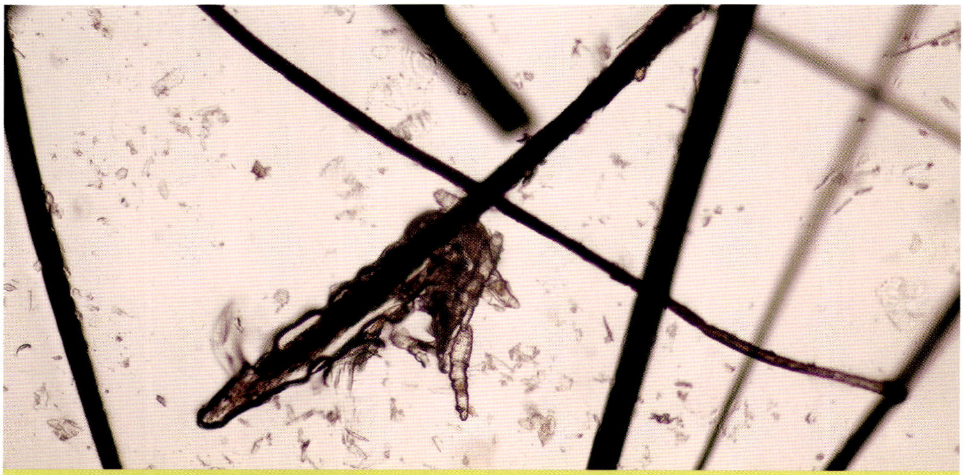

**19** Image of *Demodex canis* acquired by trichography.

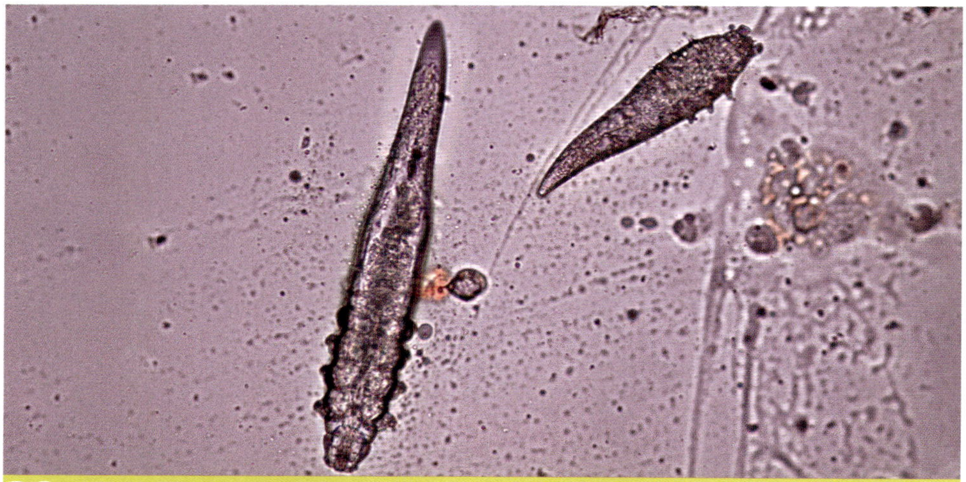

**20** *Demodex*: adult and larva.

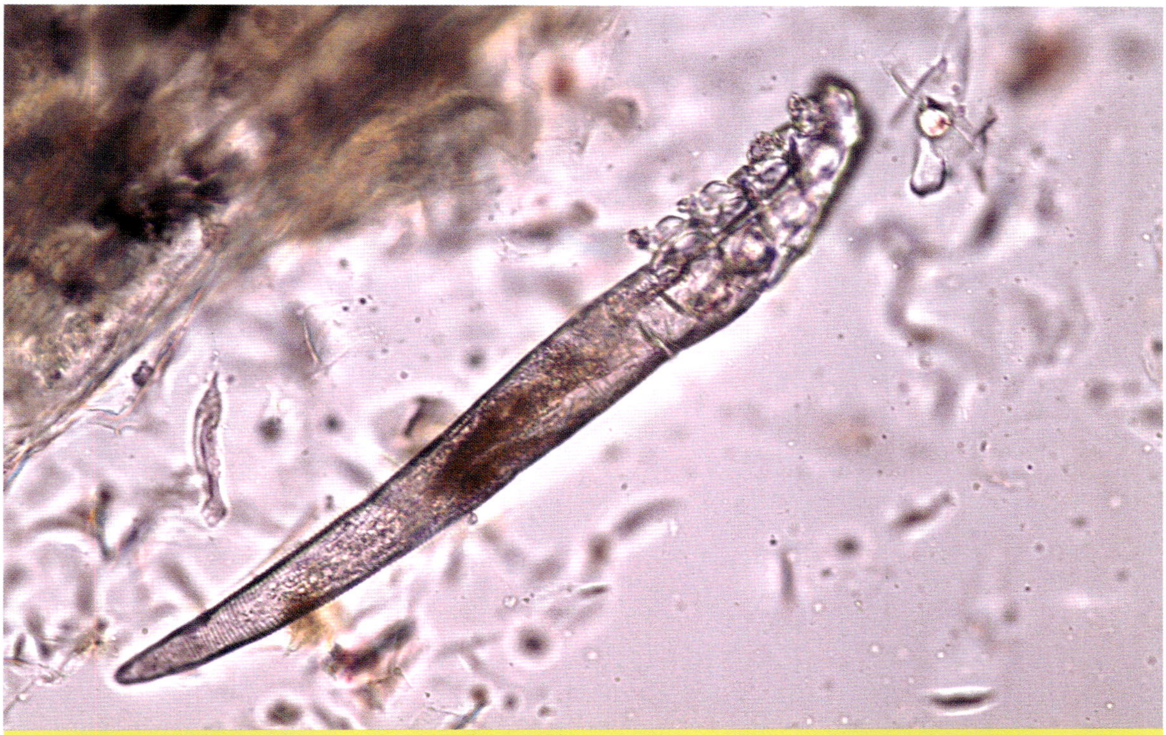

21 *Demodex injai*. Note the characteristic elongated shape.

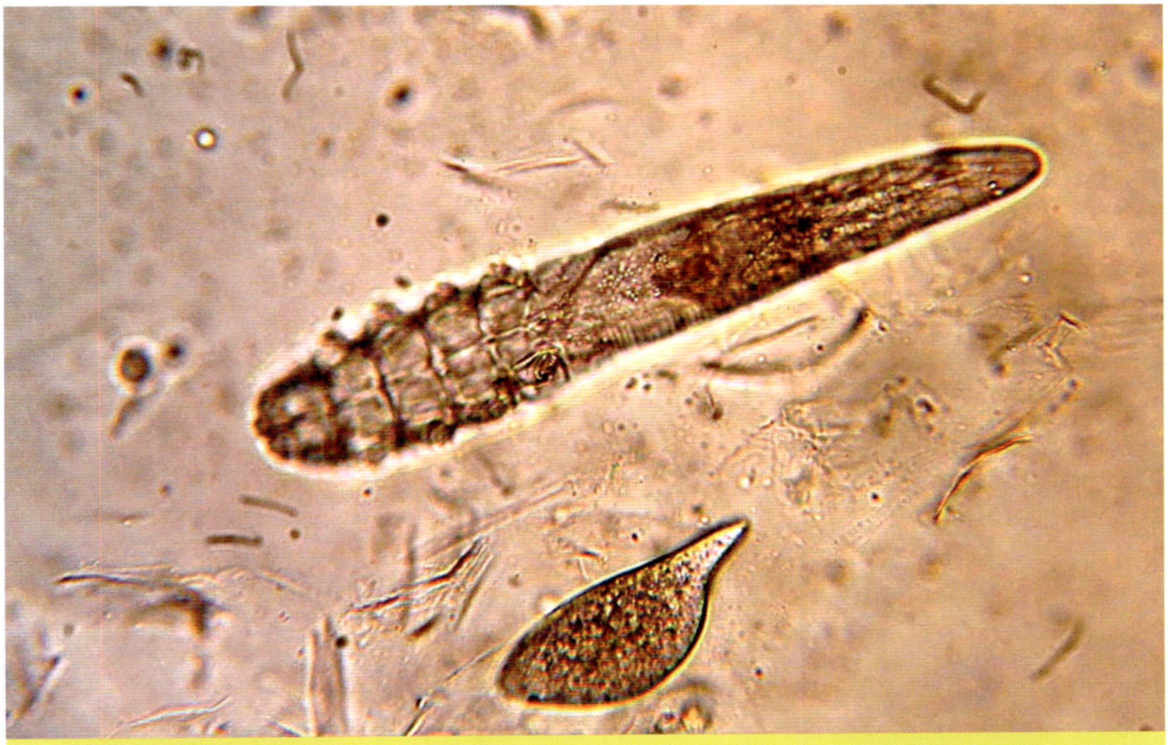

22 Adult *Demodex* with an egg.

# Feline demodicosis

## Lesion aetiology/pathogenesis and clinical picture

Dermatosis in cats caused mainly by *Demodex cati*. That caused by *Demodex gatoi* is less common. Some cases of demodicosis caused by unknown mite species have been described. This condition can result in crusted papules with folliculitis and scaling, in some cases becoming generalised, often due to immune compromise. *D. gatoi* causes a more superficial, pruritic, and contagious presentation.

## Diagnostic method

Deep scraping and adhesive tape are often the best diagnostic methods. Swabs should also be performed in case of ceruminous otitis, which can be caused by *Demodex*.

## Main differential diagnoses

- Dermatophytosis
- Otitis due to dermatophytes or mites
- Other ectoparasites

## Treatment

Macrocyclic lactones and isoxazolines are usually effective. Diseases that can cause immune compromise should not be overlooked, and should be controlled while also applying acaricidal treatment.

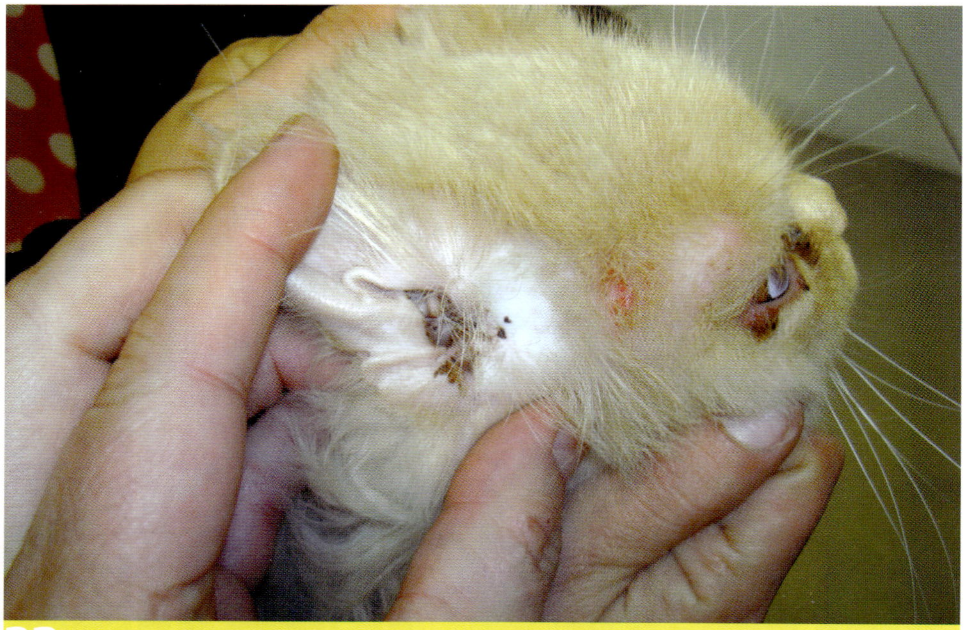

**23** Feline demodicosis due to *Demodex cati*. Note alopecia and erosion above the eye.

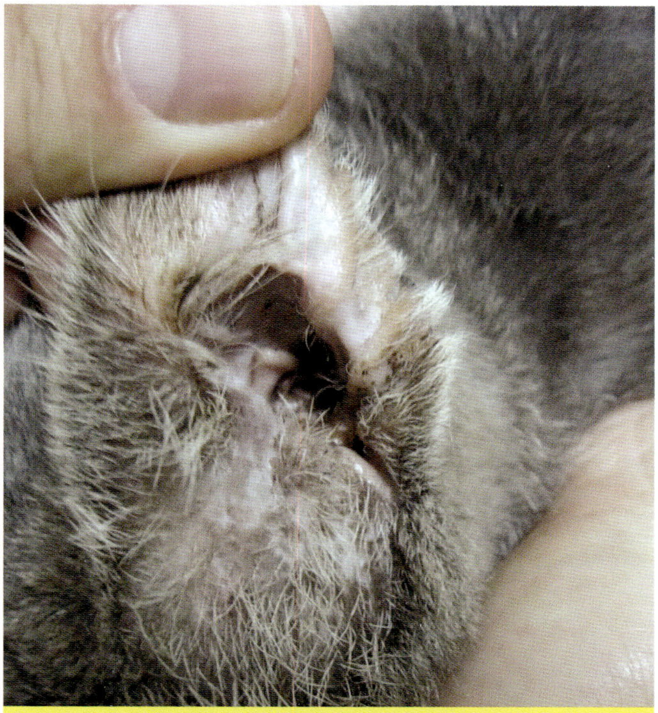

**24** Otitis caused by *Demodex cati*. Image courtesy of Julio Fariñas.

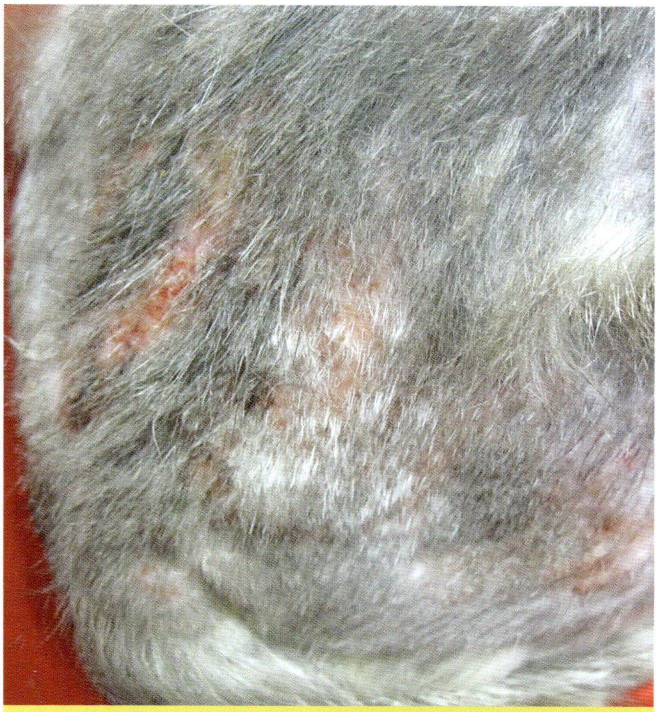

**25** Dermatosis on the back of a cat caused by *Demodex cati*. Image courtesy of Julio Fariñas.

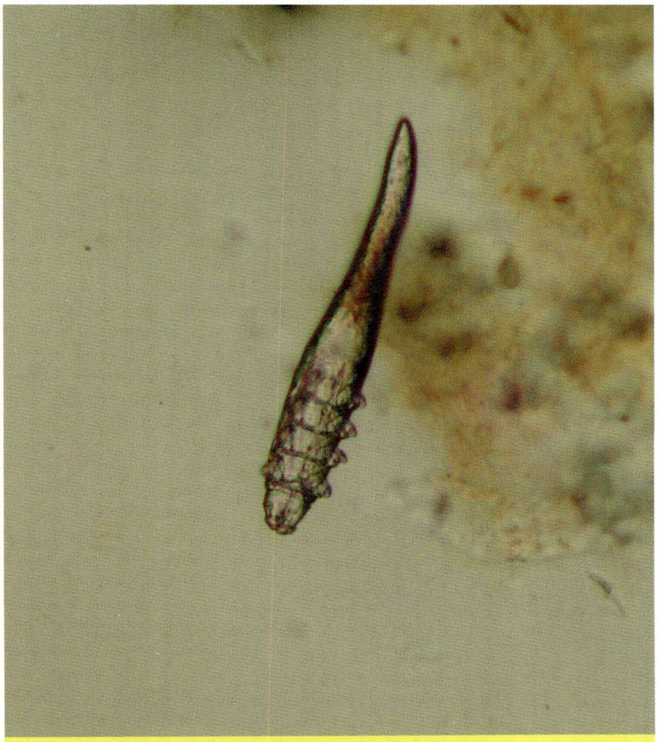

**26** *Demodex cati*.

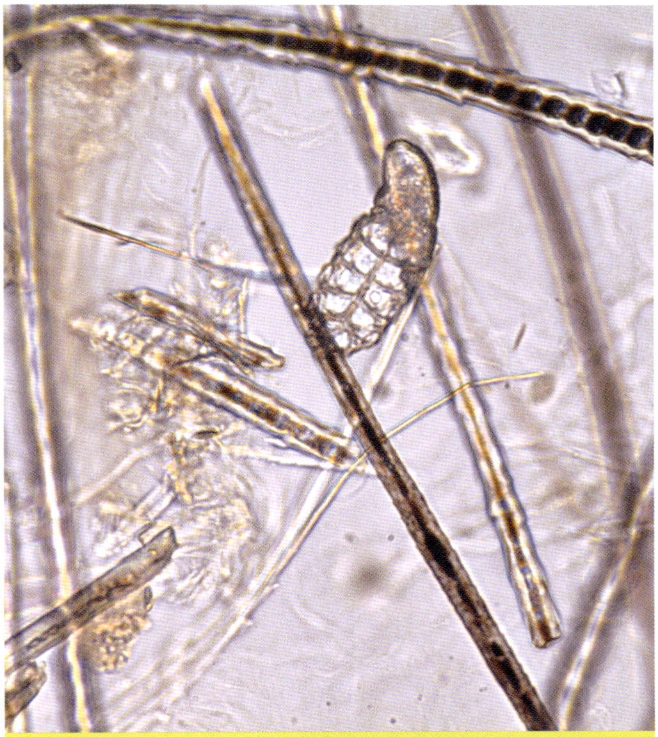

**27** *Demodex gatoi*. Image courtesy of Oriol Sanz.

# Canine scabies or sarcoptic mange

## Lesion aetiology/pathogenesis and clinical picture

This dermatitis is almost always highly pruritic and is caused by the obligate mite *Sarcoptes scabiei* var. *canis*. The mite creates extrafollicular burrows that give rise to a characteristic clinical picture, with the appearance of papules/crusts, alopecia, erythema, and seborrhoea in areas including the elbows, tarsi, periocular region, and ears, later becoming generalised and affecting the entire trunk. This parasite can cause transient, highly pruritic papules in humans.

Contagion can occur in the most unexpected ways.

## Diagnostic method

Medium-depth scrapings are usually necessary, although the parasite is not easily detected. The best places to acquire scrapings are the ear margin or any yellowish crusts. The pinnal-pedal reflex is almost always positive, and the mite should be suspected in cases of itching that does not respond to conventional treatments. It can often be difficult to distinguish from states of acute hypersensitivity. Serum IgG specific for *Sarcoptes* can be determined: this is a reliable method to detect the mite after 3 weeks of infestation and to verify treatment efficacy, as reflected by a decrease in antibody titres over time.

The use of isoxazolines can be an excellent therapeutic diagnostic method.

## Main differential diagnoses

- Allergies
- Demodicosis
- Keratinisation disorders
- Pemphigus complex

## Treatment

Isoxazolines have significantly improved the treatment of this disease. Treatment with macrocyclic lactones, repeated every 21 days, remains effective, and it should be borne in mind that all fomites should also be treated. Because this is a very contagious disease, all individuals living together should be treated.

Pruritus can be controlled with oclacitinib from the moment of initiation of acaricidal treatment.

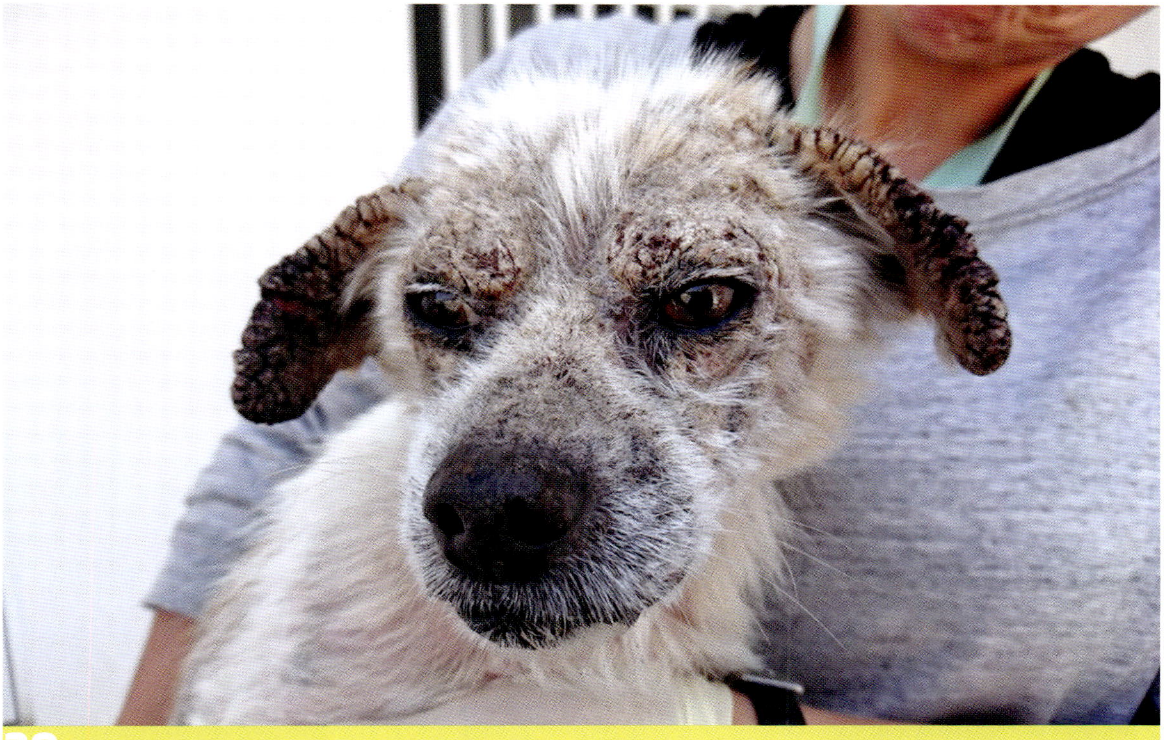

28 Crusted papular and erythematous facial alopecia in a dog with sarcoptic mange.

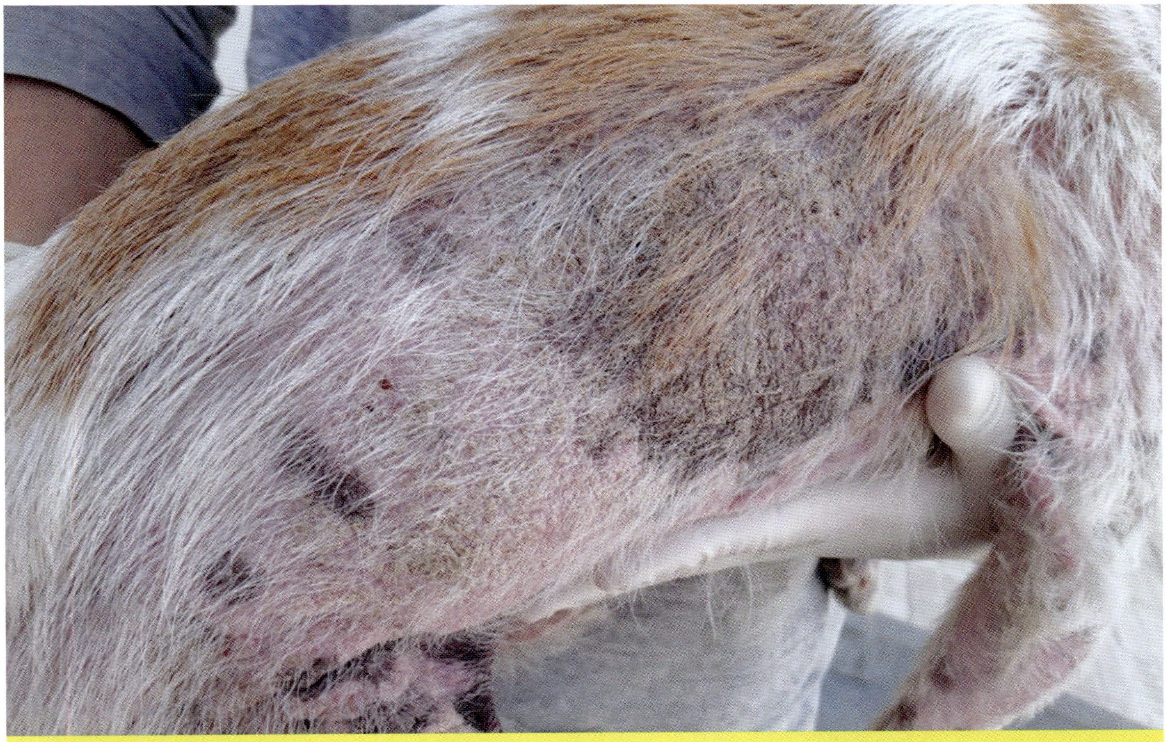

29 Same dog as in previous photo: general view of the entire body. Note the erythema and crusts.

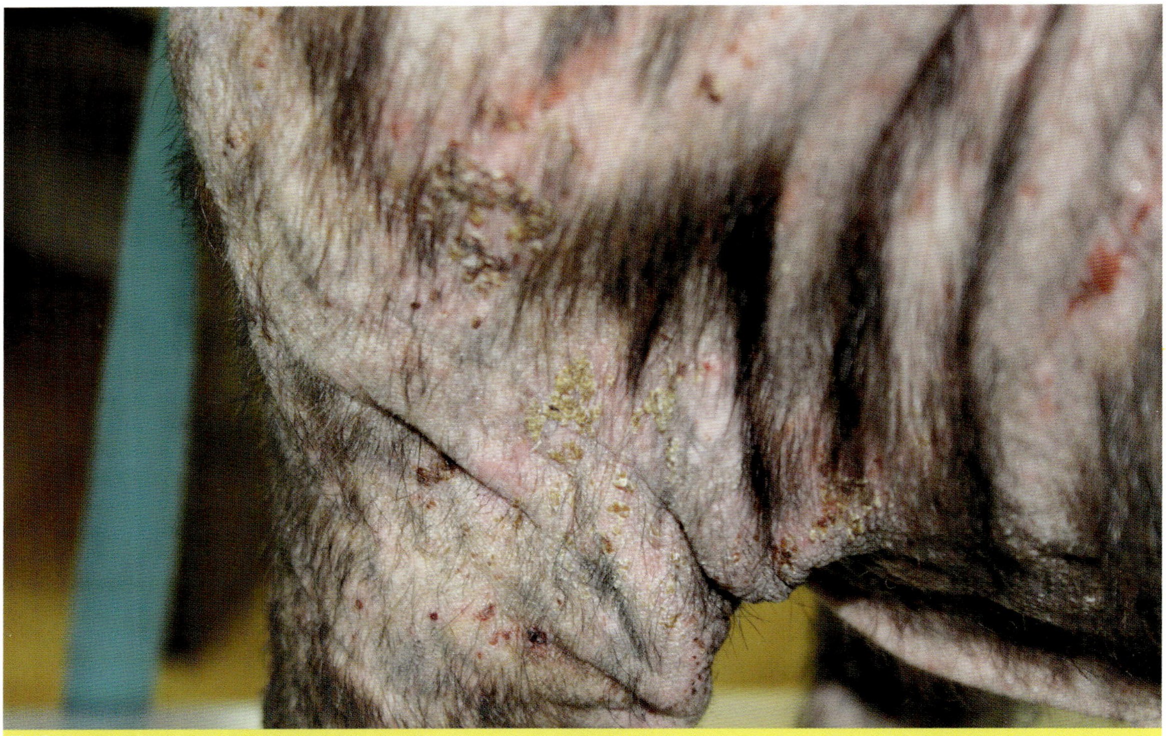

30 Elbow of a dog with sarcoptic mange. The yellow crust is highly characteristic.

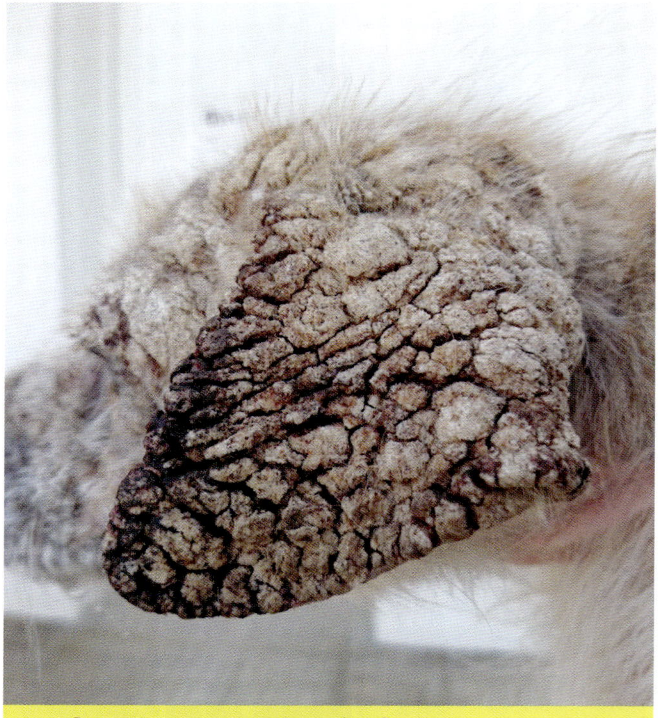

31 Sarcoptic mange several months after onset.
Ear involvement.

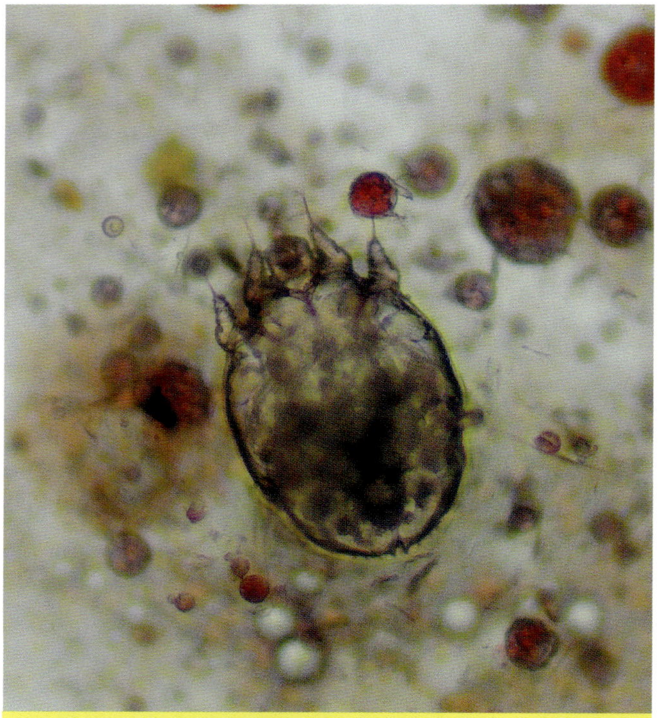

32 *Sarcoptes* scabiei var. *canis* mite.

# Feline notoedric mange or feline mange

## Lesion aetiology/pathogenesis and clinical picture

This is a highly pruritic and contagious dermatitis caused by the obligate mite *Notoedres cati*. The mite creates extrafollicular burrows that give rise to a characteristic clinical picture consisting of papules/crusts, alopecia, and erythema, with a typical lichenified and crusted appearance. The ears are usually affected first, but grooming frequently results in spread to the head and body. Transmission to owners can also occur, resulting in the development of highly pruritic papules.

It is a very infrequent disease, which occurs mainly in tropical climates.

## Diagnostic method

A medium depth skin scraping is usually necessary. The ear margin or yellowish crusts may be the best places to scrape. The clinical history is very important in order to establish a history of contacts with other animals.

## Main differential diagnoses

- Autoimmune dermatosis
- Dermatophytosis
- Other ectoparasites
- Other feline facial conditions with an erosive–ulcerative pattern

## Treatment

Treatment with macrocyclic lactones, repeated every 21 days, is highly effective, and should be accompanied by treatment of all fomites. Repeated isoxazoline treatment, following the regimen indicated on the product leaflet, is also very effective.

Because this is a highly contagious disease, all individuals living together should be treated. The use of antipruritic agents may be necessary to alleviate the severe itching.

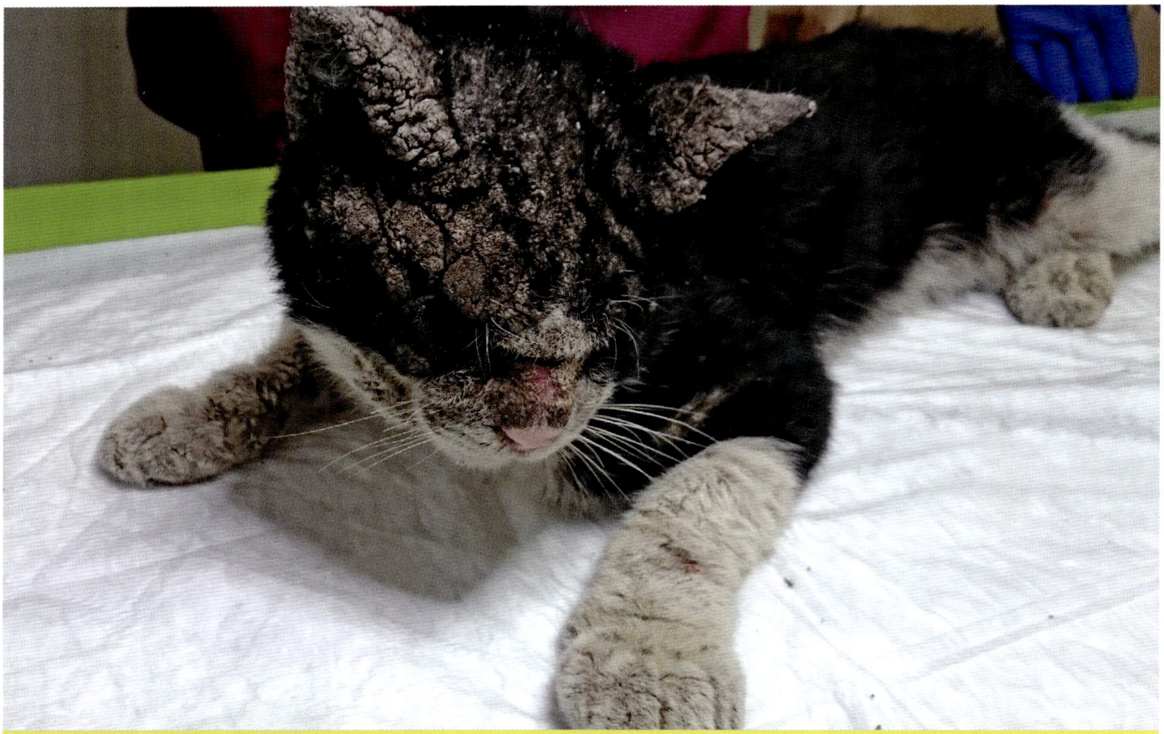

**33** Notoedric mange. Classic presentation affecting the head and paws of a cat. Image courtesy of David Sanmiguel.

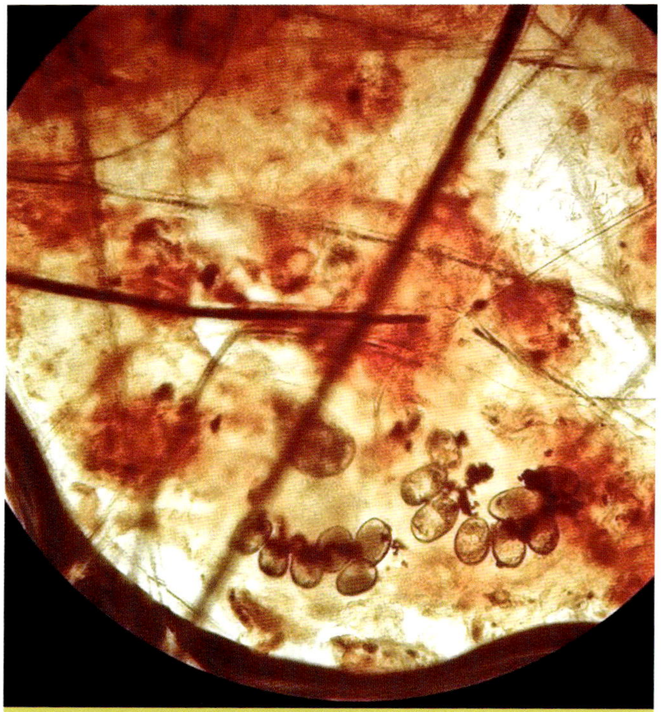

**34** Abundant eggs of *Notoedres* obtained by scraping. Image courtesy of Guillermina Maningot.

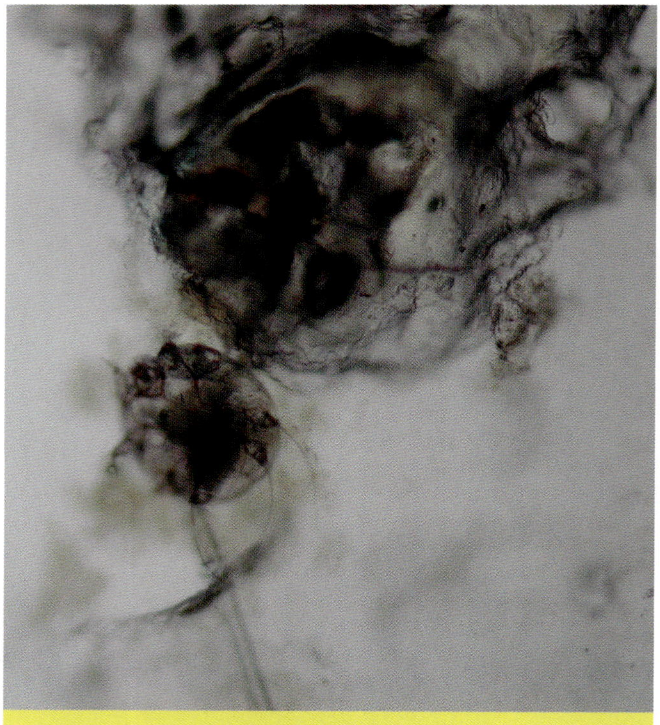

**35** *Notoedres cati*. Image courtesy of César Yotti.

# Otitis due to *Otodectes cynotis*

## Lesion aetiology/pathogenesis and clinical picture

The mite *Otodectes cynotis* is the main cause of otitis in both dogs and cats. This primarily affects puppies and kittens, although animals of any age can be affected. It is characterised by abundant secretion of dark dry wax that resembles coffee grounds. This can indicate the onset of ceruminous otitis that later becomes contaminated with secondary agents such as bacteria or yeast. The condition can spread to other parts of the body causing hypersensitivity and pruritus, mainly in cats. In many cases, it triggers miliary dermatitis and, less commonly, dermatitis of the head and neck.

## Diagnostic method

The parasite is very obvious and can be observed with the naked eye as a moving white dot in the cone of the otoscope. The best diagnostic method is take an ear swab for examination of the cerumen at low magnification under the microscope.

## Main differential diagnoses

- Other forms of otitis
- Other forms of miliary dermatitis

## Treatment

Acaricidal drops can be administered directly into the ear canal, or systemic treatment with macrocyclic lactones or isoxazolines can be applied. The oily vehicles used in ear drops can also have an acaricidal effect.

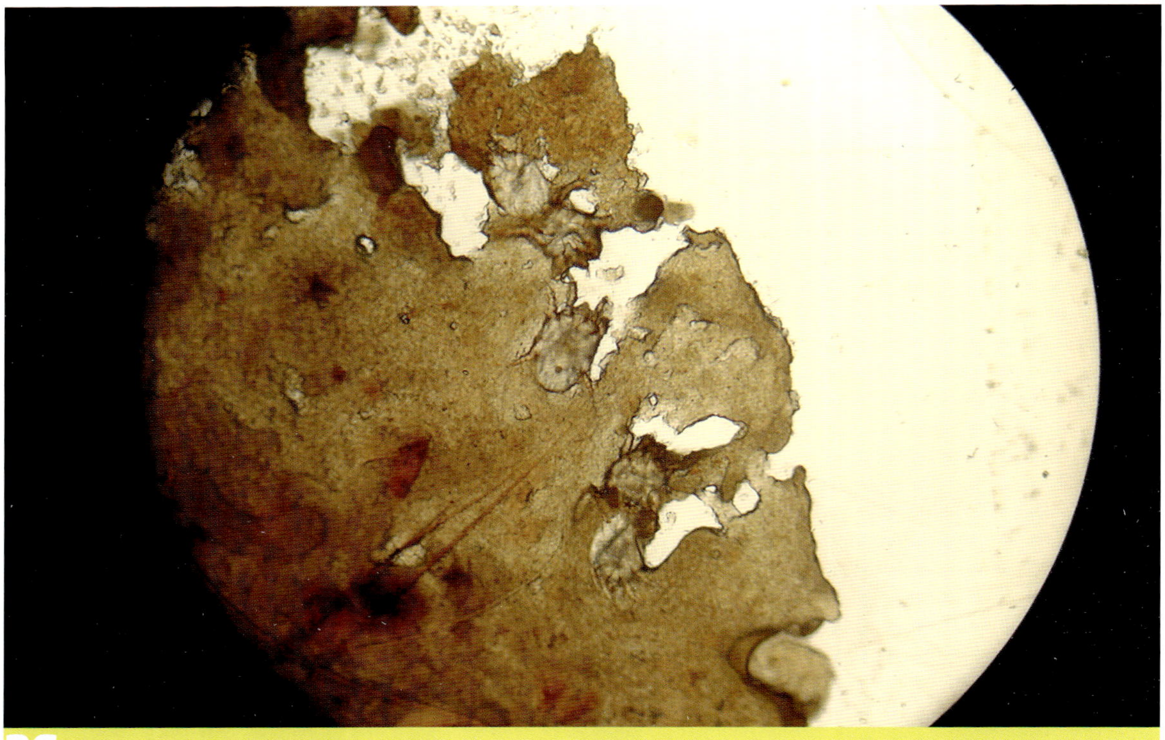

36 *Otodectes cynotis* mite.

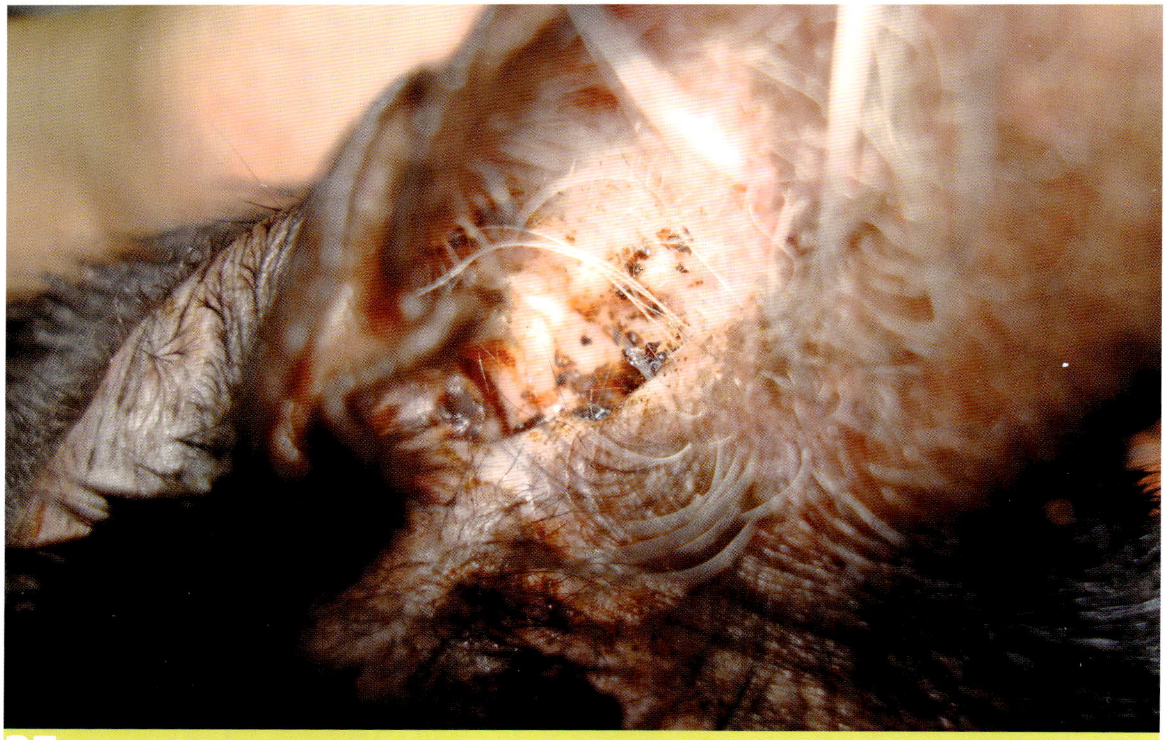

37 Otitis caused by *Otodectes cynotis* on a cat. Note the cerumen.

# Trombiculiasis

## *Neotrombicula autumnalis*

### Lesion aetiology/pathogenesis and clinical picture

This cutaneous parasitosis is caused by larvae of *Neotrombicula* spp. that ascend to the areas of skin closest to the ground, such as the limbs, head, ears, and abdomen. The mite completes part of its life cycle in the host and then the adult form falls back to the ground. It can affect dogs, cats, and humans. It causes moderate itching and scaling with papules/crusts, pustules, and excoriations. Cases of severe anaphylaxis and febrile syndrome have been described.

### Diagnostic method

Direct inspection or observation with adhesive tape or a comb are sufficient.

### Main differential diagnoses

- Other ectoparasitic diseases
- Allergies
- Anaphylaxis (in cases of hypersensitivity reaction to the parasite)

### Treatment

This parasite is sensitive to classic acaricidal treatments for dogs and cats. Infestations frequently occur during harvest time, and should be prevented.

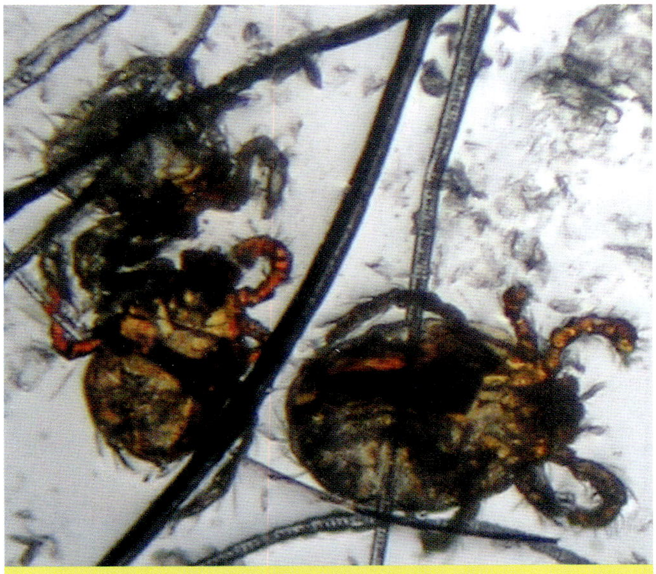

38 *Neotrombicula autumnalis*. Image courtesy of the Anida Veterinary Clinic (Spain).

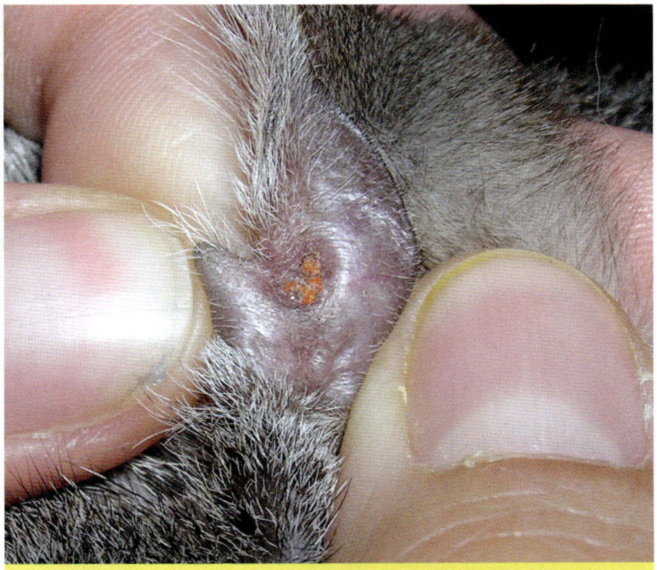

39 Appearance of *Neotrombicula* larvae in the ear. Image courtesy of the Anida Veterinary Clinic (Spain).

# *Straelensia cynotis*

## Lesion aetiology/pathogenesis and clinical picture

This relatively new cutaneous parasitosis is caused by the trombiculid mite *Straelensia cynotis*. It affects dogs living in rural areas, presumably following direct or indirect contact with foxes, which may be the mite's definitive host. It is a follicular dermatosis that produces painful papules and crusting, mainly affecting the head and back. In Europe, a higher incidence has been reported in France, Portugal, and northern Spain.

Cases have already been described in cats.

## Diagnostic method

The clinical picture, history and lesion distribution are quite characteristic. It can be difficult to detect the larvae in deep skin scrapings. A biopsy is usually necessary.

Pain in the affected area is a characteristic sign that can help establish the diagnosis.

## Main differential diagnoses

- Demodicosis
- Bacterial or dermatophyte folliculitis
- Multiple foreign bodies (grass awns or shotgun pellets)

## Treatment

This parasitosis appears to self-resolve within a variable period of several months. Therefore, it remains unclear what the most effective available treatment is. In areas in which the disease is more prevalent, macrocyclic lactones and amitraz appear to be relatively effective. These can be combined in pipette form, applied daily, or administered systemically. Some studies have reported that isoxazolines are also effective, although larger numbers of cases are required to confirm this claim.

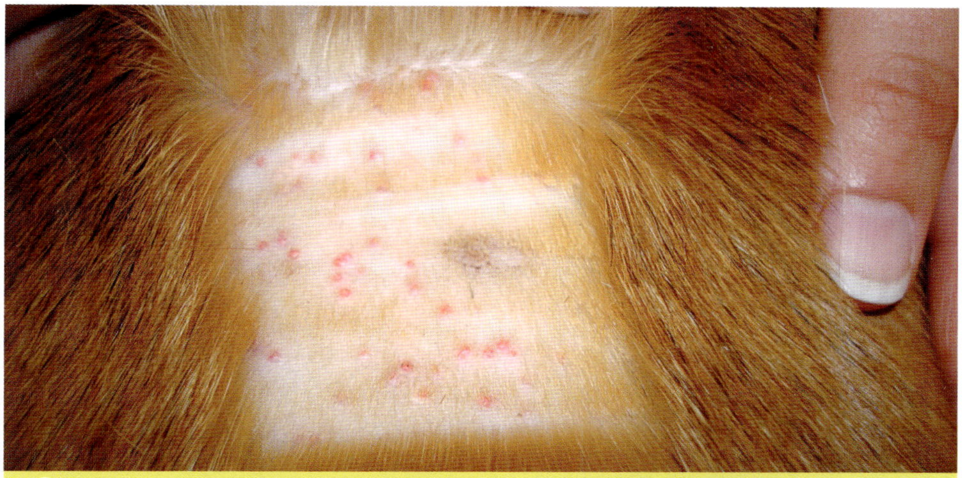

40 Serohaemorrhagic papules and pustules typical of acute straelensiosis.

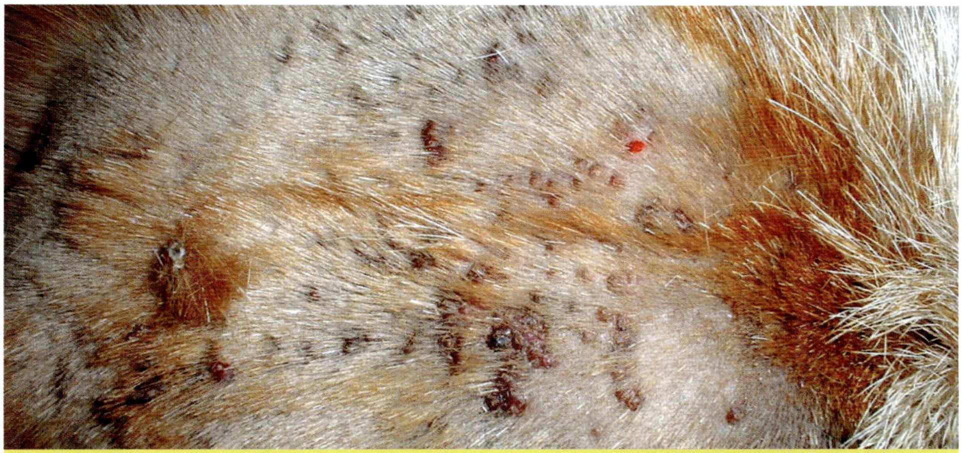

41 Clinical appearance of straelensiosis 1 month after onset. Note the more crusted presentation compared with the previous image.

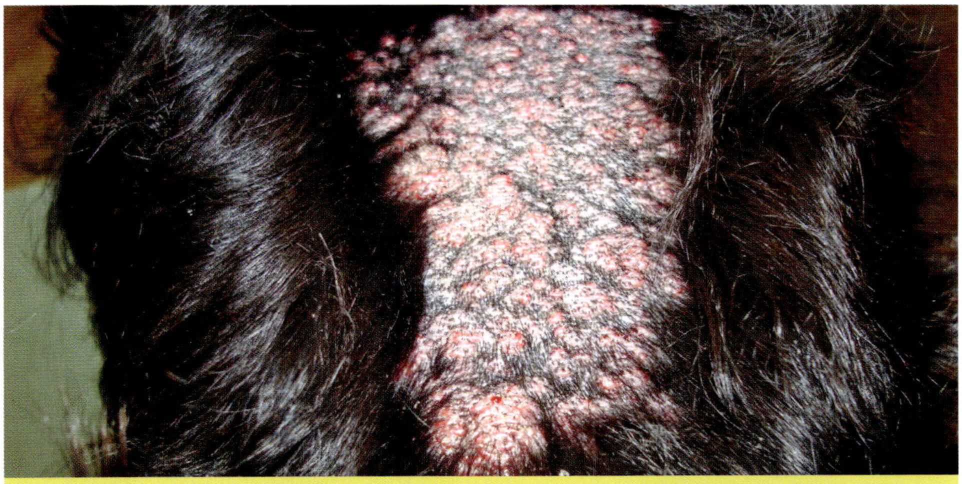

42 Straelensiosis in plaques on the back of a dog.

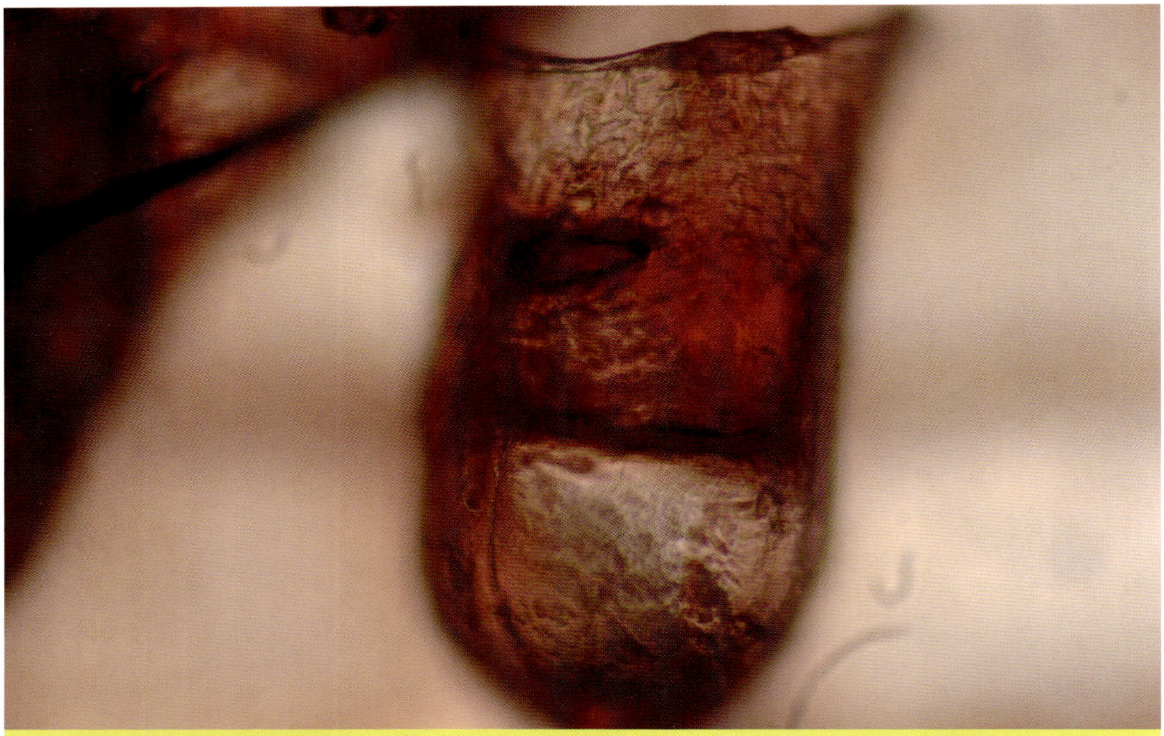

43 Cuticle of *Straelensia cynotis* larva obtained by deep scraping.

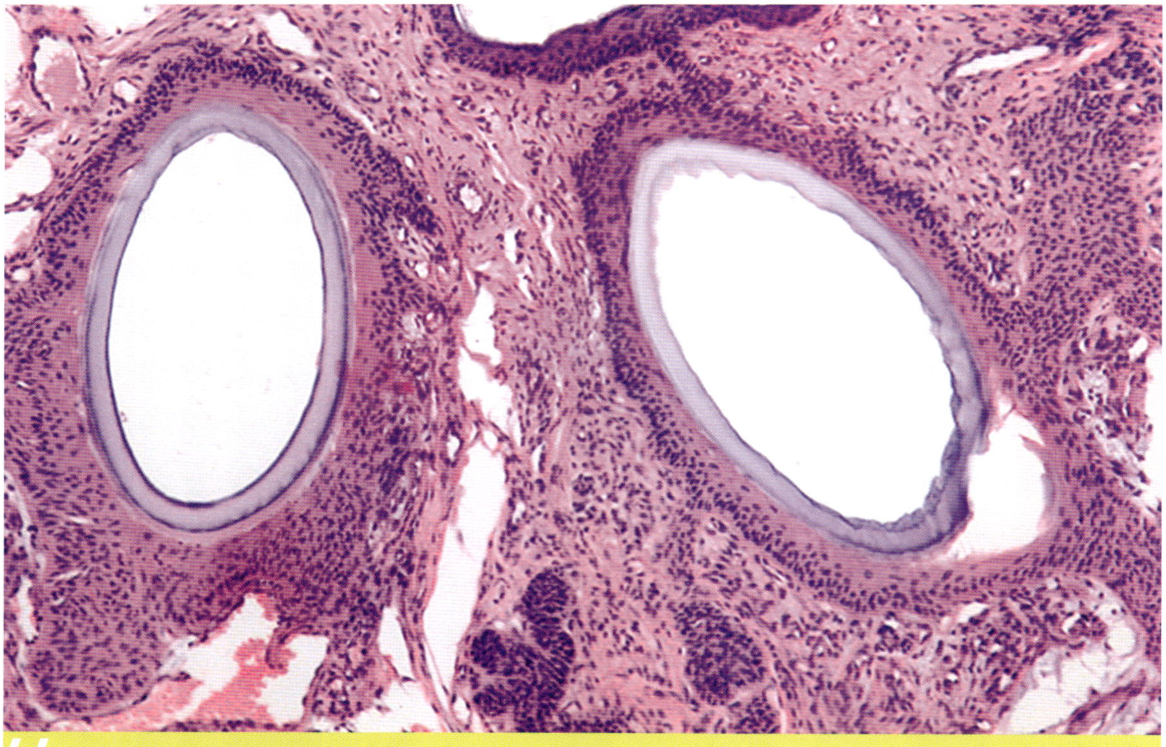

44 Histopathology of straelensiosis. Note the cuticles attached to the follicle wall.

# 05 Viral, protozoal, and algal dermatoses

# Introduction

The following viral, protozoal, and algal dermatoses are described in this chapter:

- Dermatosis due to the canine distemper virus
- Feline herpesvirus dermatosis
- Papillomavirus
- Poxvirus
- Protothecosis
- Leishmaniasis

Viral skin conditions are generally characterised by the formation of vesicles that evolve into crusts. In other circumstances, the systemic disease caused by the virus can affect the general condition of the skin and hair coat.

Protothecosis is a cutaneous and/or systemic ulcerative condition caused by *Prototheca* spp.

Leishmaniasis, which is generally a wasting disease, affects the skin and hair in a diffuse and generalised manner, although it can produce typical reactions such as chancres and granulomas.

# Canine distemper virus dermatosis

## Lesion aetiology/pathogenesis and clinical picture

This disease is caused by a paramyxovirus, which can give rise to skin lesions in some affected dogs. Clinical signs of impetigo are often observed as a result of generalised weakness and concurrent immune suppression, in some cases accompanied by hyperkeratosis of the muzzle and paw pads. The facial region, mainly the periorbital, buccal, and nasal areas, is affected.

## Diagnostic method

The clinical history usually reveals an unvaccinated animal, contact with other sick individuals, and concurrent gastrointestinal, respiratory, or neurological disorders. Generalised depression and marked hyperkeratosis of the muzzle and paw pads are quite indicative of the disease. The characteristic signs can include scaling blepharitis and epiphora.

## Main differential diagnoses

- Dermatosis due to nutritional deficiencies
- Zinc-responsive dermatosis
- Hepatocutaneous syndrome
- Senile hyperkeratosis

## Treatment

The prognosis of the disease is quite uncertain and difficult to determine. Treatment is aimed at avoiding the concomitant effects of bacterial infections and improving the general condition of the patient by adding vitamin complexes and enriching the diet.

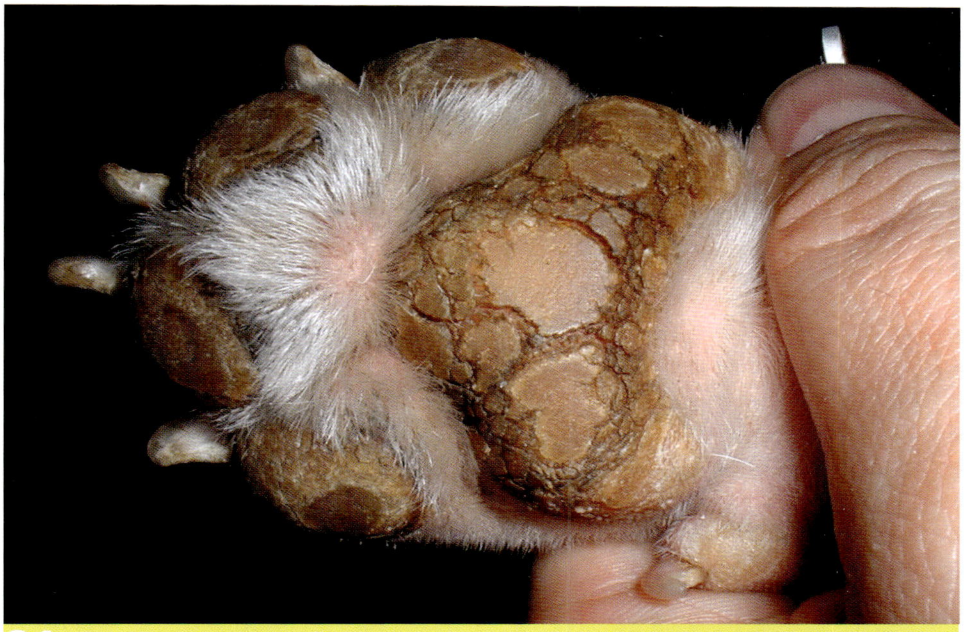

01 Hyperkeratosis with cracked paw pads in a dog with distemper.

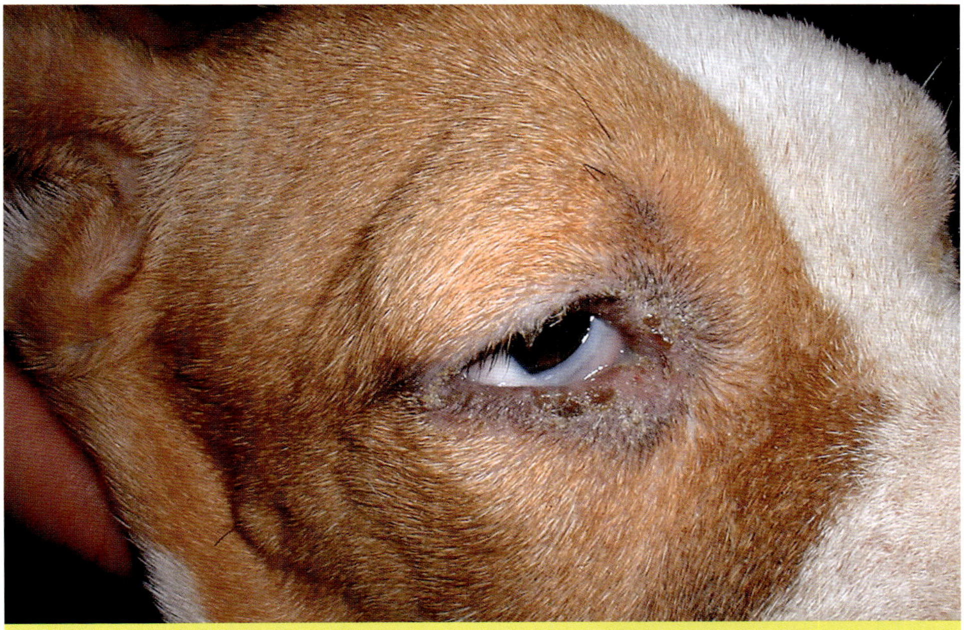

02 Diffuse alopecia and periocular scaling in a puppy with distemper.

# Feline herpesvirus dermatosis

## Lesion aetiology/pathogenesis and clinical picture

Crusted and ulcerative lesions are usually observed, mainly on the bridge of the nose. This can be accompanied by lesions on the pinnae and around the eyes and erosions on the tongue.

## Diagnostic method

The clinical picture is quite evident, although some differential diagnoses must be taken into account. Biopsy is usually necessary to verify the presence of inclusion bodies, although these are not always easy to detect, as their presence depends on the course of the disease. Immunohistochemistry or PCR tests may be necessary.

## Main differential diagnoses

- Hypersensitivity to insect bites
- Dermatophytosis
- Pemphigus complex
- Squamous cell carcinoma
- Calicivirus infection

## Treatment

Lysine can prevent viral replication. Other options that can be helpful in certain cases include subcutaneous omega interferon, systemic famciclovir, and idoxuridine.

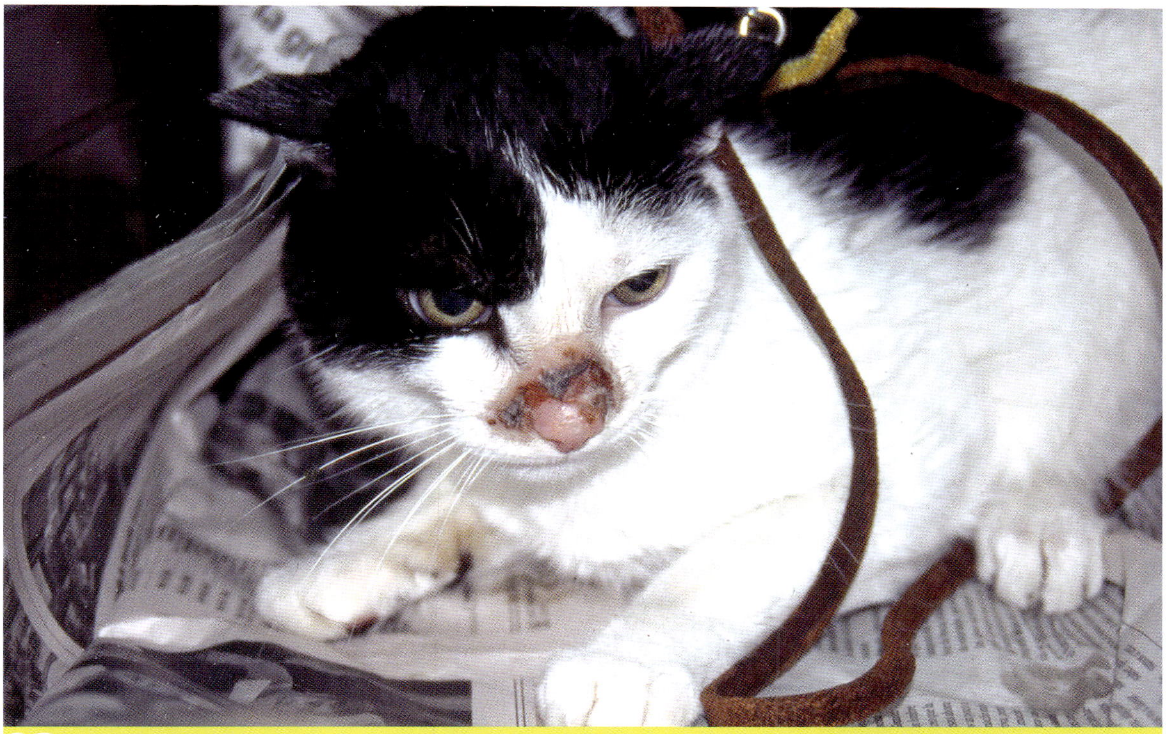

03 Involvement of the nasal bridge in a cat with feline herpesvirus.

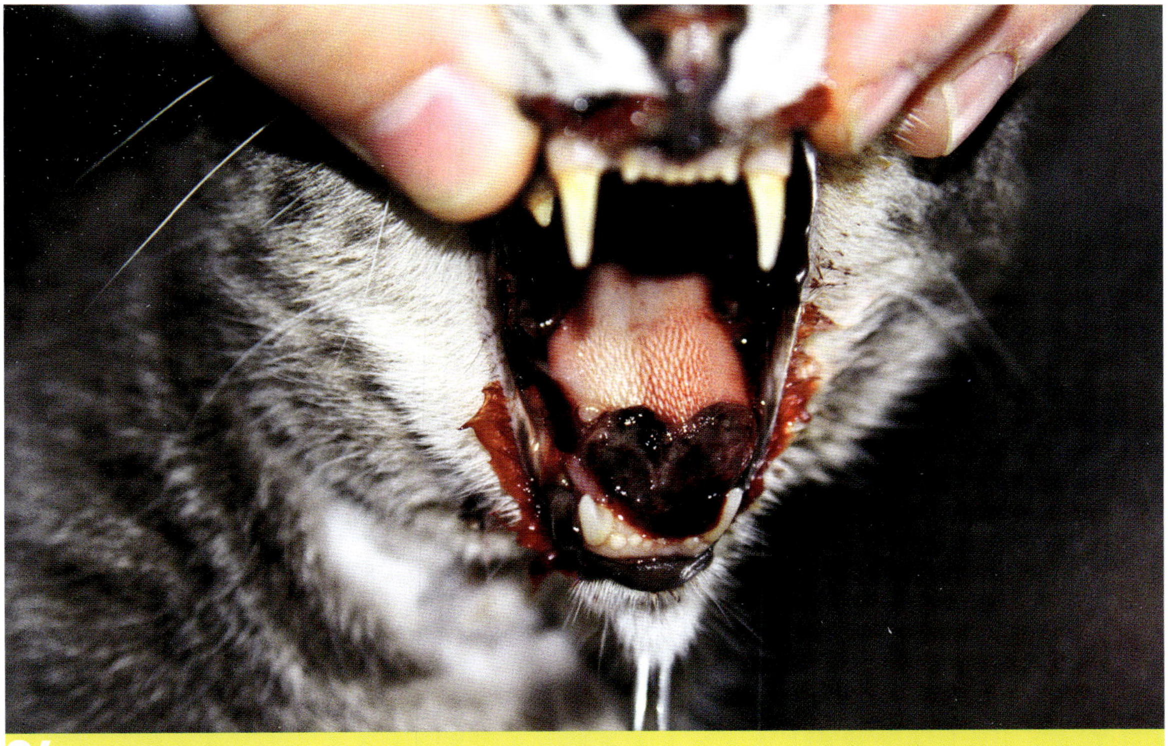

04 Necrosis and severe erosion on the tongue of a cat with herpesvirus.

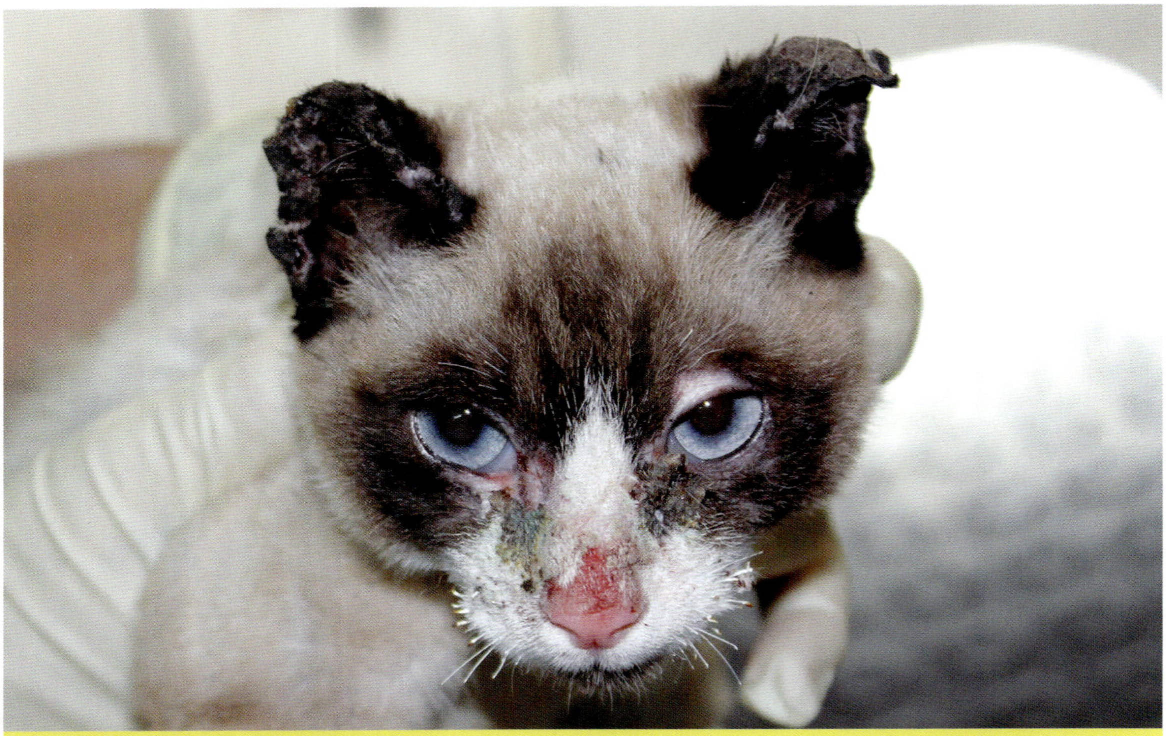

05 Ischaemic ulcerative crusting reaction in a herpesvirus-positive cat.

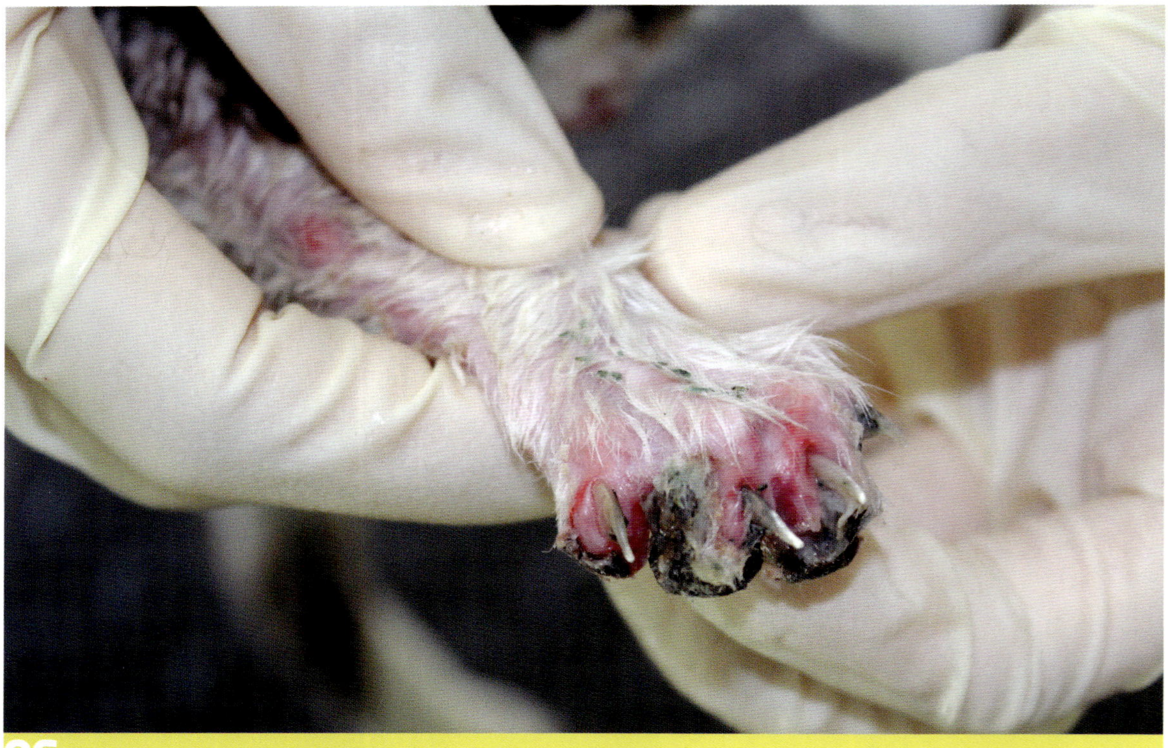

06 Ischaemic dermatosis due to herpesvirus (dorsal view of limb).

# Papillomavirus

## Lesion aetiology/pathogenesis and clinical picture

Viral papillomas usually affect young dogs or those with some form of immune compromise, and result in isolated or multiple small, highly exophytic projections, especially in the oral mucosa and the perioral region.

In cats, papillomavirus is more associated with squamous cell carcinoma in situ.

## Diagnostic method

The clinical picture is highly characteristic and histological examination is necessary to confirm diagnosis.

## Main differential diagnoses

- Nonviral papillomas
- Other tumours
- Ticks
- Cutaneous outgrowths and other pseudotumours

## Treatment

Viral papillomas usually resolve spontaneously within 3 months. Surgical resection using cryosurgery, electrosurgery, or laser surgery may be necessary in certain cases in which these lesions cause discomfort.

Successful outcomes have been described following treatment with topical imiquimod or interferon alfa. Azithromycin, administered systemically, is another useful molecule.

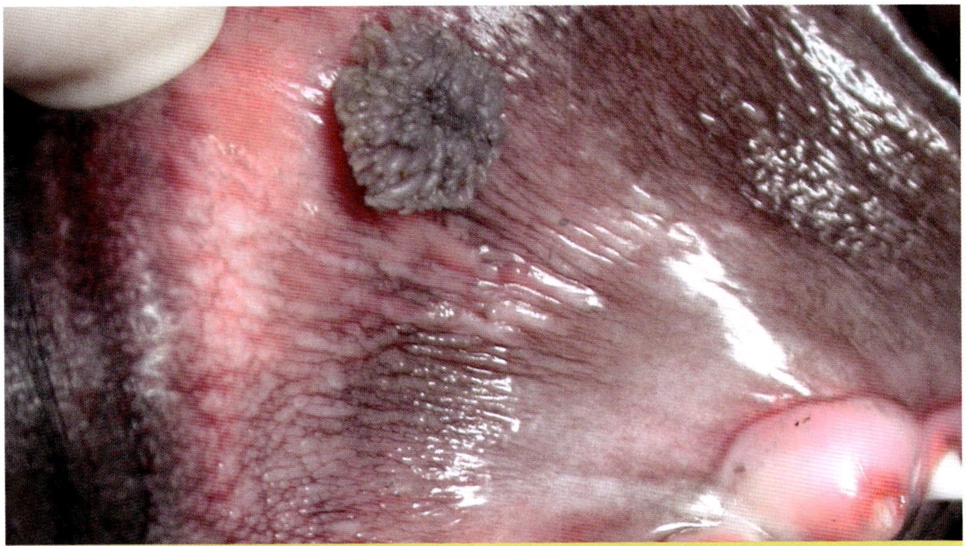

07 Involvement of the papillae of the oral mucosa in a puppy. Image courtesy of the Somaza Pérez Veterinary Clinic (Spain).

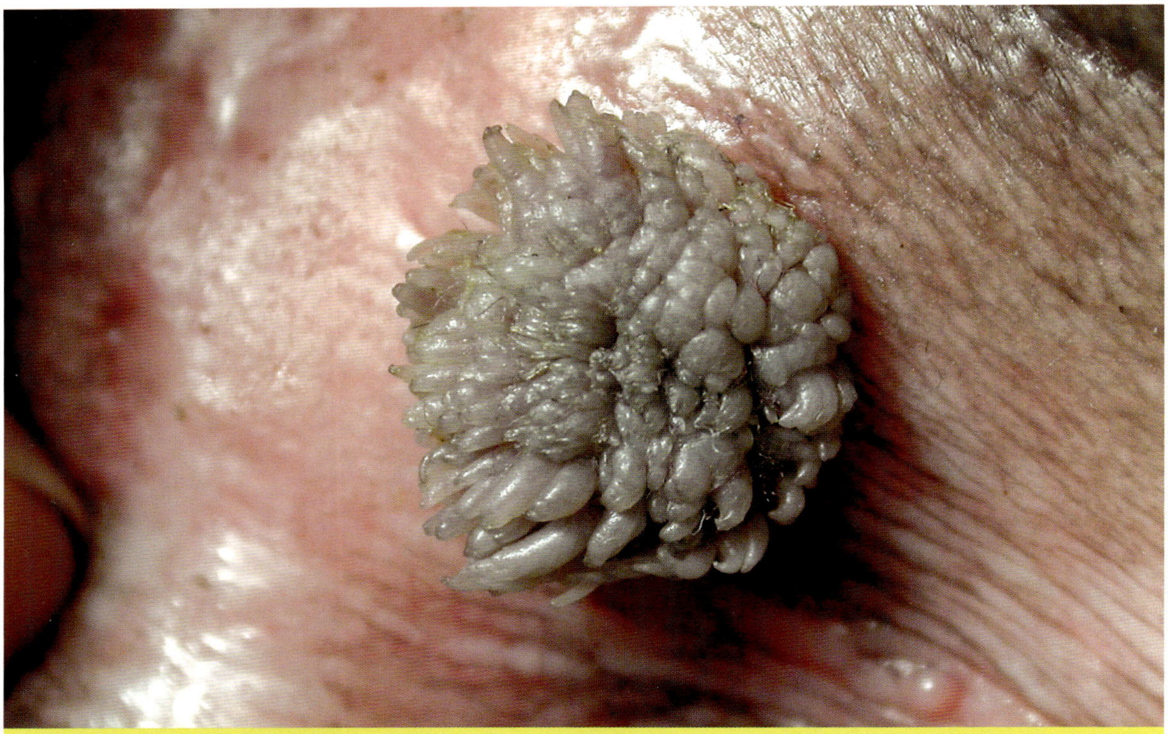

08 Close-up of the papilloma. Image courtesy of the Somaza Pérez Veterinary Clinic (Spain).

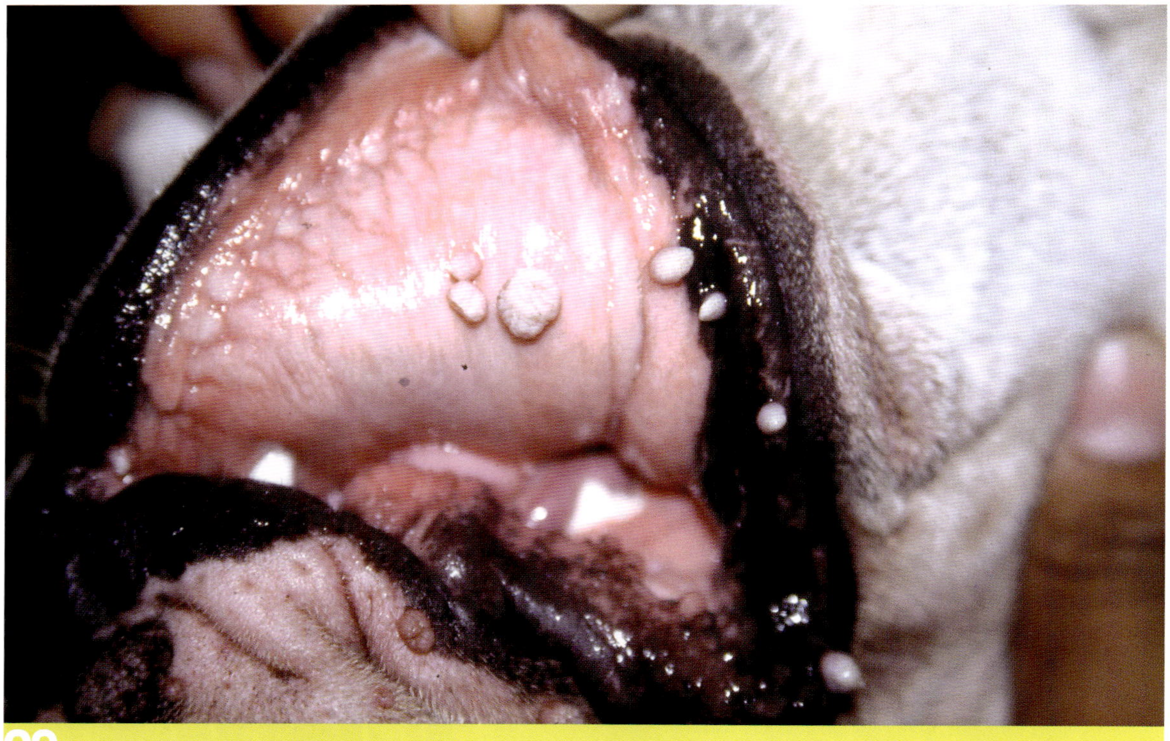

09 English Bulldog puppy with multiple papillomatosis of the oral mucosa. Oral and perioral affection.

# Poxvirus

## Lesion aetiology/pathogenesis and clinical picture

This dermatosis is caused by an *Orthopoxvirus* (cowpox) and mainly affects cats, which acquire the virus via rodent bites. The disease, which also has zoonotic potential, is more common in summer and autumn.

After being bitten, affected animals develop an initial lesion consisting of a nodule that can subsequently ulcerate and form a crater. The lesion progresses to a crust that tends to spread either due to opportunistic infections or scratching.

## Diagnostic method

The clinical picture can be ambiguous and additional tests are required to confirm the diagnosis. The presence of nodules on the owner's hands, although rare, can be indicative of potential disease.

Diagnosis can be confirmed by serology, PCR, or biopsy.

## Main differential diagnoses

- Bacterial or fungal infections
- Tumours
- Eosinophilic granuloma

## Treatment

Treatment consists of supportive care, as there is no specific treatment. Thorough disinfection of the environment is important.

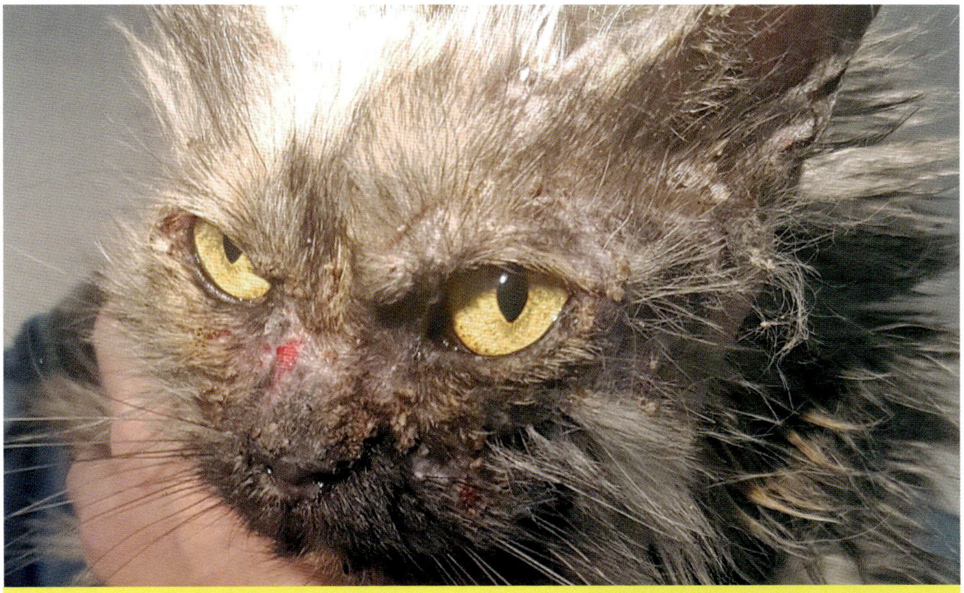

10 Facial involvement in a cat with poxvirus.

# Protothecosis

## Lesion aetiology/pathogenesis and clinical picture

Protothecosis is a rare infectious disease that can affect humans and other mammals and is caused by microscopic algae of the genus *Prototheca*. In dogs, the cutaneous form is characterised by the formation of ulcerative lesions on the paw pads, nose, mouth, and eyes.

There are only three pathogenic species described: *Prototheca wickerhamii*, *Prototheca stagnora*, and *Prototheca zopfii*.

In dogs and cats, prior immunosuppression is often required for infection to be established. The disease can be purely cutaneous and subcutaneous, or systemic, affecting internal organs and in some cases causing blindness.

In the few cases described *Prototheca wickerhamii* is considered the main cause of the cutaneous form.

## Diagnostic method

Cytology and in particular histopathology are key to establishing the diagnosis.

## Main differential diagnoses

- Bullous pustular autoimmune diseases
- Tumours
- Pyoderma

## Treatment

This disease is quite insidious and very difficult to treat. Itraconazole, fluconazole, and amphotericin B are often used, with varying degrees of success.

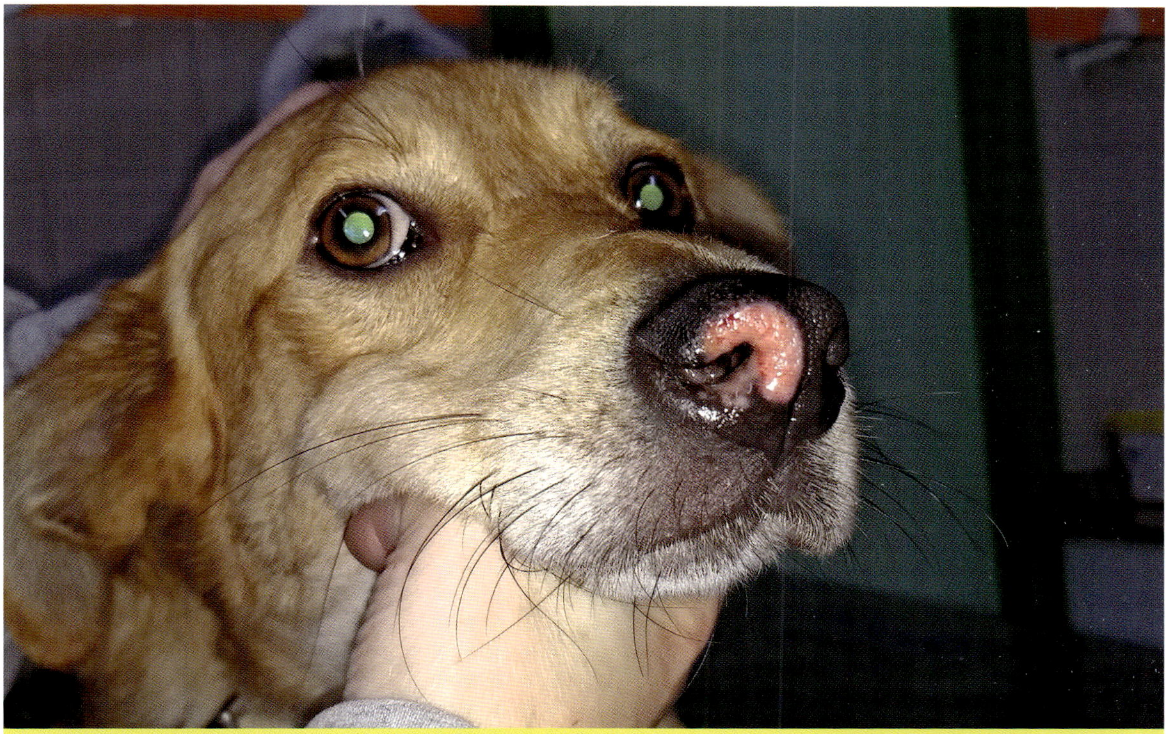

11 Protothecosis with ulceration on the muzzle of an affected dog.

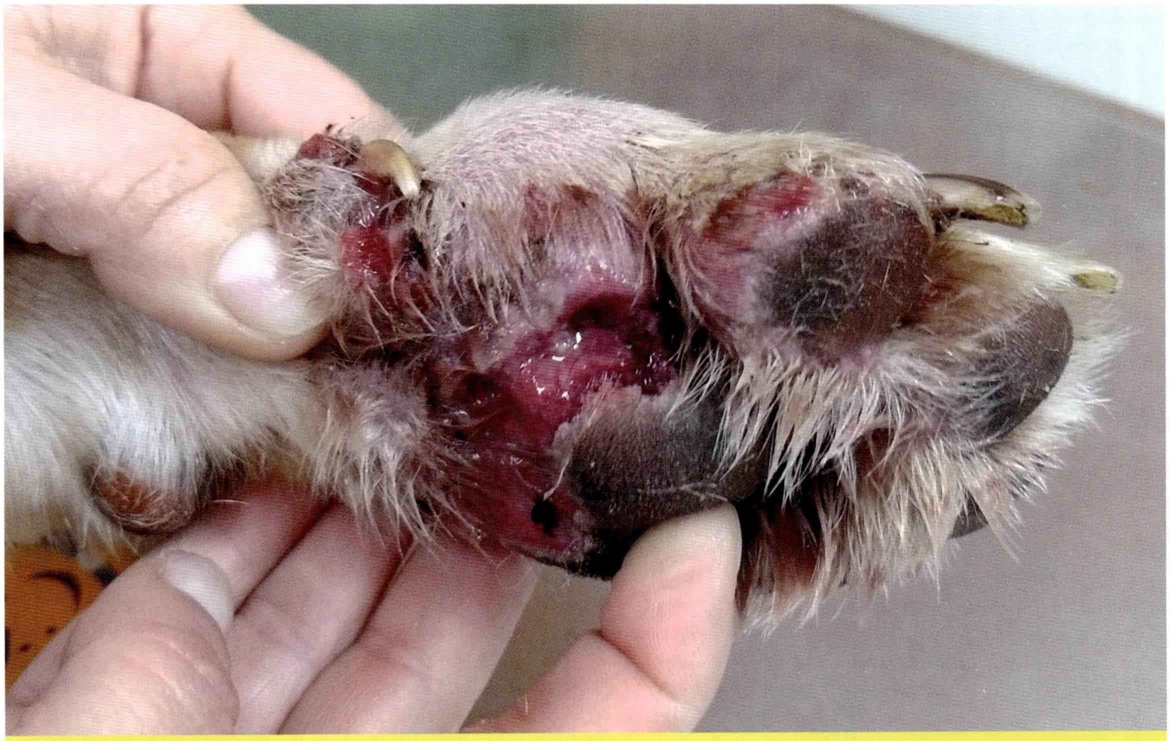

12 Ulceration in the distal part of the limb of a dog with protothecosis.

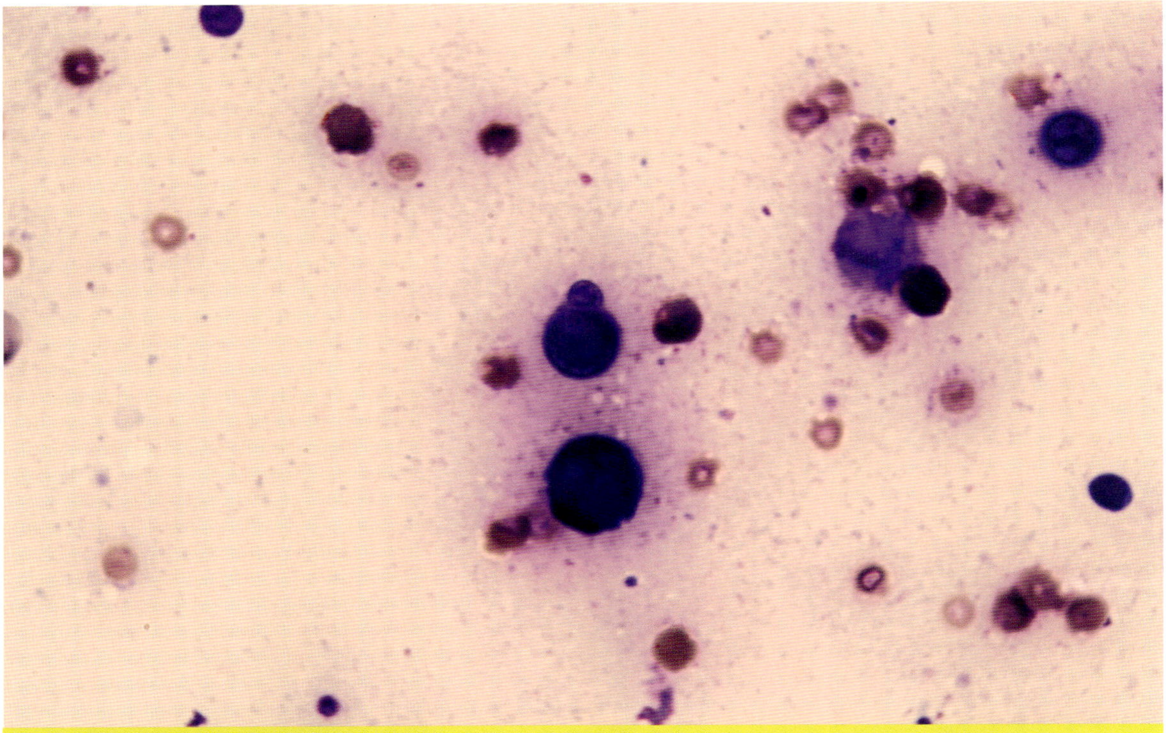

13 Ulcer cytology revealing a budding prototheque.

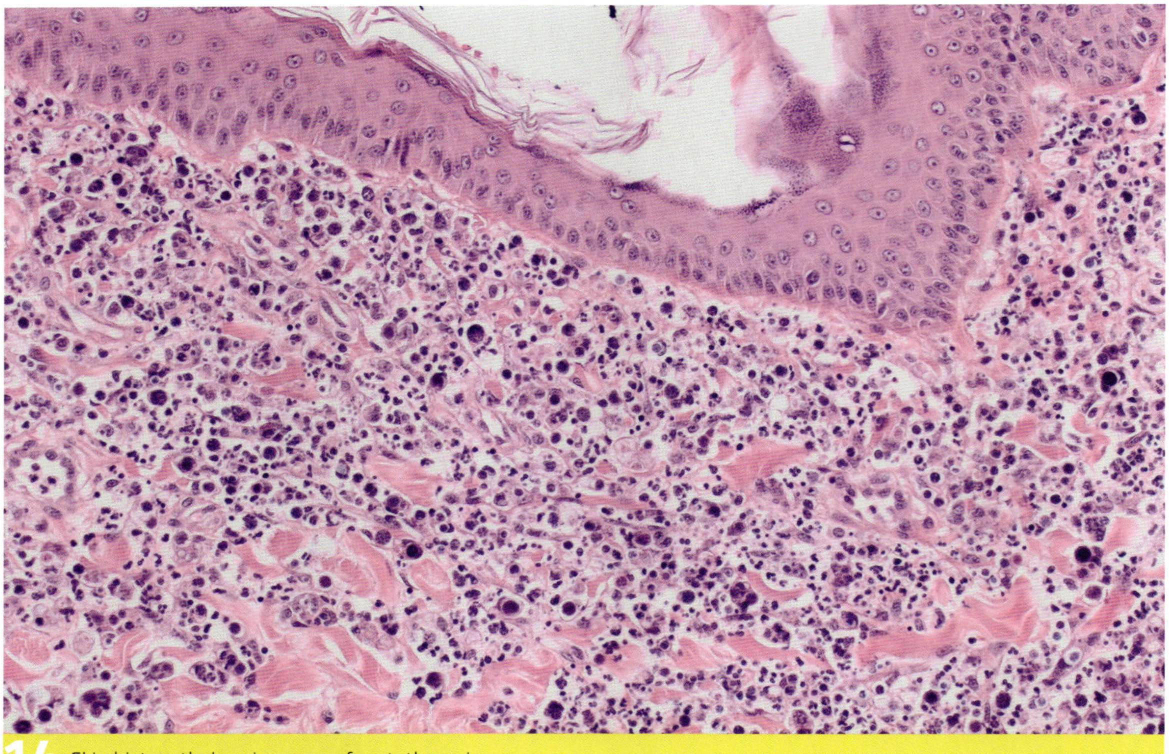

14 Skin histopathology in a case of protothecosis.

# Leishmaniasis

## Lesion aetiology/pathogenesis and clinical picture

Canine leishmaniasis is a disease caused by protozoa of the genus *Leishmania*, and is transmitted through the bite of the sandfly. The disease gives rise to variable clinical signs and mainly affects individuals with poor cellular immunity. It primarily causes tissue granulomas, vasculitis, uveitis, arthritis, and glomerulonephritis. It mainly affects dogs and is rare in cats.

The classic dermatosis manifests with scaling and diffuse alopecia that begins on the head and spreads throughout the body. Vasculitis can give rise to skin ulcers, especially on bony prominences or on the margins of the pinnae. Depigmentation of the muzzle and nasal ulcers may also be observed, accompanied by epistaxis in many cases. In resistant animals or those with good cellular immunity, papular or nodular lesions can form in various parts of the body.

## Diagnostic method

The clinical picture is highly characteristic. However, diagnosis is confirmed by fine needle aspiration cytology of the lymph nodes, bone marrow, or spleen or by imprint cytology of exudative skin lesions beneath the scales or of nodular lesions. Serology (indirect immunofluorescence) and a proteinogram are also very important. In some cases, a biopsy together with immunohistochemistry or PCR testing may be necessary. The geographical areas in which this disease is detected have expanded, possibly due to climate change.

## Main differential diagnoses

The clinical picture of leishmaniasis is highly variable, and therefore it must be distinguished from countless other skin diseases.

## Treatment

Current treatment options focus on reinforcing cellular immunity (Th1). Examples include domperidone, although this is primarily used as a preventive treatment. The classical treatment regimen consists of meglumine antimoniate with allopurinol or miltefosine. Currently available preventive agents include insecticides, immunomodulators, and vaccines. Other molecules being studied for the control of sandflies include isoxazolines.

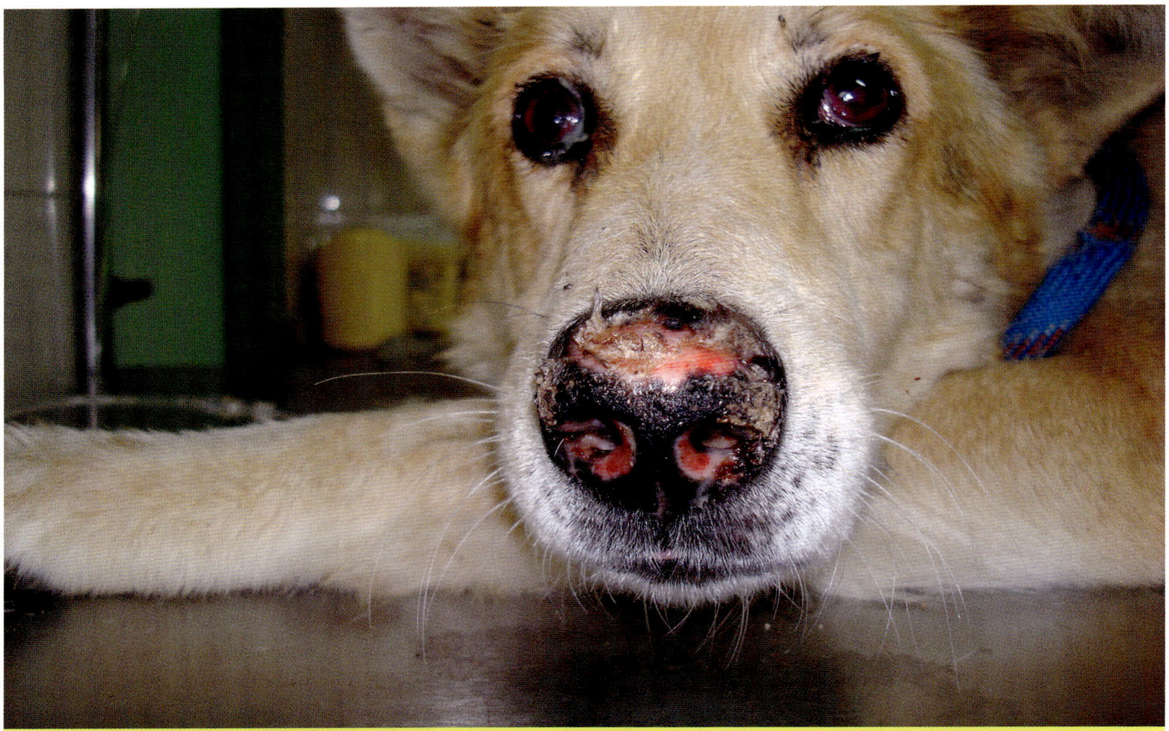

15 Dog with leishmaniasis. Uveitis due to vasculitis and ulceration of the nasal area are evident.

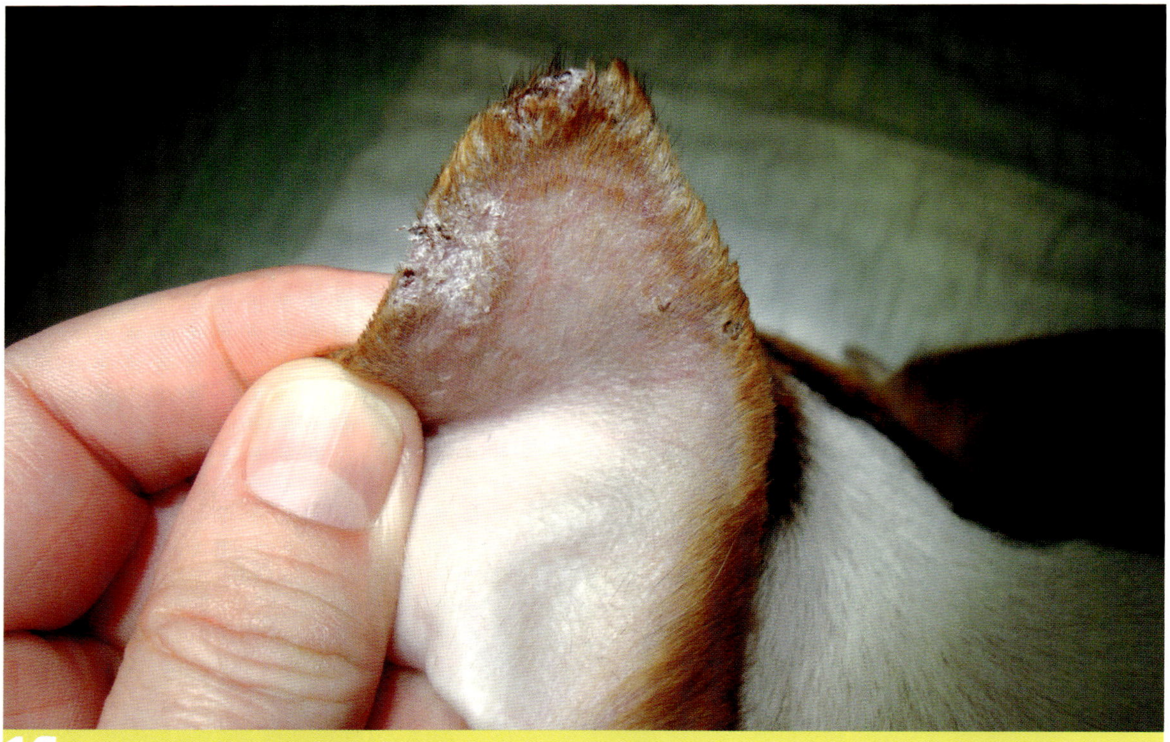

16 Dog with leishmaniasis. Necrosis of the pinnal margin caused by vasculitis.

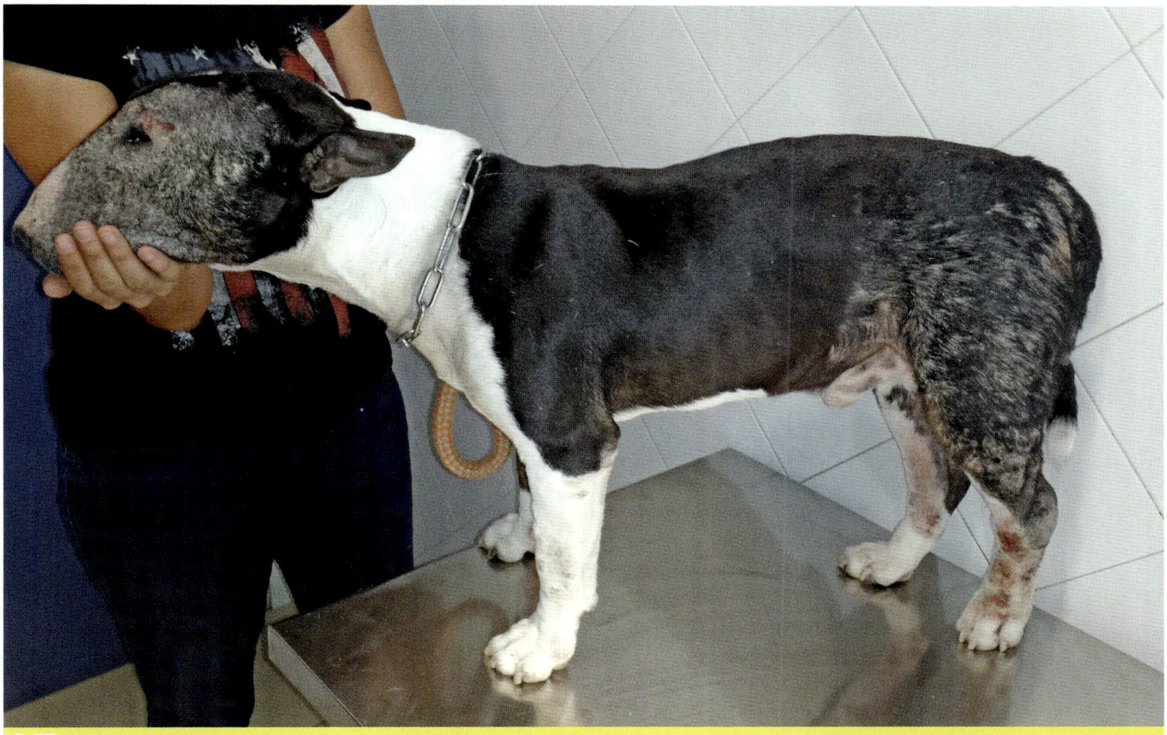

17 General appearance of a Bull Terrier with leishmaniasis.

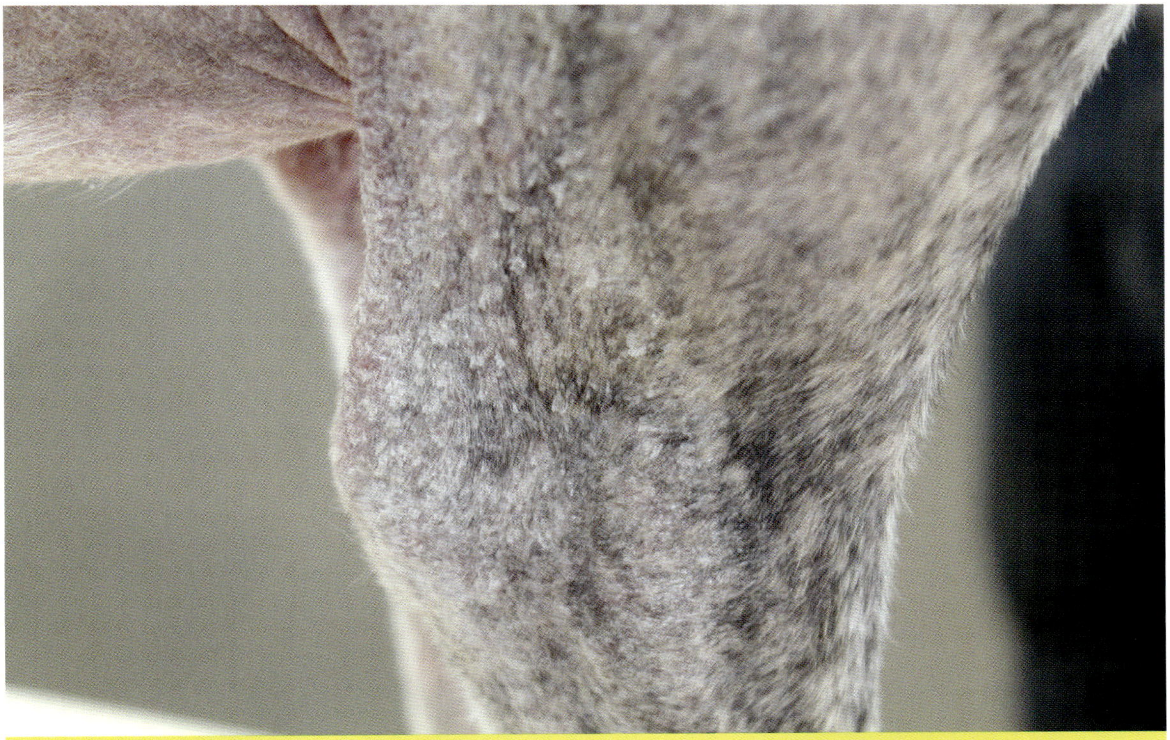

18 Close-up image of dermatosis due to *Leishmania*. Scaling and erythematous alopecia are evident.

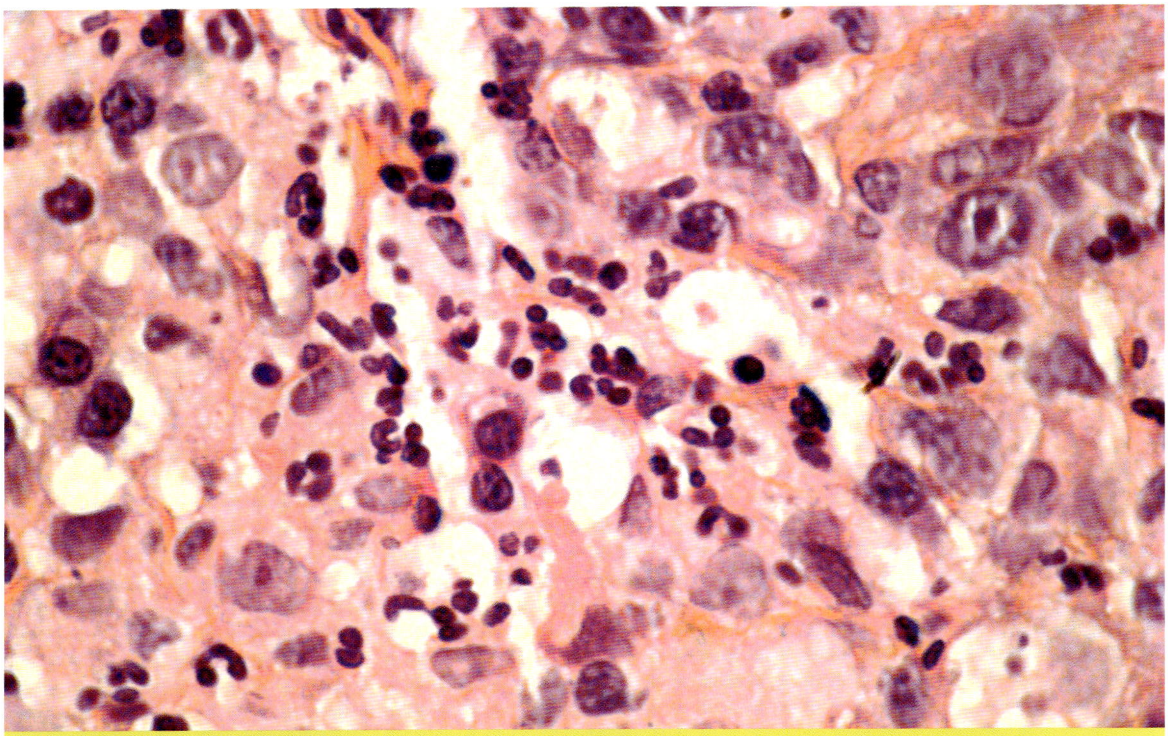

19 Histological sample in which abundant amastigotes are evident in the dermis.

# 06 Allergic dermatoses

# Introduction

The following allergic dermatoses are covered in this chapter:

- Urticaria and angioedema
- Atopy and adverse food reaction
- Contact hypersensitivity
- Flea allergy dermatitis
- Allergy to insect bites:
  - Insect allergy in cats
  - Canine facial eosinophilic furunculosis
- Manifestations of allergy in cats:
  - Miliary dermatitis
  - Self-induced alopecia
  - Erosion and ulceration of the face and cervical area
  - Eosinophilic granuloma complex:
    - Granuloma
    - Plaque
    - Indolent ulcer
  - Urticaria pigmentosa
- Drug reaction

Allergic dermatoses are generally characterised by inflammation and pruritus of variable severity.

It should be noted that this type of disease produces very different reaction patterns in dogs and cats. Scratching is much less evident in cats, in which four main clinical patterns are observed:

- Miliary dermatitis
- Symmetric alopecia
- Eosinophilic complexes
- Erosion and ulceration of the face and neck

A very particular mast cell–mediated reaction can be observed in Sphynx, Himalayan, and Devon Rex cat breeds, characterised by the formation of erythematous to brownish macules, papules, and crusts distributed throughout the body.

# Urticaria and angioedema

## Lesion aetiology/pathogenesis and clinical picture

Type I hypersensitivity reactions in animals previously sensitised to an allergen. These are usually acute or hyperacute reactions. They can be triggered by insect bites, foods, or drugs.

A predisposition has been described in Boxers.

The typical urticaria lesions are wheals, which can occur in widespread outbreaks and cause profuse pruritus. If the oedema affects the muzzle and eyelids it is known as angioedema.

Many cases resolve within a few hours.

In cats this reaction is much less common and can be related to poisoning. Urticaria in Sphynx cats manifests as a breed-specific reaction pattern with wheals or plaques that can form pigmented crusts. This is usually related to hypersensitivity states.

## Diagnostic method

The clinical picture and sudden onset are highly characteristic.

## Main differential diagnoses

- Juvenile cellulitis
- Demodicosis
- Bacterial folliculitis
- Muzzle pyoderma
- Blepharitis

## Treatment

A good response is usually observed following treatment with corticosteroids and, in some cases, antihistamines. It is very important to avoid allergens, identification of which can be difficult.

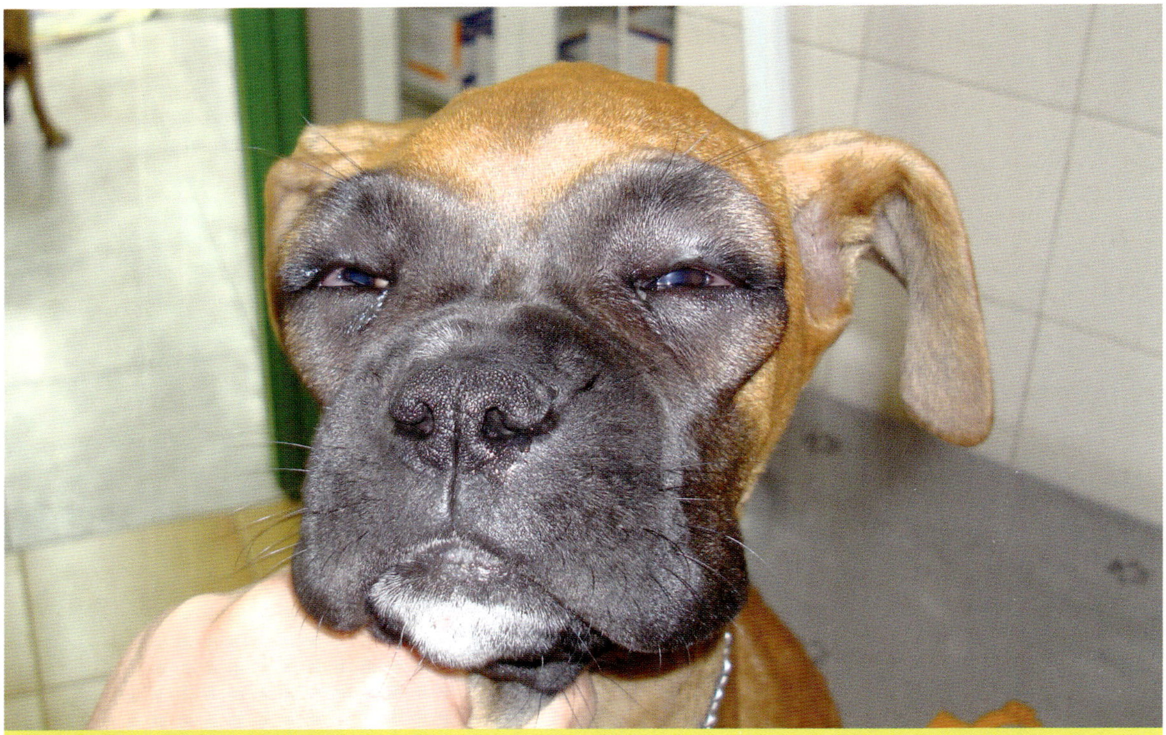

01 Angioedema in a Boxer puppy, mainly affecting the eyelids.

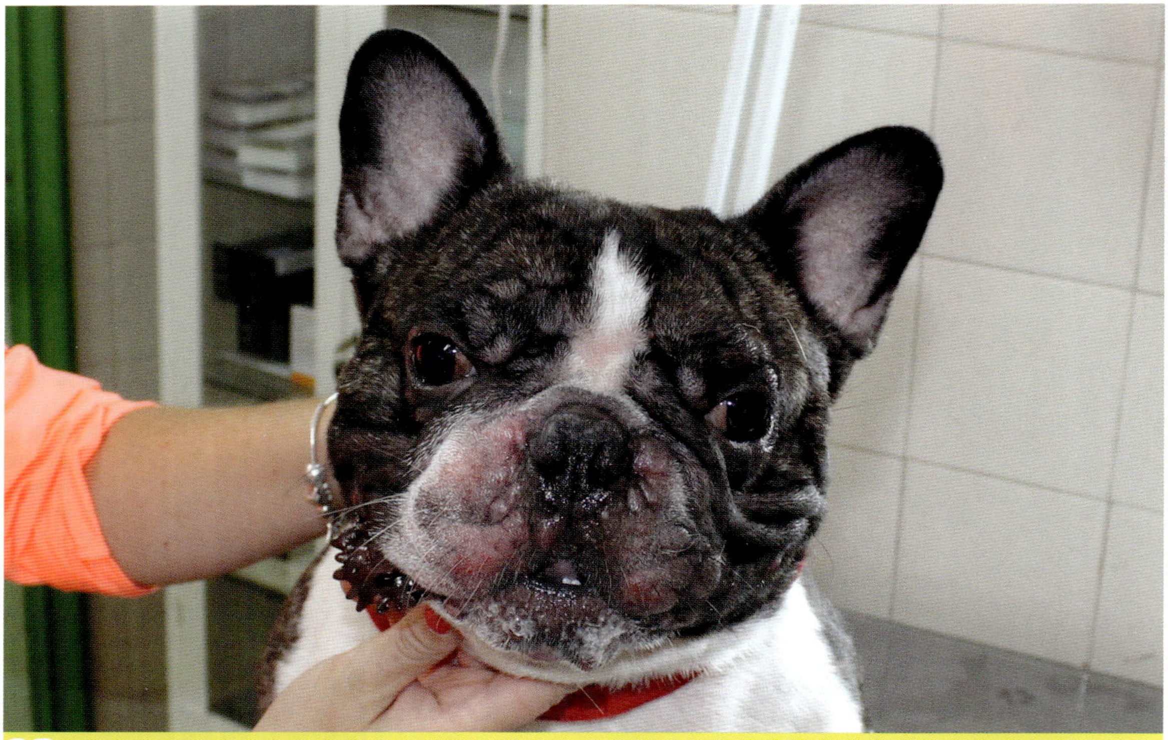

02 Facial involvement with multiple wheals in a dog stunk by a *Hymenoptera* insect.

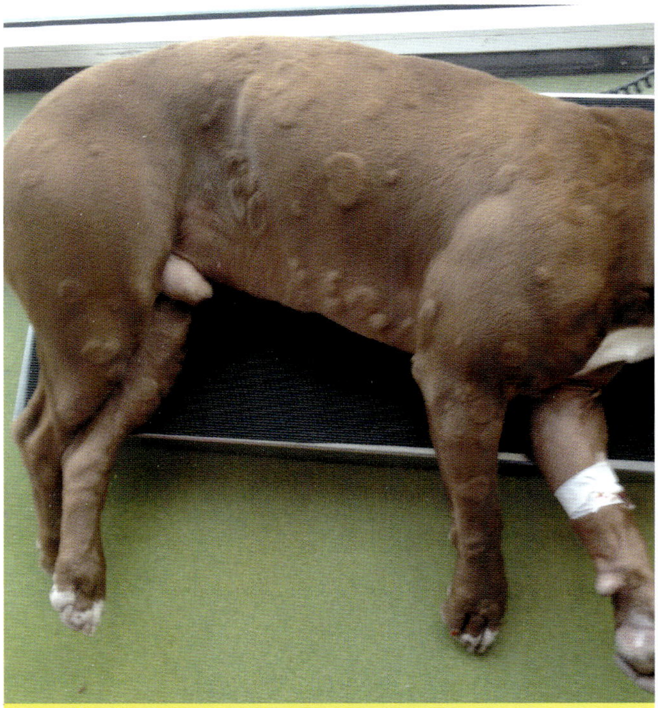

03 Urticaria with the formation of classic wheals all over the body.

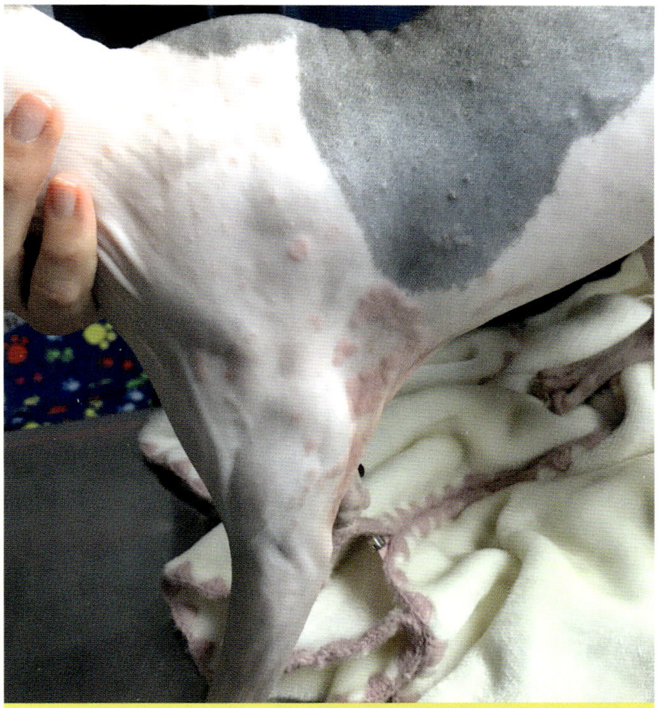

04 Wheals in a Sphynx cat. Classic pattern observed in this breed, characterised by wheals and not-yet-pigmented plaques.

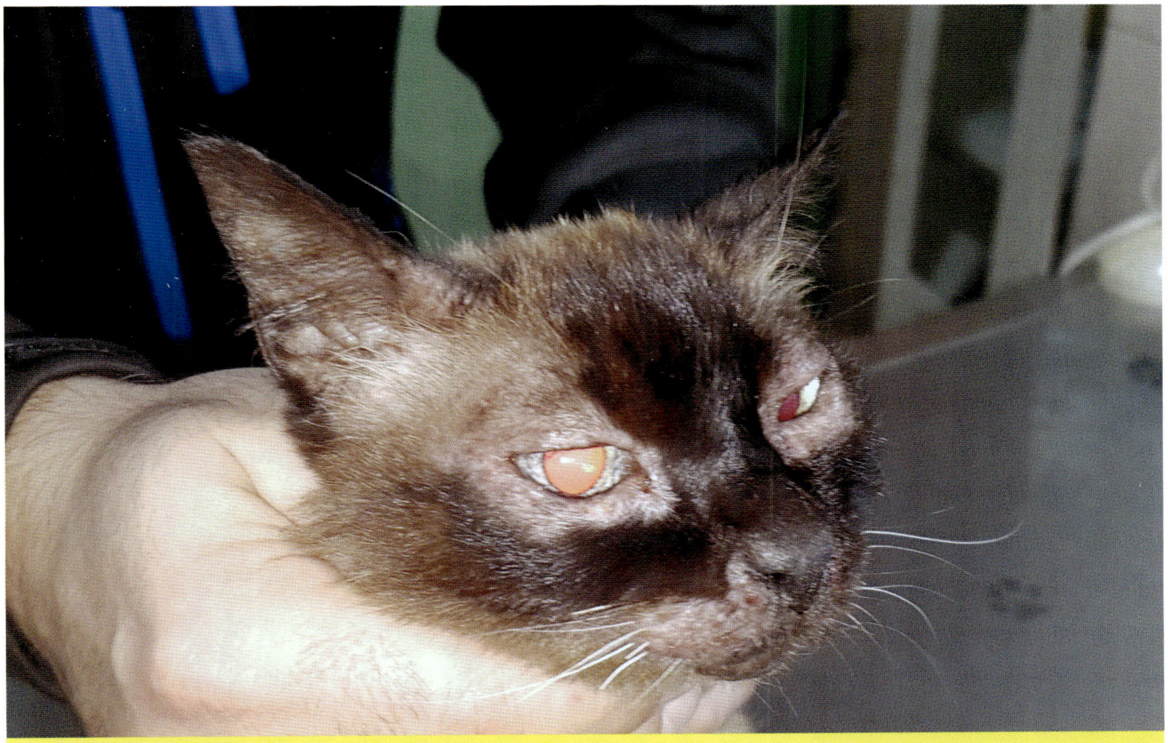

05 Rare facial oedema due to hypersensitivity in a cat.

# Atopy and adverse food reaction

## Lesion aetiology/pathogenesis and clinical picture

Both forms of type I hypersensitivity reaction are included in the same description: from a dermatological point of view both cause clinical atopic dermatitis.

The clinical picture consists of essential pruritus, without lesions, which can later progress to secondary lesions and become chronic due to excoriations and the presence of opportunistic bacteria and yeasts. Different body regions can be affected in different breeds, although the paws, axillae, groin, head, and periocular and perioral areas are commonly affected. Recurrent otitis is also common.

The associated dermatosis usually begins with erythema, progressing to papules/pustules and crusts, and ultimately to lichenification, hyperpigmentation, and seborrhoea.

This disease is much better defined in dogs than in cats. In cats, the corresponding condition is more accurately described as feline atopic syndrome, caused by allergies to food or fleas. This gives rise to the reaction patterns characteristic of cats, which include miliary dermatitis, erosion ulceration of the face and neck, eosinophilic reactions, and self-induced alopecia. It is important to remember that feline atopic syndrome can also manifest as feline asthma.

## Diagnostic method

This group of diseases is mainly diagnosed clinically. Certain criteria must be fulfilled to establish diagnosis. The origin of atopic dermatitis (environmental or food allergens) can be determined by beginning an elimination diet. Subsequently, environmental allergens can be identified by serological or intradermal reaction tests. Certain clinically atopic cases test negative in serological or intradermal reaction tests. This disease is defined as atopy-like dermatitis. Serology to identify food allergens can have a high negative predictive value, which is useful when designing an elimination diet.

## Main differential diagnoses

- Sarcoptic mange
- Flea allergy dermatitis
- Primary seborrhoea
- Dermatophytosis (mainly in cats)
- Contact allergy

## Treatment

Environmental allergen immunotherapy to desensitise the animal is the only truly curative treatment. Clinical signs can be controlled with lokivetmab, oclacitinib, cyclosporine, or corticosteroids. It is important to ensure a good diet with high levels of omega-3 and omega-6 fatty acids, combined with the use of hydrating, emollient, and antiseptic shampoos. The use of topical products containing lipid complexes and sphingosines can markedly improve the quality of the intercellular substance. Any implicated food allergens should be avoided.

Systemic treatment with dietary supplements such as zinc, fatty acids, vitamin E, nucleotides, and hyaluronic acid can be very useful to improve skin structure. Palmitoylethanolamide is a cannabinoid nutraceutical that can act as a mast cell stabiliser.

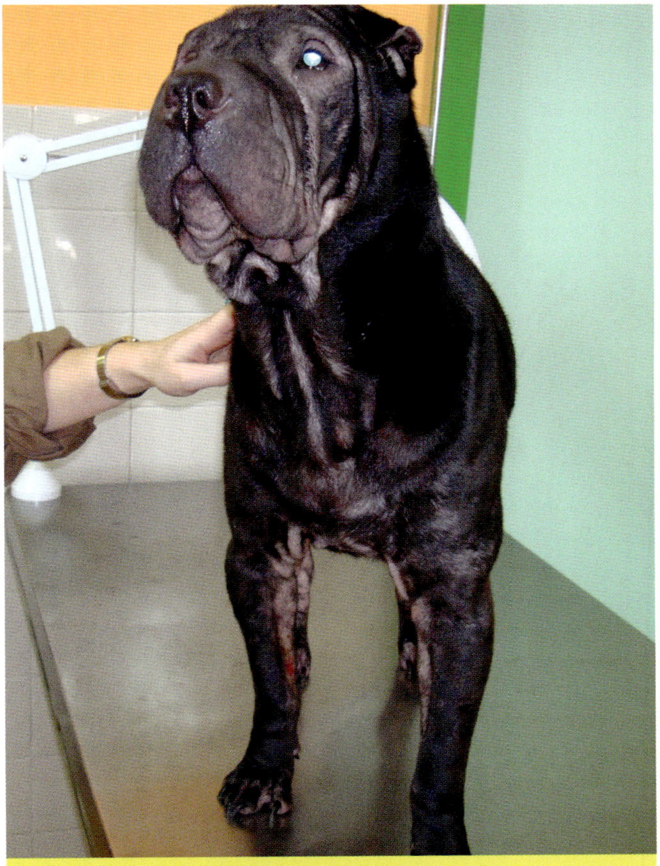

06 Shar Pei with atopic dermatitis. The face, cervical area, and feet are primarily affected.

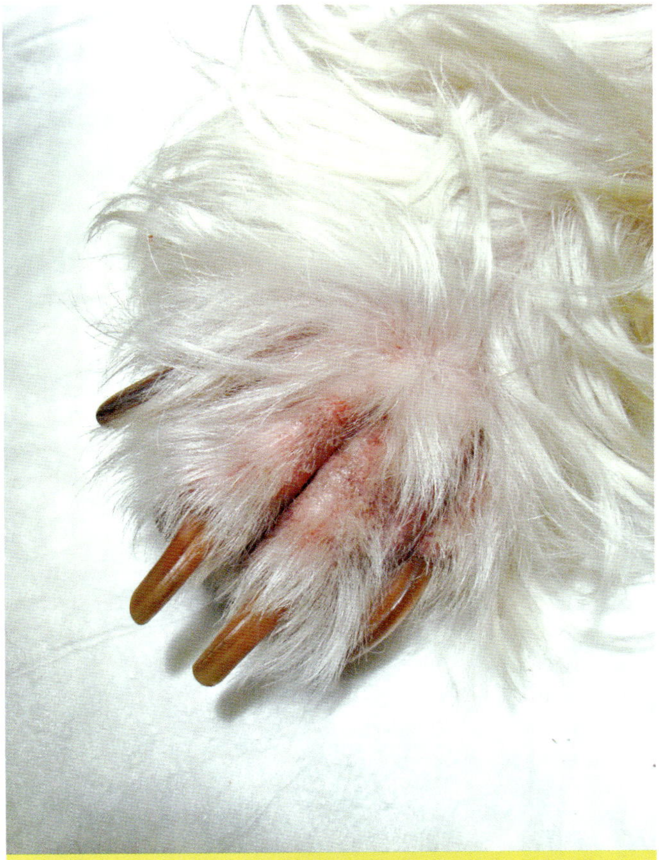

07 Dog with atopic dermatitis affecting the feet.

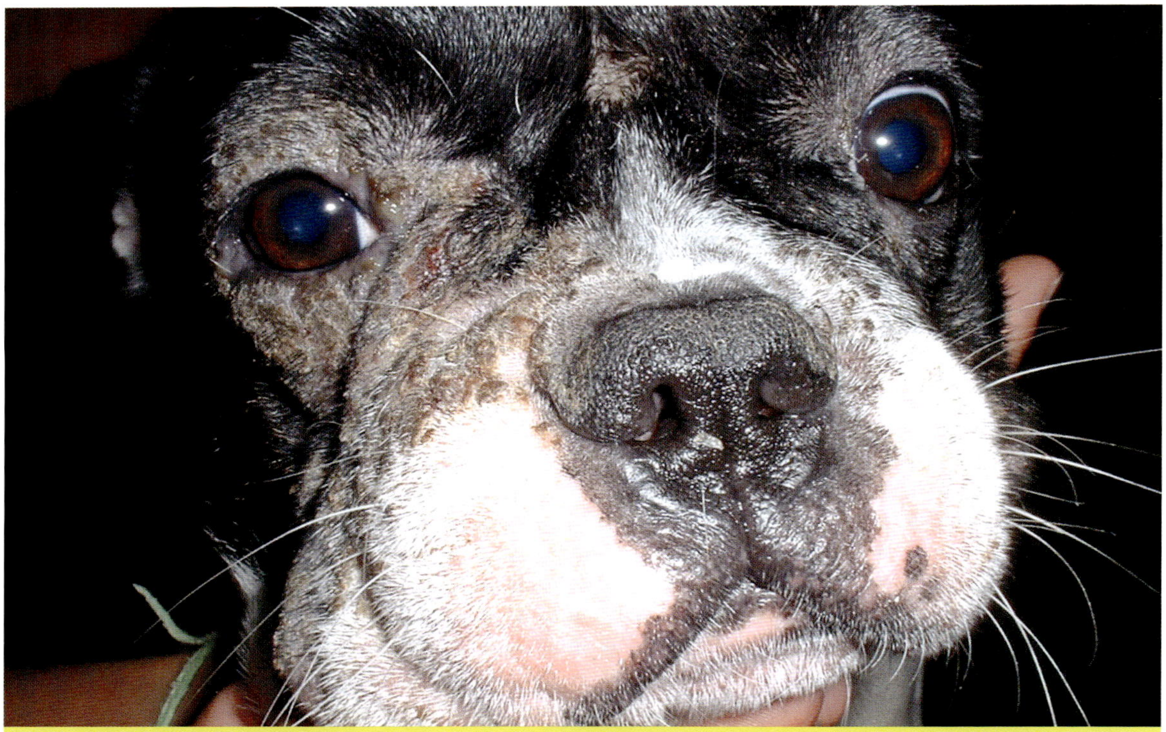

08 Facial involvement (blepharitis and cheilitis) in a dog with atopic dermatitis.

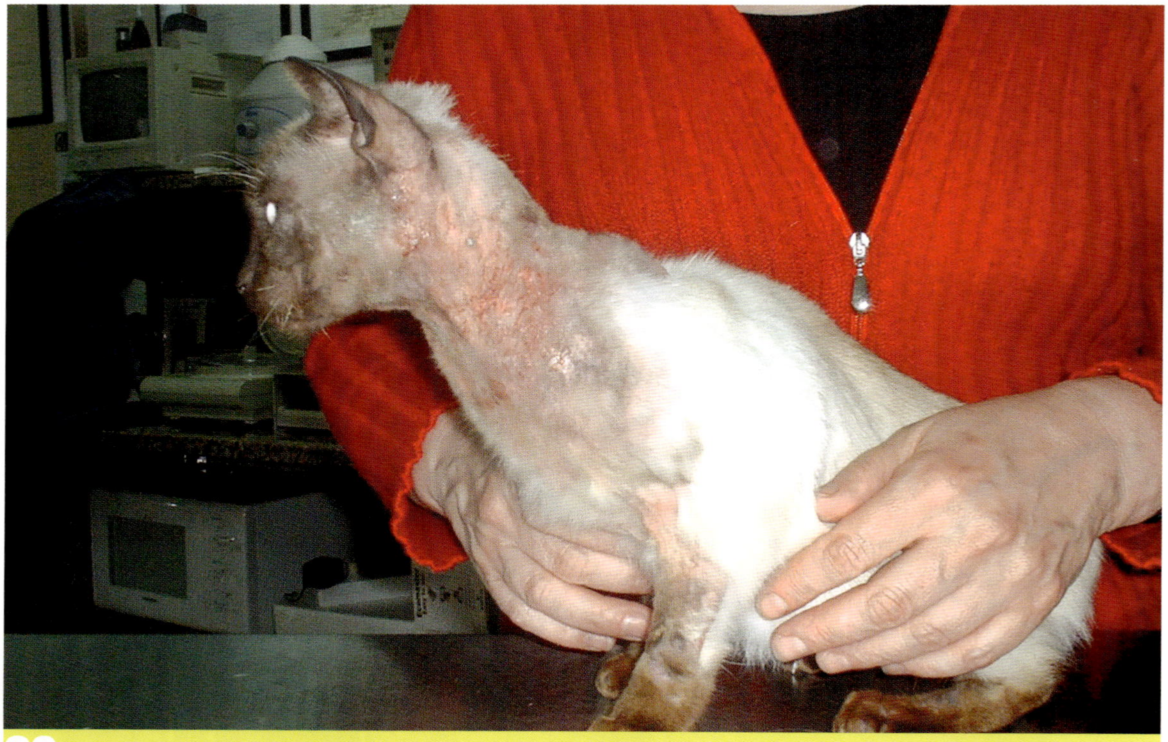

09 Cat with erosion and ulceration on the face and neck due to hypersensitivity.

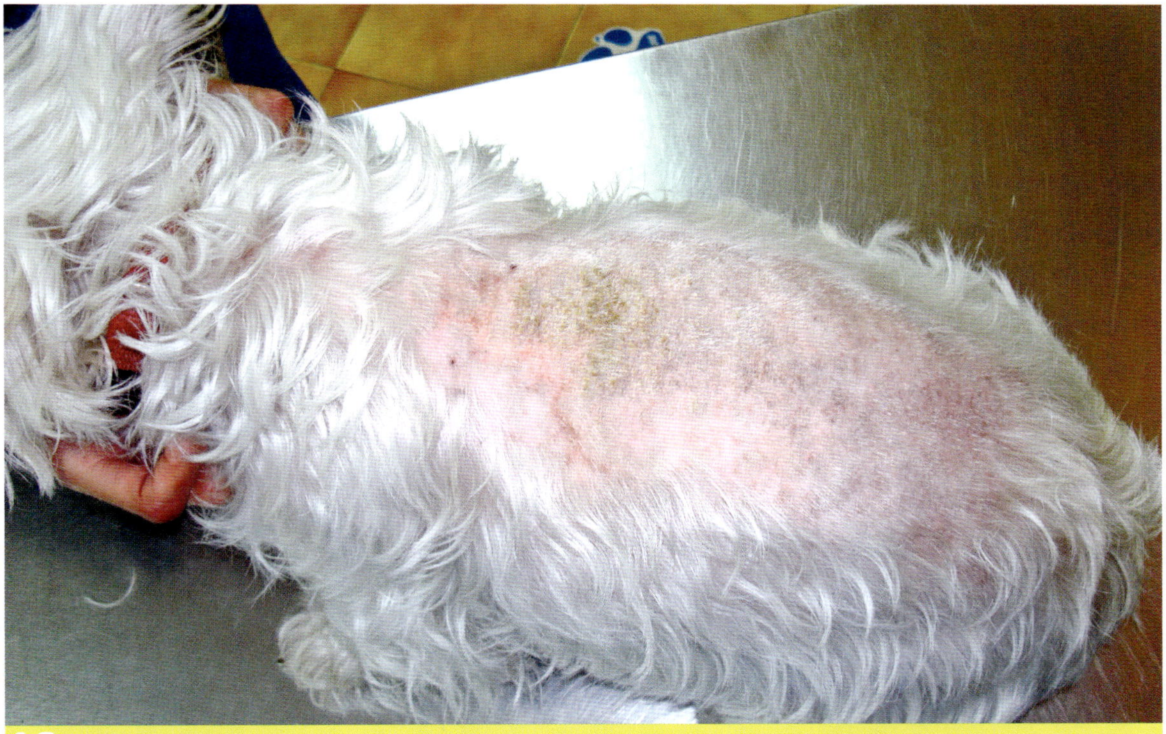

10 West Highland White Terrier with atopic dermatitis and a plaque due to *Malassezia* overgrowth.

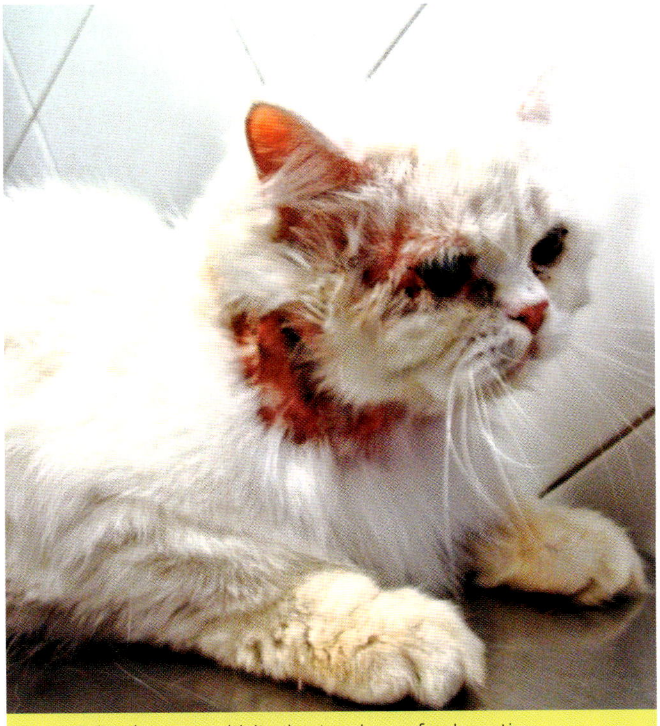

11 Feline hypersensitivity due to adverse food reaction.
Head and neck involvement.

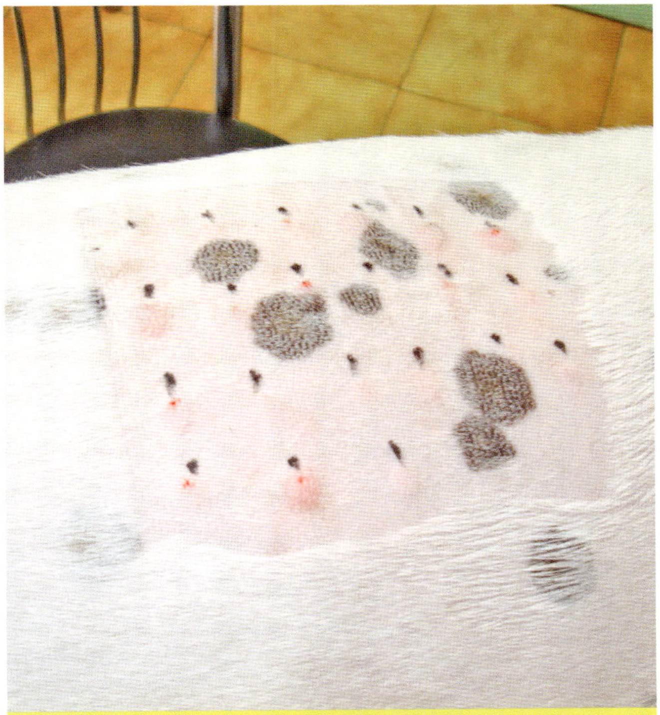

12 Intradermal reaction. Note the positive reactions.

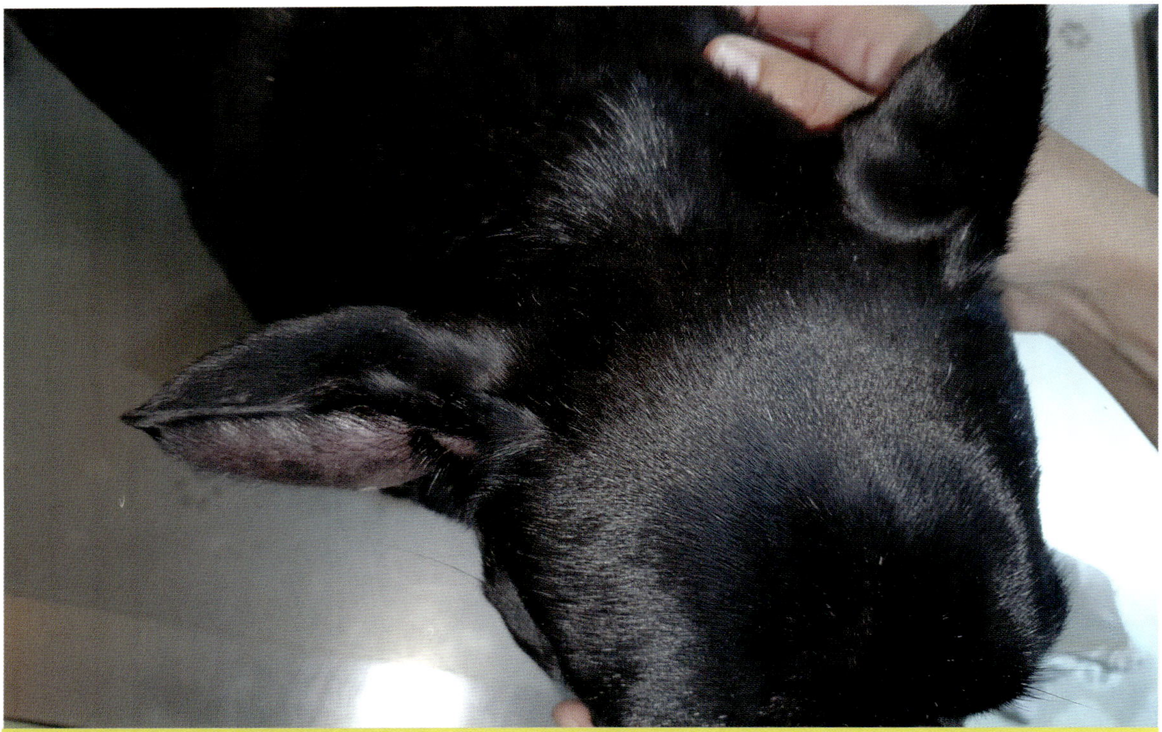

**13** Haematoma in the right ear of a dog with ear pruritus caused by canine atopic dermatitis.

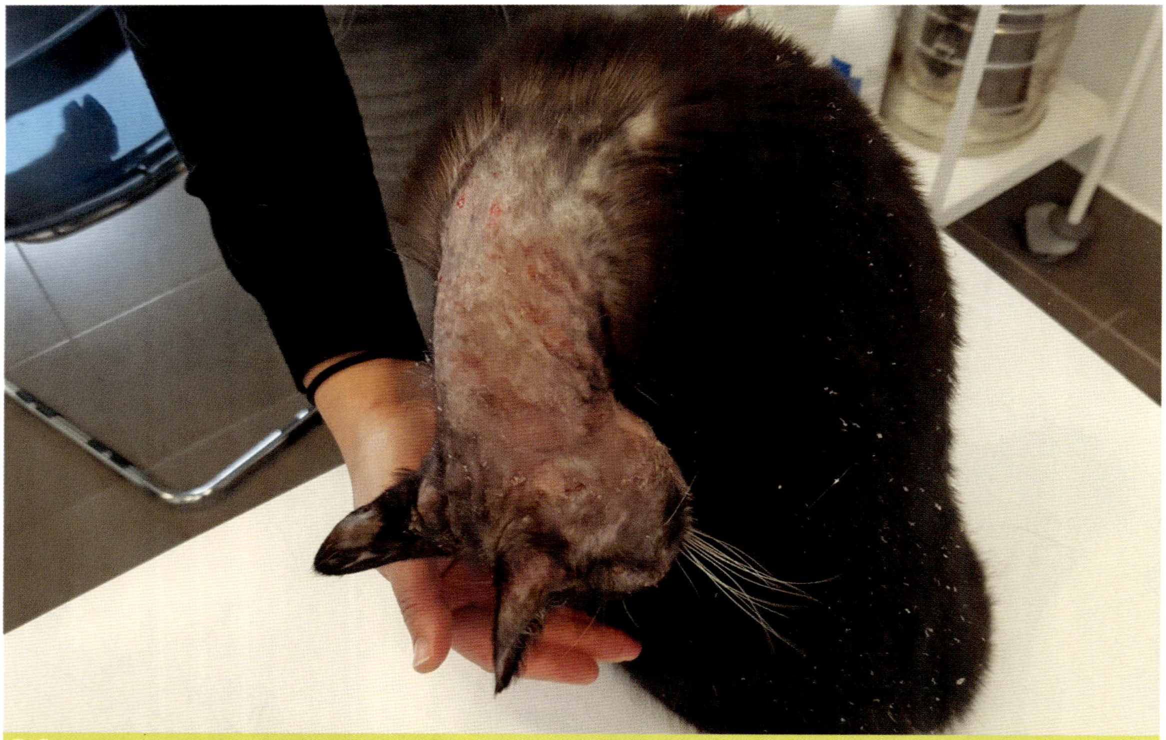

**14** Dermatosis of the face and neck, affecting a large portion of the latter area, in a cat that responded to a restriction diet.

# Contact hypersensitivity

## Lesion aetiology/pathogenesis and clinical picture

This is a process that can be caused by an allergic reaction or by a nonallergic irritative reaction.

Contact dermatitis of allergic origin is caused by sensitisation to allergens such as dyes, plastics, collars, and topical drugs. Irritant contact dermatitis occurs in the presence of substances that can cause chemical irritation, such as detergents, antiparasitics, disinfectants, and plants.

Affected areas are those that have had contact with the aforementioned substances, and tend to be the most exposed regions of the body (e.g. scrotum, legs, muzzle, abdomen, neck). Erythema develops and, due to pruritus, progresses to excoriations, alopecia, and skin hyperplasia. Chronification of the lesions can lead to lichenification and scaling.

Allergic contact dermatitis tends to be more pruritic and irritant contact dermatitis more ulcerative and painful.

## Diagnostic method

Diagnosis is not easy to establish and is made based on the clinical history and the observation of improvements after avoidance of the suspected allergen. Diagnosis should be confirmed with subsequent provocation tests, although in reality these are not usually performed.

## Main differential diagnoses

- Intertrigo
- Mucocutaneous pyoderma
- Other forms of hypersensitivity
- Leishmaniasis (scrotal affection)
- Cutaneous lupus

## Treatment

Treatment consists of avoiding contact with the suspected allergen, topical application of corticosteroids or, in some cases, tacrolimus, avoidance of bacterial infections, and the use of hypoallergenic washes. Pentoxifylline can be helpful in some cases. Itching can be controlled with oclacitinib, lokivetmab, or corticosteroids.

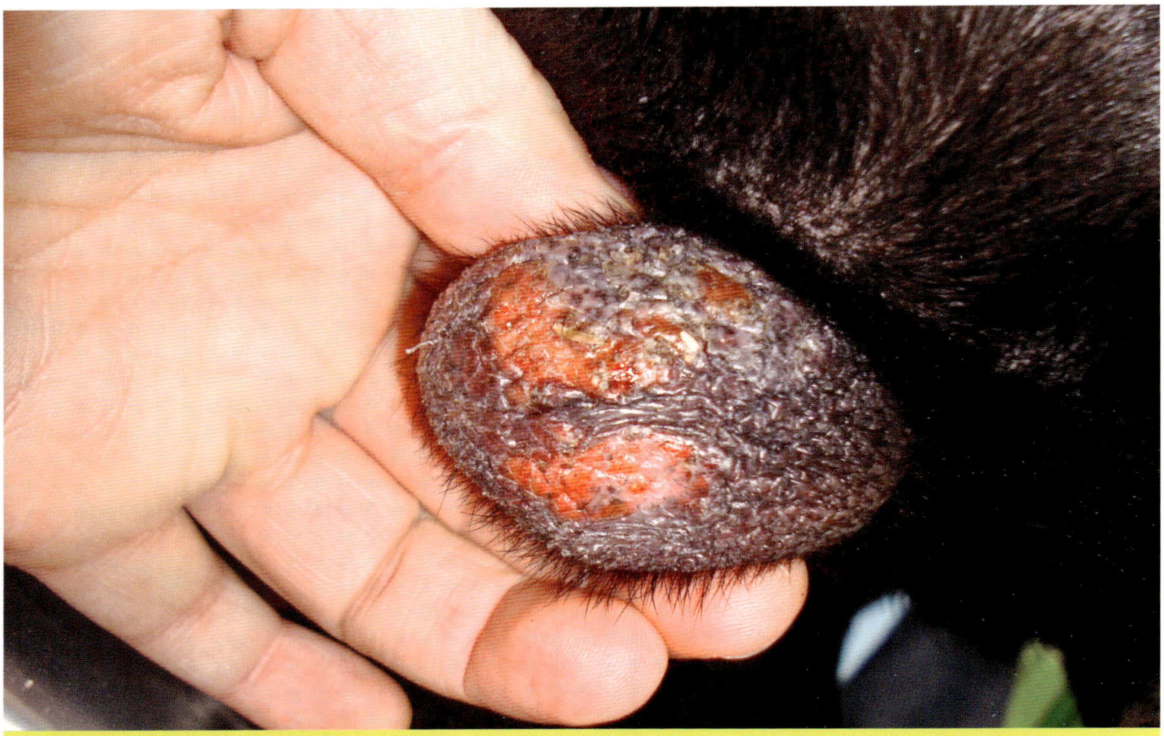

15 Contact dermatitis of the scrotum caused by irritant substances.

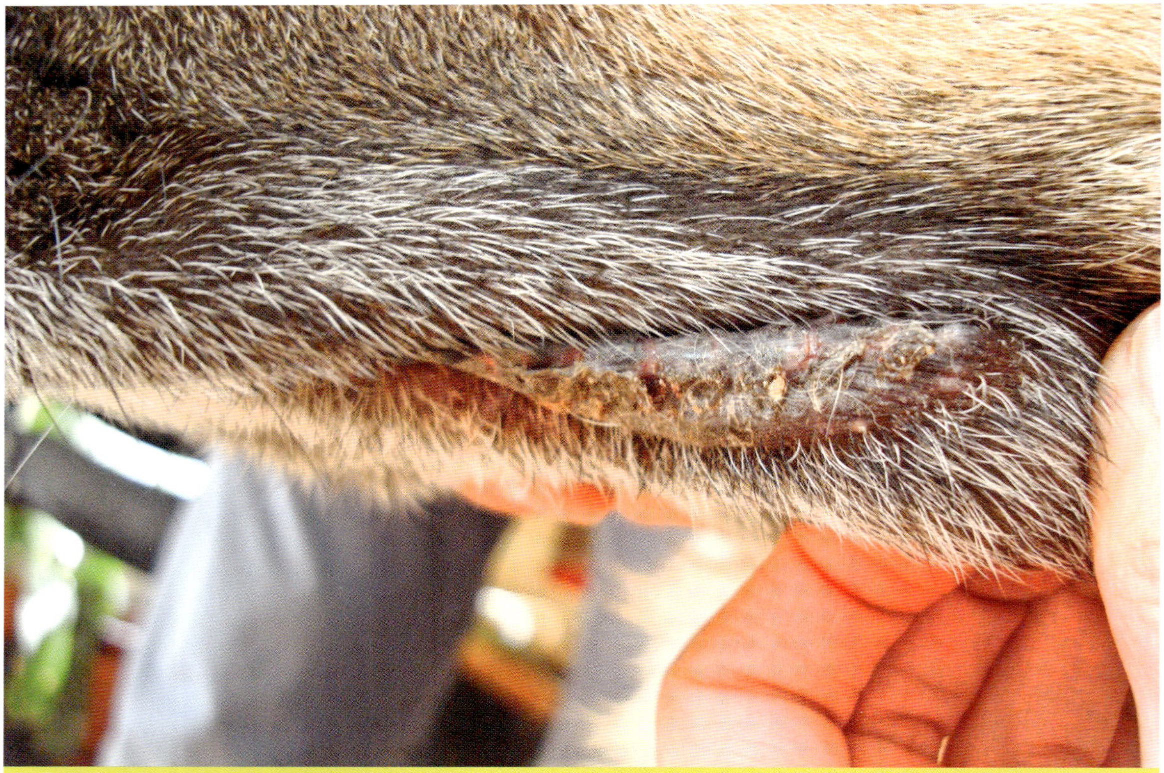

16 Contact dermatitis in the labial area.

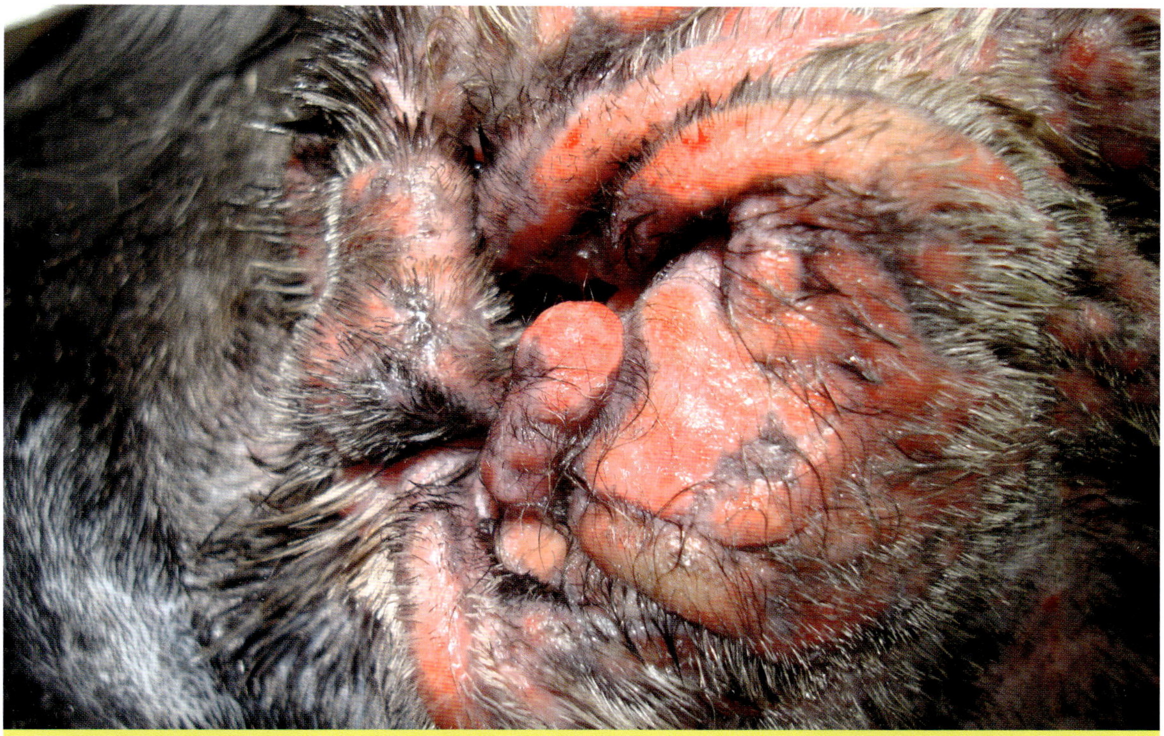

17 Irritant contact dermatitis in one ear caused by a reaction to topical medication.

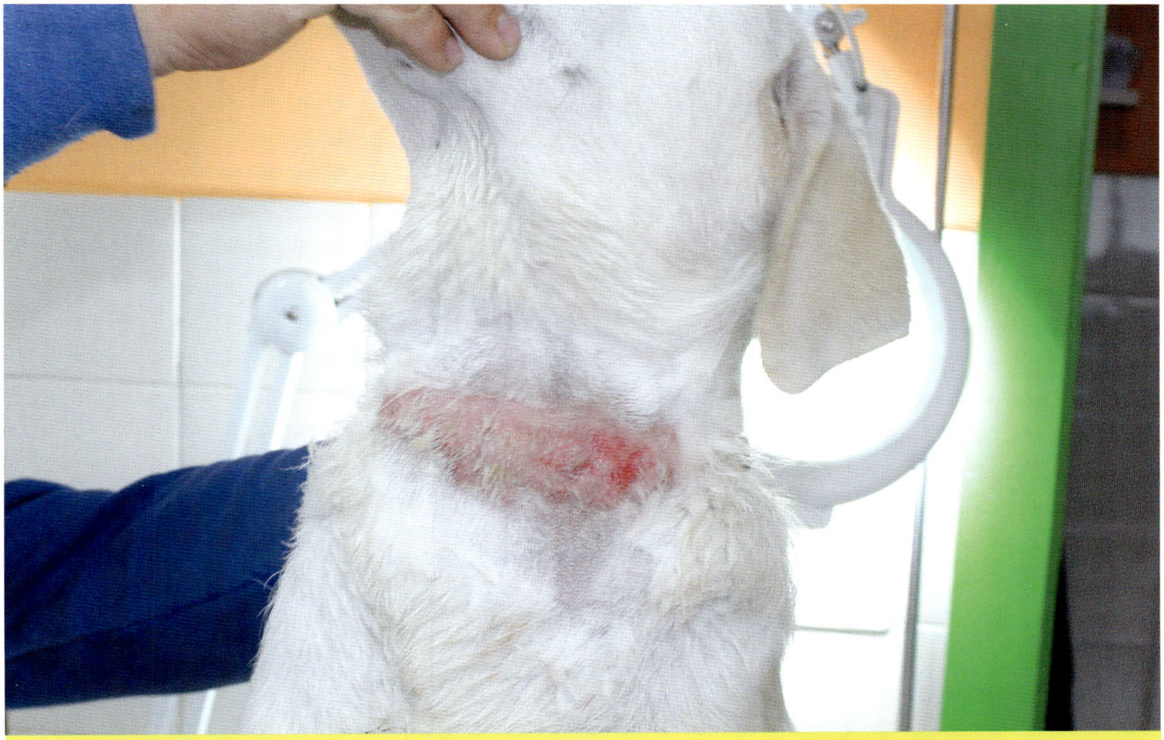

18 Irritant contact dermatitis caused by a citronella-based insecticide collar.

# Flea allergy dermatitis

## Lesion aetiology/pathogenesis and clinical picture

Fleas can affect dogs and cats simply by biting, which produces papules and wheals or, in sensitised or hypersensitive individuals, by causing a much more exaggerated reaction consisting of crusts/papules with scaling or, in some cases, seborrhoeic alopecia. Pruritus is the common denominator in this dermatosis. If not controlled, the lesions progress to hyperpigmentation and lichenification. This picture is a little more characteristic in dogs. In cats, the main reactions triggered are miliary dermatitis, eosinophilic dermatitis, and self-induced alopecia.

The lesions are usually concentrated in the lumbar, inguinal, abdominal, and perianal areas. Pruritus typically occurs in sudden bouts, and the affected animal will often nibble at itself using its incisors as if searching for the flea.

Hypersensitivity occurs in animals over 1 year of age and is more frequent during flea season (i.e. spring and summer). However, diagnosis and treatment are somewhat more complicated in animals that live indoors (where the temperature is much more stable, providing an ideal habitat for the maintenance of juvenile forms of the insect).

## Diagnostic method

The presence of flea droppings, the clinical picture, *Dipylidium* infestation, and the response to treatment are all taken into consideration when diagnosing this condition.

In the clinical history it is important to note the presence of bites on the owner.

## Main differential diagnoses

- Canine atopic dermatitis
- Cheyletiellosis
- Pediculosis
- Sarcoptic mange
- Other causes of reaction patterns in cats

## Treatment

Eradication of the insect requires treatment of all the individuals that live together (especially cats) and elimination of juvenile forms of the flea in the environment. Several effective treatments are available in collar, pipette, spray, and tablet formulations. Many affected animals also suffer from atopic dermatitis and require frequent bathing. In these cases, the use of systemic flea treatments such as isoxazolines or certain macrocyclic lactones may be recommended.

The environment must also be treated, either directly using development inhibitors in the form of pipettes or sprays to eradicate adult parasites, or indirectly using tablets administered to the animal.

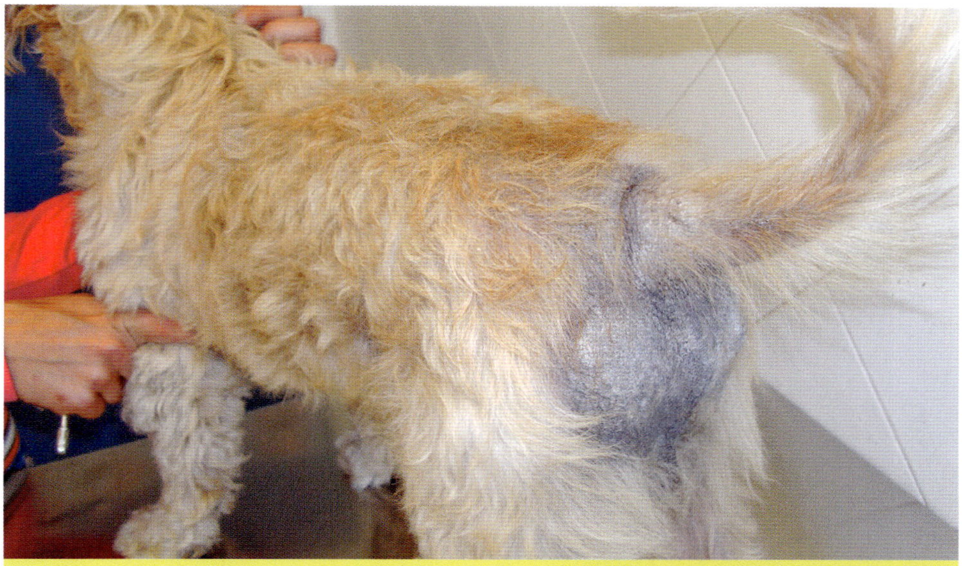

19 Classic appearance of a dog with flea allergy dermatitis. Note the alopecia with hyperpigmentation and lichenification.

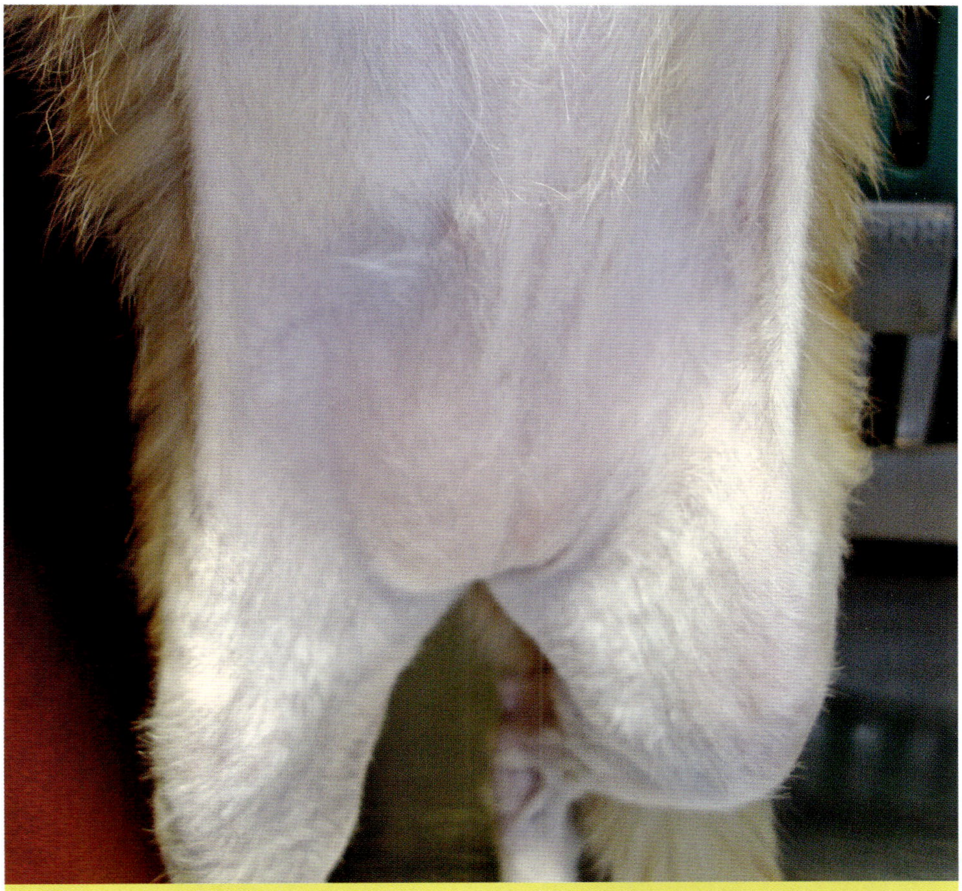

20 Self-induced symmetric alopecia in the abdominal area and hindlimbs of a cat with flea allergy dermatitis.

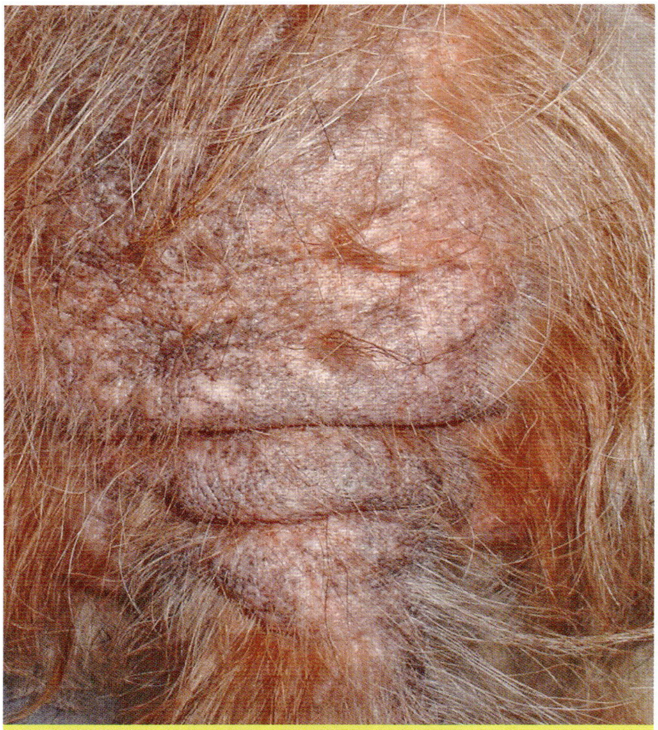

**21** Close-up view of the lower back of a dog with flea bite allergy.

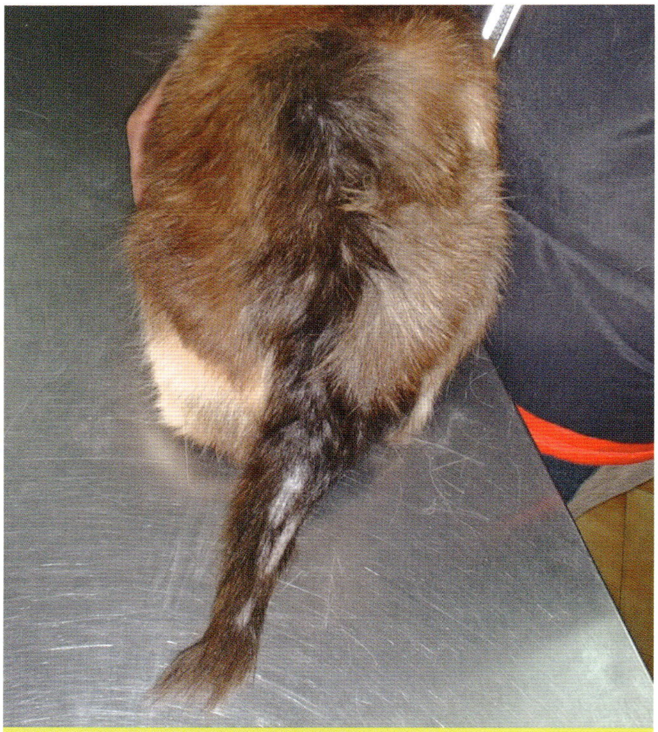

**22** Dorsolumbar view of a cat with flea allergy dermatitis.

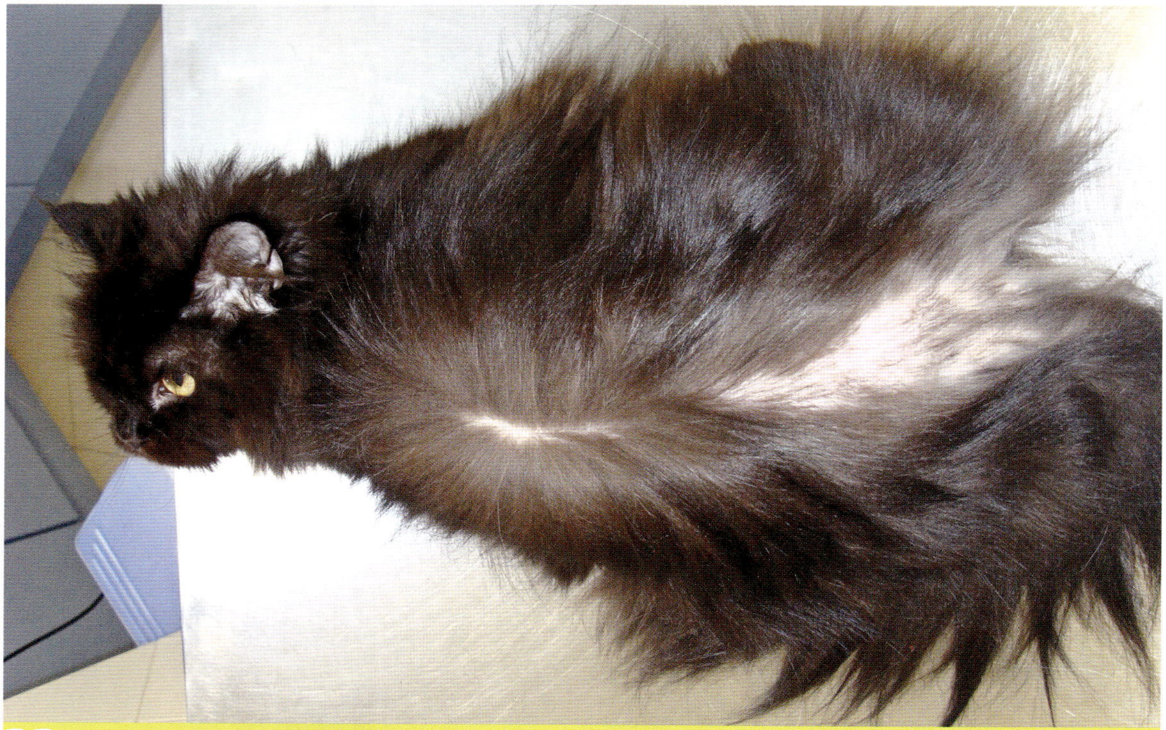

**23** Cat with self-induced alopecia on the back caused by flea allergy.

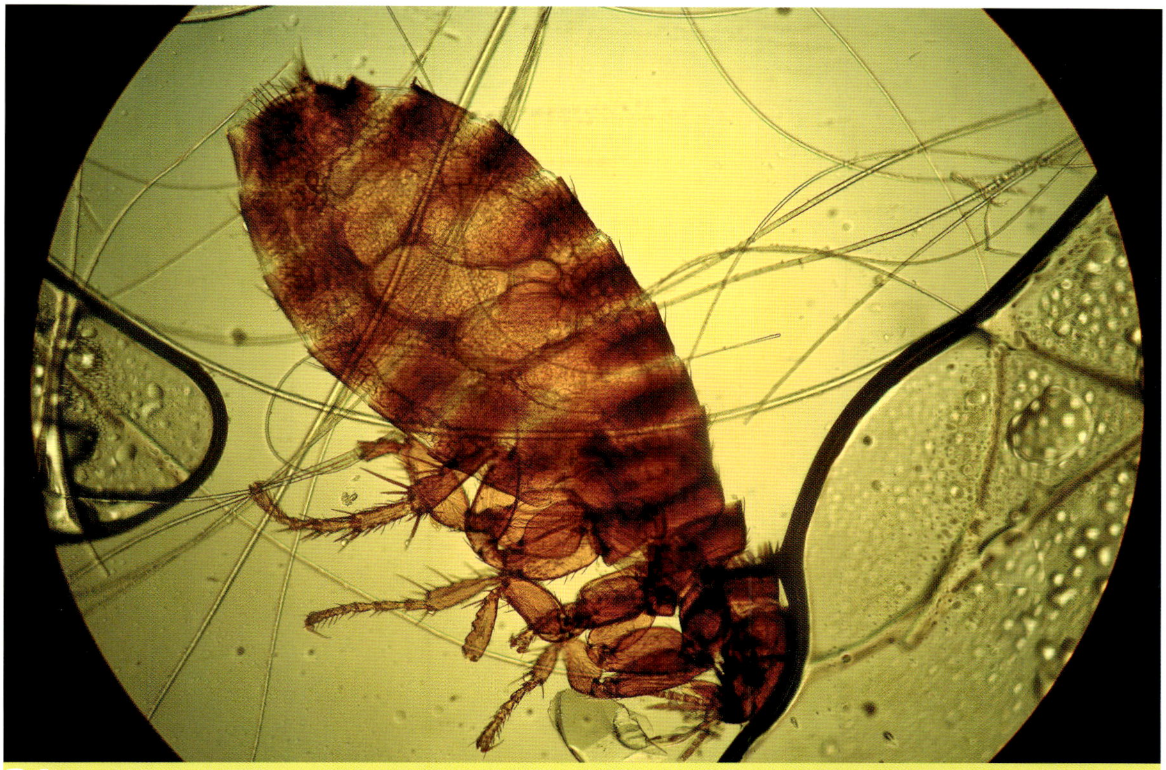

24 Microscopic image of a cat and dog flea.

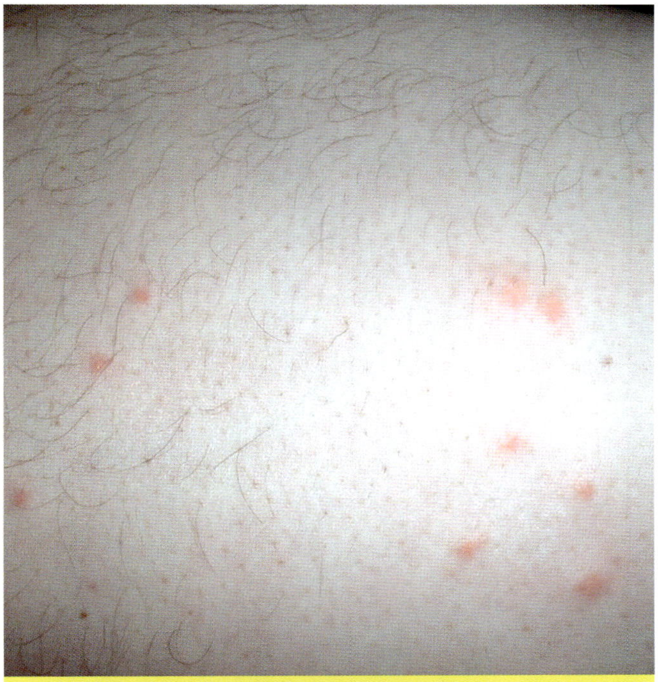

25 Papules caused by flea bites on a person's thigh. The presence of surrounding papules is characteristic.

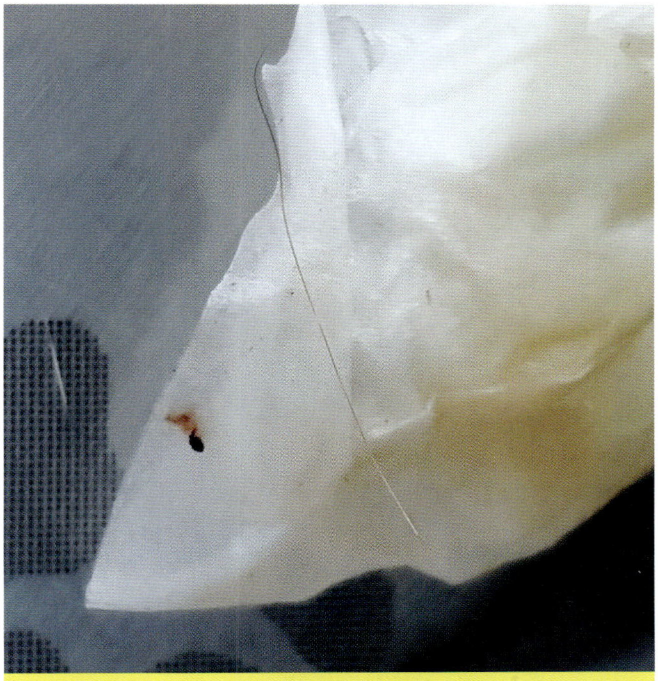

26 Flea faeces collected by brushing and placed on a damp paper. Note how the blood in the faeces stains the paper.

# Allergy to insect bites

## Insect allergy in cats

### Lesion aetiology/pathogenesis and clinical picture

Cats can display a hypersensitivity reaction in response to the bite of insects (mainly mosquitoes). Erythematous papular lesions are usually observed on the bridge of the nose and the pinnae. In some cases this condition can spread to the paw pads and digits.

These lesions can progress to form crusts and erosions with marked pruritus, as evidenced by the presence of excoriations. If the condition is not controlled, furunculosis with marked alopecia may appear.

### Diagnostic method

Strong indicators of the possible presence of this disease include onset during seasons of the year in which mosquitoes are present and an outdoor lifestyle. Cytology and histology reveal a predominantly eosinophilic reaction.

### Main differential diagnoses

- Feline herpesvirus
- Dermatophytosis
- Squamous cell carcinoma
- Pemphigus foliaceus

### Treatment

Animals generally respond very well to corticosteroids. Insects should be eliminated, mainly by changing the animal's environment or using creams or protective lotions suitable for cats.

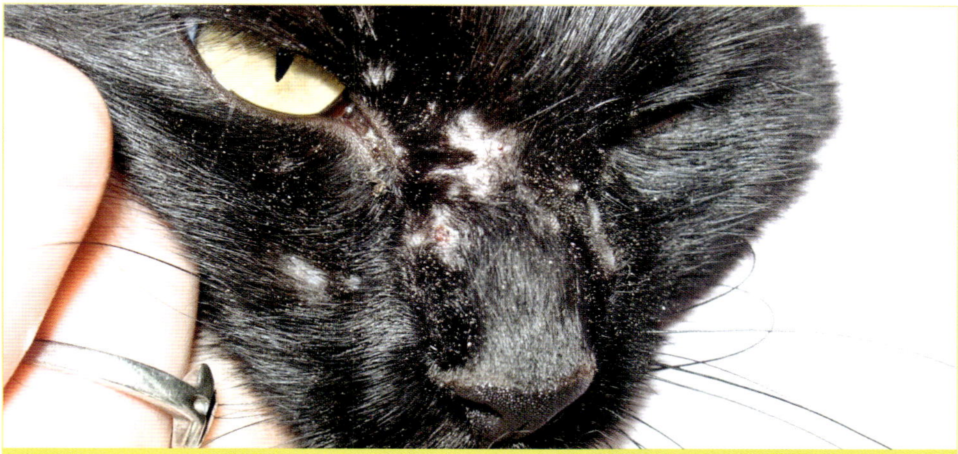

27 Alopecia, papules, and crusting caused by mosquito bites on a cat's face. Image courtesy of Frédéric Lanot.

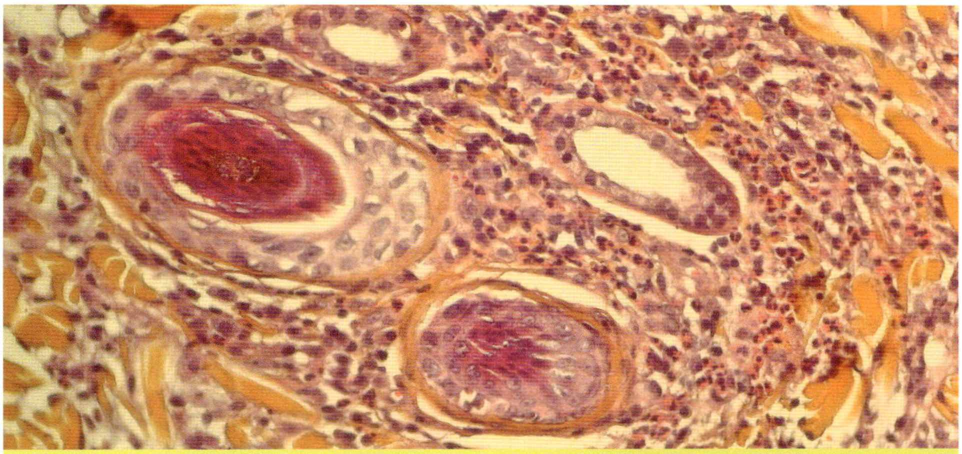

28 Eosinophilic infiltration around the follicles and collagen fibres caused by mosquito bite. Image courtesy of Didier Carlotti (RIP).

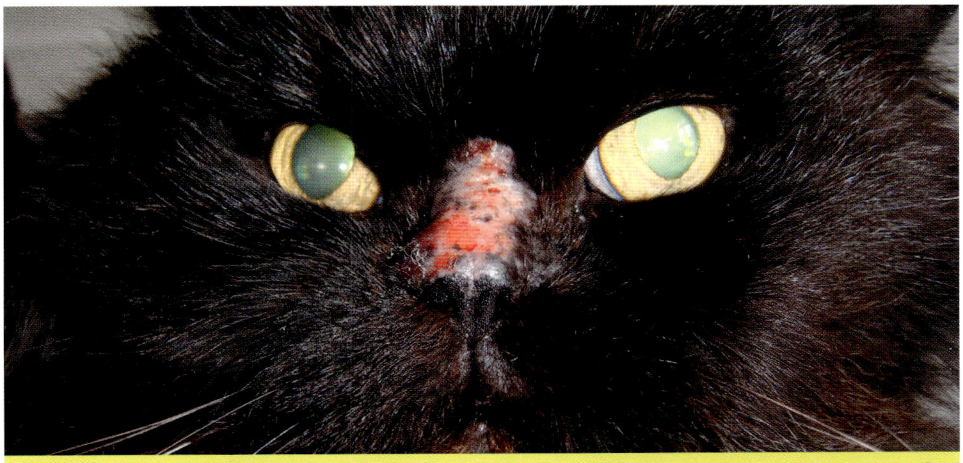

29 Involvement of the nasal bridge in a patient with mosquito bite hypersensitivity. Image courtesy of Ana Cabrero.

# Canine facial eosinophilic furunculosis

## Lesion aetiology/pathogenesis and clinical picture

The underlying aetiology appears to involve the bite of certain insects such as wasps, bees, and ants. Lesions occur on the nasal bridge and upper lip, with the appearance of alopecia, clusters of papules that form plaques, erosion, erythema, and crusts. The plaques can often ulcerate due to the concomitant pruritus.

## Diagnostic method

Establishing the diagnosis is not always easy, although it can be facilitated by the clinical picture and knowledge of the dog's lifestyle. Cytology confirms an eosinophilic picture.

## Main differential diagnoses

- Dermatophytosis
- Pyoderma
- Pemphigus complex
- Lupus with facial involvement

## Treatment

In general, animals respond very well to corticosteroids. Elimination of insects should be attempted, mainly by changing the animal's environment or by applying repellents authorised for use in dogs.

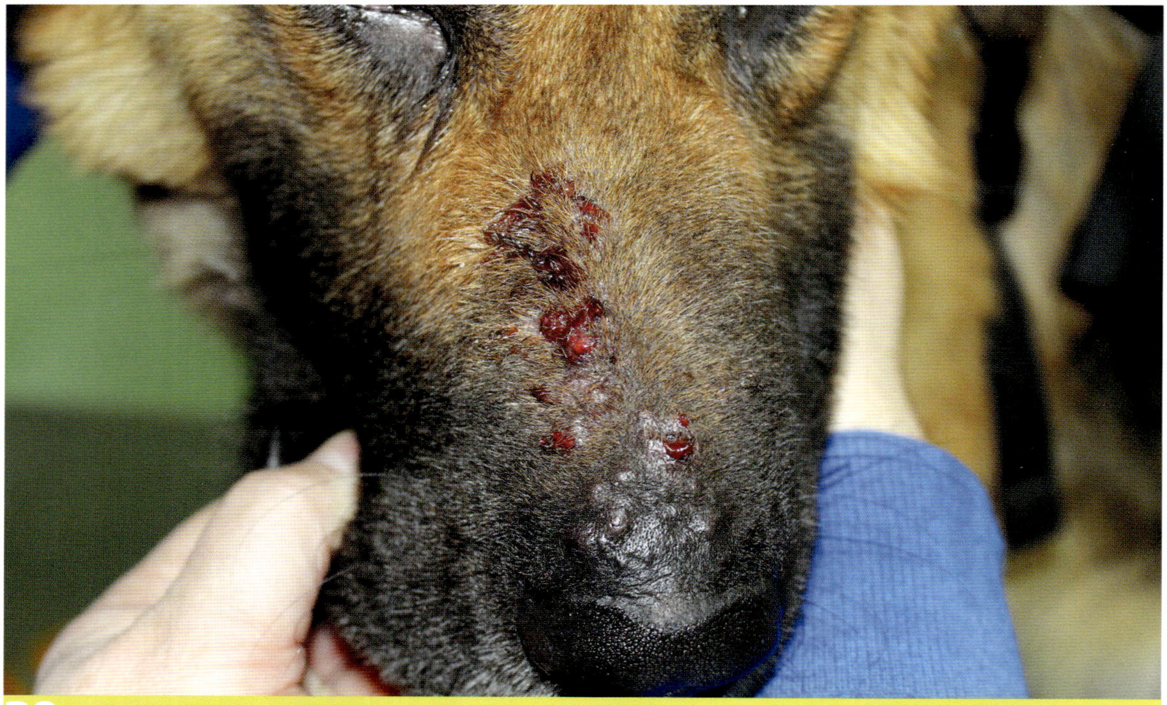

30 Facial eosinophilic furunculosis in a German Shepherd.

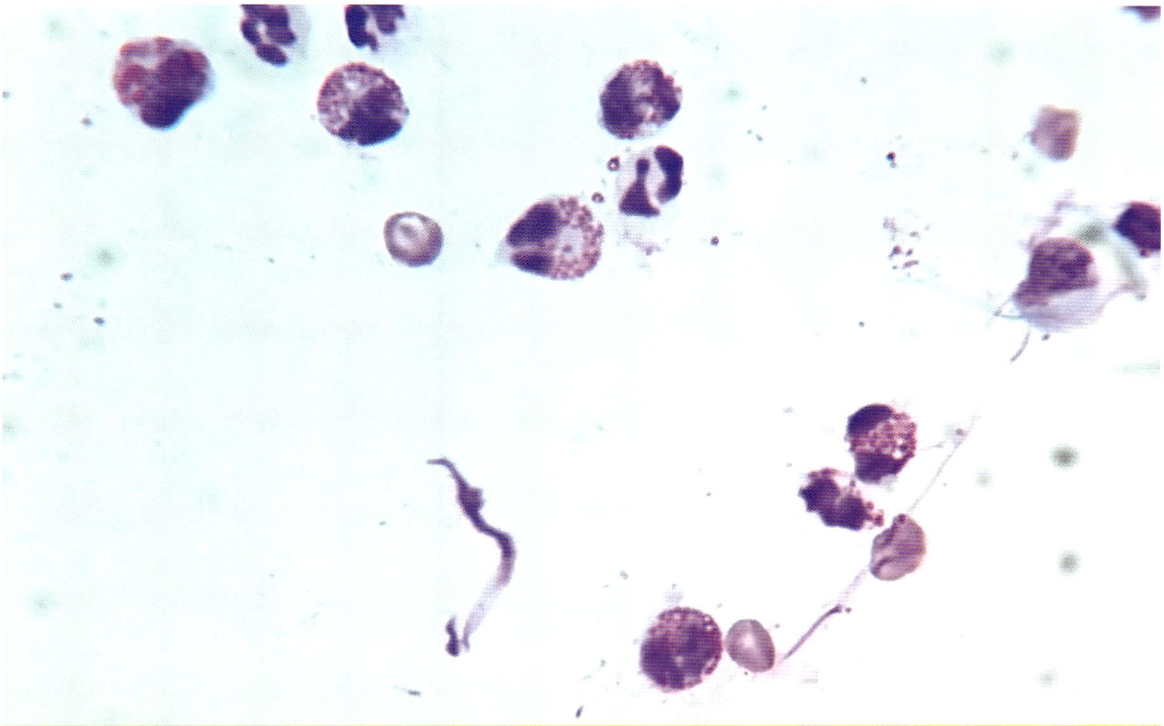

31 Cytology of eosinophilic furunculosis.

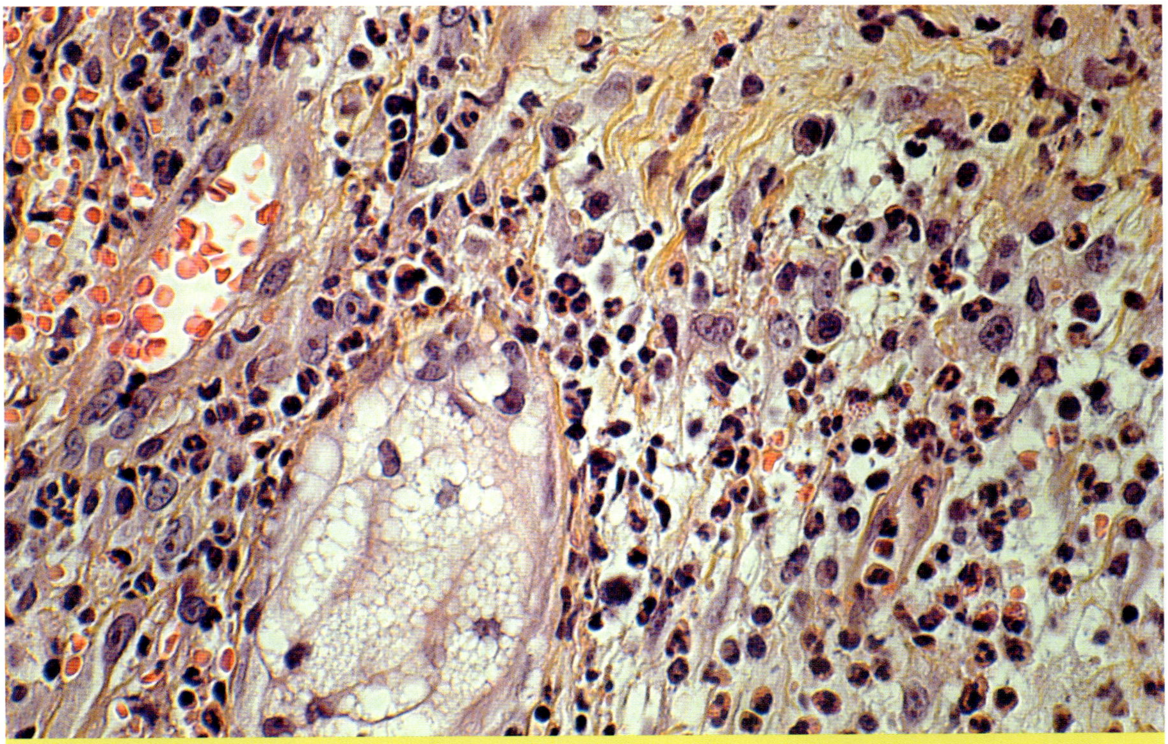

32 Histopathology of facial eosinophilic furunculosis.

# Manifestations of allergy in cats

## Miliary dermatitis

### Lesion aetiology/pathogenesis and clinical picture

Miliary dermatitis is one of four typical cutaneous reaction patterns observed in cats. Its appearance usually indicates a hypersensitivity reaction, dermatophytosis, or a cutaneous parasitic disease. The characteristic lesions are small crusts distributed throughout the body that feel like grains of sand on palpation. Miliary dermatitis can occur alone or in association with other patterns, which increases the likelihood of environmental hypersensitivity.

### Diagnostic method

The clinical picture is quite characteristic and cytology of the lesions usually reveals abundant eosinophilic infiltrate.

### Main differential diagnoses

Causes of miliary dermatitis:

- Hypersensitivity
- Dermatophytosis
- Ectoparasites
- Pemphigus complex

### Treatment

A good response to corticosteroids is usually observed, although it is important to try to determine the origin, as corticosteroids may be contraindicated in cases of dermatophytosis. We must control the primary cause, especially in the case of fleas. Cyclosporine may be indicated in recurrent cases and, in certain circumstances, oclacitinib may be effective at a dose slightly higher than that used in dogs.

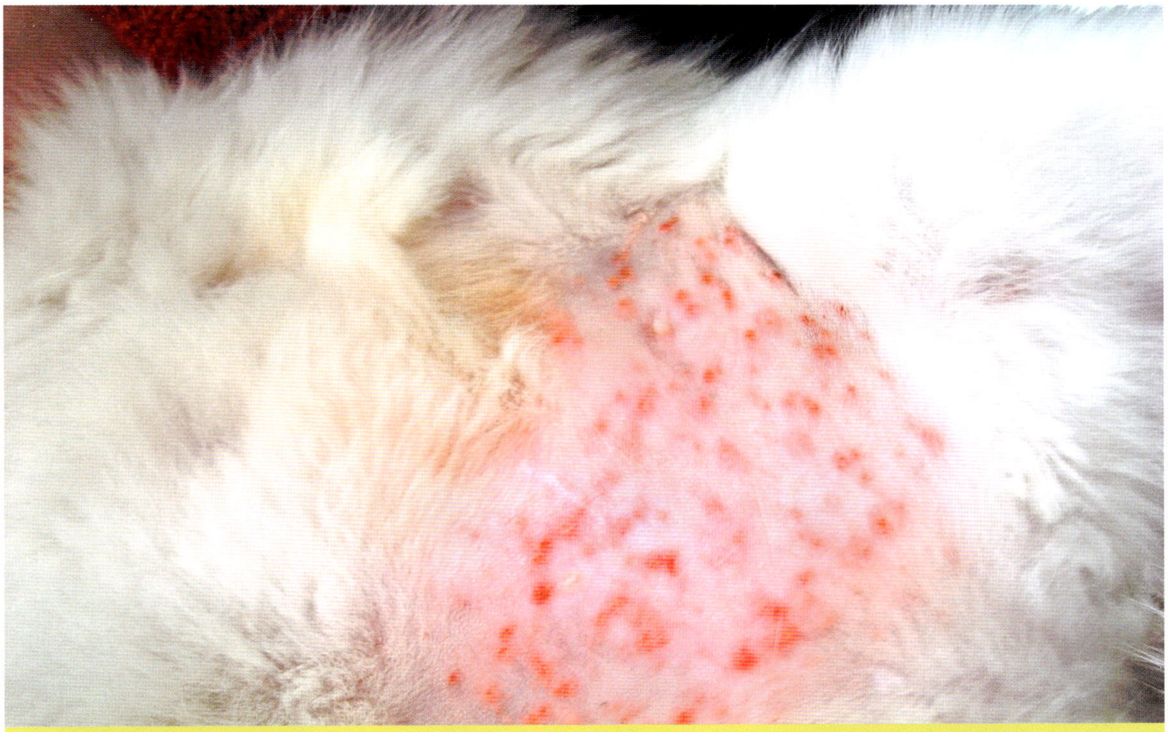

33 Miliary dermatitis on the abdomen.

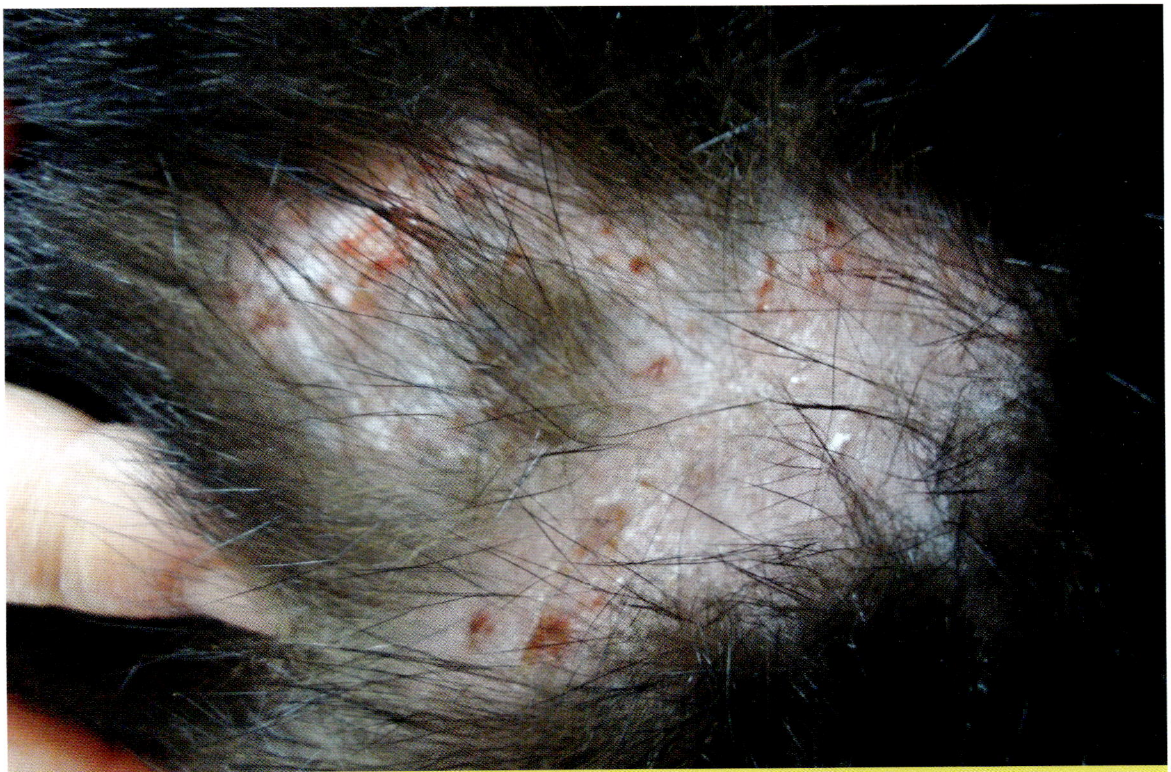

34 Close-up view of miliary dermatitis.

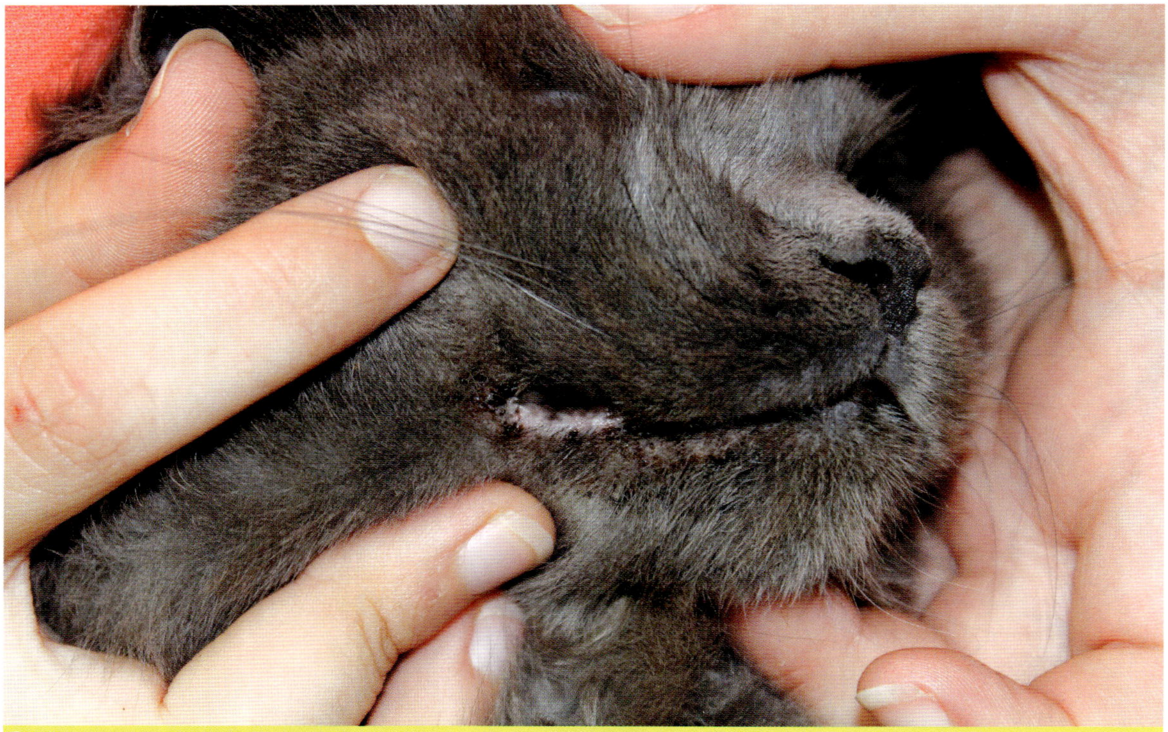

35 Perioral miliary dermatitis. Note the crusting around the lips.

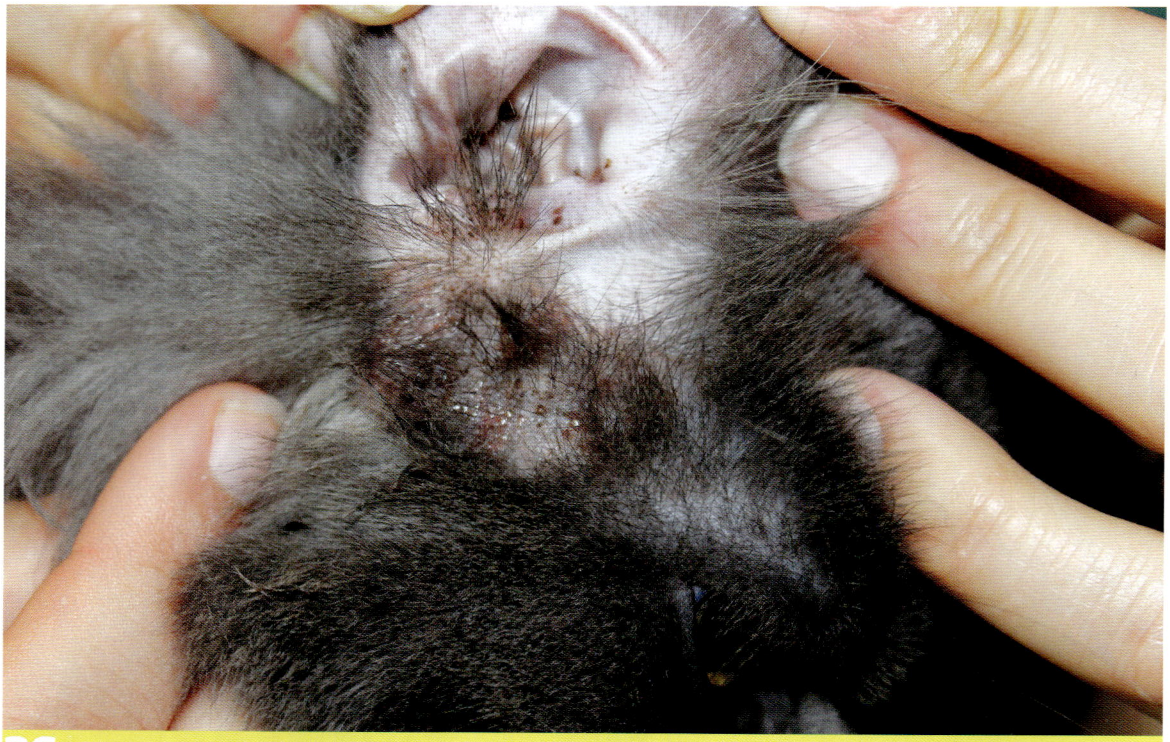

36 Periauricular miliary dermatitis. Note the crusting at the base of the ear and on the pinna.

# Self-induced alopecia

## Lesion aetiology/pathogenesis and clinical picture

This is another reaction pattern in cats. In most cases it results from excessive licking triggered by parasitic or allergic pruritus. In a very small number of cases it is caused by pathological grooming of psychogenic origin. Strikingly, skin lesions can be few or totally absent, and hairs are perfectly rooted but broken. In certain circumstances organic and behavioural causes can contribute to this condition.

It should be borne in mind that the papillae of the feline tongue make it a powerful tool in circumstances in which overgrcoming occurs.

## Diagnostic method

Diagnosis is based on the clinical picture, a clinical history indicating pruritus, trichogram findings, and the presence of abundant faecaliths. The presence of any of the other feline reaction patterns is a good indicator of hypersensitivity.

The response to corticosteroids may orient the diagnosis towards a hypersensitivity problem.

## Main differential diagnoses

- Ectoparasites
- Hypersensitivity
- Behavioural causes
- Other rare forms of noninflammatory alopecia in cats

## Treatment

Obviously, it is essential to eliminate the cause of the allergy or to look for other possibilities.

Therapeutic diagnosis is often used as it may not be possible to precisely determine the origin of the problem. Corticosteroids and flea treatments are commonly used.

In cases in which a behavioural disorder is confirmed, the environment should be enriched using pheromones and drugs indicated for this purpose. There are different types of pheromones indicated for problems with environmental adaptation or interactions between cats. Commercial forms that combine the two types are also available.

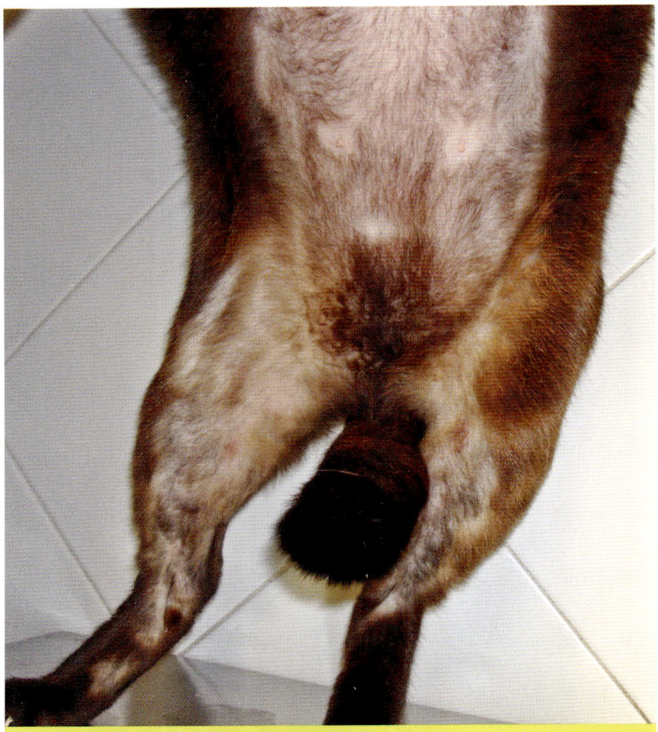
37 Self-induced alopecia. Note the abdomen and medial thighs.

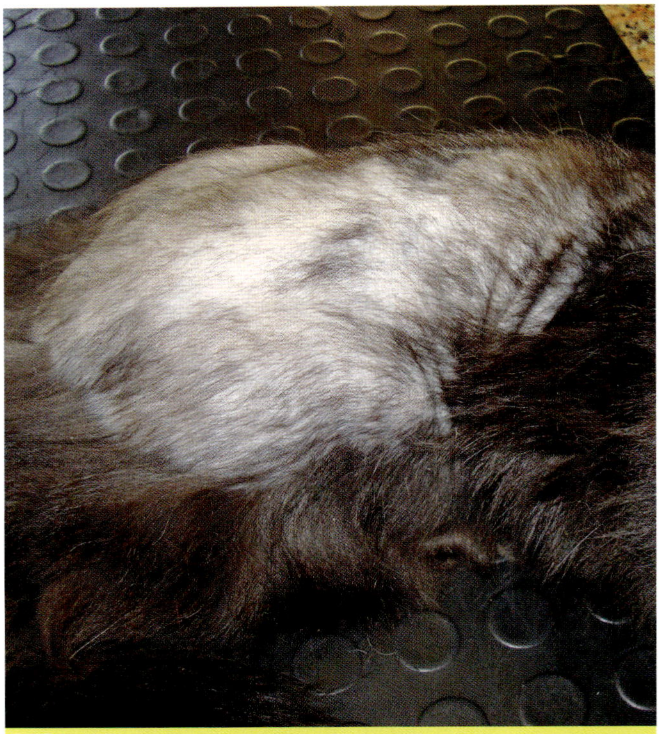
38 Self-induced alopecia in the dorsal and lumbar areas.

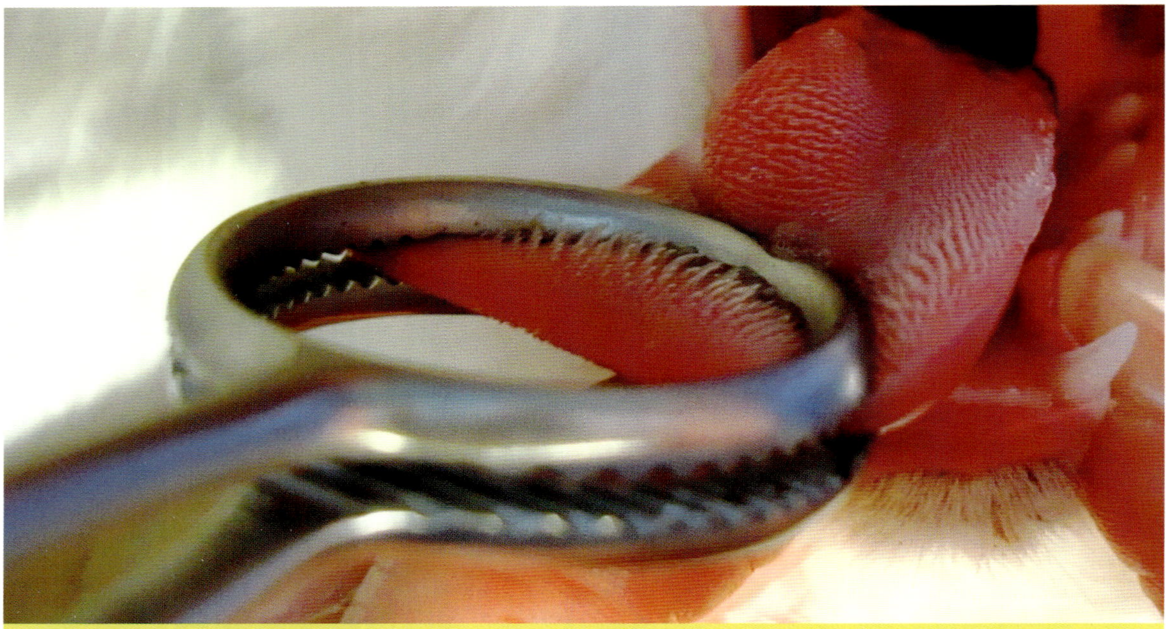
39 Papillae on the dorsal aspect of a cat's tongue.

# Erosion and ulceration of the face and cervical area

## Lesion aetiology/pathogenesis and clinical picture

This is a feline reaction pattern characterised by occasionally severe lesions consisting mainly of excoriations, erosions, and alopecia, often complicated by bacterial or yeast overgrowth.

The face and neck are primarily affected, with lesions as deep as ulcers. Pruritus of allergic origin is usually the predominant cause. Food allergens are thought to be implicated. Behavioural disorders have also been described as a cause of this pattern.

## Diagnostic method

Diagnosis is difficult and is usually confirmed therapeutically using an elimination diet. If this origin is ruled out, the response to corticosteroids can confirm a non-food-related aetiology.

Environmental enrichment and the use of pheromones may also be indicated.

## Main differential diagnoses

- Hypersensitivity states
- Ectoparasites
- Dermatophytosis
- Dirty face syndrome in Persian and Himalayan cats

## Treatment

The therapeutic arsenal includes elimination diets, corticosteroids, cyclosporine, oclacitinib, pyoderma control, and antiparasitics. Some cases can be very frustrating, and it can be difficult to allay the owner's concerns. It is essential to ensure appropriate enrichment of the patient's environment.

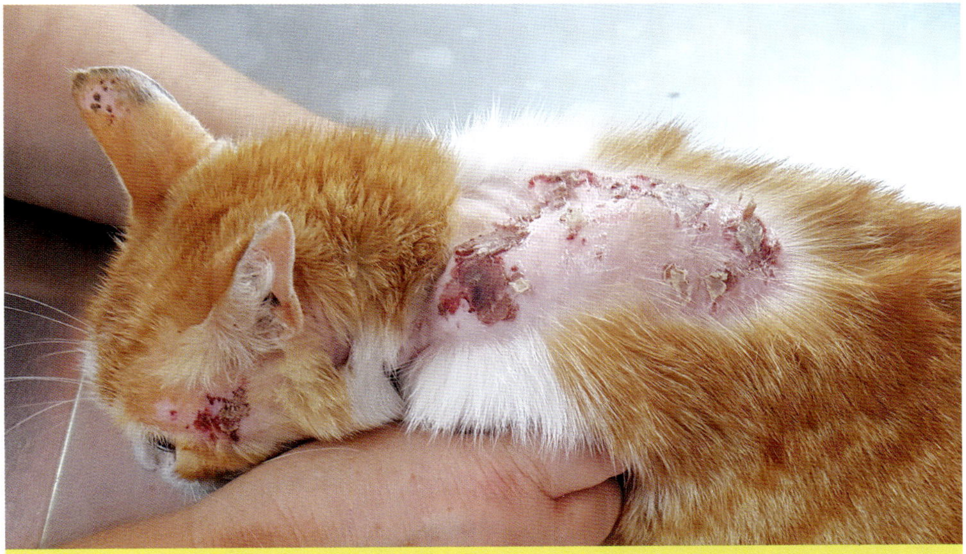

40 Lesions caused by pruritus on the face and cervical area.

# Eosinophilic granuloma complex

## Lesion aetiology/pathogenesis and clinical picture

This complex of feline reaction patterns includes granuloma, plaques, and labial ulcer. It is more appropriate to treat these entities separately, as they have distinct origins and characteristics. They can be considered reactions of the cat's skin to different aggressions, including excessive licking, allergies, and parasites. Cases in which it is impossible to determine the underlying cause are considered idiopathic.

- Granulomas are characteristic lesions ranging in colour from pinkish-yellowish to dark red, and often give rise to raised lesions due to the coalescence of multiple small granulomas. These lesions can progress to ulcers surrounded by a clear background. They can occur in a linear pattern on the caudal aspect of the hindlimbs, in the labial commissure, above the eyes, inside the mouth, or around the paw pads.
- Eosinophilic plaques are closely associated with excessive licking, and can occur on the abdomen, accompanied by alopecia, and in the interdigital spaces.
- Labial or indolent ulcers commonly recur, and the underlying aetiology can be difficult to determine. They often respond to antibiotics, and therefore may be associated with bacterial infections, although the relationship with allergies is undeniable. The corresponding lesion consists of an ulcerative plaque on the upper lip, often at the point where the adjacent canine tooth rests.

## Diagnostic method

Suspicion is usually confirmed based on the clinical picture, cytology, and the response to classical treatments with anti-inflammatory drugs and antibiotics. In certain stubborn cases all differential diagnoses must be meticulously ruled out.

## Main differential diagnoses

- Tumours
- Infections
- Other hypersensitivity states

## Treatment

The arsenal of drugs commonly used to treat this condition includes corticosteroids, antibiotics, cyclosporine, palmidrol derivatives, antiparasitics, and oclacitinib.

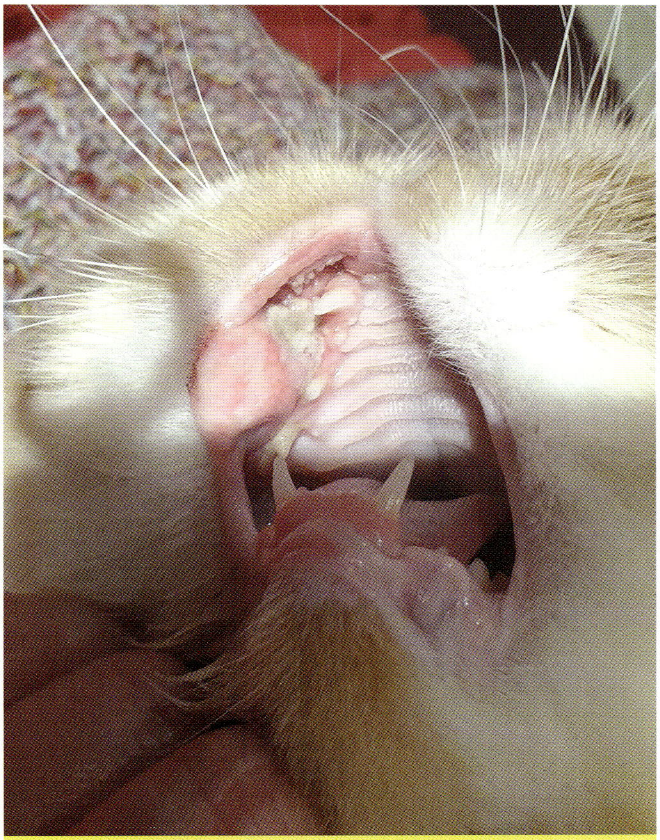

41 Eosinophilic granuloma in the mouth of a cat.

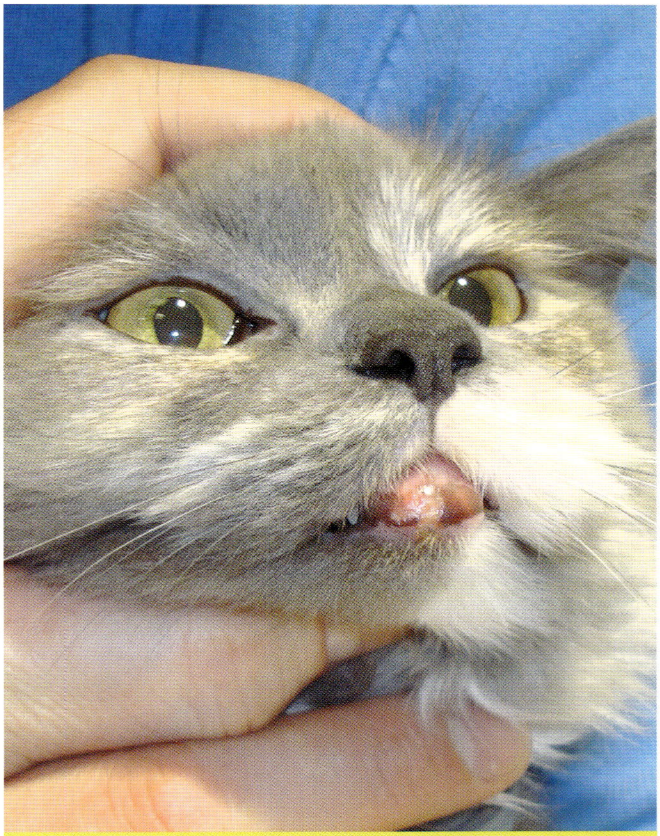

42 Eosinophilic granuloma on the lower lip of a cat.

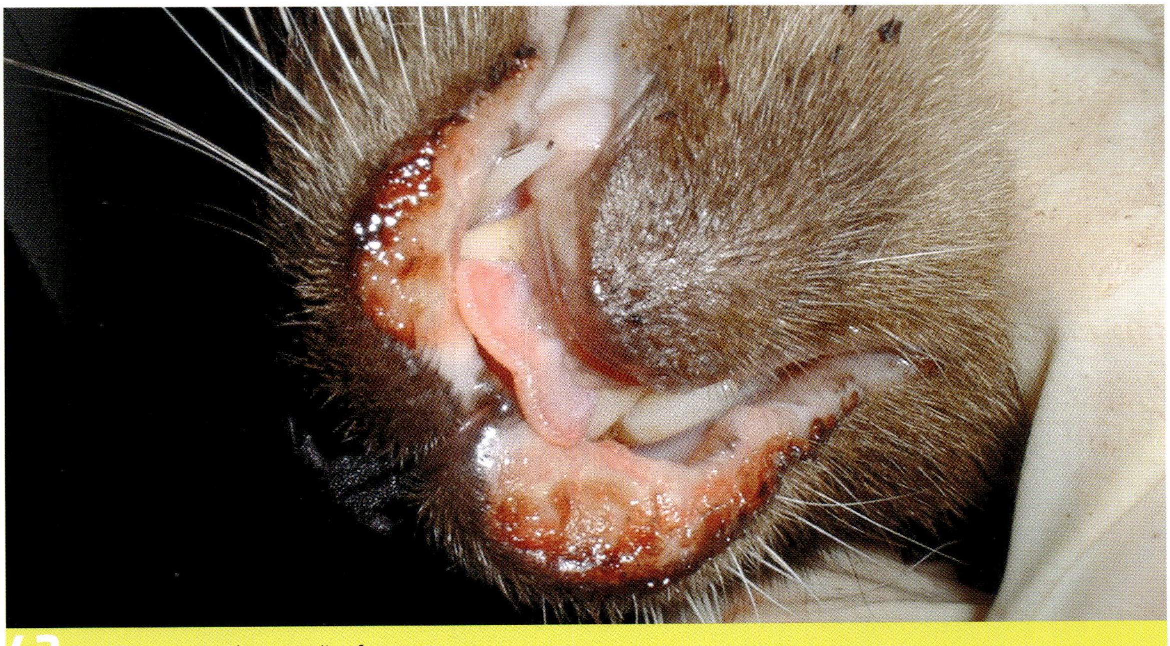

43 Indolent ulcer on the upper lip of a cat.

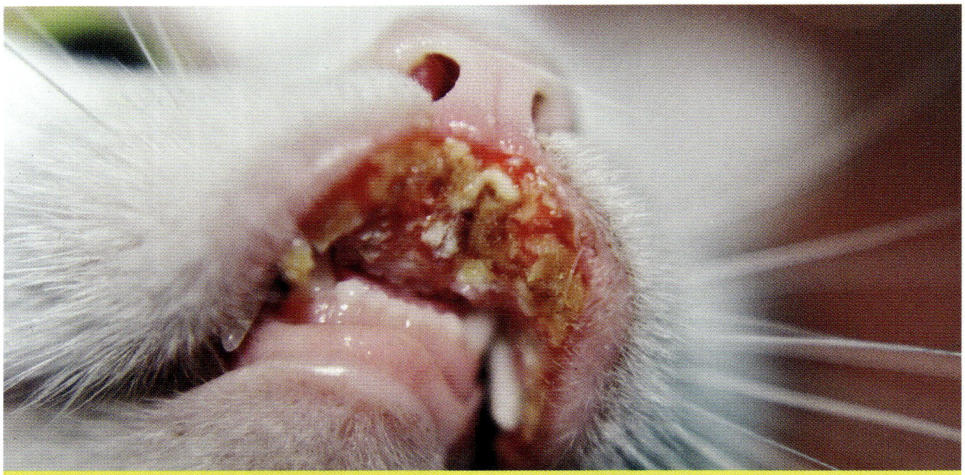

44 Indolent ulcer with infection. Note the characteristic yellowish colouration.

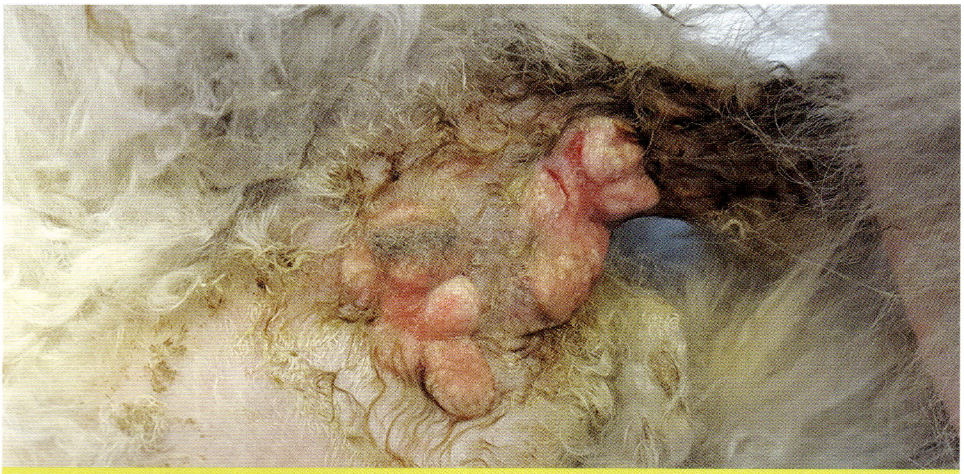

45 Exuberant eosinophilic granulomas on the groin of a Persian cat.

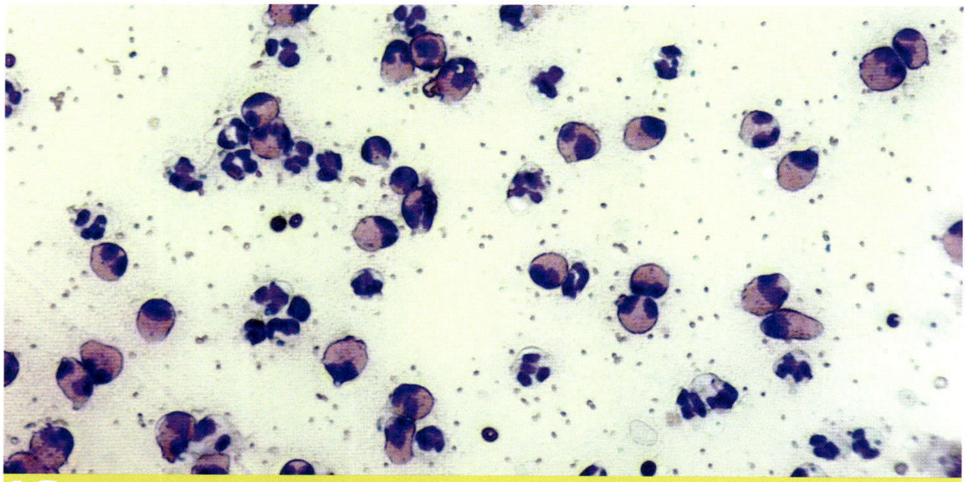

46 Cytology of an eosinophilic plaque from an affected cat. Note the characteristic eosinophils.

# Urticaria pigmentosa

## Lesion aetiology/pathogenesis and clinical picture

This is a mast cell reaction that usually occurs in cats and is characterised by the formation of small yellowish or reddish macules or papules. It more frequently occurs in the Sphynx, Himalayan, and Devon Rex breeds.

The lesions are not always accompanied by pruritus.

It is usually associated with allergic or parasitic conditions.

## Main differential diagnoses

- Miliary dermatitis of other aetiology
- Pigment disorders

## Treatment

It is very important to identify the primary cause of this reaction. If this is achieved, it may be sufficient to prevent the reaction.

Treatment options include corticosteroids, antihistamines, and oclacitinib.

In the case of very frequent recurrence, control can be achieved using cyclosporine, palmitoylethanolamide, or oclacitinib.

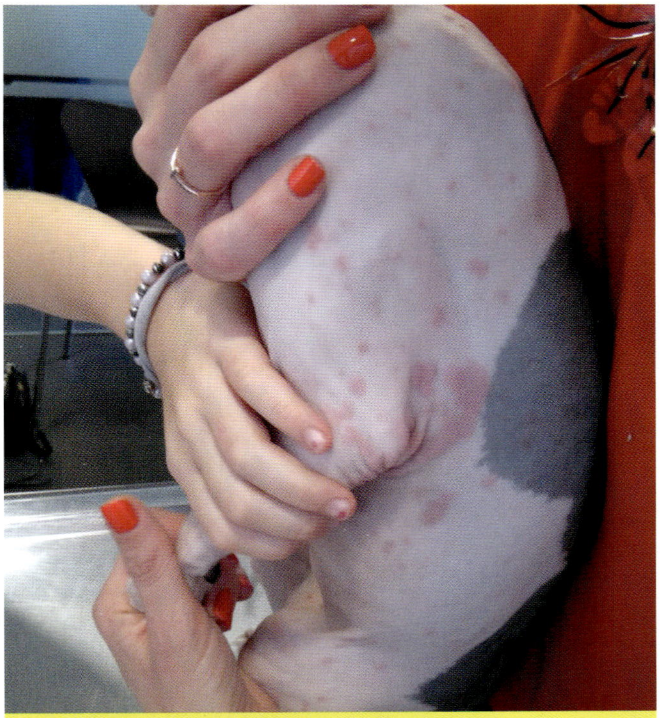

47 Initial stage of urticaria pigmentosa in a Sphynx cat.

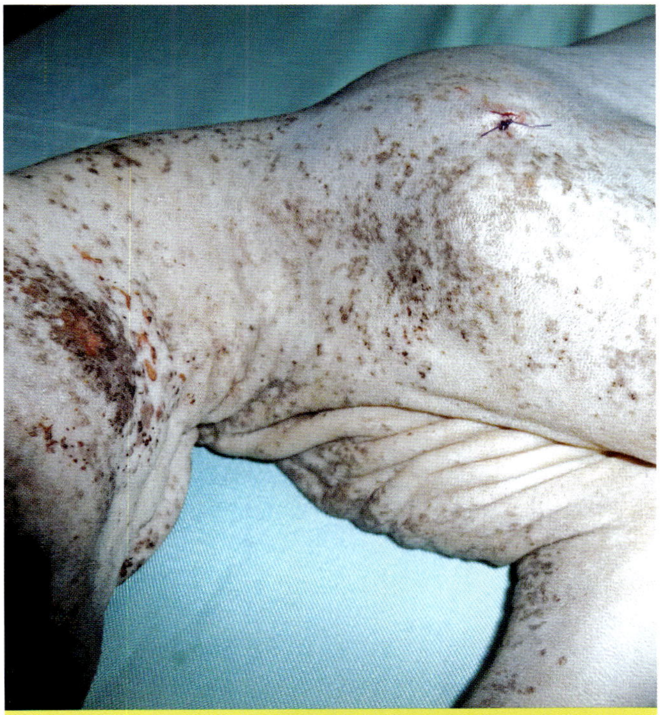

48 Advanced crusting stage of urticaria pigmentosa in a Sphynx cat. Image courtesy of Marino Moro.

# Drug reactions

## Lesion aetiology/pathogenesis and clinical picture

These can include cutaneous reactions to different substances. They can be caused by hypersensitivity (often type III hypersensitivity, as in erythema multiforme) or drug-specific reactions, or can be idiopathic (i.e. of unknown aetiology). The lesions can appear acutely or gradually, and the clinical picture can vary considerably, ranging from simple itching with scaling, erythroderma, nodules, and macules to erosions and ulcers. Underlying vascular processes are more common in dogs, and in severe cases can give rise to toxic epidermal necrolysis. Pruritic dermatosis is more common in cats, often accompanied by scaling and shedding of hair.

## Diagnostic method

Diagnosis is not always easy to establish, and is based on the clinical history and clinical signs, after ruling out other diseases. When the condition coincides with application of a topical substance it is easier to diagnose, but in some cases, mainly those involving vasculitis, lesions can take several weeks to appear.

## Main differential diagnoses

- Tumours
- Deep infections
- Vasculitis due to other causes
- Necrosis due to extravasation of irritant medications
- Burns

## Treatment

Treatment is based on removal of the causative substance and administration of the most innocuous drugs possible (unrelated to those administered previously). Fluid therapy and administration of pentoxifylline and, occasionally, immunosuppressants can be useful.

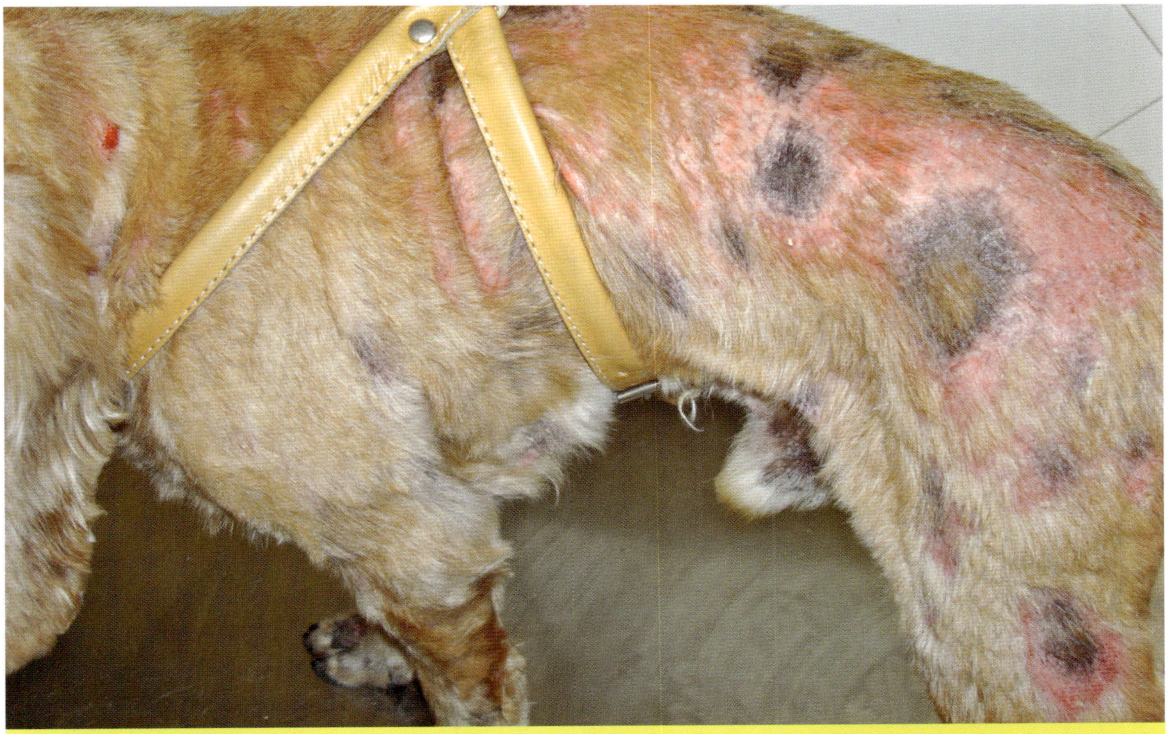

49 Severe erythroderma in a dog after ingestion of an antiparasitic agent.

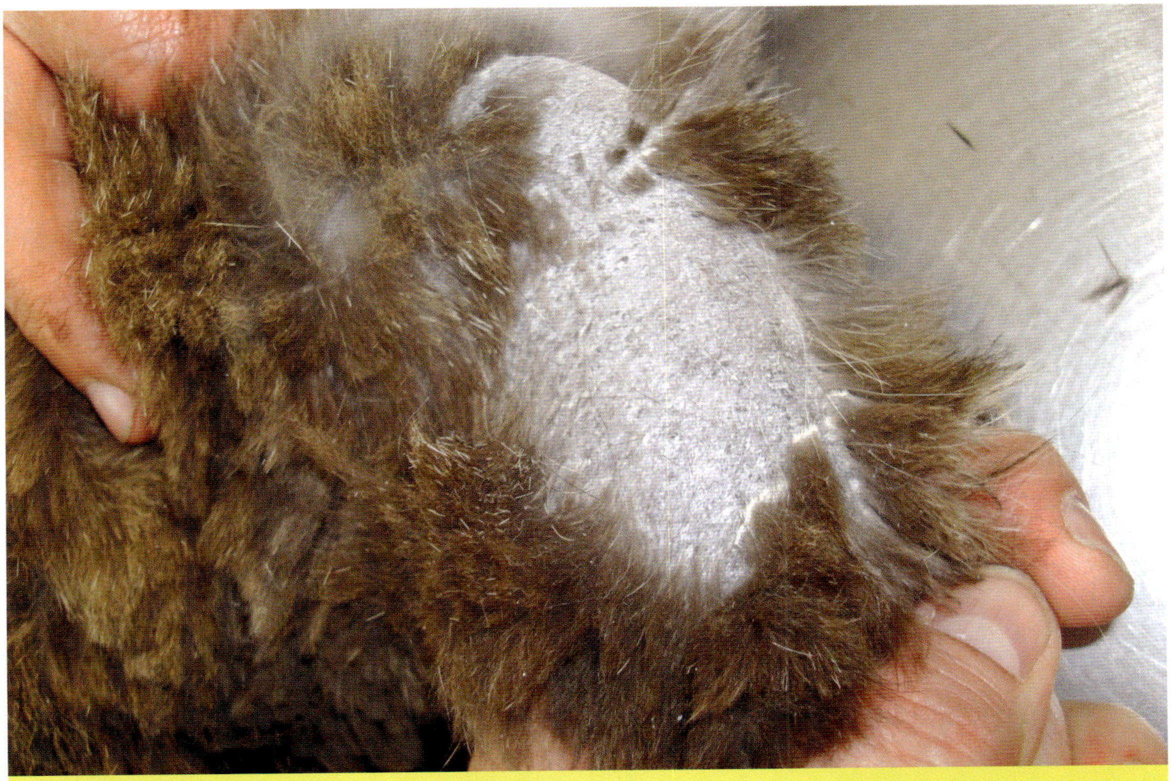

50 Cat with skin reaction following application of a solvent.

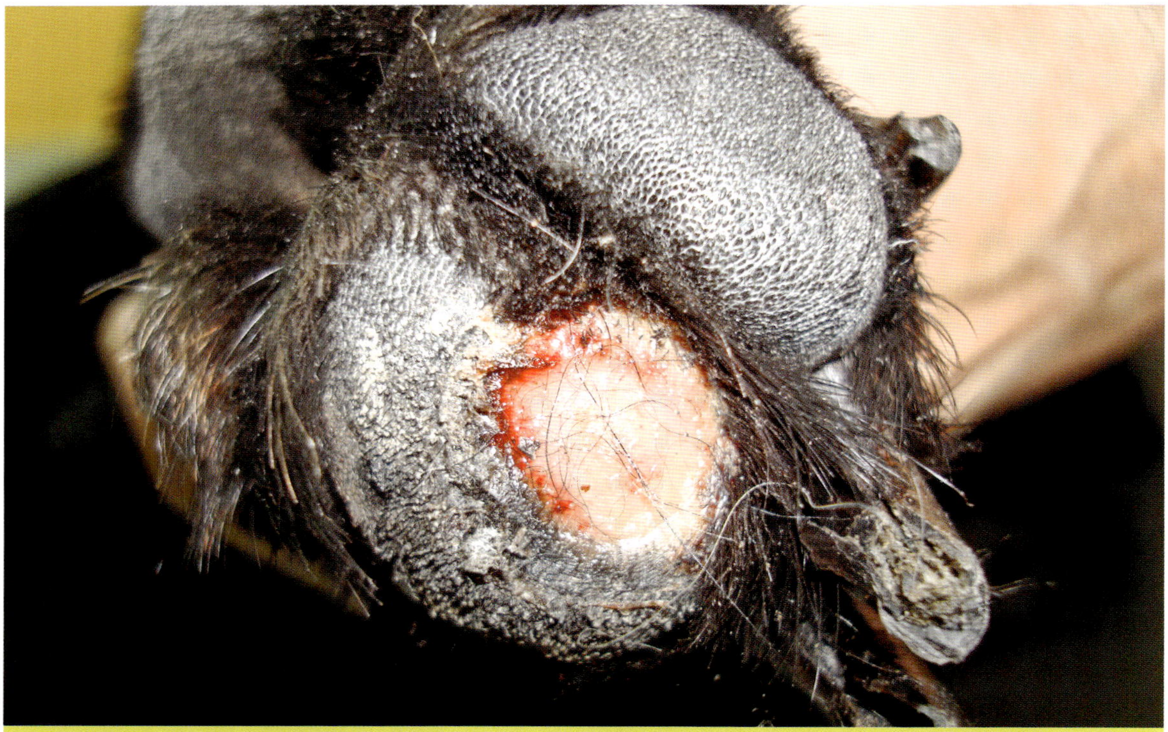

51 Paw pad ulcer due to postvaccinal vasculitis.

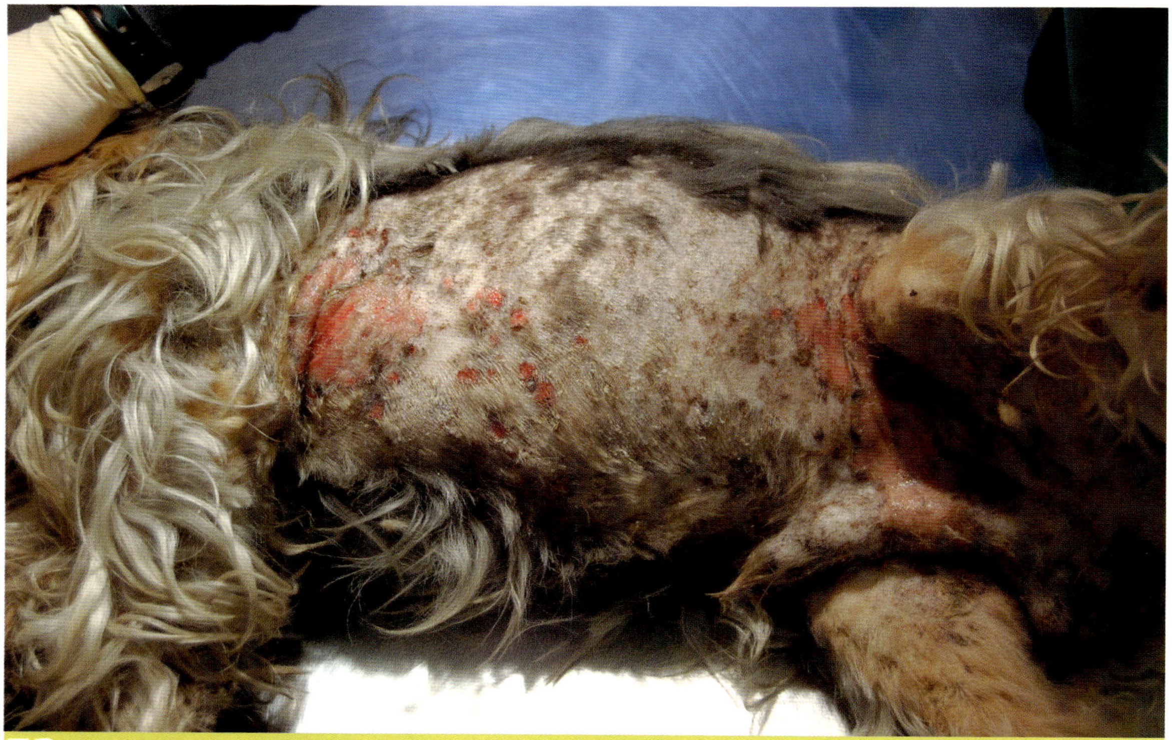

52 Severe erythema multiforme. Image courtesy of the Fauna Veterinary Clinic (Spain).

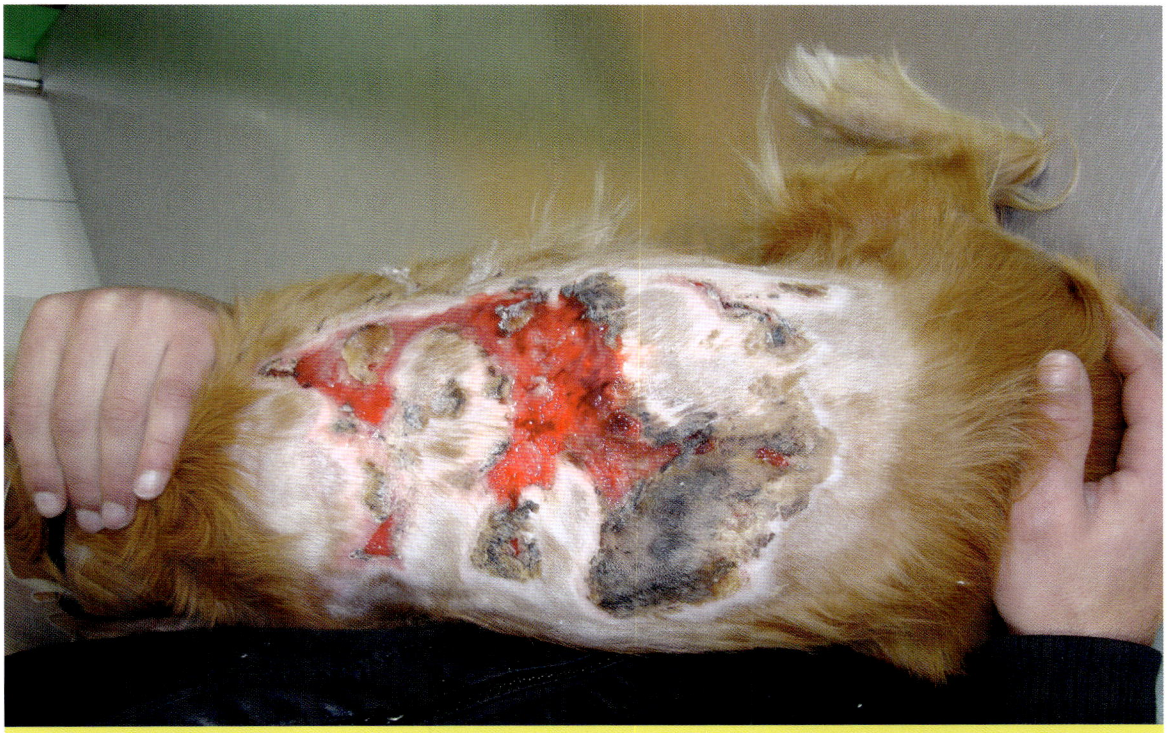
53 Close-up view of skin ulcers in a dog with toxic epidermal necrolysis.

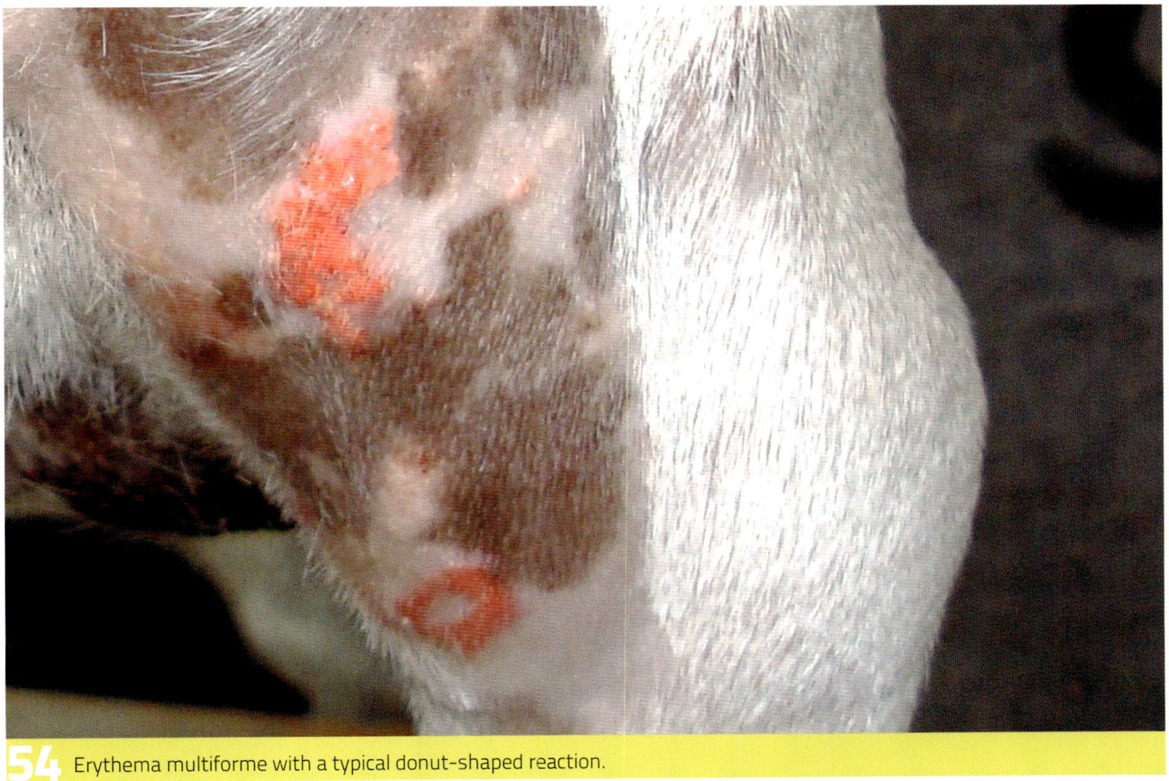
54 Erythema multiforme with a typical donut-shaped reaction.

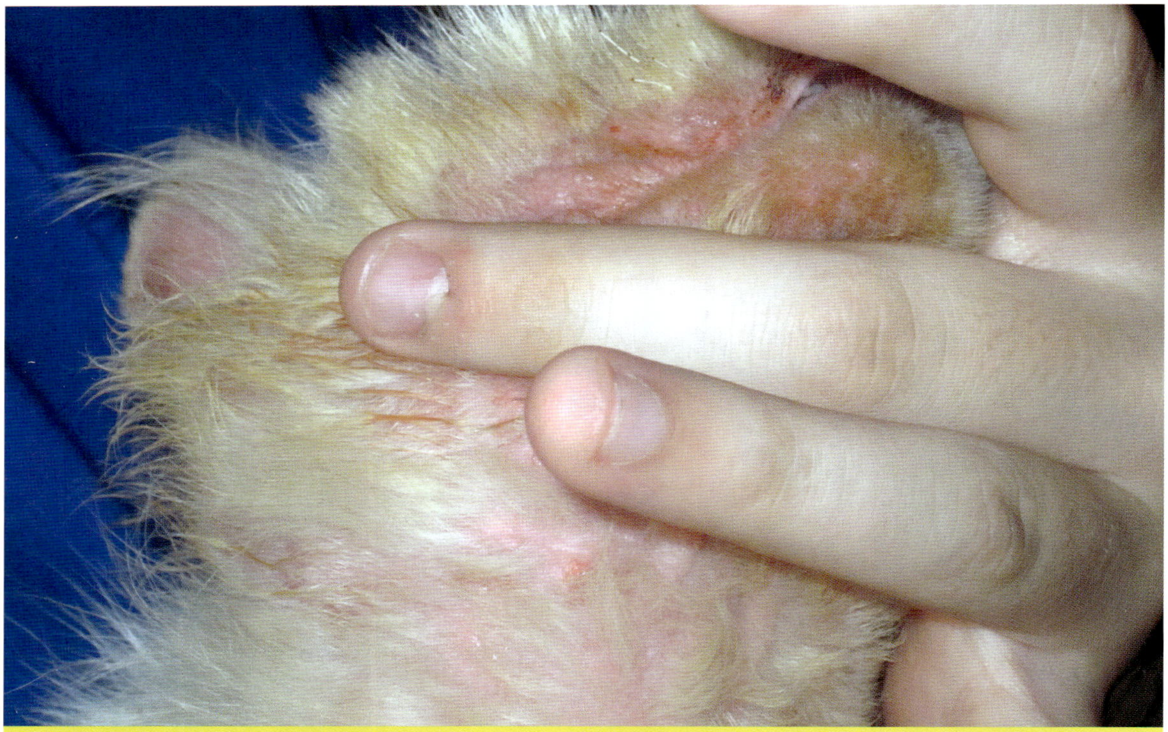
55 Very marked erythema on the neck of a cat after administration of medication for hyperthyroidism.

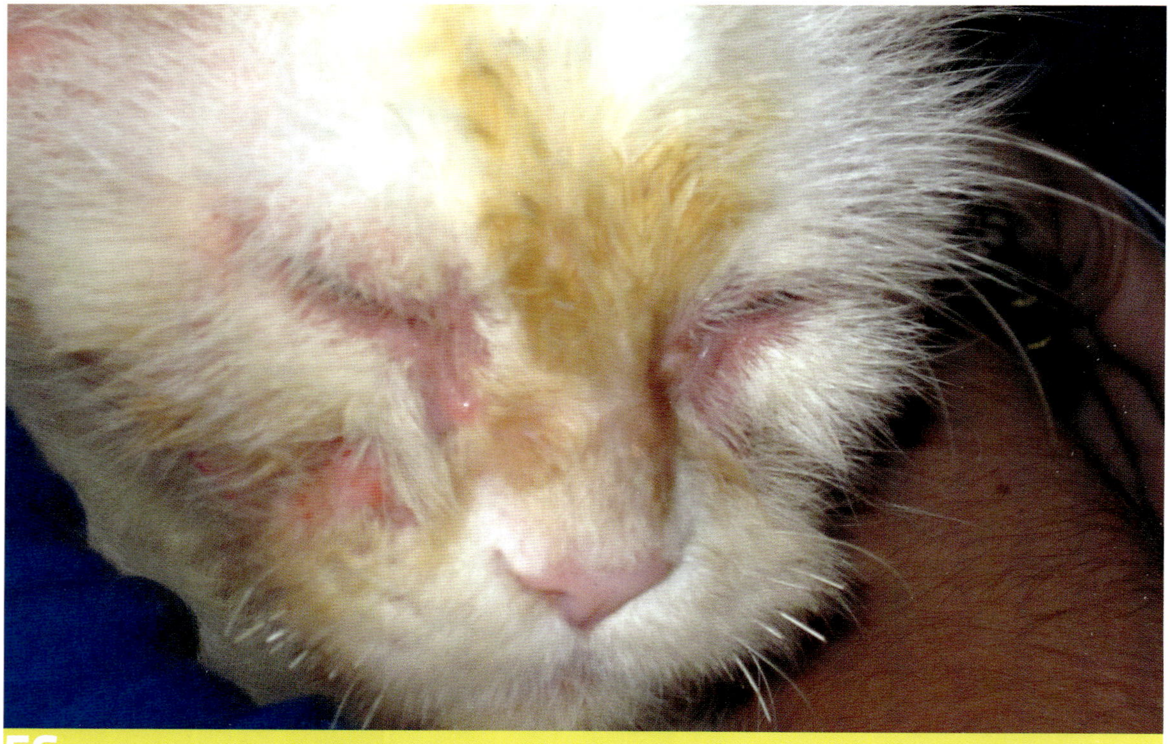
56 Face of the cat with a drug reaction from the previous photo.

# 07

# Dermatoses of endocrine and metabolic origin

# Introduction

The following skin conditions of endocrine and metabolic origin are covered in this book:

- Hypothyroidism
- Feline hyperthyroidism
- Hyperadrenocorticism
- Growth hormone disturbances
- Sex hormone dermatoses:
  - Hyperoestrogenism in females
  - Hyperoestrogenism in males
- Alopecia X
- Hepatocutaneous syndrome
- Shar Pei mucinosis
- Calcinosis circumscripta

Poor hair coat condition and diffuse and symmetric alopecia are clinical signs common to endocrine and metabolic dermatoses. These conditions tend to entail deterioration of the animal's general condition, except in the case of alopecia X, which is merely a cosmetic problem and is classified by some authors as a nonendocrine noninflammatory form of alopecia.

Hepatocutaneous syndrome is thought to be caused by metabolic alterations of hepatic or pancreatic origin. Often it is associated with a tumour, in which case it can be considered a form of paraneoplasia.

Shar Pei mucinosis can be considered a metabolic alteration in mucin production, while calcinosis may be linked to altered calcium metabolism.

Zinc-responsive dermatoses can be included in this group, although they are generally classified as a form of keratinisation disorder.

# Hypothyroidism

## Lesion aetiology/pathogenesis and clinical picture

This is a highly overdiagnosed endocrine disease caused by a lack of thyroxine production by the thyroid gland. It is the second most prevalent endocrine disease in dogs. By contrast, it is very rare in cats. It usually occurs in dogs over 4 years of age, mainly in medium- or large-sized breeds.

The clinical picture is highly variable, although diffuse alopecia with coarse hair, a tendency towards obesity, and recurrent otitis and bacterial and yeast dermatoses are common. Alopecia is more common on the bony prominences, flanks, and tail.

## Diagnostic method

Diagnosis is established based on the clinical picture and measurement of thyroxine ($T_4$) and thyrotropin (TSH) levels. The likelihood of diagnosis increases if hypercholesterolaemia, hypertriglyceridaemia, mild anaemia, drowsiness, and inappetence are also present. It is important to bear in mind the possibility of encountering euthyroid sick syndrome, which can complicate the diagnosis.

Chronic hypothyroidism can sometimes be accompanied by low $T_4$ levels and TSH at borderline or normal levels due to pituitary fatigue.

## Main differential diagnoses

- Other endocrinopathies
- Follicular dysplasia

## Treatment

Treatment consists of specific thyroxine supplementation. In addition, bacteria and yeast overgrowth should be controlled and shampoos used to combat dry hair coat.

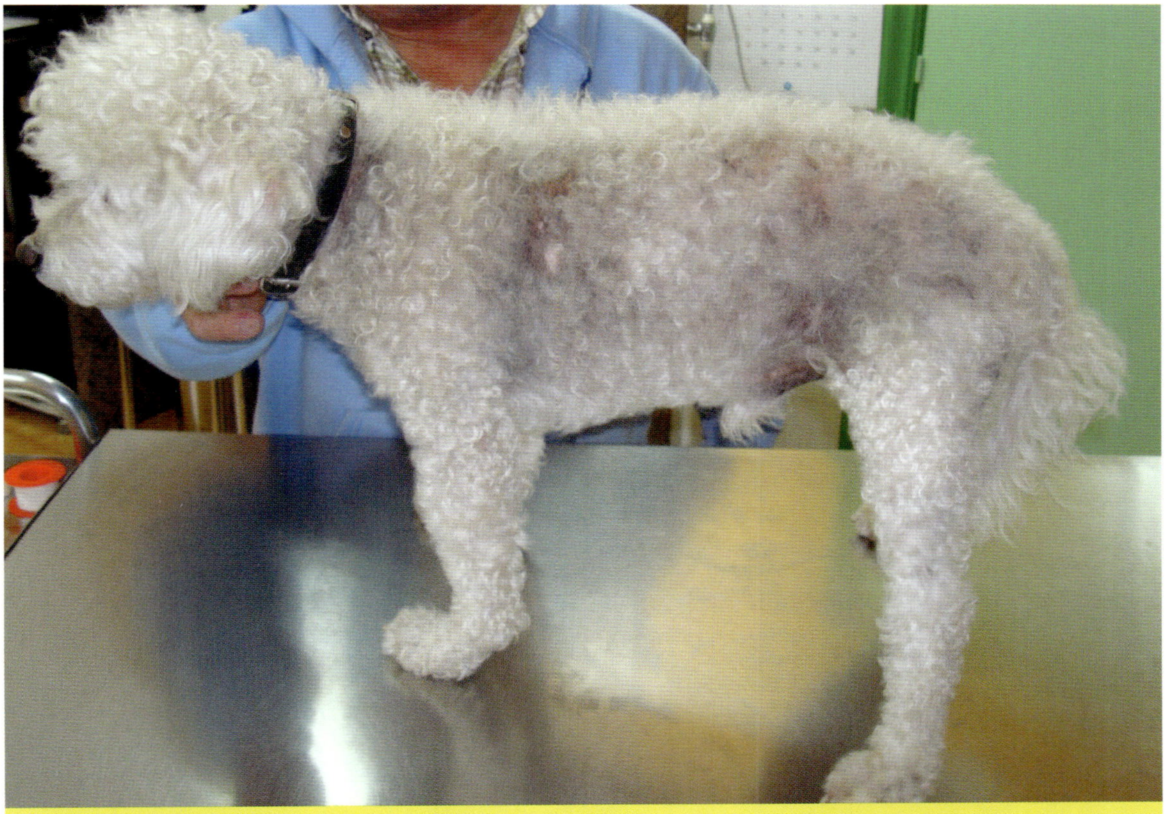

01 Poor hair coat appearance and hyperpigmentation in a dog with hypothyroidism.

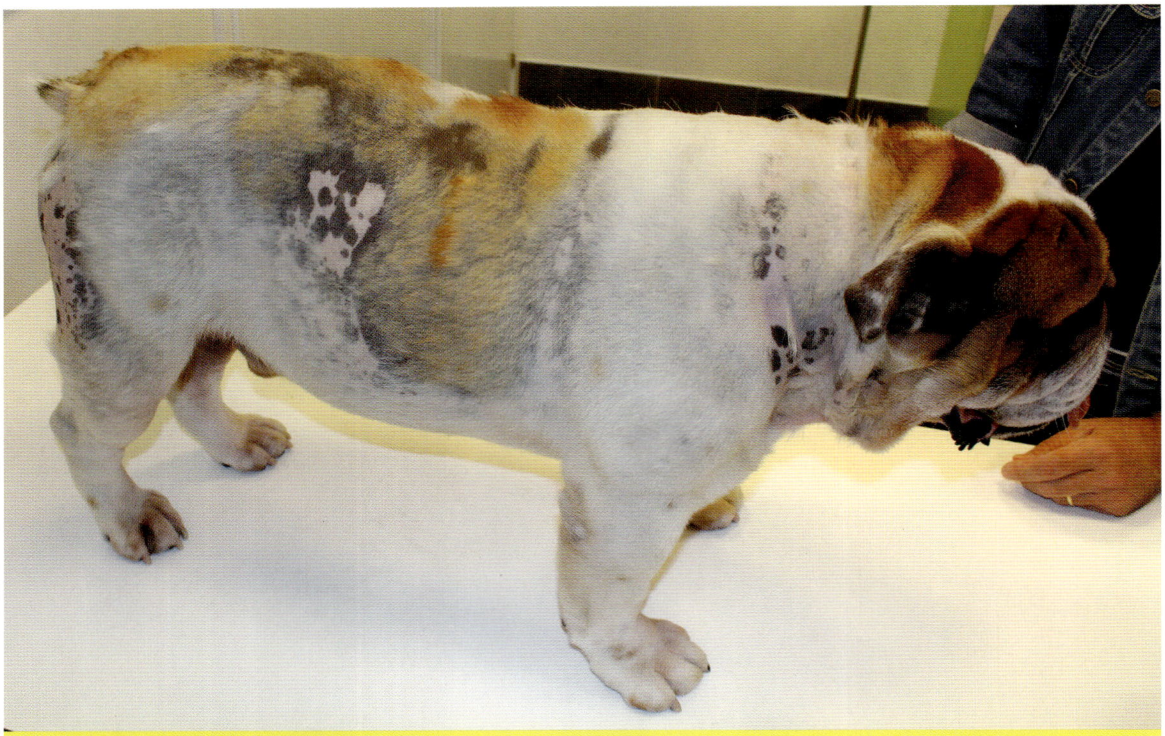

02 Diffuse alopecia and coarse hair in an English Bulldog with hypothyroidism.

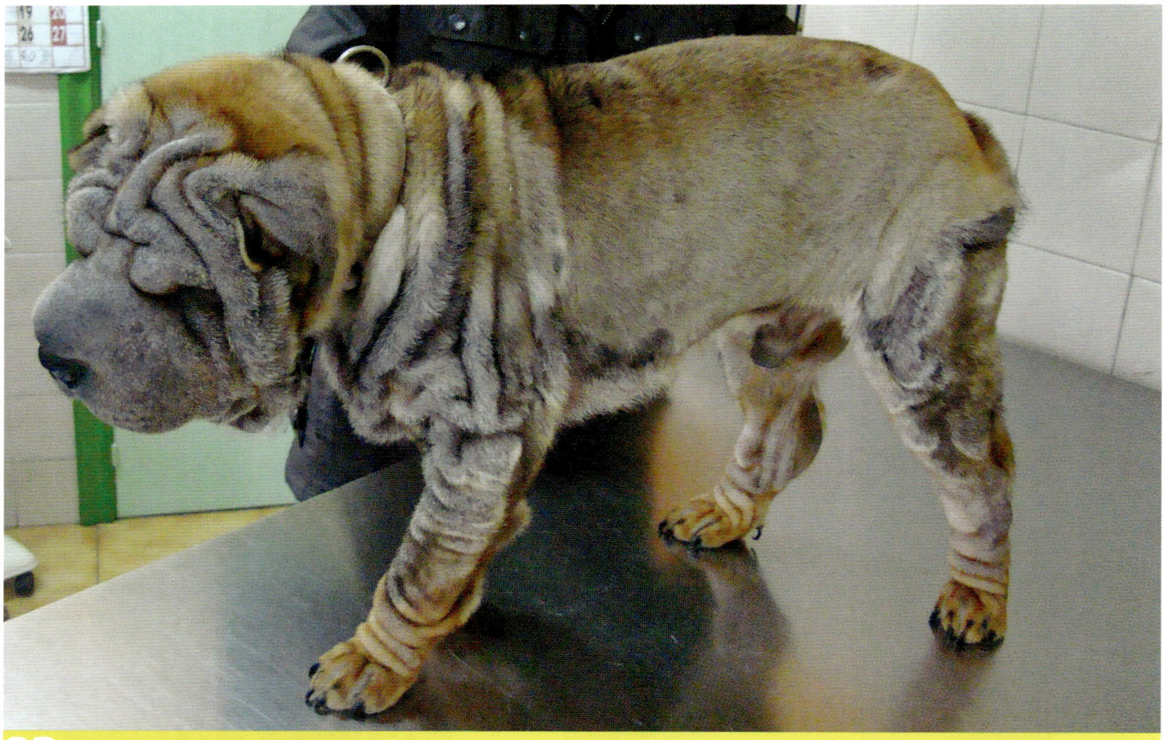

03 Shar Pei with hypothyroidism and myxoedema.

# Feline hyperthyroidism

## Lesion aetiology/pathogenesis and clinical picture

This disease does not always manifest with cutaneous clinical signs, but the patient's state of anxiety often leads to exaggerated grooming, which, together with weight loss, leads to a dishevelled, alopecic appearance with prominent bones.

Elderly animals are typically affected.

## Diagnostic method

A definitive diagnosis can be established based on palpation of an enlarged thyroid in the cervical area, tachycardia, and a clinical history revealing weight loss and excitation, together with the measurement of $T_4$ levels.

## Main differential diagnoses

- Self-induced alopecia of other aetiology
- Other wasting diseases

## Treatment

Treatment with methimazole or carbimazole is usually effective. Other options include a low-iodine diet, thyroidectomy, and administration of radioactive iodine.

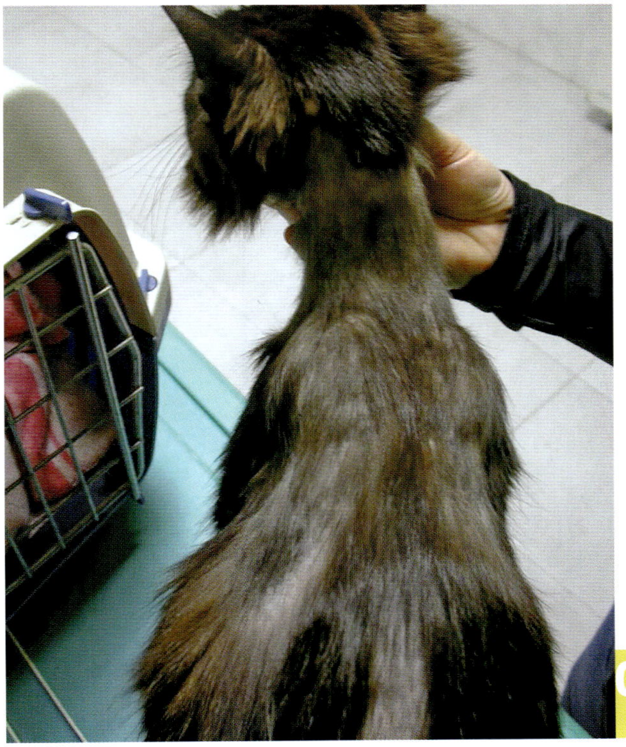

04 Cat with hyperthyroidism. Note the marked weight loss and self-induced alopecia.

# Hyperadrenocorticism

## Lesion aetiology/pathogenesis and clinical picture

Hyperadrenocorticism (HAC), also known as Cushing's syndrome, is the most prevalent endocrine disease in dogs. An excess of cortisol is caused by tumours in the pituitary gland, which secretes more corticotropin (ACTH), or in the adrenal gland. An excess of corticosteroids can also be caused by treatment errors when these drugs are indiscriminately administered either systemically or topically. However, iatrogenic HAC is less common nowadays with the availability of newer antipruritic molecules such as oclacitinib and lokivetmab.

HAC tends to occur more frequently in dogs of over 8 years of age, and primarily affects small breeds and Boxers. It is very rare in cats.

Cutaneous clinical signs include very thin skin with visible telangiectasias, a barrel-shaped abdomen, abundant comedones, diffuse alopecia mainly affecting the trunk, and cutaneous calcinosis. Recurrent pyodermas can also occur, together with characteristic systemic clinical signs including polyuria/polydipsia, panting, polyphagia, and muscle atrophy. Generalised adult demodicosis is another potential complication of this disease. A paradox that must be taken into account is that despite the excess of cortisol, cutaneous calcinosis can make this disease highly pruritogenic due to fissures and infections caused by calcium accumulation.

This disease is very rare in cats, although the iatrogenic form, which may be accompanied by fragile skin, can occur with a slightly higher incidence in this species.

## Diagnostic method

Confirmation of the diagnosis is based on the clinical picture, in some cases accompanied by a stress leukogram, elevated alkaline phosphatase levels, hypersecretion of cortisol upon stimulation with ACTH, or a nonresponse in the dexamethasone suppression test. An ultrasound of the adrenal glands often reveals hyperplasia. Iatrogenic Cushing's syndrome is diagnosed by measuring basal cortisol levels in the blood, which are usually very low and do not respond to ACTH stimulation. In such cases the adrenal glands are usually atrophic.

## Main differential diagnoses

- Other endocrinopathies
- Other keratinisation disorders
- Cutaneous calcinosis of other aetiology
- Other diseases that cause polyuria–polydipsia

## Treatment

Classic treatments with mitotane or ketoconazole have been replaced in many countries with trilostane, which is usually effective. Surgery may be an option in patients with resectable tumours.

In cases of iatrogenic HAC, administration of corticosteroids should be gradually discontinued.

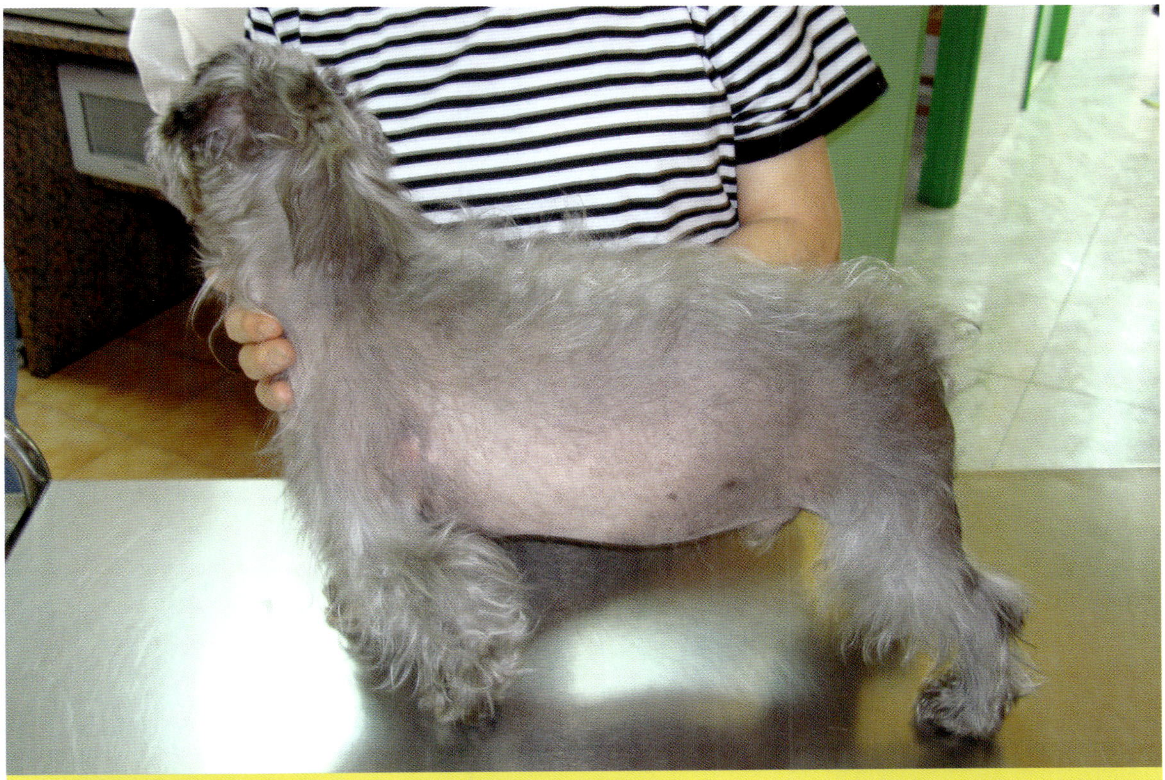

05 Cushing's syndrome of pituitary origin in a 10-year-old Schnauzer mix.

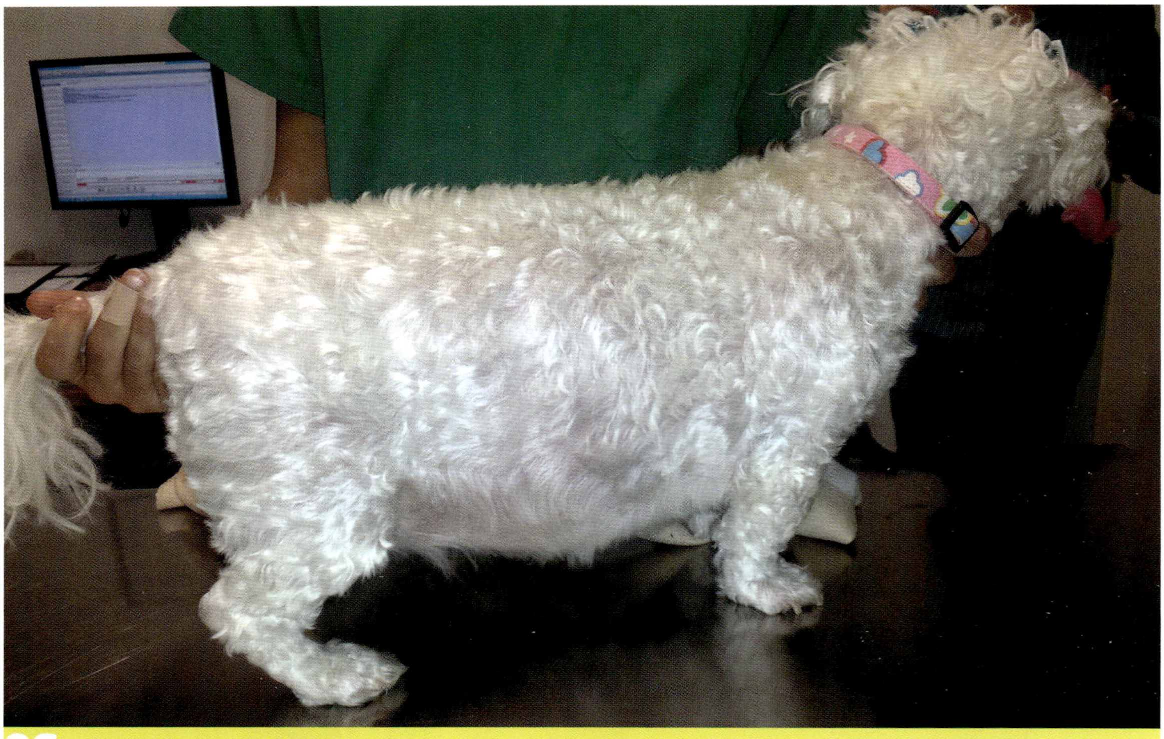

06 Cushing's syndrome with abdominal dilation, without clear skin manifestations.

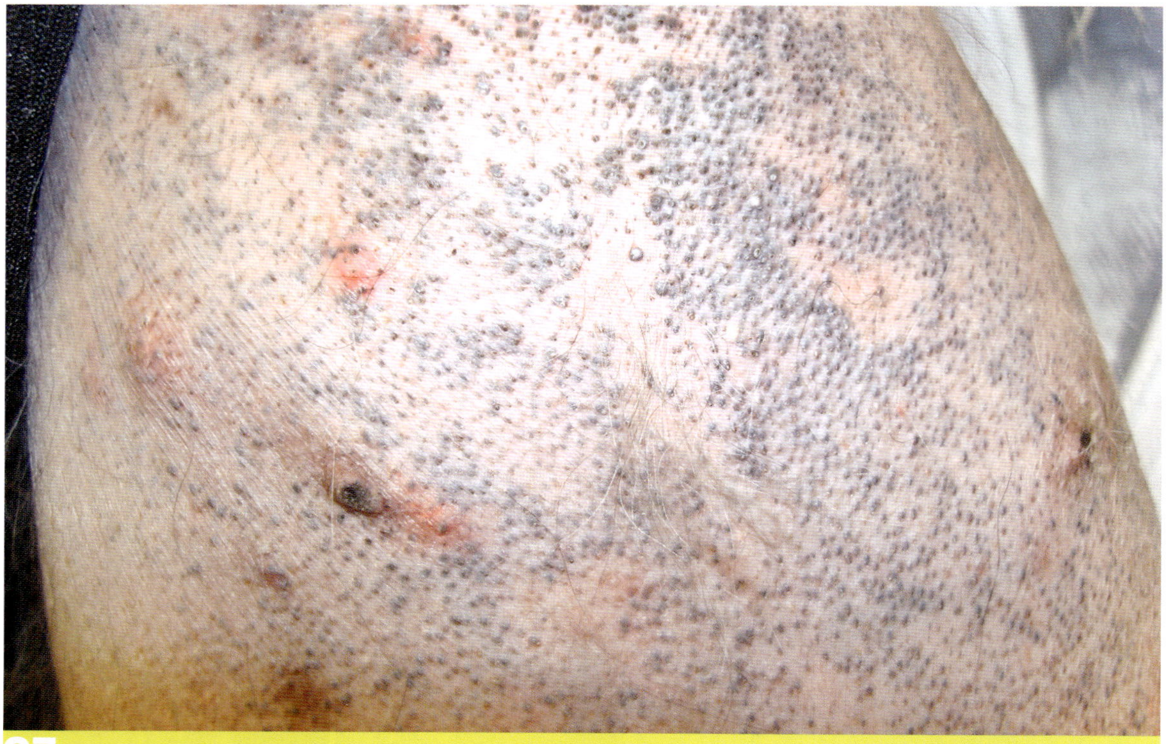

07 Abundant comedones on the skin of the dog from Figure 5.

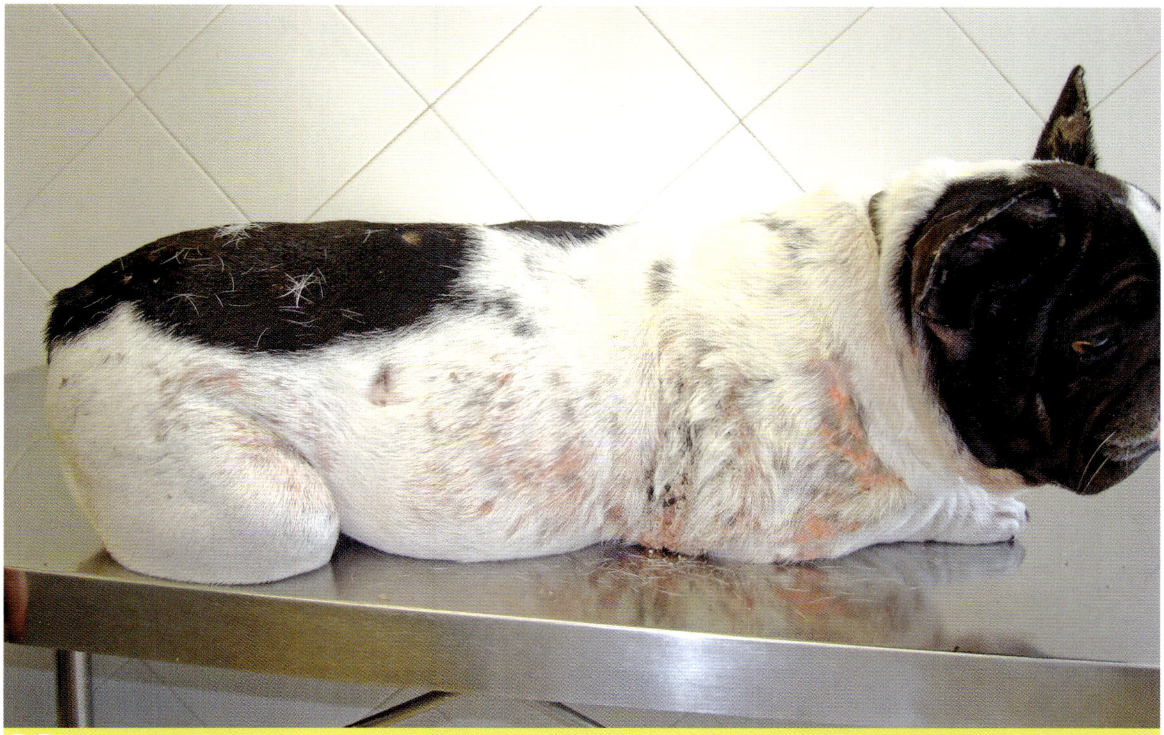

08 Cutaneous calcinosis in a French Bulldog with iatrogenic Cushing's syndrome.

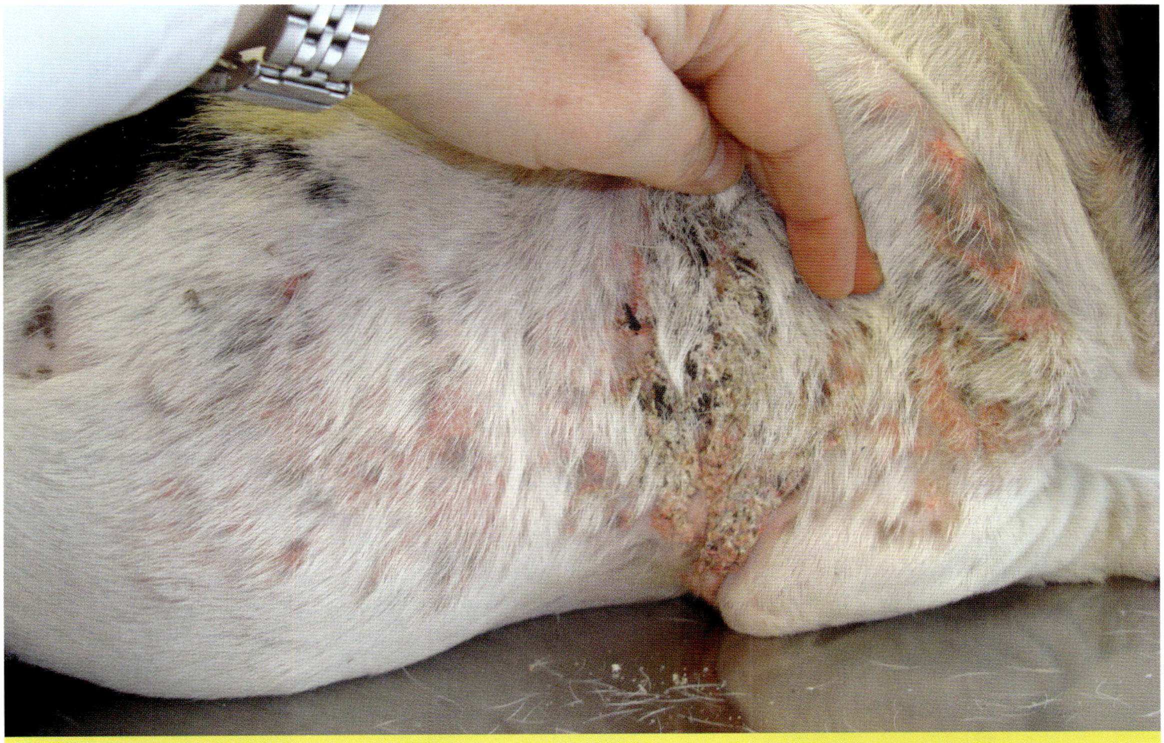

09 Close-up image showing the accumulation of calcium salts in the skin of the dog from the previous image.

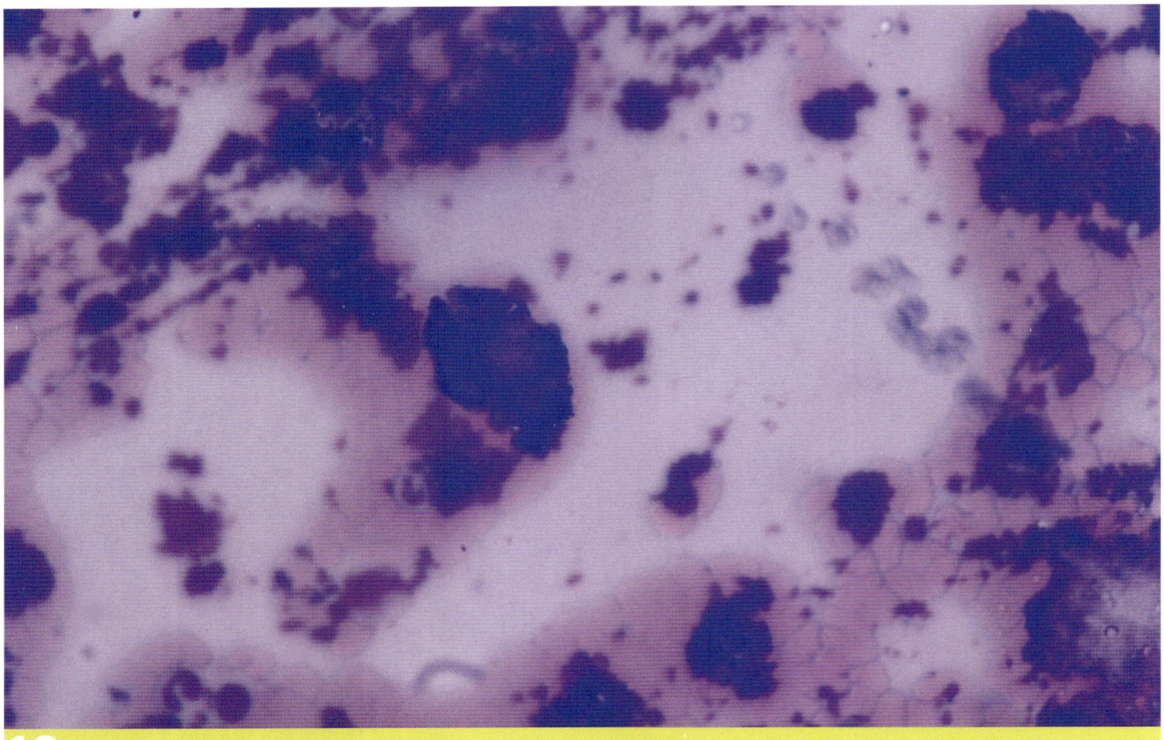

10 Cytology in a case of calcinosis, in which the bluish colouration verifies the presence of calcium salts.

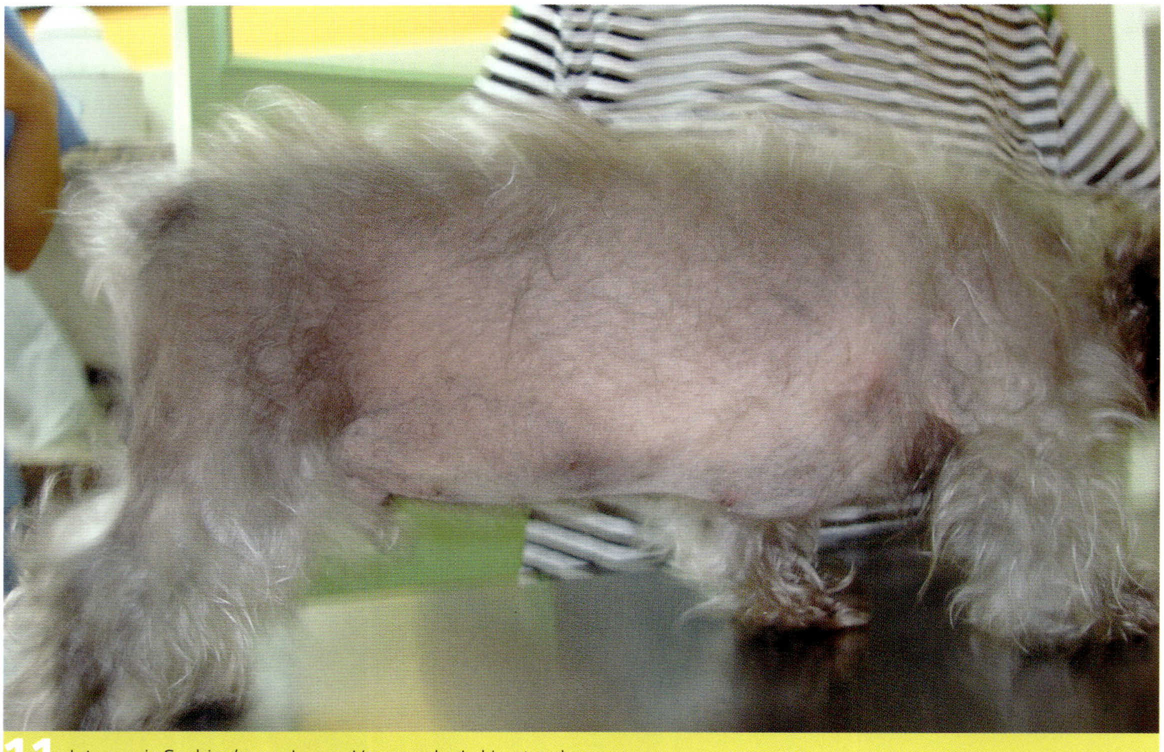

11 Iatrogenic Cushing's syndrome. Very marked skin atrophy.

# Growth hormone disturbances

## Lesion aetiology/pathogenesis and clinical picture

- **Hyposecretion:** a rare adenohypophyseal hormonal deficiency, mainly in growth hormone (GH), results in growth impairment, which manifests with hair development disorders due to the persistence of puppy hair, progressing to symmetric alopecia in the cervical area, thighs, and trunk. Skin infections, hyperpigmentation, and scaling are common. This disorder is more frequent in German Shepherds and is inherited in a simple autosomal recessive manner. The cutaneous picture is usually accompanied by characteristic growth retardation, with altered TSH and prolactin production. ACTH secretion is usually maintained. There are very few reports of this condition in cats.
- **Hypersecretion:** conversely, excess GH in dogs, also known as acromegaly or hypersomatotropism, is almost always caused by hypersecretion of GH induced by progesterone in the mammary gland. Cutaneous signs include poor hair coat, oedema, and general thickening of the skin. Feline acromegaly is a very rare disease, and most commonly affects middle-aged and older neutered cats. No breed predisposition has been described. Cats with acromegaly often have insulin-resistant diabetes mellitus (insulin doses dependent on the type of insulin) with concurrent weight gain rather than weight loss. Fragile skin and a poor hair coat may be observed.

## Diagnostic method

- **Hyposecretion:** the clinical presentation together with the clinical history are quite conclusive. There is usually a decrease in plasma levels of total and free $T_4$, and TSH levels are usually at the lower limit. Insulin-like growth factor (IGF-1), which indirectly reflects GH levels, can be measured in plasma.
- **Hypersecretion:** in dogs this can be diagnosed based on the clinical presentation, a history indicating previous administration of progestogens, and measurement of IGF-1. Measurement of serum IGF-1 is the most widely used diagnostic test for feline acromegaly. Unlike growth hormone, IGF-1 concentrations are less likely to fluctuate throughout the day, as most IGF-1 is bound to proteins, meaning it has a longer half-life in the body. Insulin resistance in diabetes is also a good indicator.

## Main differential diagnoses

- Other endocrine disorders
- Malnutrition
- Liver or kidney disease

## Treatment

In animals with hyposecretion, treatment should be initiated as soon as possible, although it is difficult to achieve normal growth because the bone growth plates seal early. Bovine GH can be used to improve hair and skin condition, although there is a risk of developing hypersensitivity or diabetes. Progestogens can also be relatively effective, stimulating the production of growth hormone in the mammary gland, although there is a risk of adverse effects. Attempts should be made to normalise levels of thyroid and adrenal hormones.

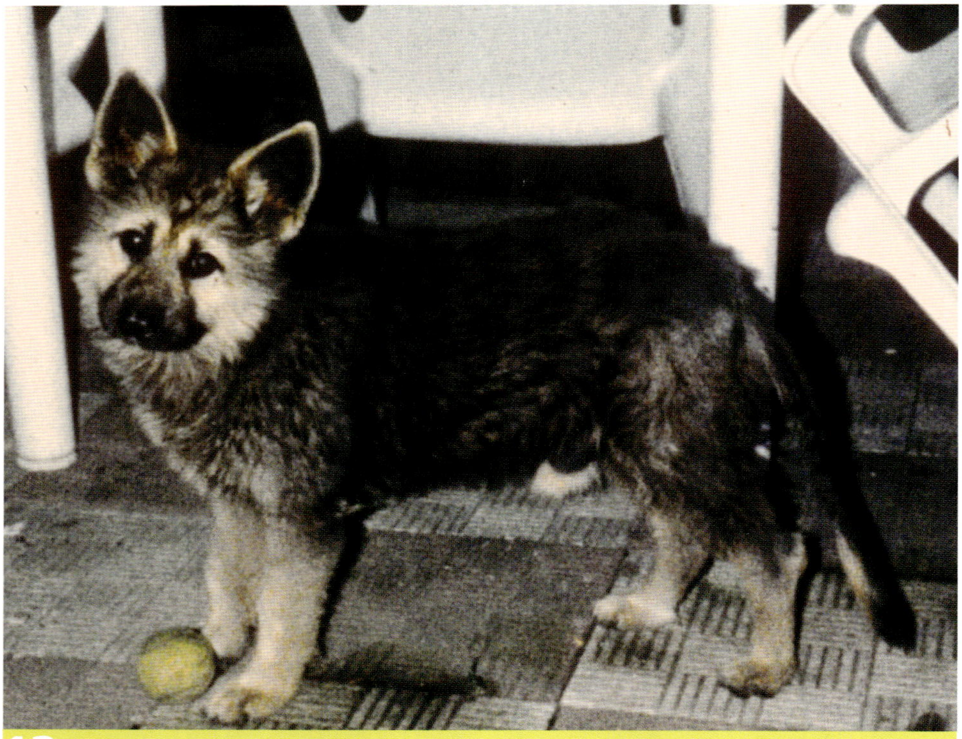

12 Pituitary dwarfism.

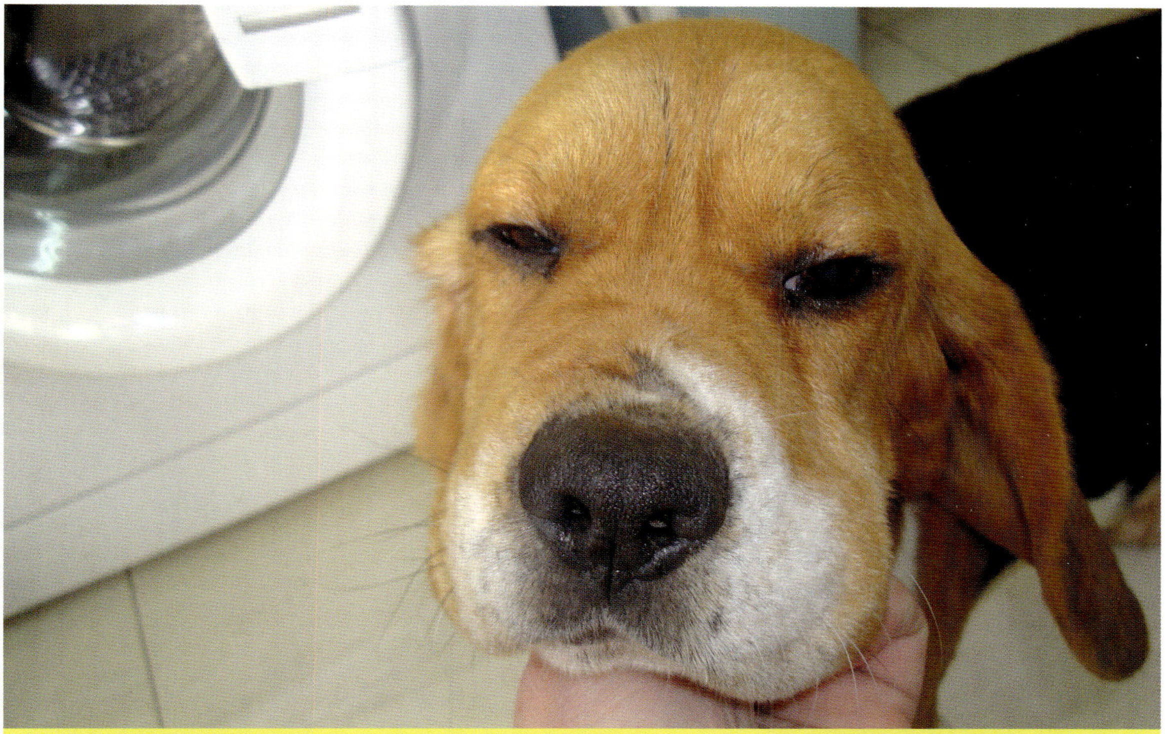

13 Acromegaly induced by excessive use of progestogens. Note the thickening of the skin on the face.

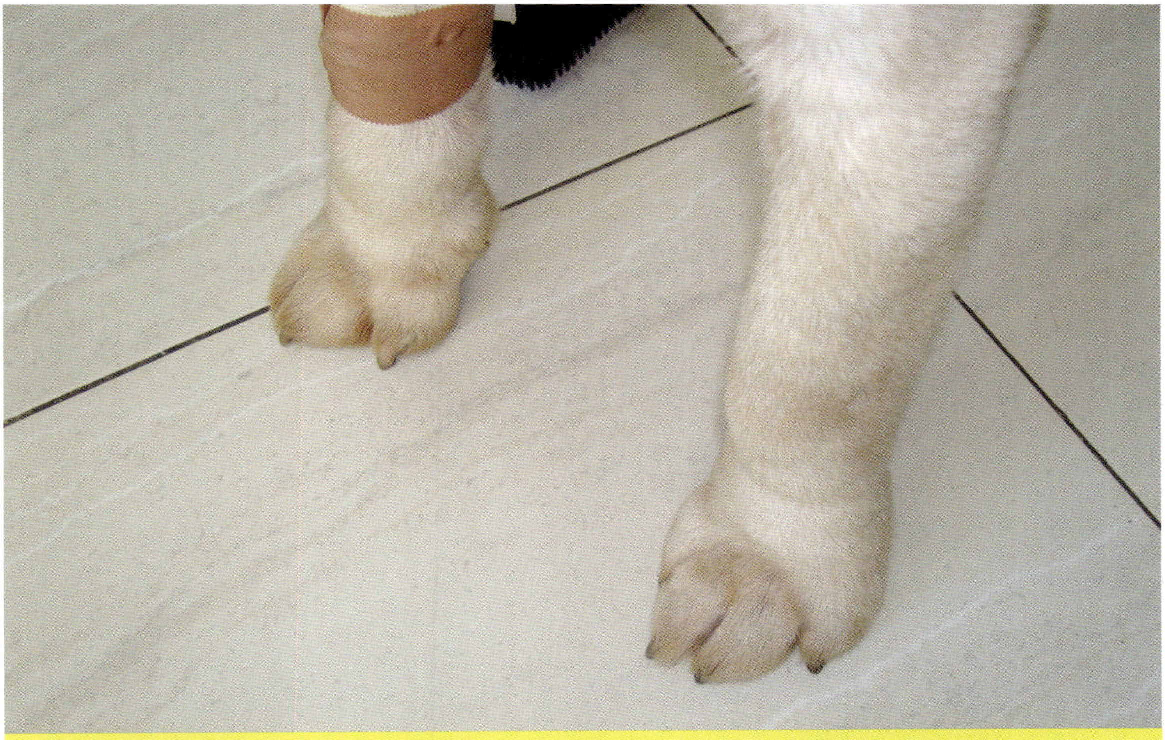

14 Acromegaly induced by excessive use of progestogens. Note the thickening of the skin in the distal portion of the limbs.

# Sex hormones dermatoses

## Hyperoestrogenism in females

### Lesion aetiology/pathogenesis and clinical picture

This is a rare disorder that occurs in female dogs, usually due to ovarian cysts, ovarian tumours, or oestrogen therapy. Progressive alopecia usually occurs on the flanks, perineum, and ventral area of the abdomen. Seborrhoea and ceruminous otitis may also be present. Vulvar and nipple hyperplasia is very common.

Alopecia has also been described in some dogs due to contact with oestrogen supplementation patches used by women with menopausal syndrome.

### Diagnostic method

This condition must be differentiated from other endocrinopathies, for which vulvar and nipple enlargement, together with ovarian ultrasound findings, are very useful. Measurement of oestrogen is not usually necessary, as in many cases levels are within normal limits. In some cases, diagnosis is confirmed based on response to neutering.

### Main differential diagnoses

- Other endocrinopathies
- Other keratinisation disorders
- Chronic cutaneous hyperplasia in allergic females

### Treatment

Ovariohysterectomy results in improvements with 3–4 months. Shampoo therapy is very important to control skin imbalances.

All external oestrogen supplementation should be avoided.

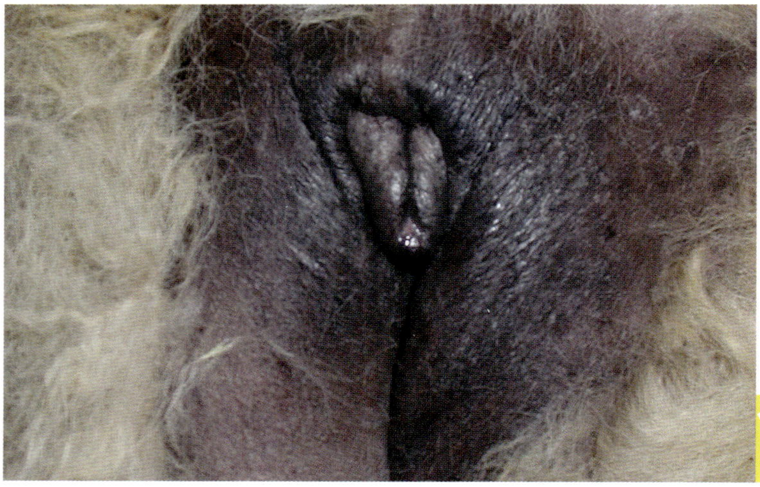

15 Hyperoestrogenism in a female. Note the size of the vulva and the perineal alopecia.

# Hyperoestrogenism in males

## Lesion aetiology/pathogenesis and clinical picture

Testicular tumours, which are usually oestrogen-producing Sertoli cell tumours, can occur in older male dogs. Cryptorchidism is a predisposing factor. The cutaneous presentation is quite characteristic, with diffuse alopecia on the trunk, neck, and hindquarters; coarse, easily epilated hair; seborrhoea; and, frequently, *Malassezia* overgrowth. Gynecomastia and the presence of an erythematous line along the medial raphe of the foreskin are features typical of this anomaly. Testicular asymmetry, attraction to other males, and behavioural changes are also usually present.

The alopecia described above may also occur due to contact with therapeutic oestrogen patches.

## Diagnostic method

Diagnosis is established based on the clinical picture, testicular ultrasound, and clinical history. Measurement of oestradiol levels in blood may be helpful, assuming that the individual's previous physiological levels are known.

Swab cytology of the preputial mucosa shows keratinised cells similar to those observed in vaginal smears from female dogs in oestrus.

## Main differential diagnoses

Other endocrinopathies.

## Treatment

Castration of both testicles is curative. Metastasis occurs in a small percentage of affected animals, sometimes manifesting as a non-response to surgery.

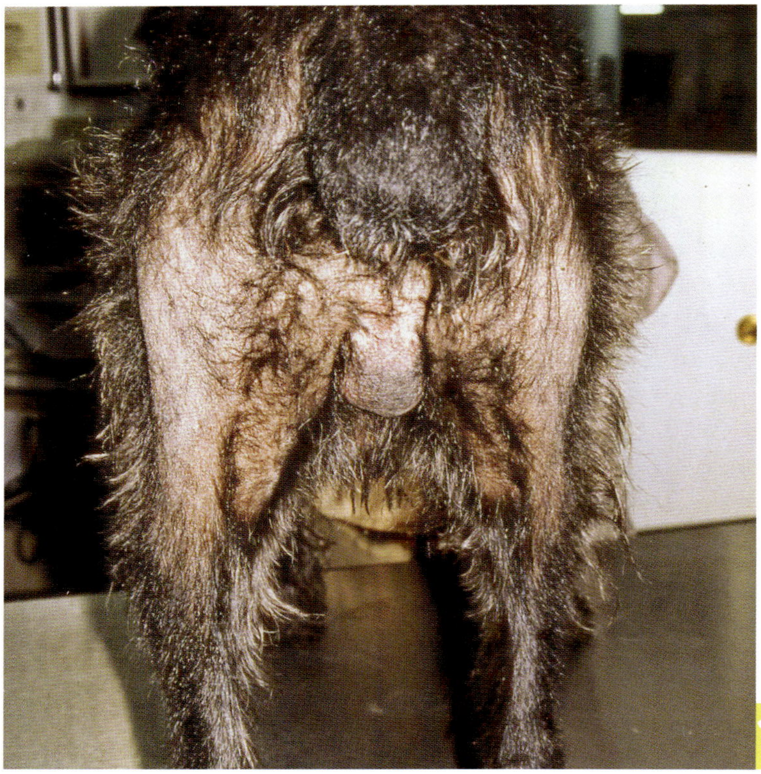

16 Alopecia on both hindlimbs of a dog with a Sertoli cell tumour.

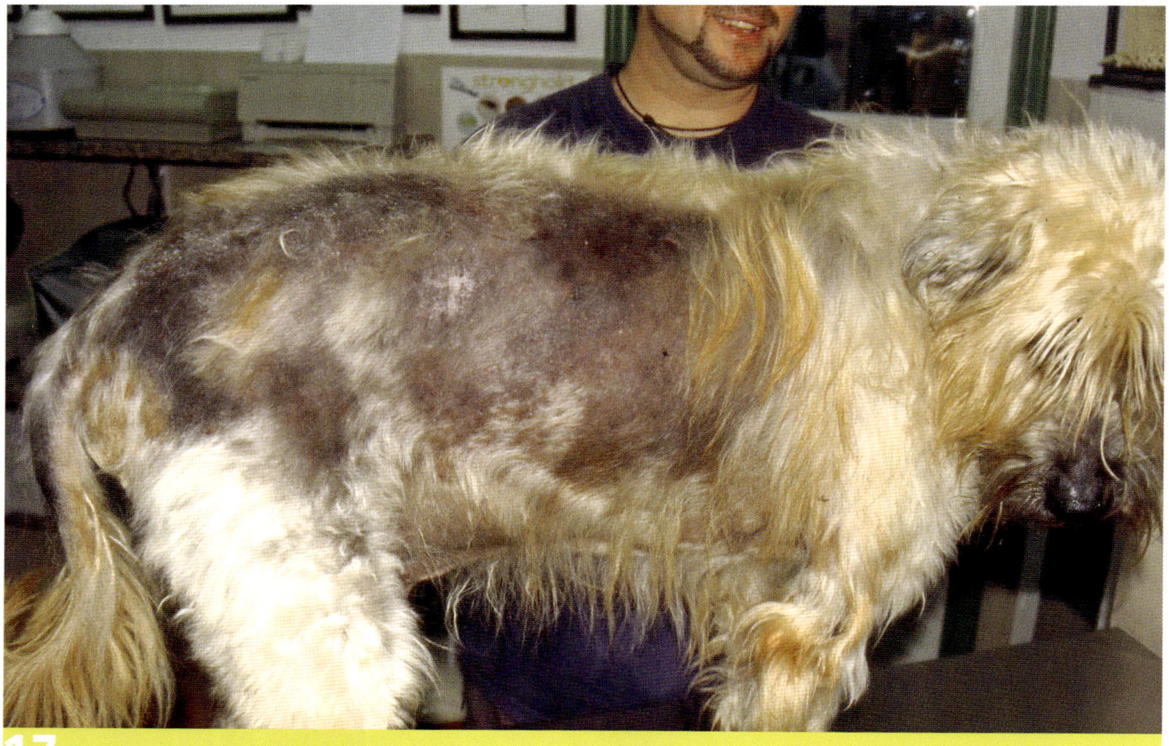

17 Appearance of the trunk of another dog with a testicular tumour. Note the poor hair coat quality.

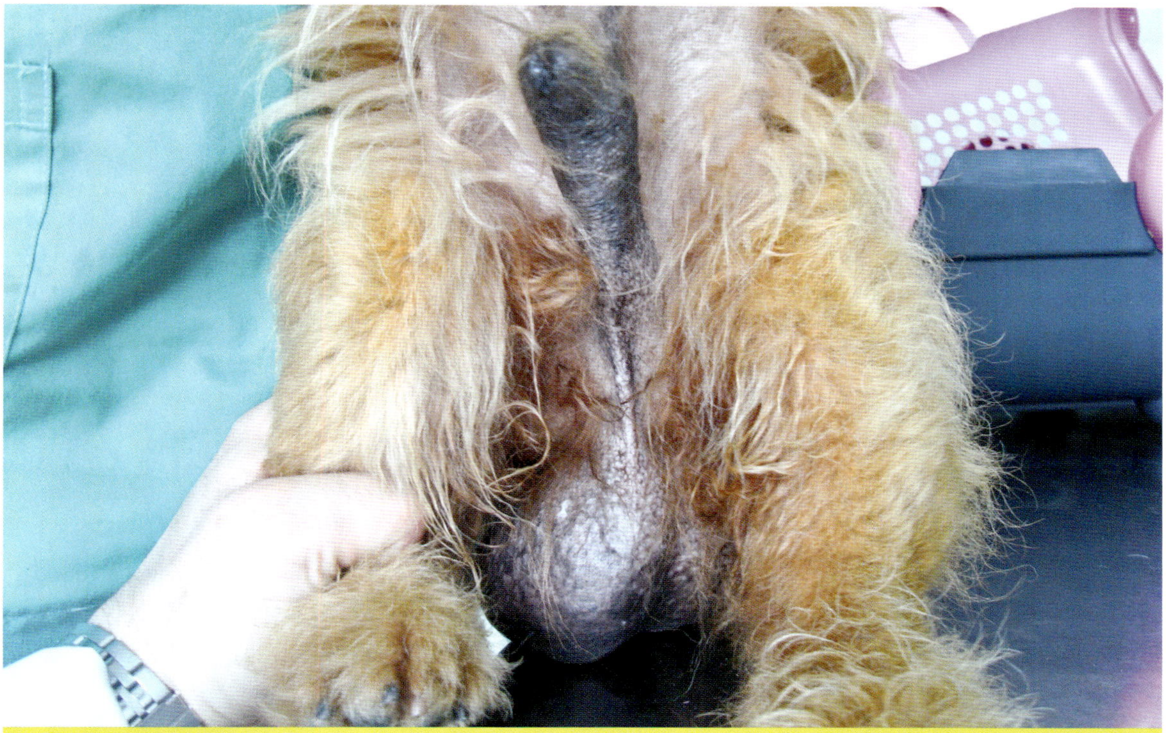

18 Testicular asymmetry and gynecomastia with hyperpigmentation in a dog with a Sertoli cell tumour.

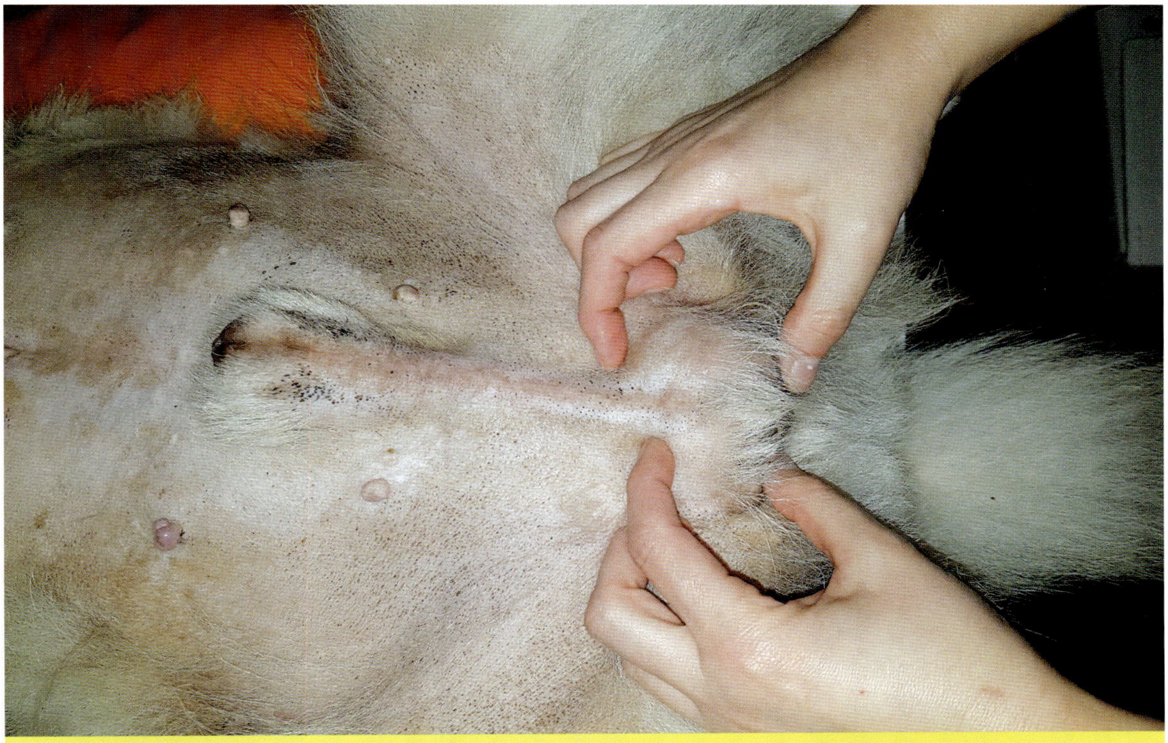

19 Erythematous line along the prepuce and testicular asymmetry in a dog with a Sertoli cell tumour.

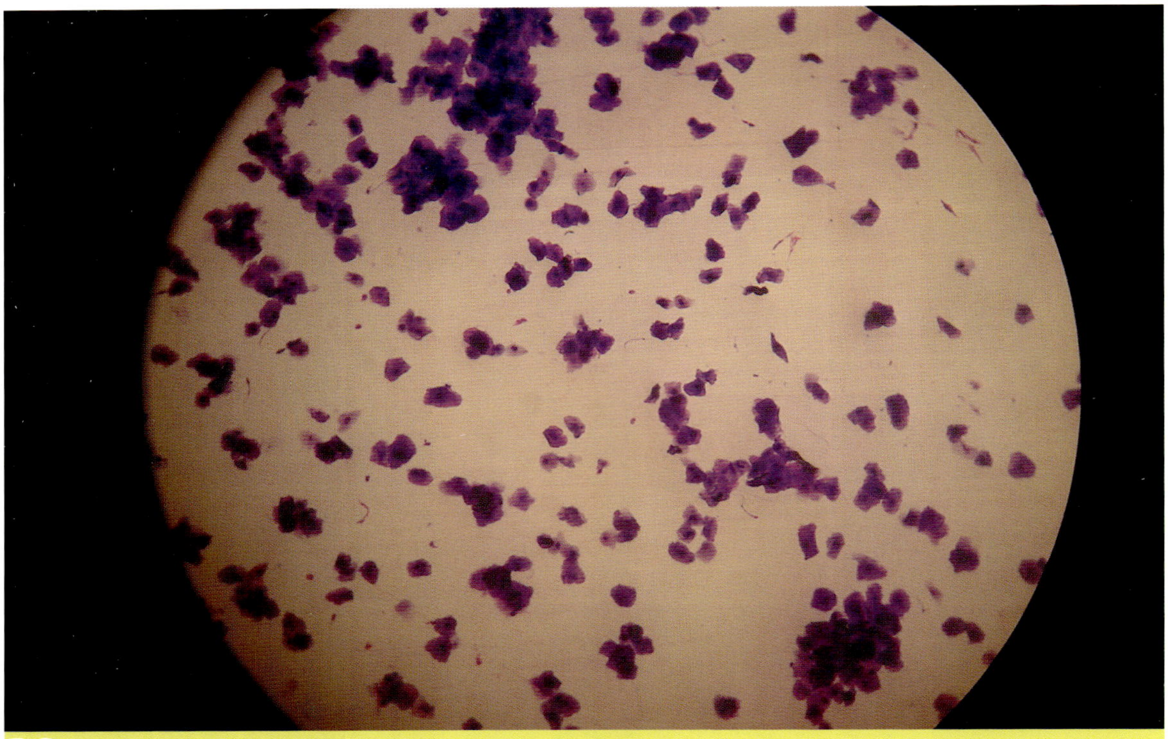

20 Preputial cytology in a dog with a Sertoli cell tumour.

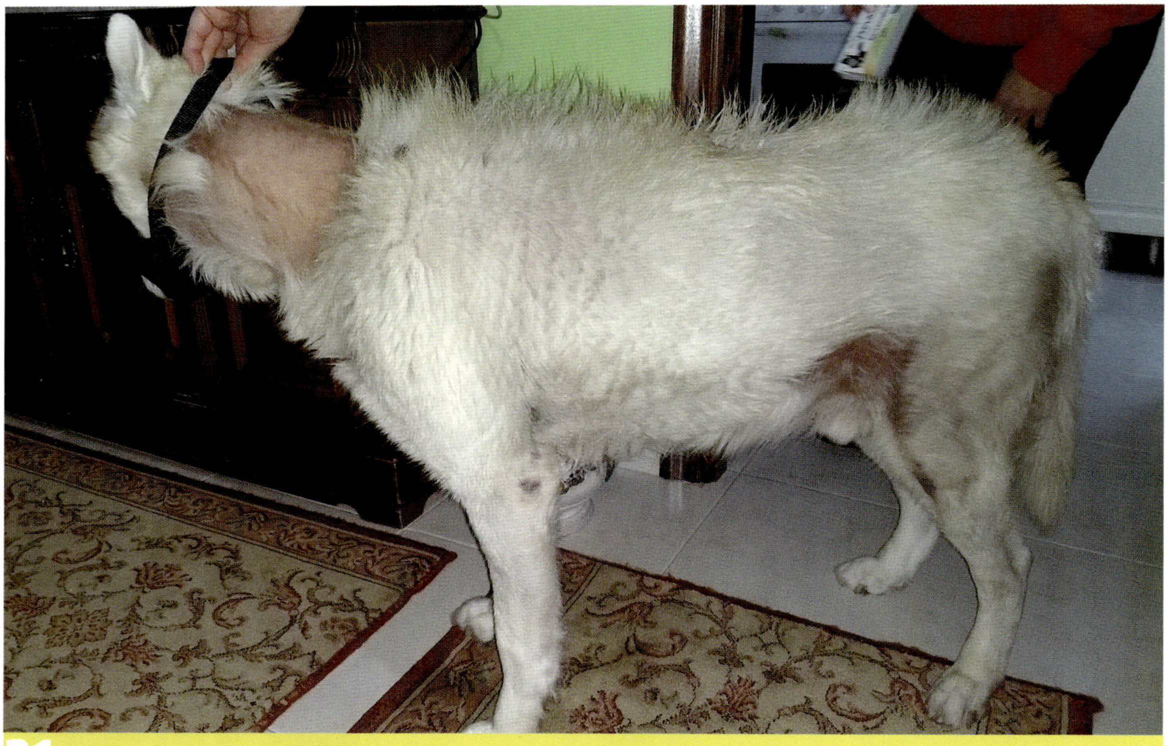

21 Coarse hair and cervical alopecia due to collar friction in a dog with a testicular tumour.

# Alopecia X

## Lesion aetiology/pathogenesis and clinical picture

Although in this book alopecia X is classified as a hormonal disease, it could also be a consequence of a follicular problem caused by alterations in hormonal receptors and in the hair growth cycle, which is arrested in the telogen phase.

It is a form of symmetric alopecia that may be associated with an imbalance in adrenal hormones or growth receptors. This hypotrichosis, characterised by woolly hair, can occur between 1 and 10 years of age, and mainly affects the trunk, neck, rump, and perineum in certain breeds, including the Spitz, Samoyed, Chow Chow, and Pomeranian. This condition, which is primarily cosmetic, can also affect Poodles and any other breed, albeit much less frequently. The skin feels cold to the touch and is hyperpigmented and dry.

The paradox of this follicular cycle disorder is that stimulation of the area (e.g. some form of trauma) induces hair growth. Castration or administration of hormones that alter metabolism (e.g. sex hormones, melatonin, somatotropin) and certain drugs (e.g. trilostane, mitotane) can also trigger hair growth.

## Diagnostic method

The clinical appearance and the breed of the affected dog are good indicators of this condition. Biopsy is useful, as it reveals an excess of trichilemmal keratin in the form of characteristic "flame follicles".

## Main differential diagnoses

- Other endocrinopathies
- Follicular dysplasia

## Treatment

As this is mainly a cosmetic problem and the aetiology is not fully known, the decision to begin treatment must be discussed with the owner.

Treatment usually begins with the safest drugs and different options are tested according to the level of concern of the pet owner. Treatment options include castration and the administration of melatonin, thyroxine, or trilostane. Hair growth can be stimulated by application under anaesthesia of a rotating cylinder with microneedles, which cause micro-injuries that trigger hair growth.

Spontaneous recovery within several months has been described.

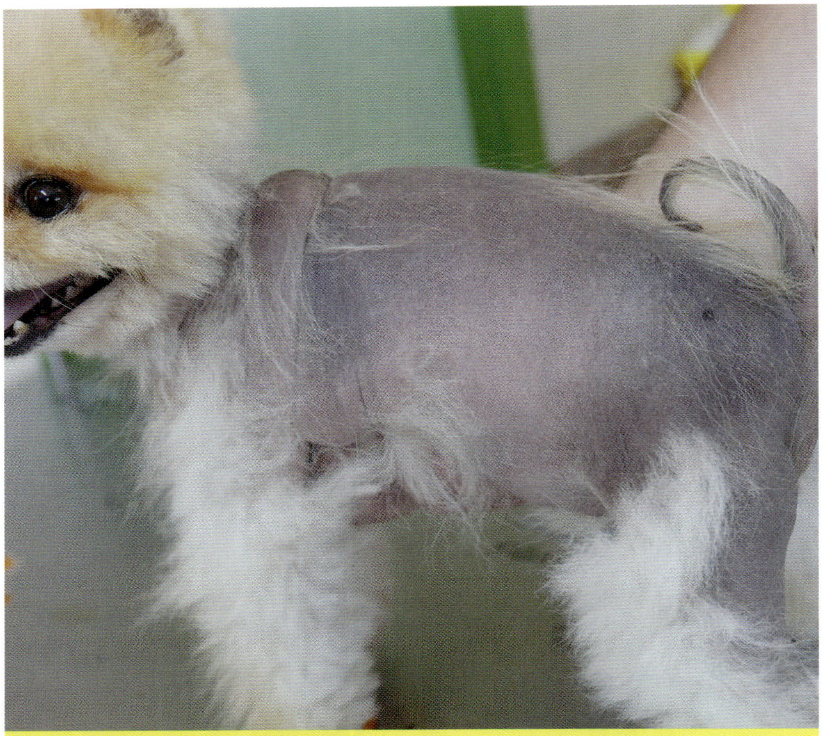

22 Extensive alopecia X without the persistence of woolly hair.

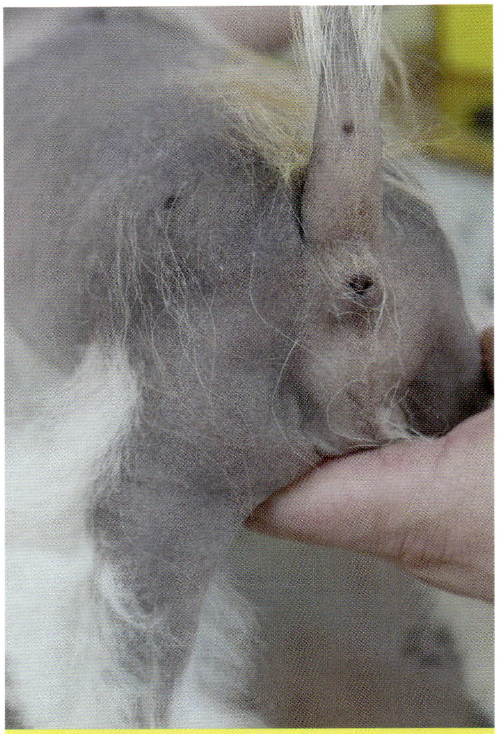

23 Appearance of the hindquarters of the dog from the previous image.

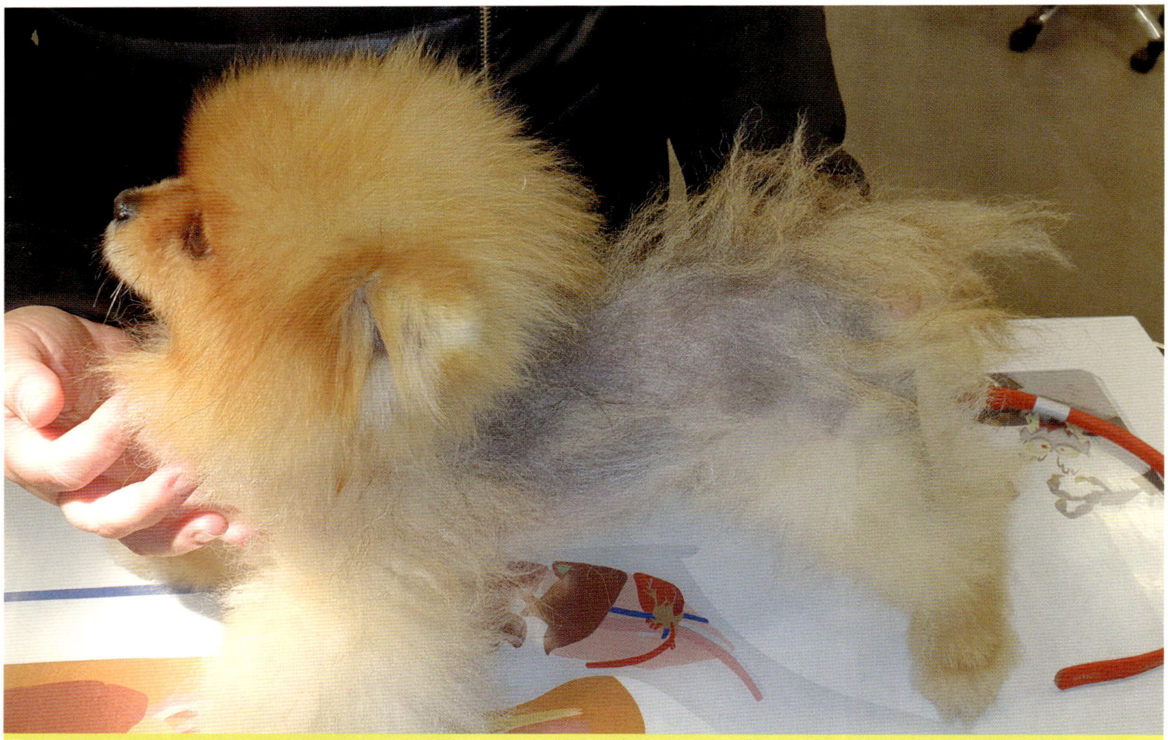

24 Alopecia X with persistence of some woolly hair.

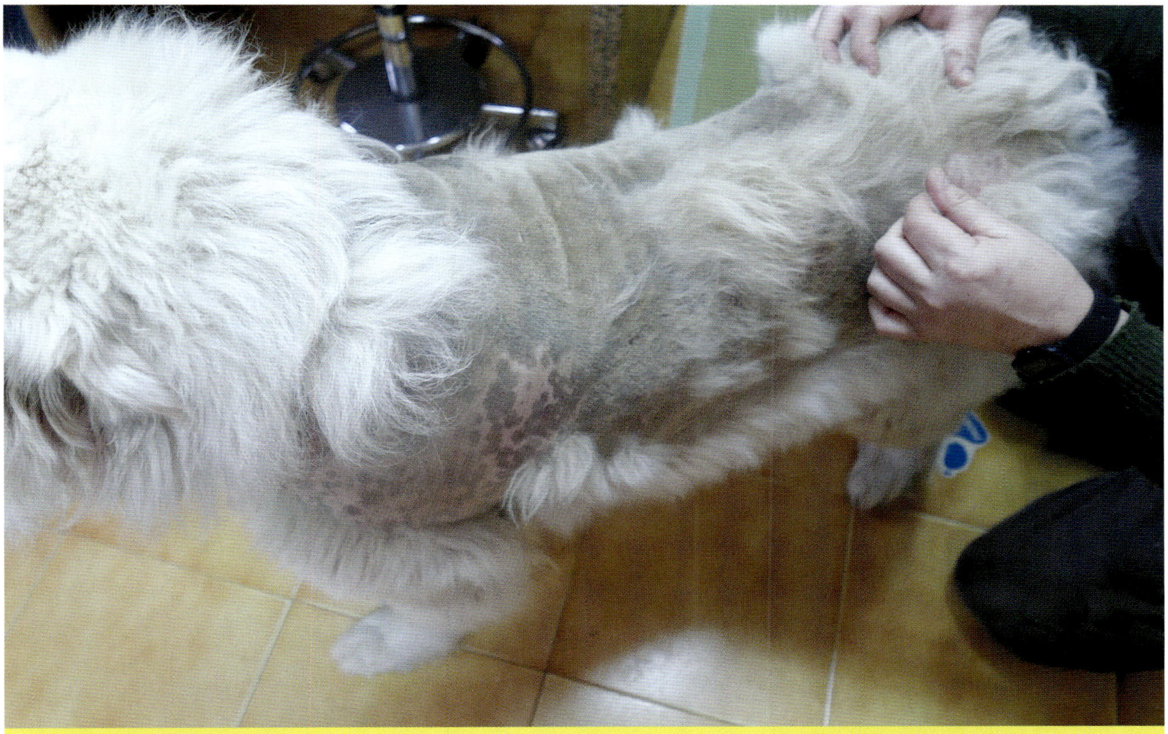

25 Alopecia X in a Samoyed.

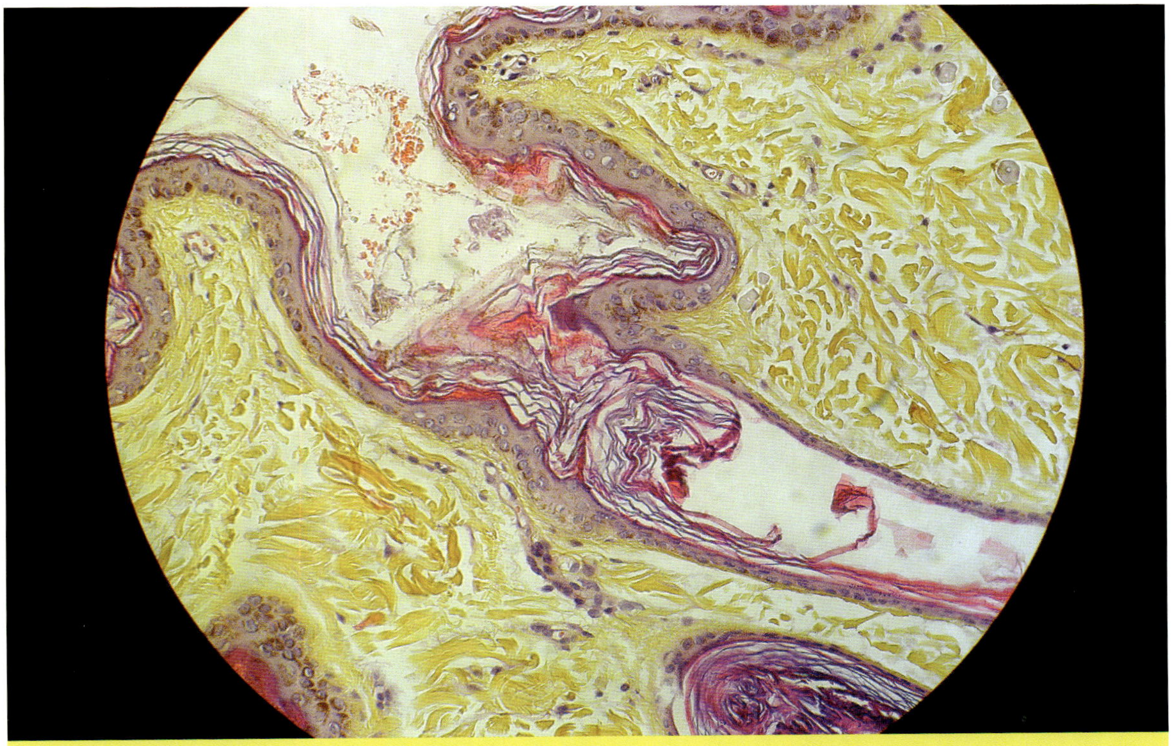

26 Histopathology of alopecia X with trichilemmal keratin accumulation in the follicle.

# Hepatocutaneous syndrome

## Lesion aetiology/pathogenesis and clinical picture

Hepatocutaneous syndrome, also known as superficial necrolytic dermatitis, is a dermatosis associated with neoplastic or degenerative disorders of the liver or pancreas. The aetiology of this disease is unclear, although it appears to involve a nutritional problem at the level of the keratinocytes, to which protein supply is altered. This is a disease of older animals, and is much more frequent in dogs than cats, in which it is extremely rare.

It can be considered a paraneoplasia. The predominant lesions are crusts, erosions, ulcers, hyperkeratosis, and fissures. The mucocutaneous junctions of the periocular, perianal, and perigenital areas are primarily affected, as well as the paw pads and the muzzle. Hyperkeratotic lesions predominantly appear on the abdomen and bony prominences.

## Diagnostic method

Diagnosis is established based on the clinical picture, abdominal ultrasound, and the characteristic "French flag" finding on examination of the skin biopsy.

## Main differential diagnoses

- Deep pyodermas
- Cushing's syndrome
- Nasodigital hyperkeratosis of older dogs
- Other metabolic disorders

## Treatment

Surgical resolution of the tumour is curative, although in most cases treatment is palliative and the prognosis guarded. Nutrition should be improved to increase protein supply to keratinocytes.

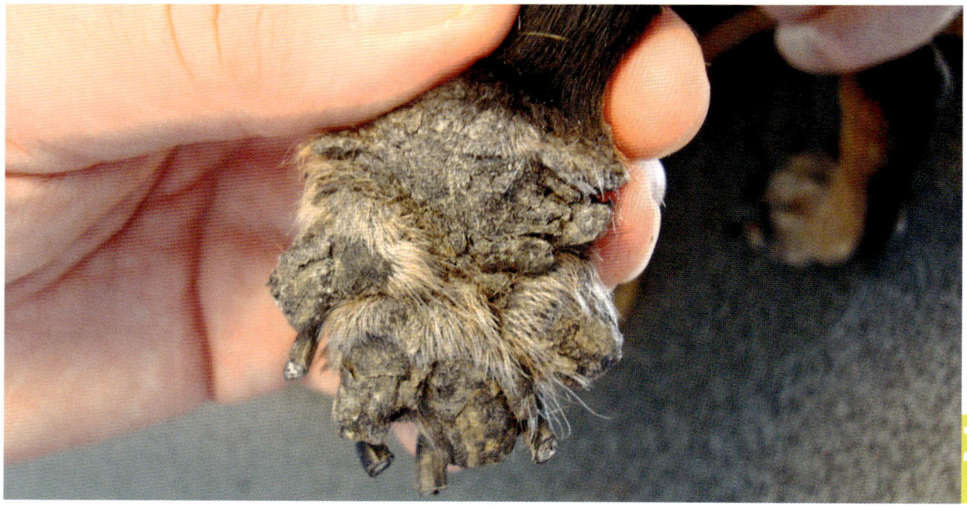

27 Typical paw pad hyperkeratosis in a dog with hepatocutaneous syndrome.

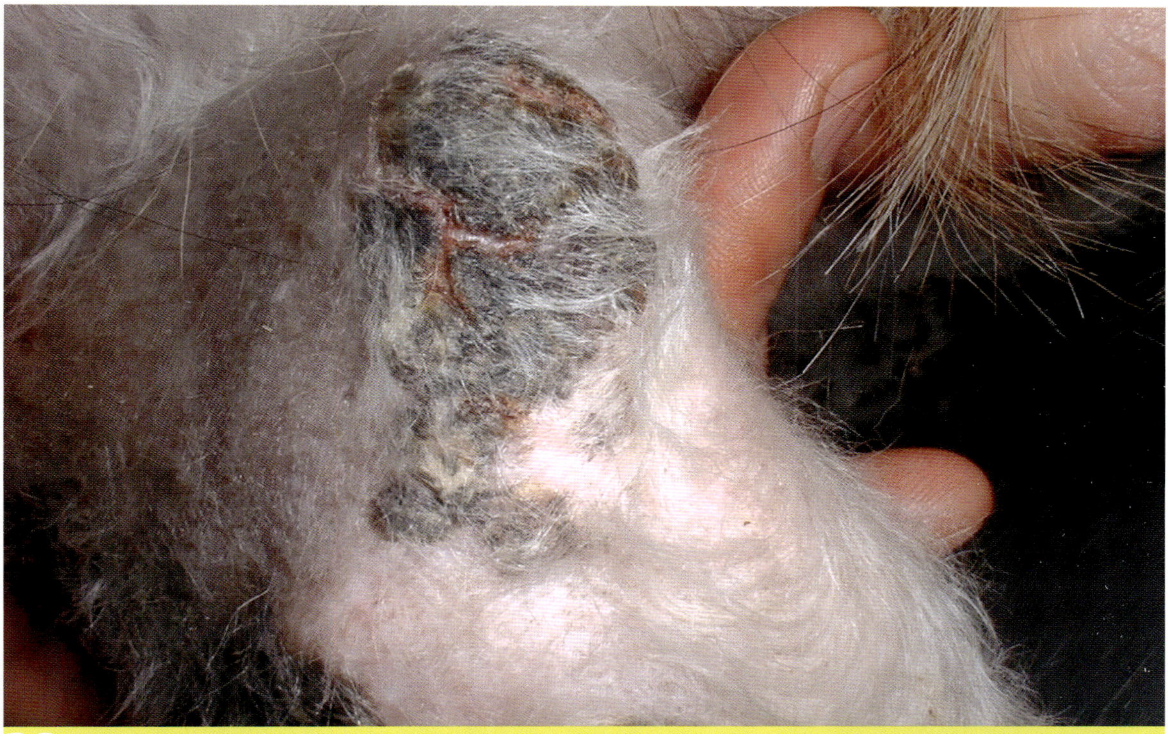

28 Appearance of the elbow of a dog with hepatocutaneous syndrome. Image courtesy of the Fauna Veterinary Clinic (Spain).

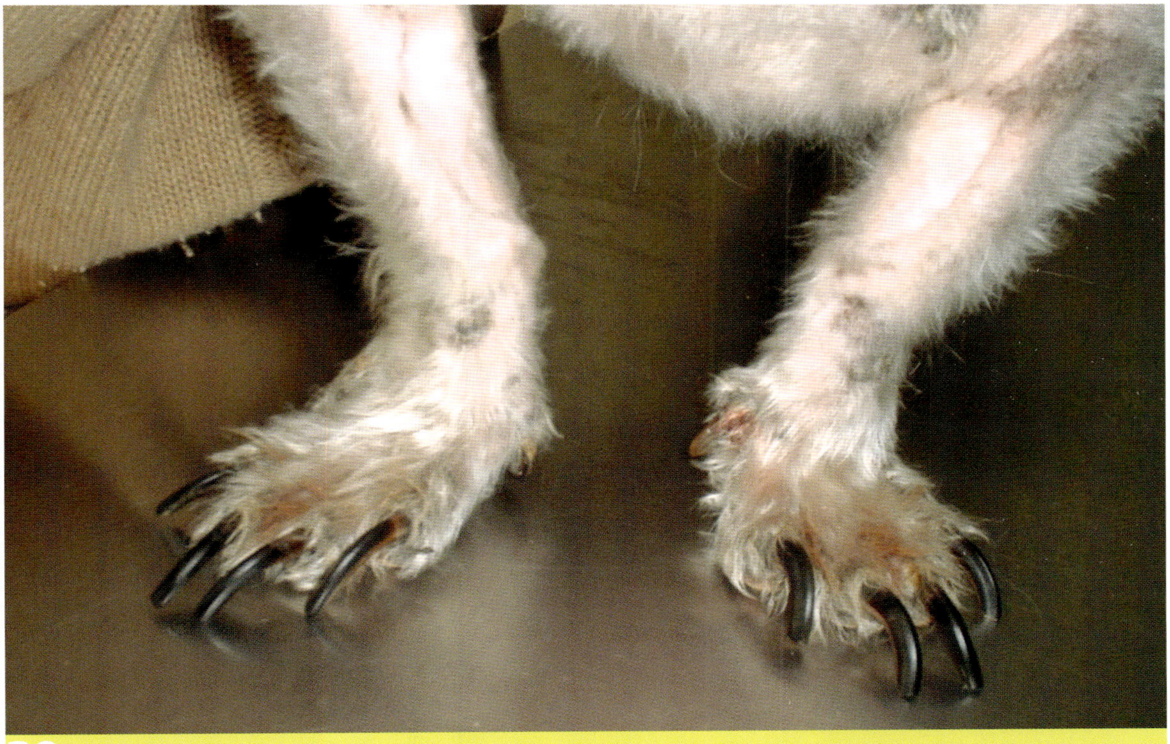

29 Onychogryphosis in a dog with hepatocutaneous syndrome. Image courtesy of the Fauna Veterinary Clinic (Spain).

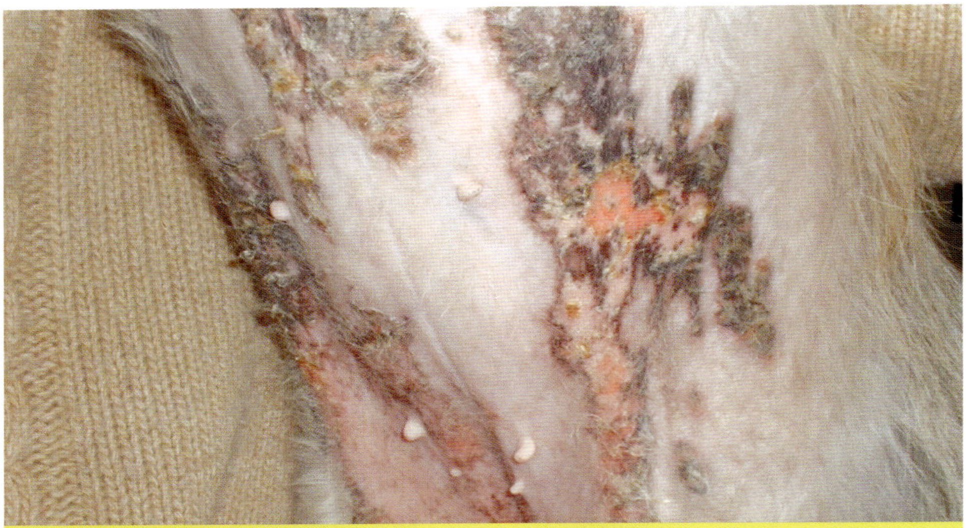

30 Abdomen of a dog with hepatocutaneous syndrome. Image courtesy of the Fauna Veterinary Clinic (Spain).

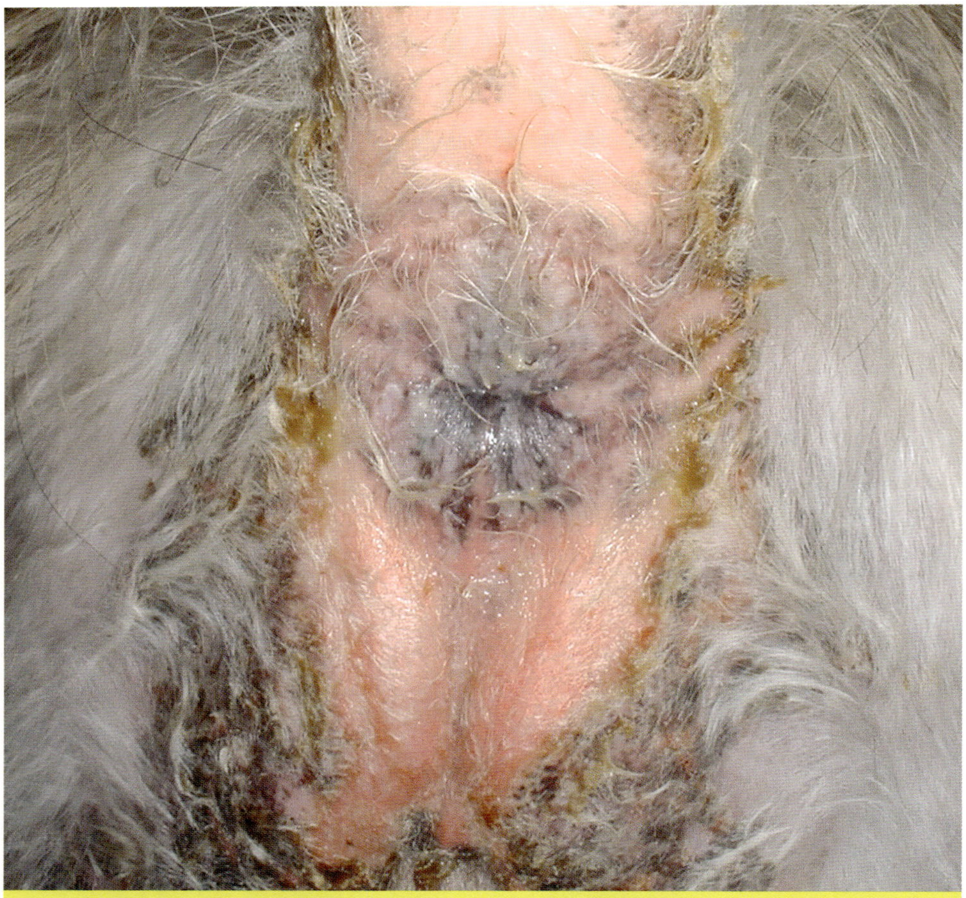

31 Perianal area of a dog with hepatocutaneous syndrome. Image courtesy of the Fauna Veterinary Clinic (Spain).

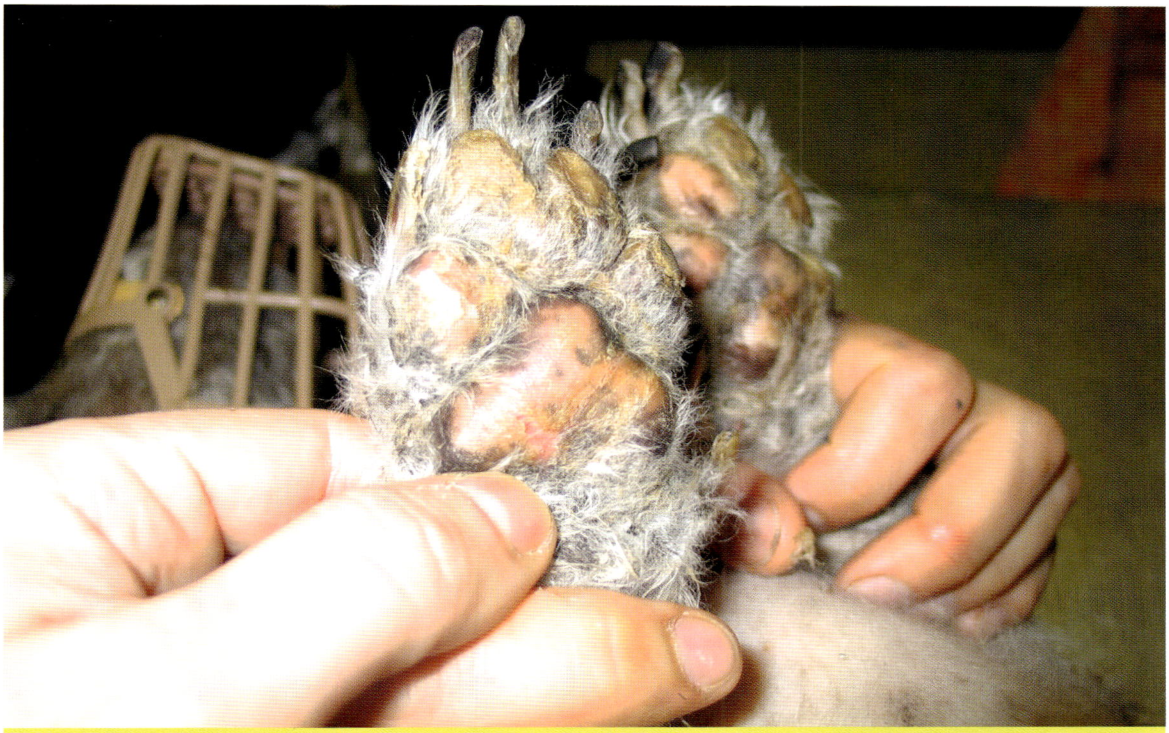

32 Jaundiced paw pads in a dog with hepatocutaneous syndrome.

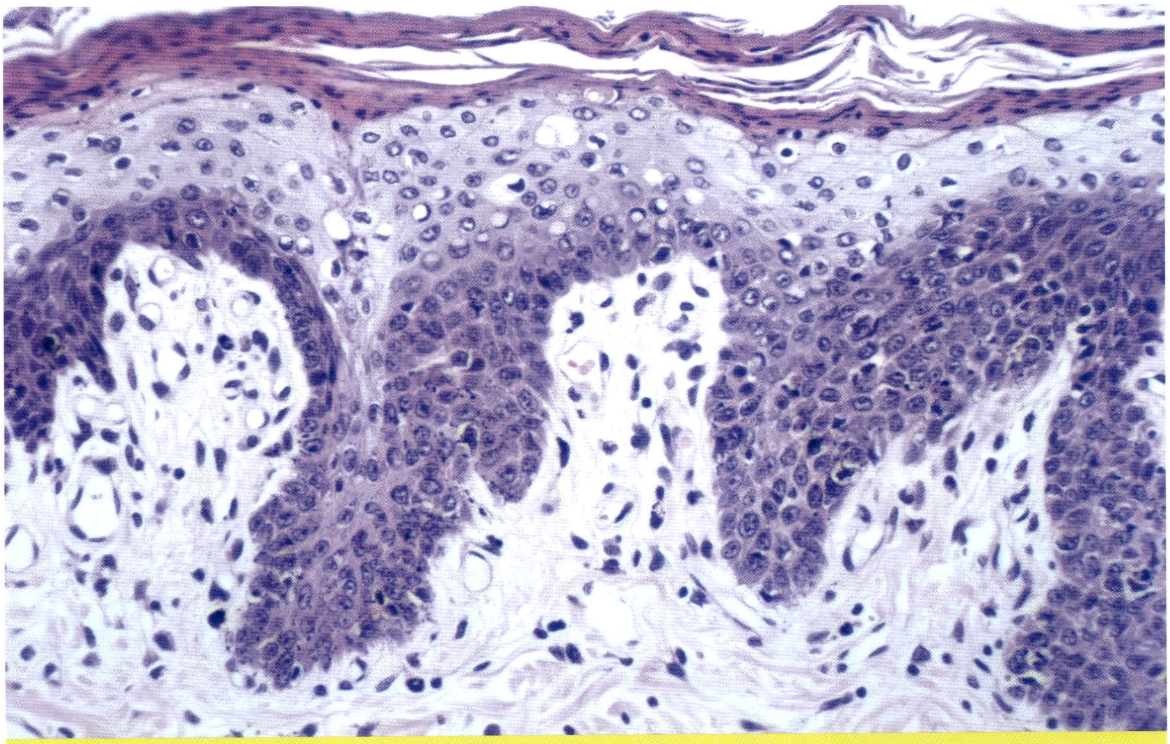

33 Classic histopathology findings of hepatocutaneous syndrome. French flag pattern.

# Shar Pei mucinosis

## Lesion aetiology/pathogenesis and clinical picture

This is a rare idiopathic form of the disease that occurs almost exclusively in Shar Peis. The accumulation of mucin, which is typical of this breed, manifests with thickened, folded skin with abundant mucin-containing vesicles or bullae in the epidermis. The clinical picture is quite striking, and owners may be alarmed when these vesicles rupture, releasing a filamentous fluid.

Skin disorders caused by some parasites, allergies, or endocrinopathies in this breed can trigger an increase in mucin production.

## Diagnostic method

Diagnosis is based on the characteristic clinical picture, after ruling out other differential diagnoses to confirm that the condition is truly idiopathic.

## Main differential diagnoses

- Hypothyroidism
- Hypersensitivity
- Acromegaly
- Demodicosis
- Familial Shar Pei fever

## Treatment

Some presentations can resolve spontaneously. The primary cause, if identified, should be treated.

Corticosteroids are effective, although the problem may recur once their administration is discontinued. Lokivetmab can help treat mastocytosis.

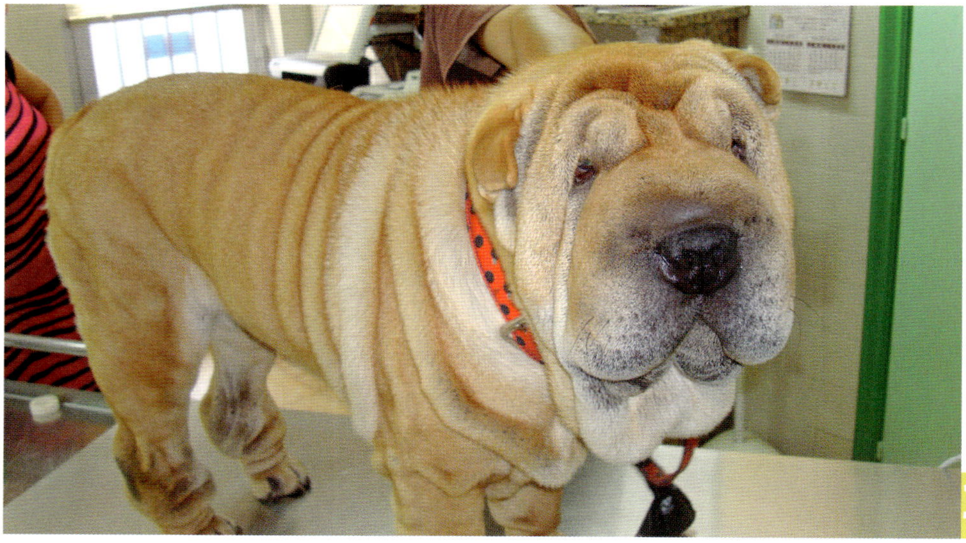

34 Shar Pei with generalised mucinosis. Note the skin folds.

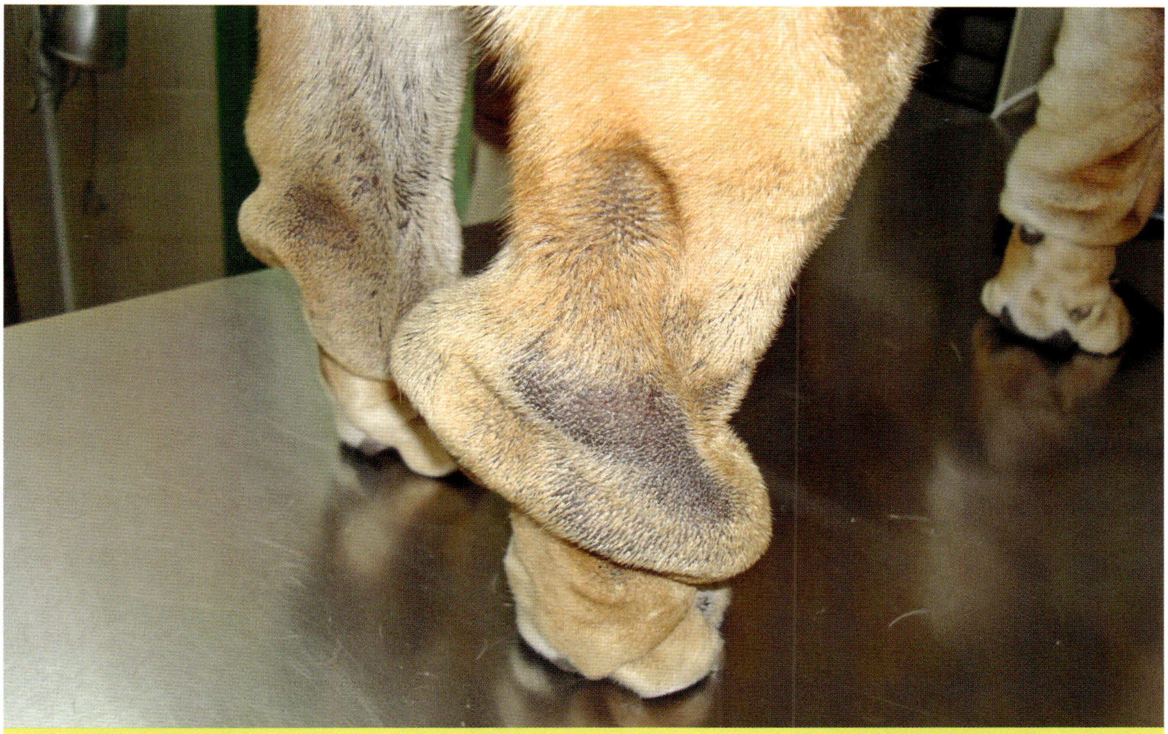

35 Skin fold in the tarsal area in the dog from the previous image.

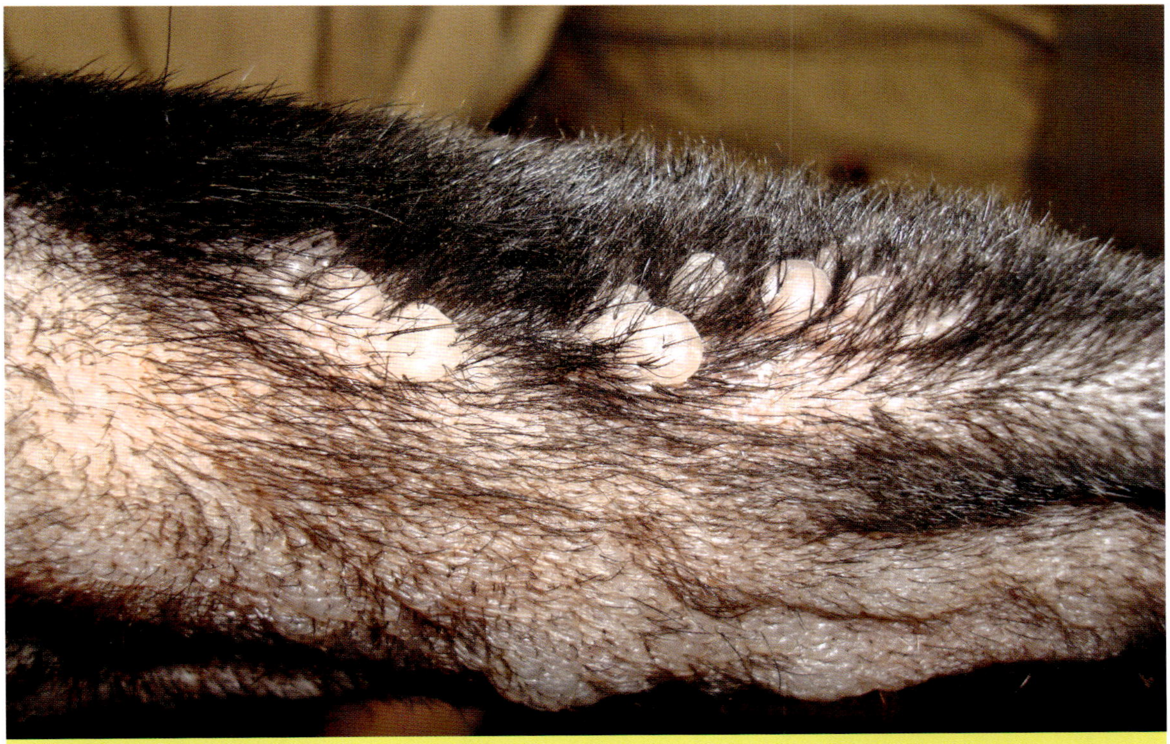

36 Mucin vesicles in a Shar Pei with mucinosis.

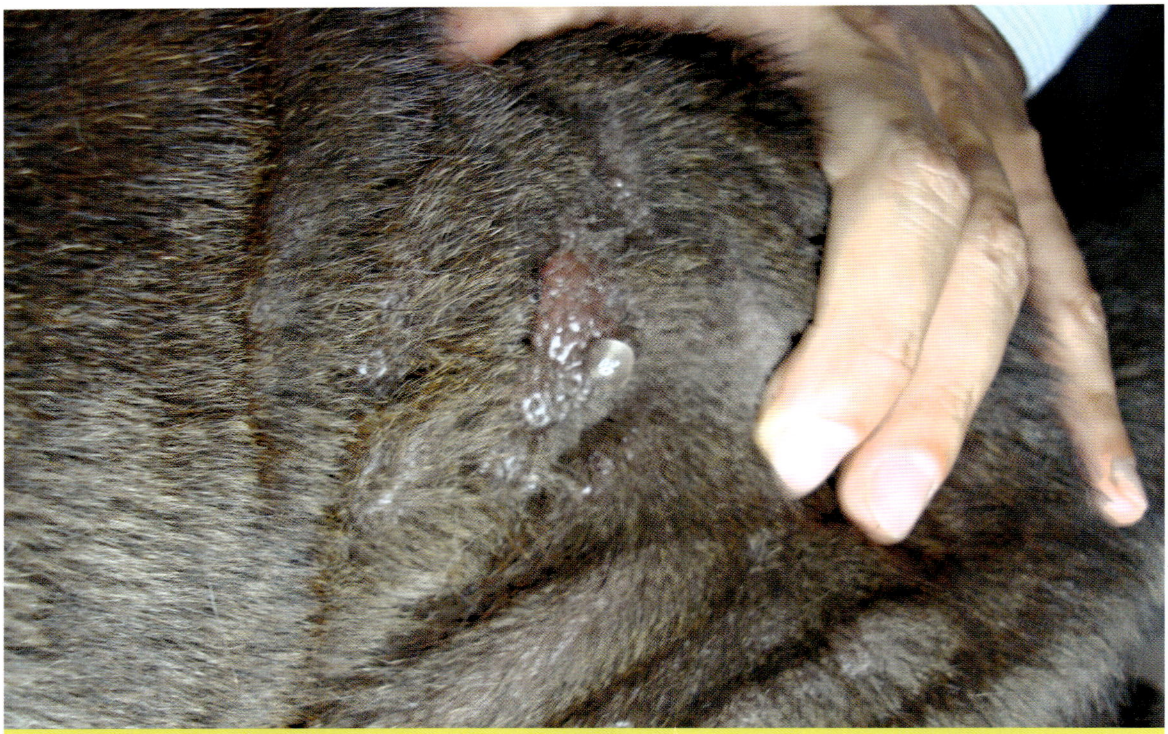

37 Compression of a mucin vesicle.

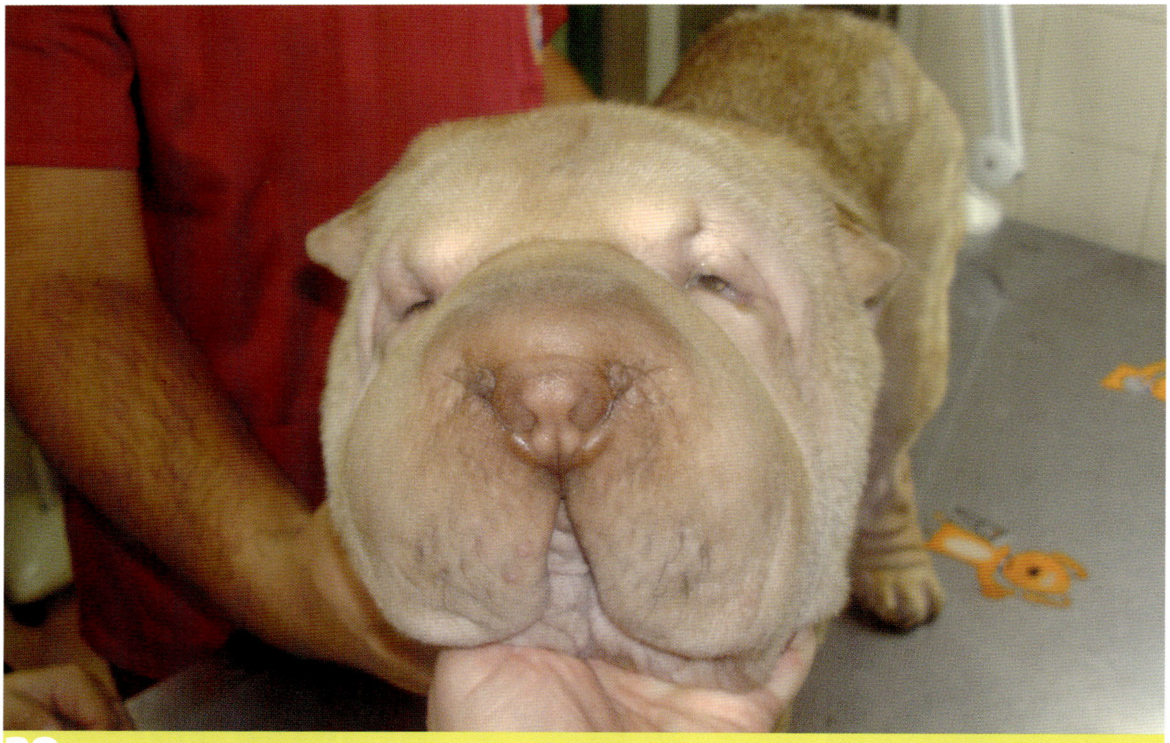

38 Appearance of the face of a dog with severe mucinosis.

# Calcinosis circumscripta

## Lesion aetiology/pathogenesis and clinical picture

This condition is caused by focal deposition of calcium salts in the subcutaneous tissue that tend to form nodules. Although the aetiology is not well understood, it is thought to involve dystrophic calcification caused by repeated trauma to pressure points or areas subjected to surgery, perhaps due to irritation of sutures. Fast-growing dog breeds, perhaps due to their accelerated calcium metabolism, tend to be more susceptible. This condition is very rare in cats.

## Diagnostic method

Diagnosis is based on the presence of nodules that release chalk-like content when punctured. Biopsy is confirmatory.

## Main differential diagnoses

- Calcinosis of other aetiology, such as that which occurs in Cushing's syndrome, osteodystrophy, kidney problems, and osteoarthritis
- Tumours

## Treatment

Surgery.

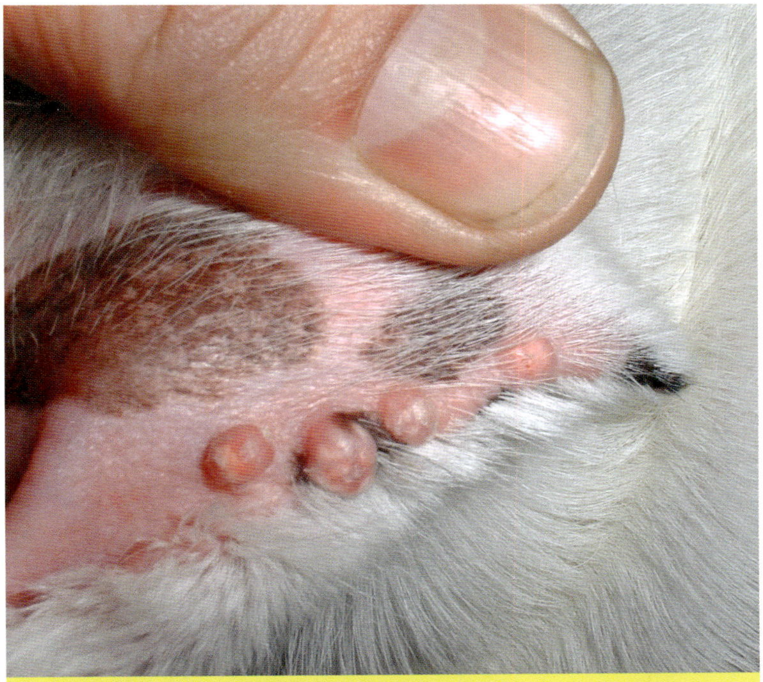

39 Calcinosis circumscripta on the ear margins of a puppy that has undergone surgery.

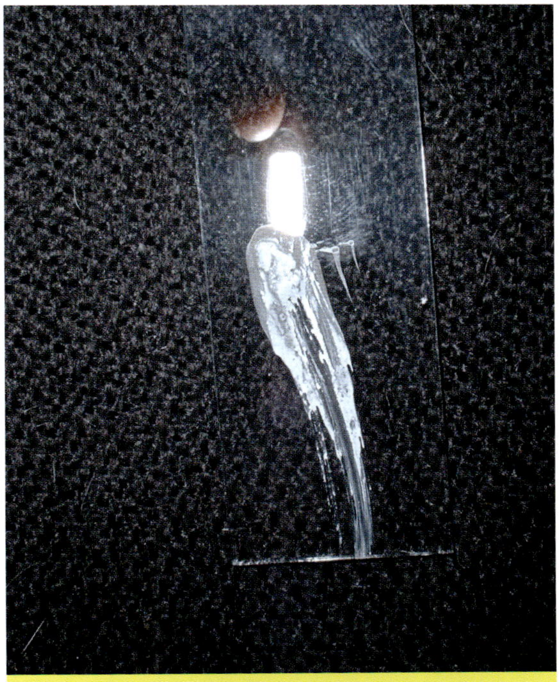

40 Content extracted from nodules on the dog from the previous image.

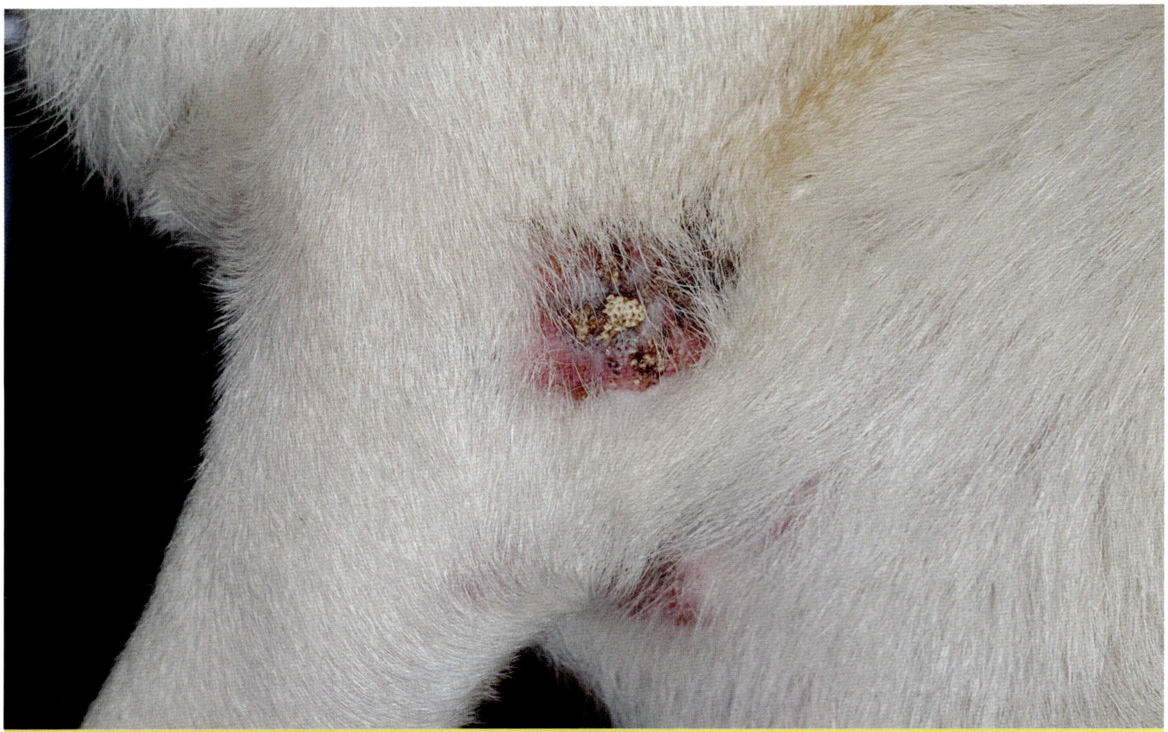

41 Calcinosis circumscripta at a pressure point on the elbow.

# 08

# Autoimmune or immune-mediated dermatoses

# Introduction

The following dermatoses of autoimmune or immune-mediated origin are discussed in this chapter:

- Juvenile cellulitis or sterile granulomatous dermatitis with lymphadenitis
- Pemphigus complex
- Subepidermal bullous diseases
- Cutaneous lupus erythematosus
- Lupoid onychodystrophy or idiopathic onychomadesis
- Sterile nodular panniculitis
- Sterile granuloma–pyogranuloma syndrome
- Sebaceous adenitis
- Ischaemic dermatopathies
- Uveodermatologic syndrome
- Fistulas:
  - Perianal
  - Metatarsal or metacarpal
- Plasma cell pododermatitis

This group of dermatoses is characterised by immune-mediated reactions directed against skin structures. While this aetiology has not been demonstrated for all types, they are included in this group owing to their response to immunosuppressive treatments.

These conditions appear to be caused by insufficient activity of the T cells that regulate the production of interleukin 10 (IL-10), which become unable to control autoreactive T cells.

For some of these autoimmune diseases the target antigen has been identified. These include:

- Desmocholine 1: in pemphigus foliaceus
- Desmoglein 3: in pemphigus vulgaris
- Nuclear antigens: in lupus
- Collagen XVII: in bullous pemphigoid
- Collagen XVII and laminin 332: in mucous membrane pemphigoid
- Collagen VII: in epidermolysis bullosa acquisita and bullous systemic lupus erythematosus

# Juvenile cellulitis or sterile granulomatous dermatitis with lymphadenitis

## Lesion aetiology/pathogenesis and clinical picture

This is a sterile pyogranulomatous reaction that exclusively affects dogs (mainly puppies). The underlying aetiology is immunological, and lesions mainly affect the dermis and hypodermis. Any breed can be affected, although the prevalence is higher in Labrador Retrievers, Golden Retrievers and Dachshunds. It can be accompanied by a febrile syndrome and submandibular lymph node enlargement that often results in fistula formation. Typical lesions include oedema, erythema and furuncles on the lips, eyelids and sometimes at the genital mucocutaneous junctions. Purulent bilateral otitis can also develop, mainly due to involvement of the pinnae and the entrance to the vertical canal.

## Diagnostic method

The clinical picture is evident and initial cytology is characterised by the absence of bacteria and abundant macrophages and neutrophils.

## Main differential diagnoses

- Angioedema
- Facial acne
- Pyoderma
- Demodicosis
- Carré's disease

## Treatment

Immunosuppressive doses of prednisone tend to produce a response. In some cases, administration of antibiotics may be necessary.

A response may be observed to tetracycline/doxycycline-nicotinamide, although caution should be exercised in the case of puppies owing to the dental problems it can cause and the risk of selecting for resistant strains of staphylococci.

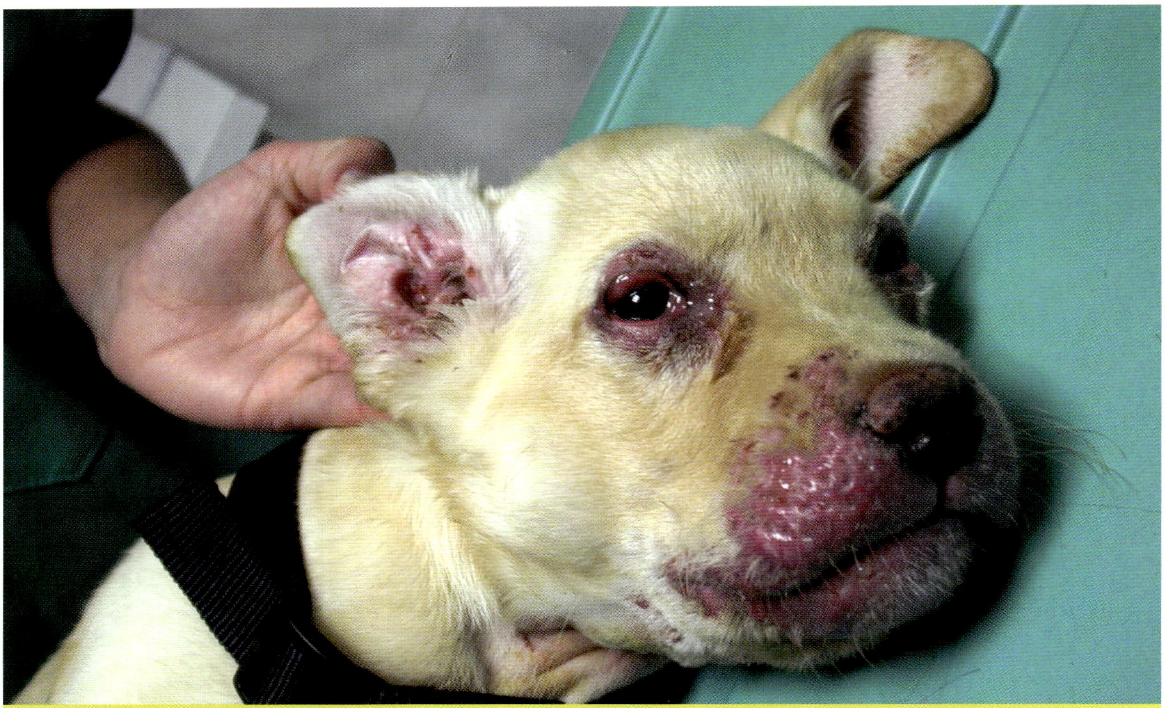

01 Lip, eyelid, and ear involvement in a puppy with juvenile cellulitis. Image courtesy of the Somaza Pérez Veterinary Clinic (Spain).

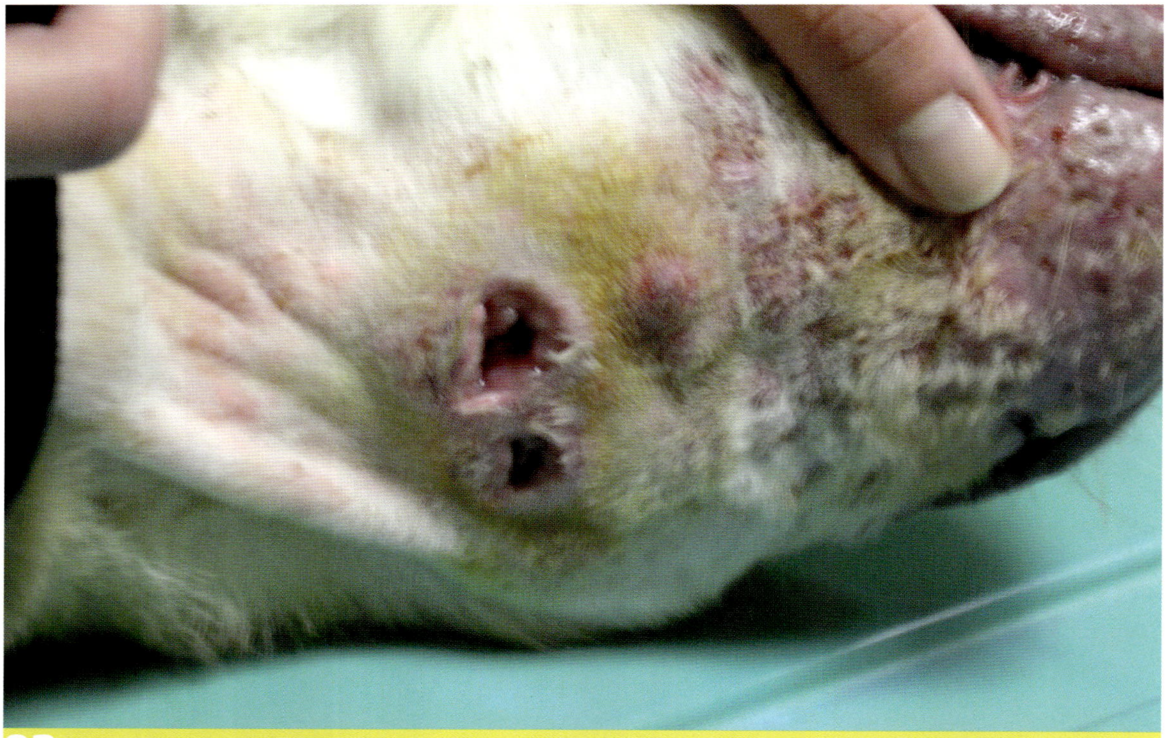

02 Submandibular fistula in a puppy with juvenile cellulitis. Image courtesy of the Somaza Pérez Veterinary Clinic (Spain).

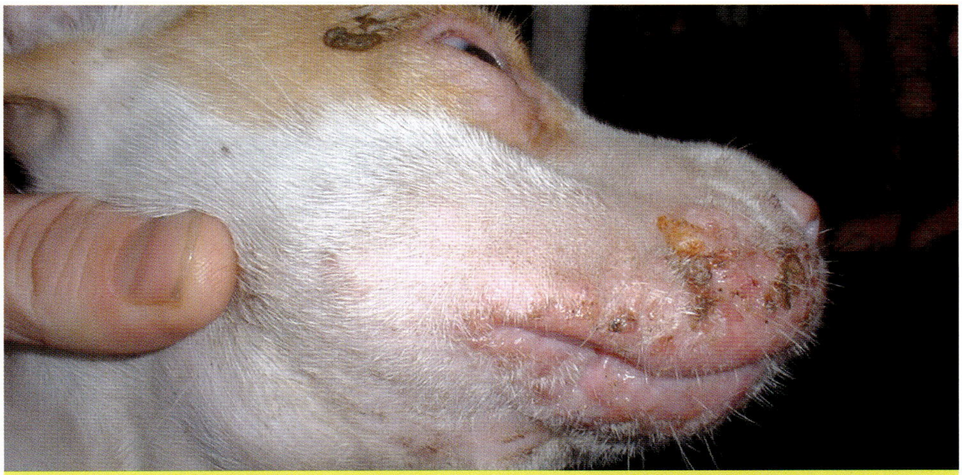

03 Juvenile cellulitis in a dog. Note the lymphadenopathy and lip and eyelid involvement.

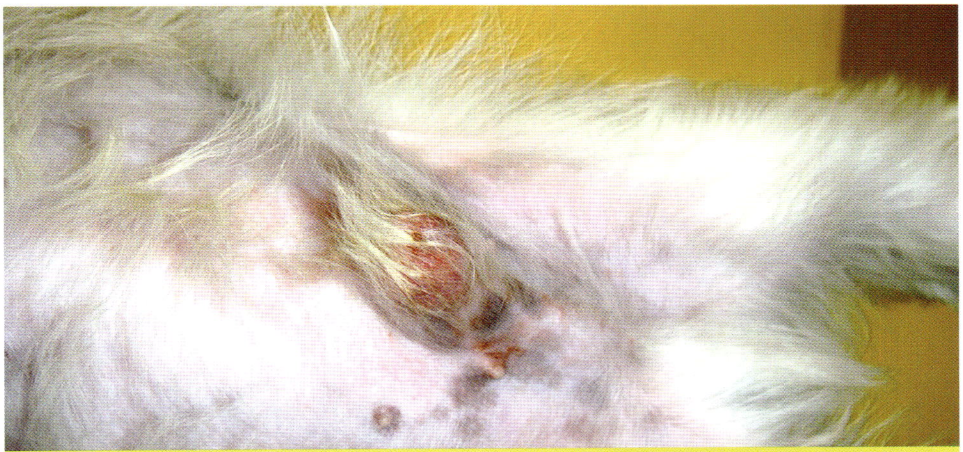

04 Preputial mucocutaneous involvement in a puppy with juvenile cellulitis. Image courtesy of the Lúa Veterinary Clinic (Spain).

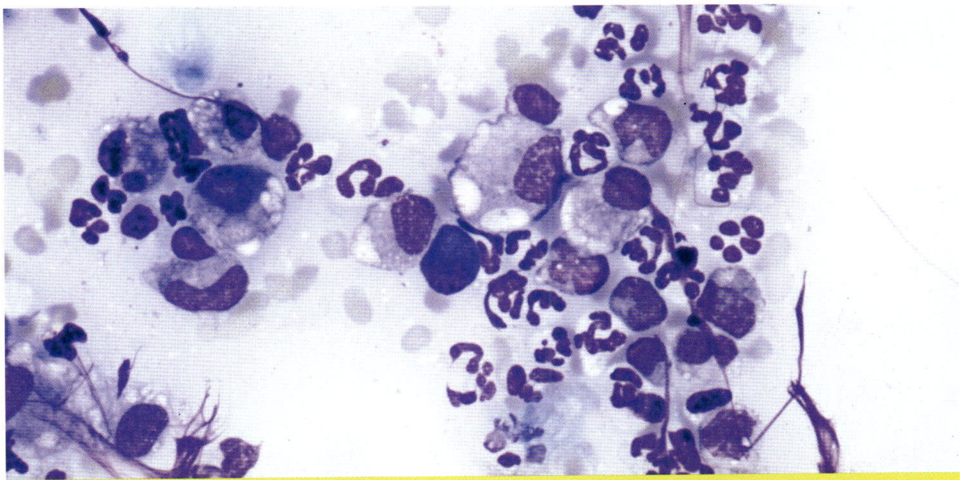

05 Cytology characteristic of pyogranuloma showing macrophages and neutrophils. Juvenile cellulitis.

# Pemphigus complex

## Lesion aetiology/pathogenesis and clinical picture

This complex consists of a series of autoimmune diseases, the aetiology of which involves the production of autoantibodies against desmosomal antigens at different sites in the epidermis. These diseases are: pemphigus foliaceous, pemphigus vulgaris, panepidermal pemphigus, and erythematous pemphigus. If the condition affects the subepidermis, it is known as bullous pemphigoid.

Both dogs and cats can be affected.

This autoimmune process results in separation of keratinocytes from one another or from the basement membrane and the formation of pustules at different levels of the epidermis with a characteristic cellular content (due to the presence of free cells called acanthocytes), surrounded by abundant neutrophils. In most cases the trigger is unknown, although known triggers include paraneoplastic situations and drug reactions. This disease is also often diagnosed in association with leishmaniasis.

The characteristic lesions are macules, large pustules, crusts, and itching. Secondary pyodermas are frequent and, depending on the depth of the process and its severity, erosions, ulcers, and abundant exudation may be observed. In dogs, the condition can be generalised, involving the paw pads or mucocutaneous regions, depending on the type of pemphigus. The formation of pustules and crusts on the medial aspect of the pinnae can be an important characteristic distinguishing this condition from pyoderma.

In cats, it tends to affect the face and digits more, resulting in production of a characteristic exudate in the nail folds. Intact pustules are very difficult to find in cats. Crusting and alopecia are common, complicating the diagnosis.

## Diagnostic method

Diagnosis can be established based on cytology, which reveals acanthocytes and neutrophils, as well as the clinical picture and biopsy findings. Some cases with marked pyoderma can be misdiagnosed macroscopically, as well cytologically and histologically.

Clear observation of acanthocytes is less common in cats.

## Main differential diagnoses

- Distinct forms of pemphigus
- Drug reaction
- Pyoderma
- Leishmaniasis
- Dermatophytosis
- Cutaneous lupus erythematosus
- Tumours

## Treatment

Treatment is based on initial immunosuppression. Once the condition is controlled, the objective is to find the minimum dose necessary to maintain remission. The main drugs used are glucocorticoids, azathioprine (not in cats), chlorambucil, tetracycline-nicotinamide, mycophenolate mofetil, and cyclosporine. Oclacitinib has also been confirmed as a potentially effective molecule.

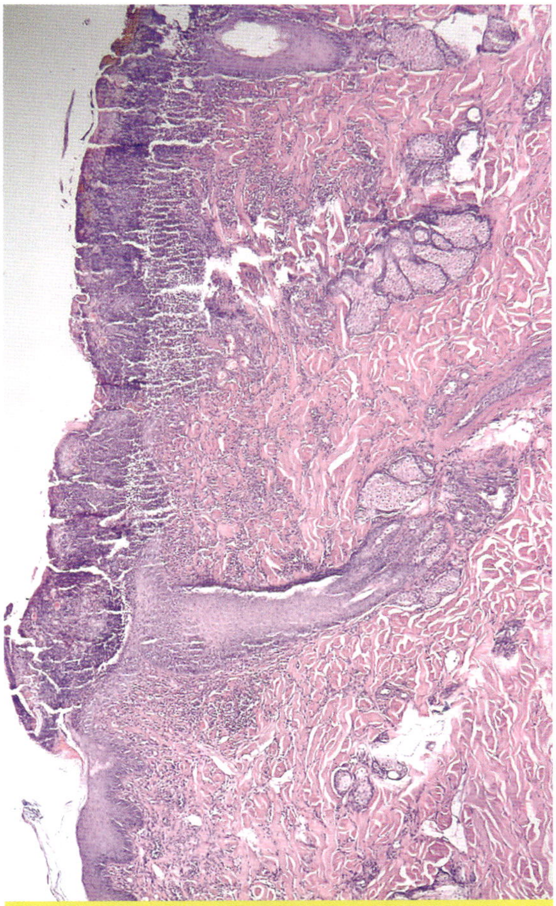

06 Histopathology of pemphigus foliaceus. Note the pustule and crusting, which encompasses the follicles.

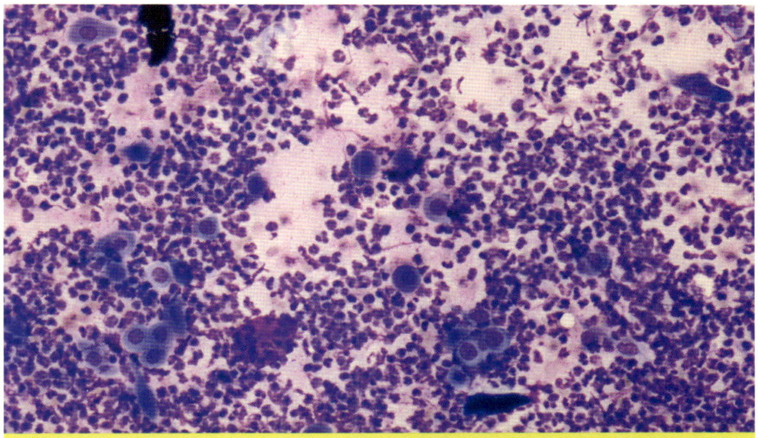

07 Pemphigus cytology showing abundant acanthocytes and neutrophils.

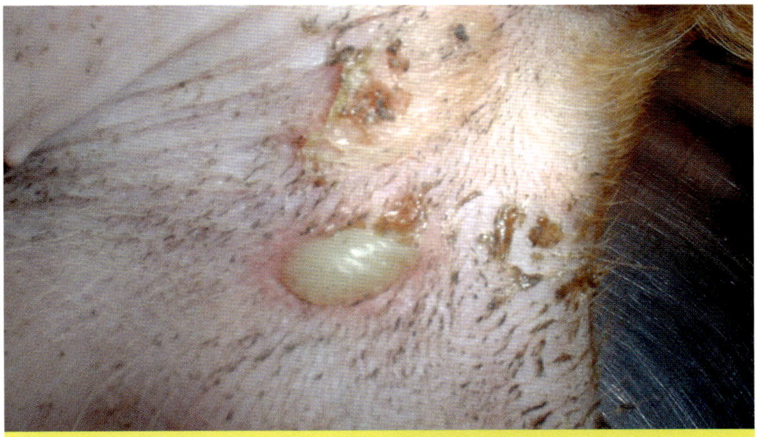

08 Classic pemphigus foliaceus pustule. Large, elongated, and flaccid.

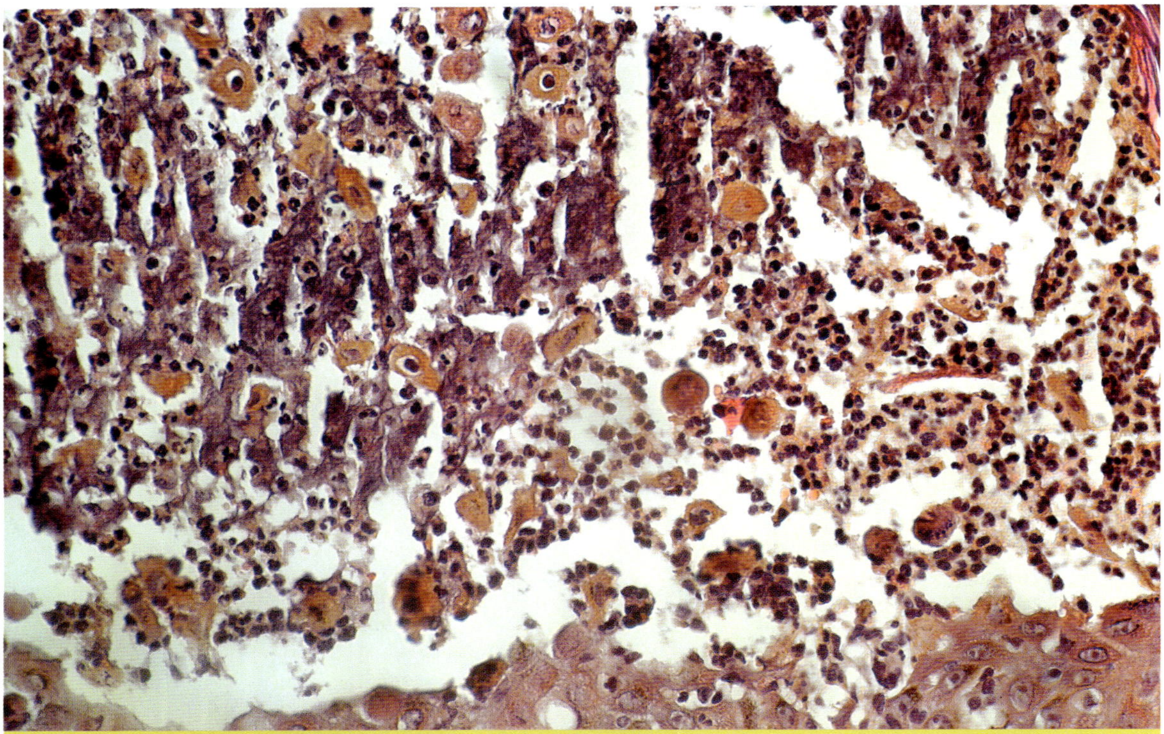

09 Release of acanthocytes in a histological image from a pemphigus foliaceus patient.

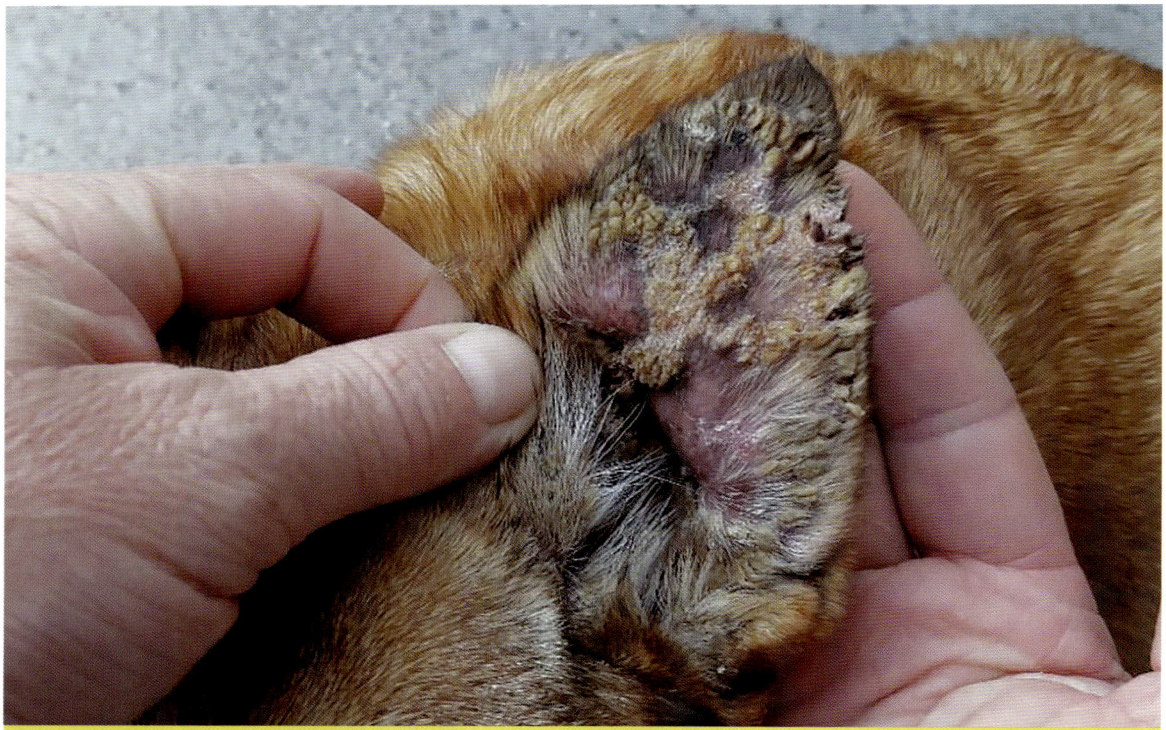

10 Involvement of the pinna in a dog with pemphigus foliaceus.

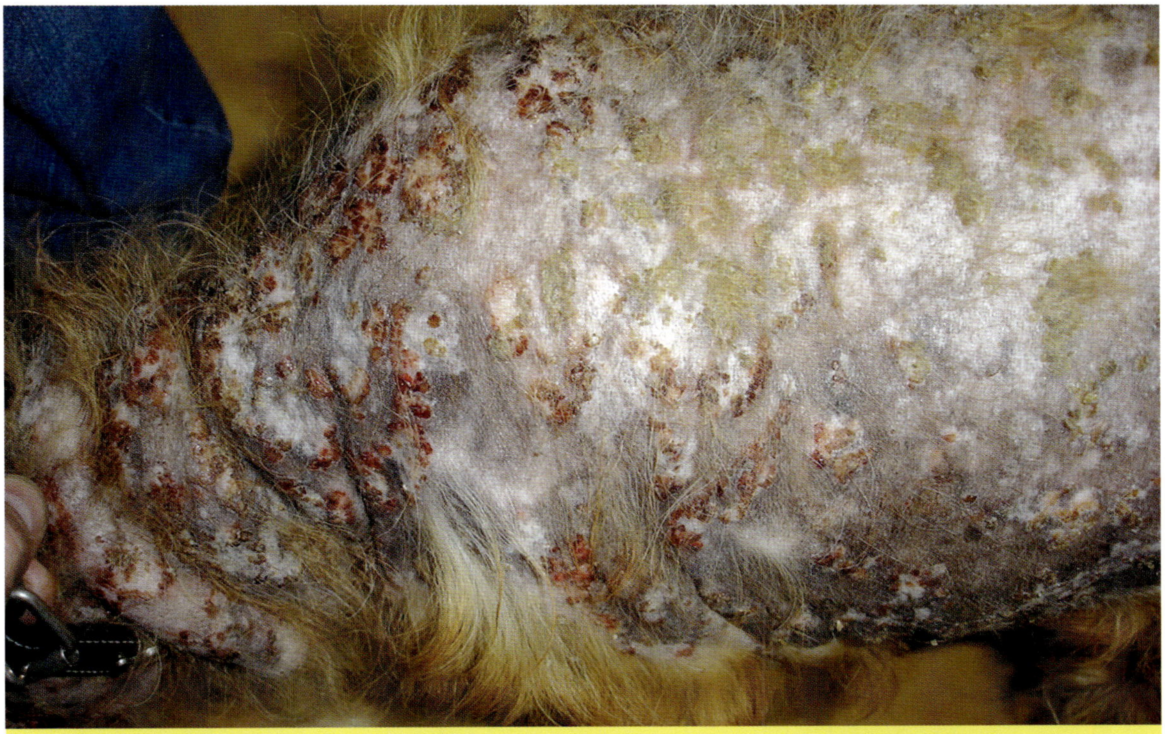

11 Generalised crusting appearance in a patient with pemphigus foliaceus.

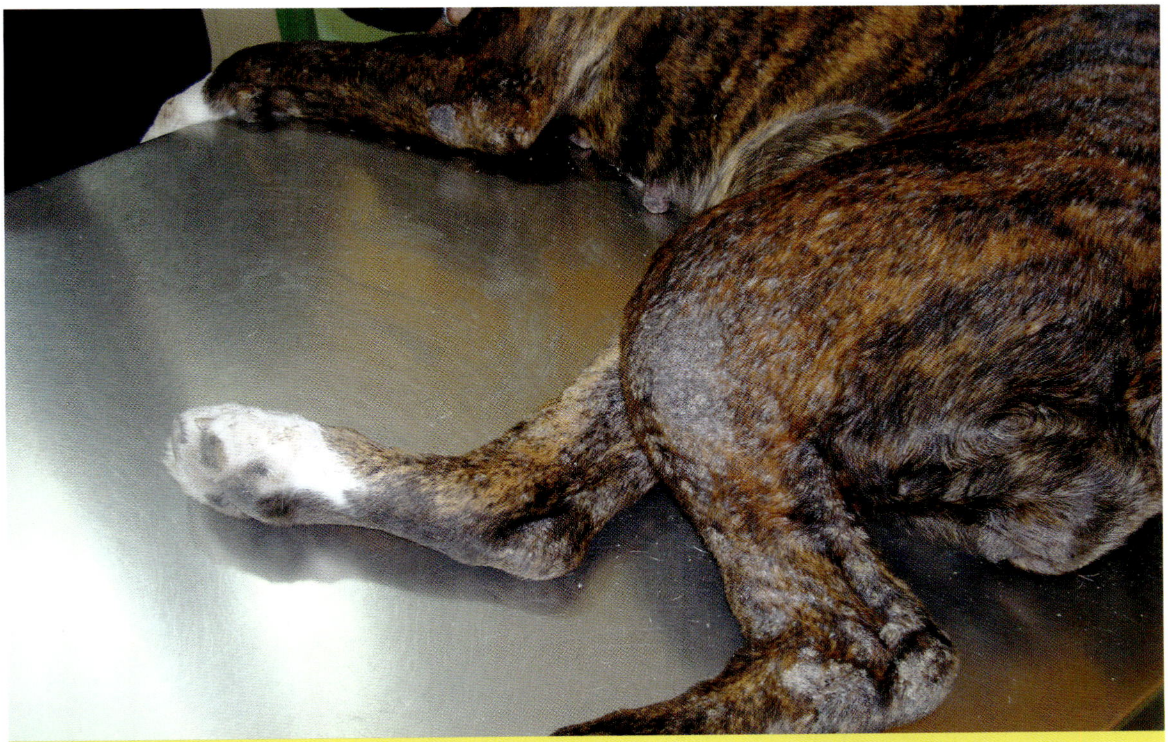

12 Crusting pattern affecting the hindlimb of a Boxer with pemphigus foliaceus.

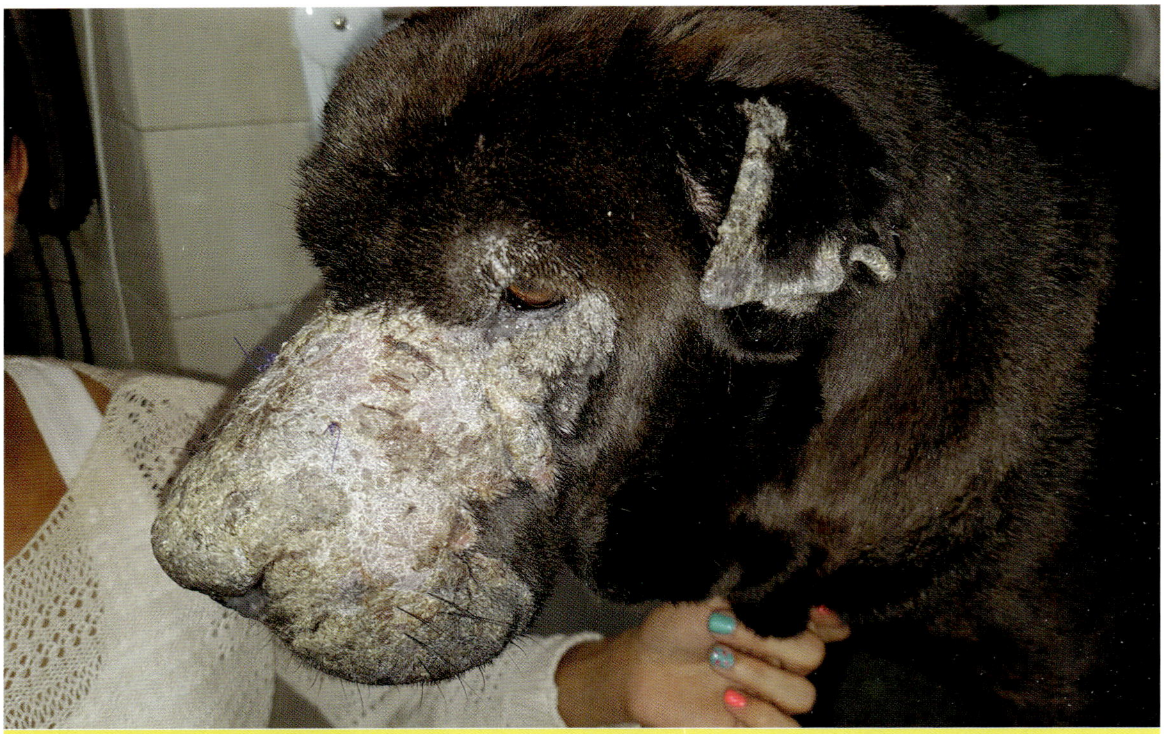

13 Severe facial involvement in a dog with pemphigus.

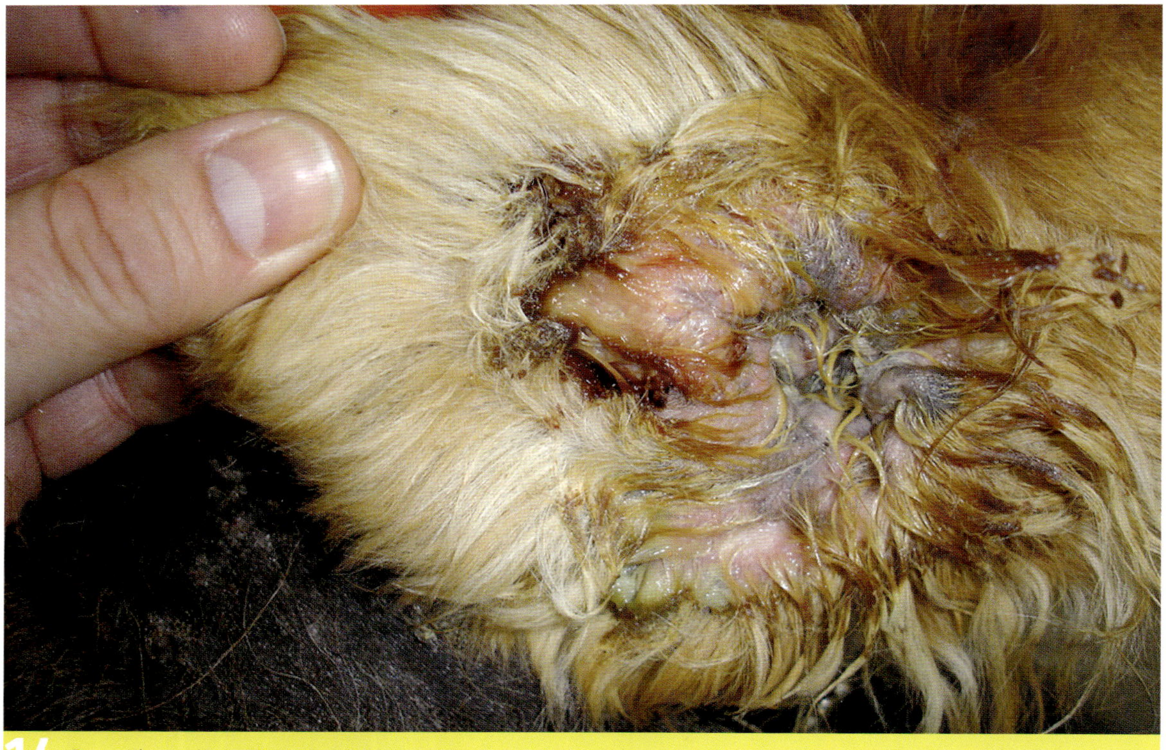

14 Dog with purulent otitis induced by pemphigus pustular disease.

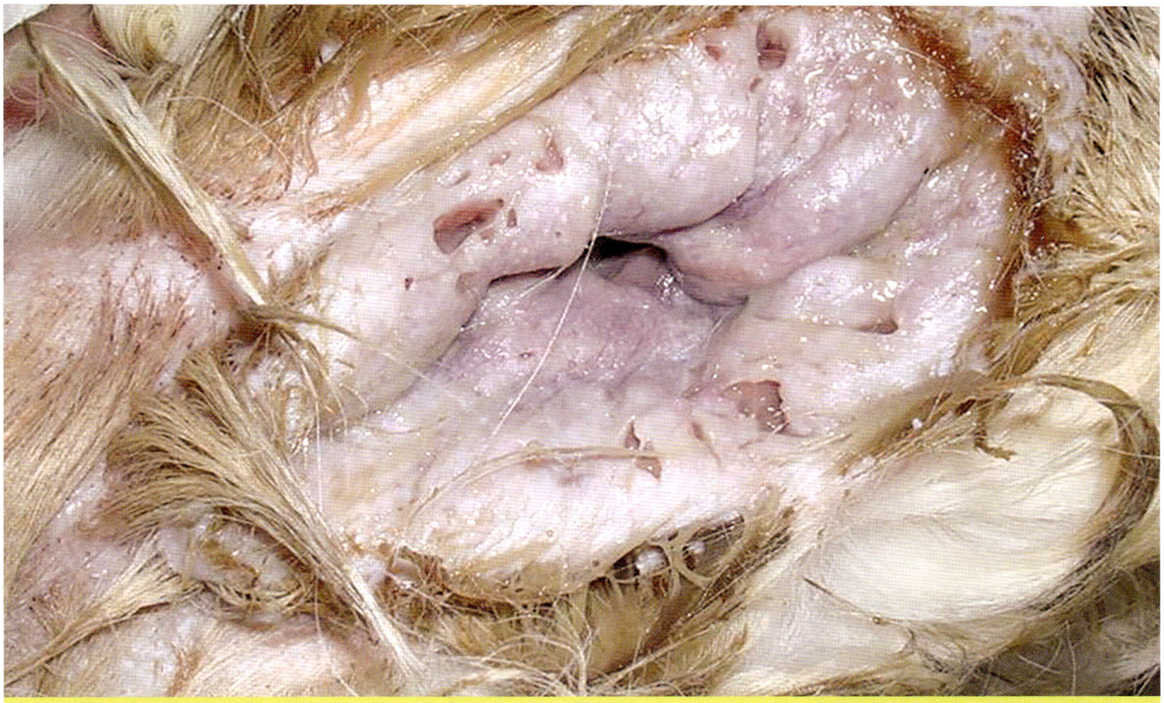

15 Detachment of the anal mucocutaneous junction in a case of pemphigus vulgaris.

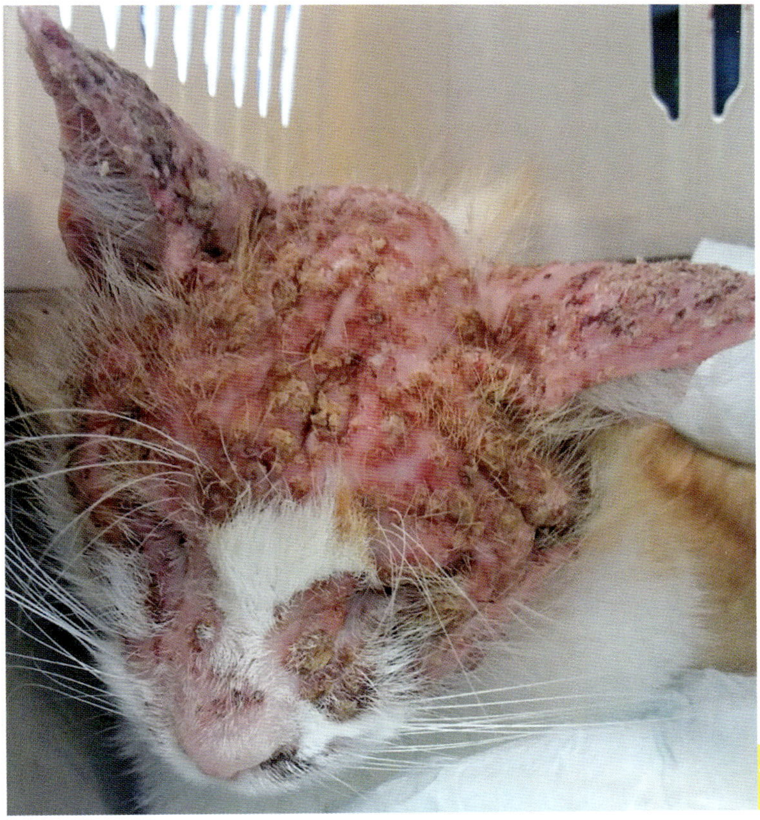

16 Pemphigus foliaceus in a cat. Image courtesy of Haridian Cachon.

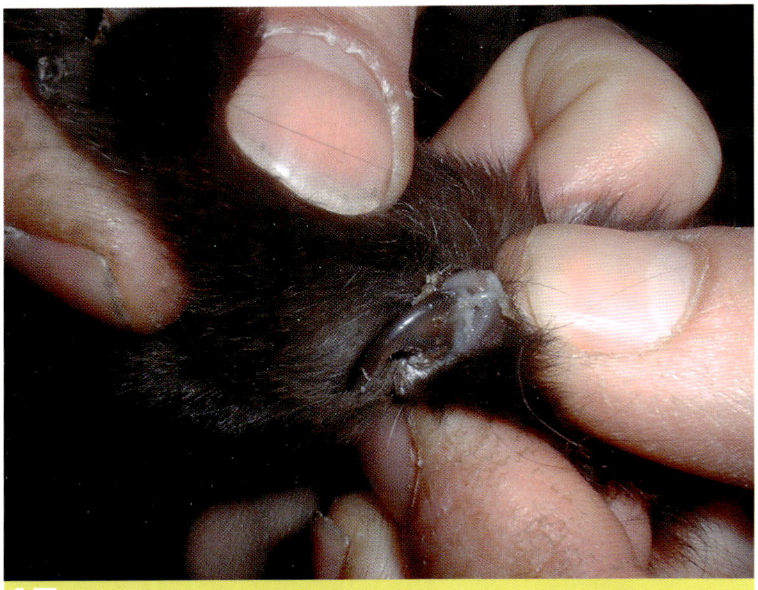

17 Exudate in the nail bed of a cat with pemphigus foliaceus.

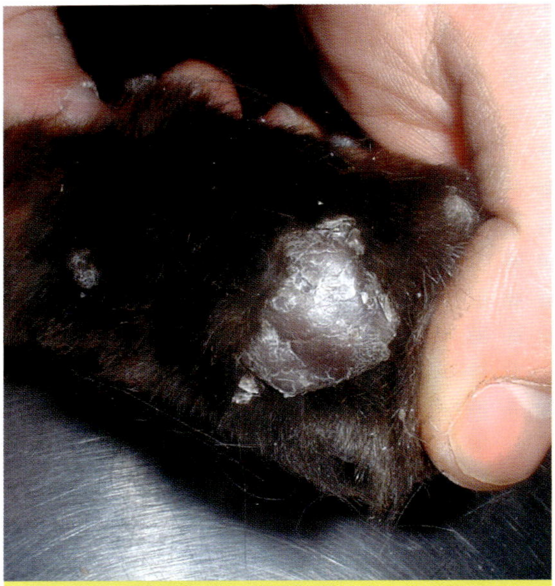

18 Paw pads of the cat from the previous image.

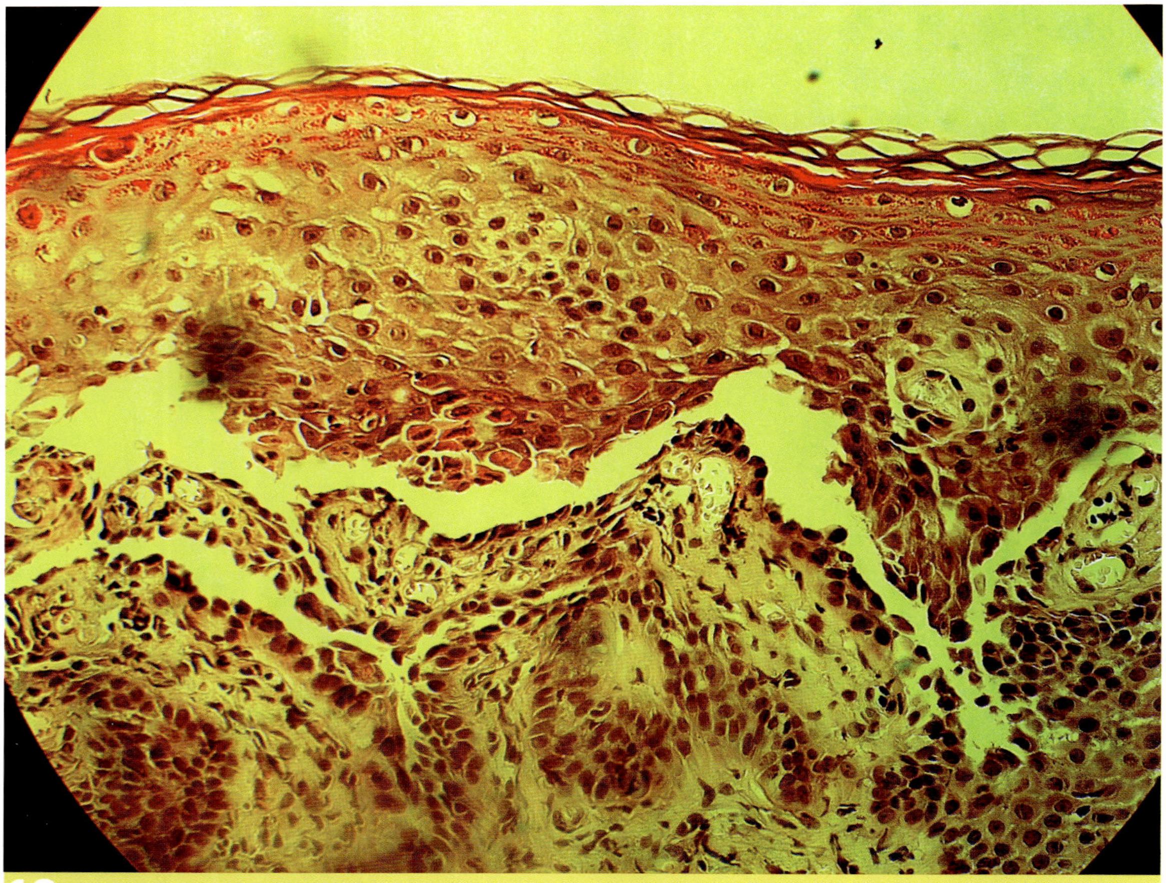

19 Histology image showing basal keratinocyte detachment near the basement membrane in a case of pemphigus vulgaris.

# Subepidermal bullous diseases

## Lesion aetiology/pathogenesis and clinical picture

This is a group of diseases that share an autoimmune reaction that targets basement membrane antigens. Their incidence is very low and they are characterised by erosions, ulcers, de-epithelialisation, vesicles, and crusts. Lesions usually appear in mucocutaneous junctions, the oral mucosa, paw pads, and the skin of the groin and axillae.

This group of diseases includes:

- Bullous pemphigoid (the most common, affects both dogs and cats).
- Epidermolysis bullosa acquisita.
- Linear IgA bullous disease.
- Mucosal pemphigoid.

## Diagnostic method

Suspicion based on the clinical picture is confirmed by histology.

## Main differential diagnoses

- Distinct autoimmune diseases
- Drug reaction
- Split paw pad disease
- Epitheliotropic lymphoma

## Treatment

Despite an uncertain prognosis, treatment is based on immunosuppression.

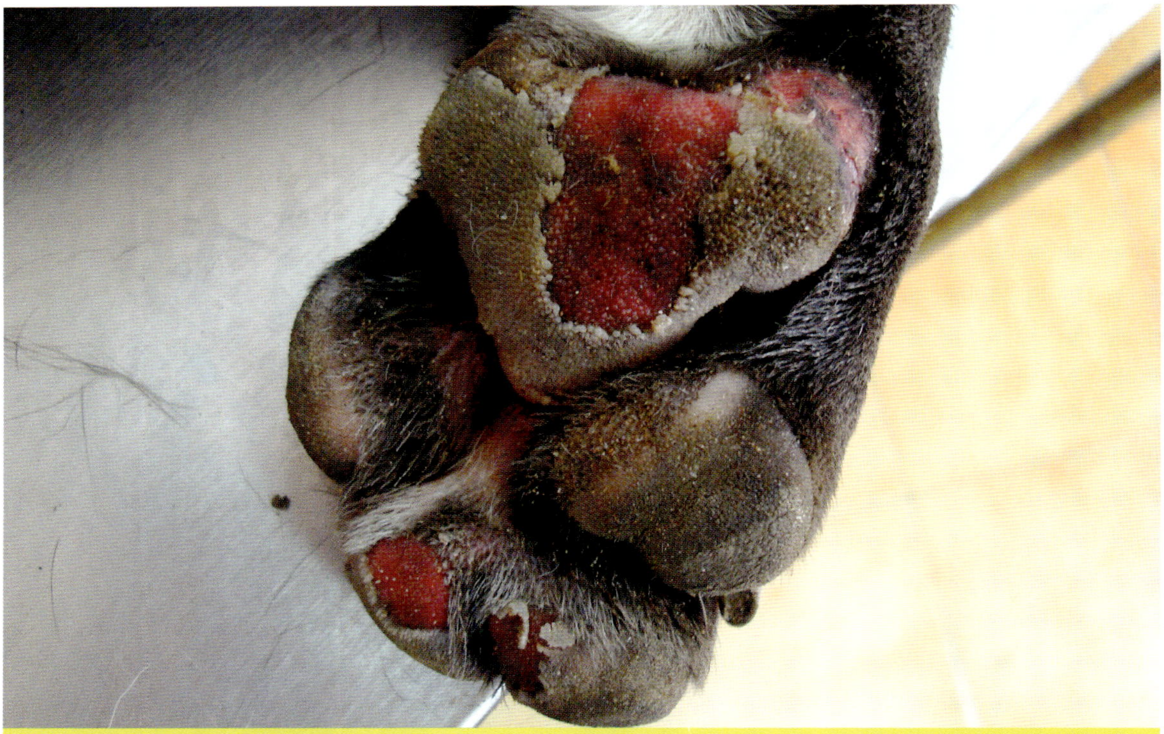

20 De-epithelialisation of the paw pads in a case of bullous pemphigoid.

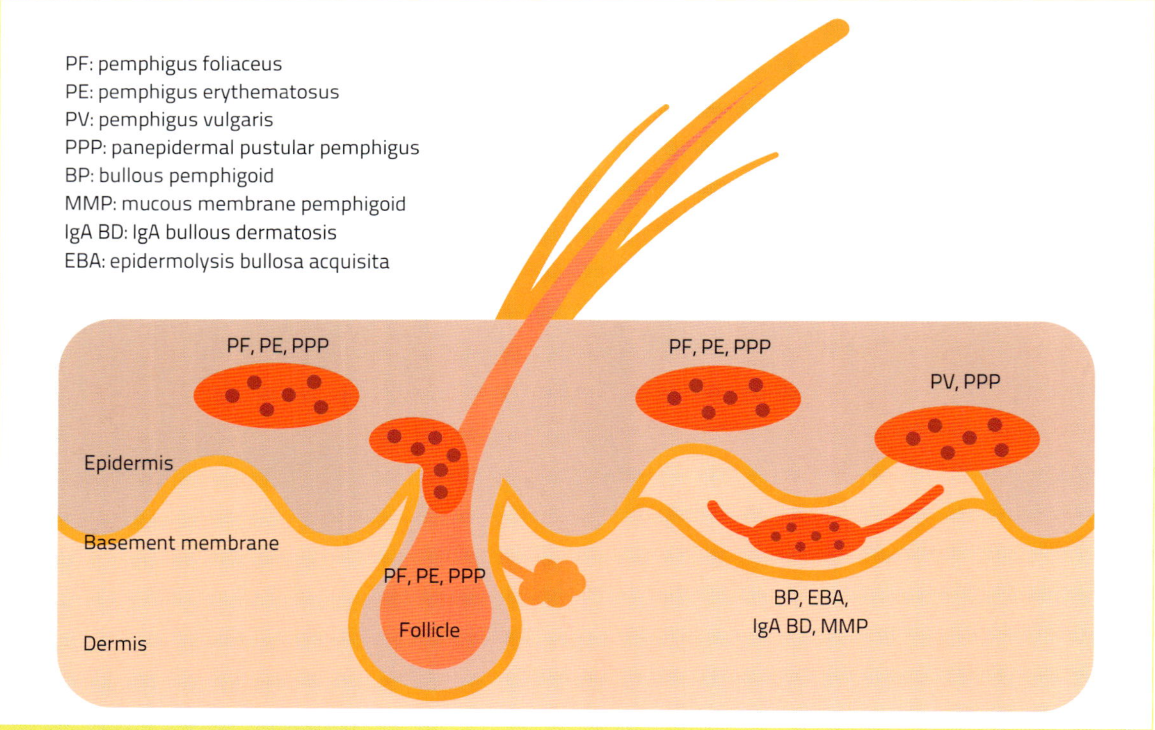


21 Types of pemphigoid disease according to depth or affected area.

# Cutaneous lupus erythematosus

## Lesion aetiology/pathogenesis and clinical picture

This skin disease is characterised by dysregulation of the immune system, and involves genetic, hormonal, and environmental factors. T cell dysfunction, polyclonal B cell activation, and cytokine disturbance are implicated.

Two forms can be distinguished based on the mean duration of the lesions:

- **Subacute cutaneous lupus erythematosus**: mainly vesicular, primarily affecting glabrous areas such as the axillae and groin.
- **Chronic cutaneous lupus erythematosus**, which encompasses several distinct forms, including:
  - Discoid lupus erythematosus, predominantly affecting the face (nose, eyelids, and pinna).
  - Generalised discoid lupus erythematosus (plaques on the neck, back, and lateral thorax).
  - Mucocutaneous lupus erythematosus, which affects the different mucocutaneous junctions with an erosive–ulcerative pattern.
  - Exfoliative cutaneous lupus erythematosus, which affects young dogs with an exfoliative alopecia pattern in areas on the muzzle, ears, extremities, and ventral region.

No sex or age predisposition is described and dogs are more commonly affected than cats.

Sunlight can be an aggravating factor, especially in the variant that affects the transitional skin above the muzzle.

It is characterised by generally slow progression with characteristic lesions such as depigmentation, erythema, ulcerations, erosions, and crusts. These lesions mainly occur on the nose, eyelids, scrotum and mucocutaneous labial junctions, and the border of the muzzle.

Any breed can be affected but the incidence is higher, depending on the type, in the German Shepherd, Belgian Shepherd, Rough Collie, and Shetland Sheepdog.

## Diagnostic method

The clinical picture can be confused with various other diagnoses. Histopathological study of an area without bacterial alterations is necessary to confirm the diagnosis. Evidence of improvement after avoidance of sunlight should be taken into account.

In certain circumstances, the so-called mucocutaneous variant of lupus can be very difficult to differentiate from mucocutaneous pyoderma.

## Main differential diagnoses

- Other autoimmune diseases
- Mucocutaneous pyodermas
- Contact dermatitis
- Leishmaniasis
- Vitiligo
- Canine proliferative arteritis of the nasal plane
- Drug reaction
- Cutaneous epitheliotropic lymphoma

## Treatment

It is very important to use protective creams and avoid ultraviolet radiation, since in some cases this may be sufficient to control the condition.

Available therapies include immunosuppressive drugs such as corticosteroids, cyclosporine, azathioprine, chlorambucil, tetracycline-nicotinamide, and mycophenolate mofetil. Other options include omega 3 and omega 6 fatty acids, vitamin E, and topical tacrolimus.

Oclacitinib is also currently being used with some success and good tolerance.

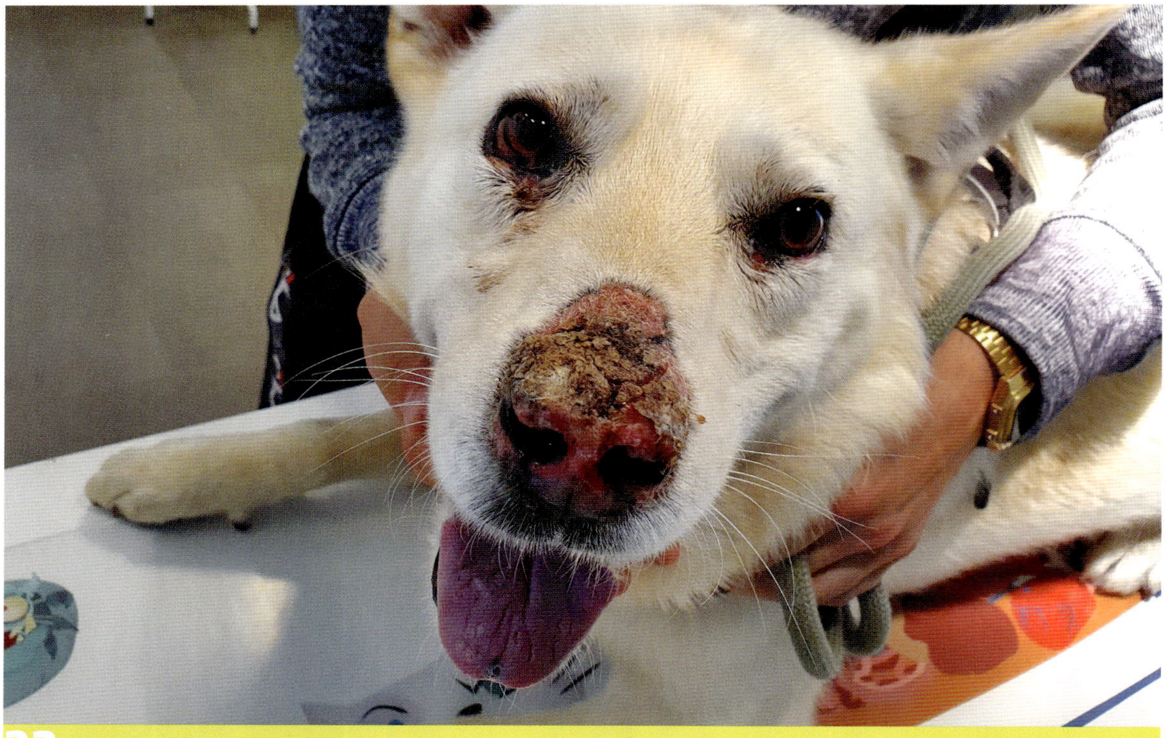

22 Nasal and eyelid involvement in a dog with predominantly facial discoid lupus erythematosus.

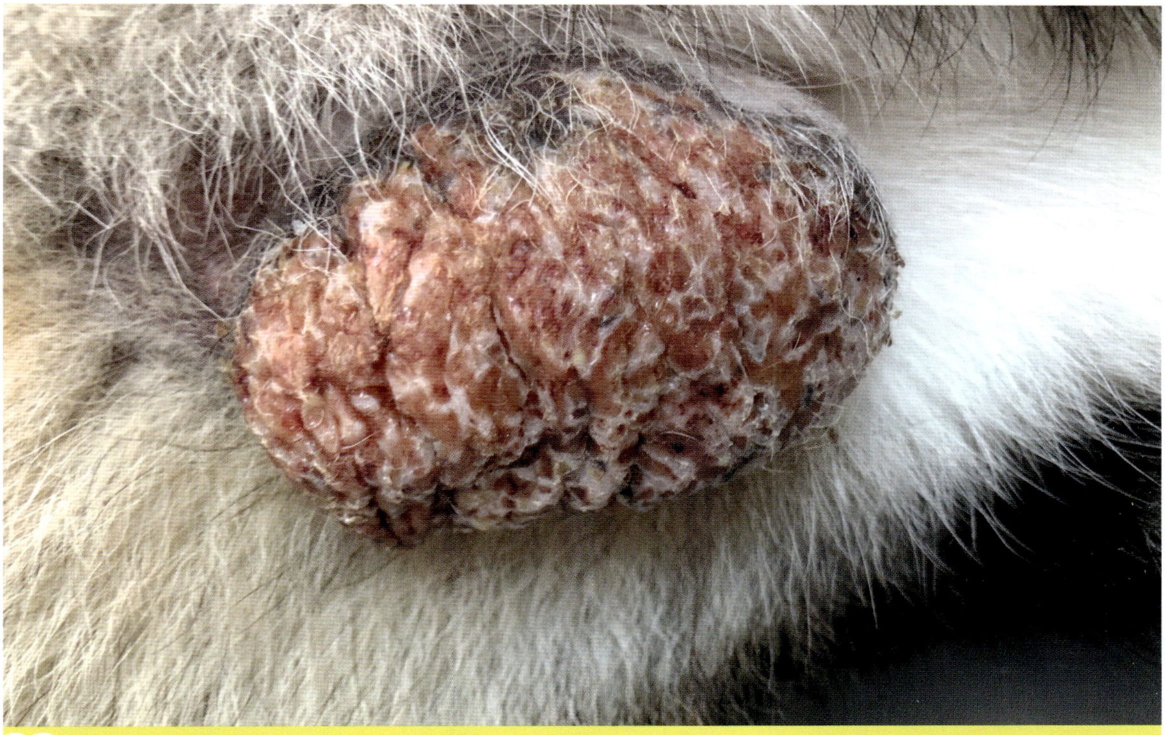

23 Severe scrotal involvement in generalised discoid lupus erythematosus.

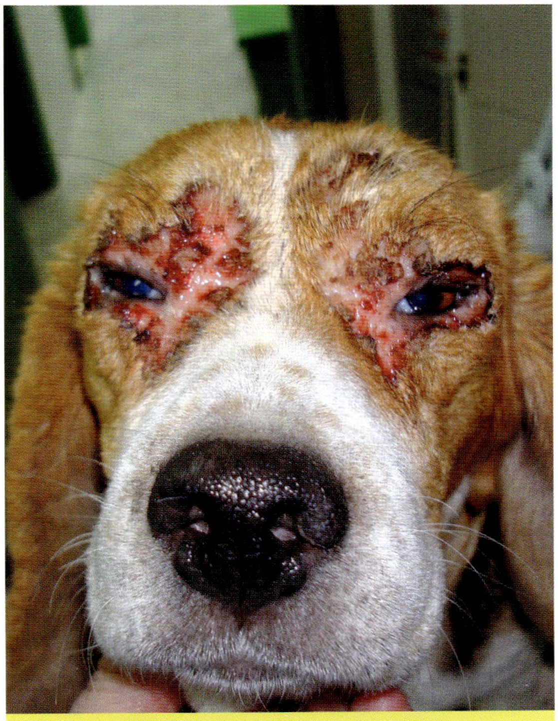

24 Severe eyelid involvement in a case of cutaneous lupus erythematosus.

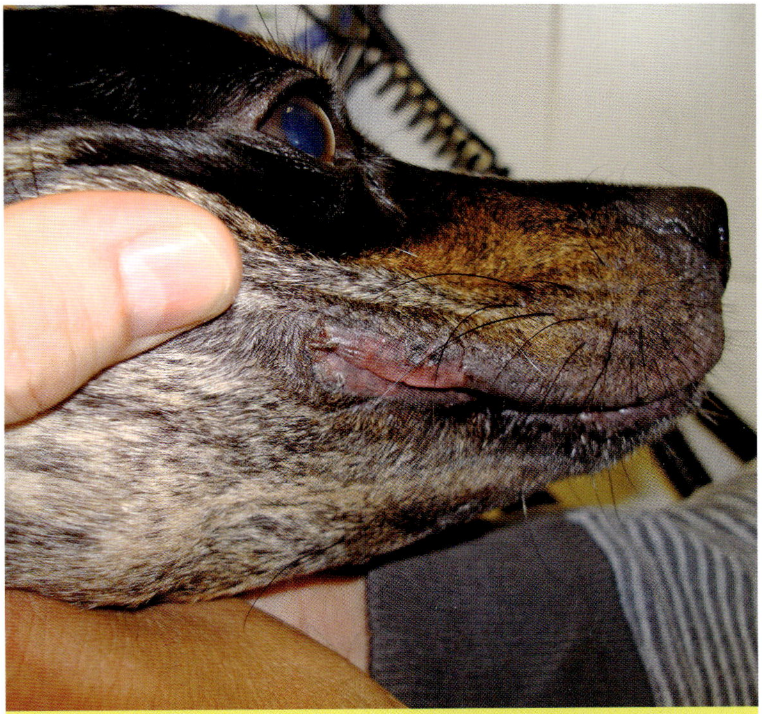

25 Mucocutaneous lupus erythematosus: involvement of the labial mucocutaneous junction.

# Lupoid onychodystrophy or idiopathic onychomadesis

## Lesion aetiology/pathogenesis and clinical picture

This is a rare disease that affects the nails. It may have an immune-mediated origin, although to date the causes are unknown. It is mainly described in dogs, although some cases of a similar disease in cats have been reported.

Despite the lupoid histopathology, the disease may constitute a reaction pattern induced by various inflammatory diseases.

No breed-, age-, or sex-related predisposition is described, although prevalence may be higher in Rottweilers, Setters, and German Shepherds.

The condition involves the gradual formation of defective nails that grow with cracks or deformations, or separate from the nail bed. It can affect some or all nails, and the animal often licks its paws and, in some cases, limps due to pain.

## Diagnostic method

The clinical picture is quite evident and must be confirmed by biopsy. It is more important to rule out other causes of onychia and then, through a process of elimination, to confirm this type of reaction pattern.

## Main differential diagnoses

- Onychomycosis and bacterial nail infections
- Cutaneous lupus erythematosus
- Leishmaniasis
- Trauma resulting in alteration of the nail matrix
- Drug reactions
- Tumours

## Treatment

Responses to treatment with antibiotics, vitamin E, pentoxifylline, essential fatty acids (mainly omega 3), biotin, immunosuppressants, and an elimination diet have been described.

Each case is distinct, and therefore treatment should start with less aggressive therapies and other options tried if no response is observed.

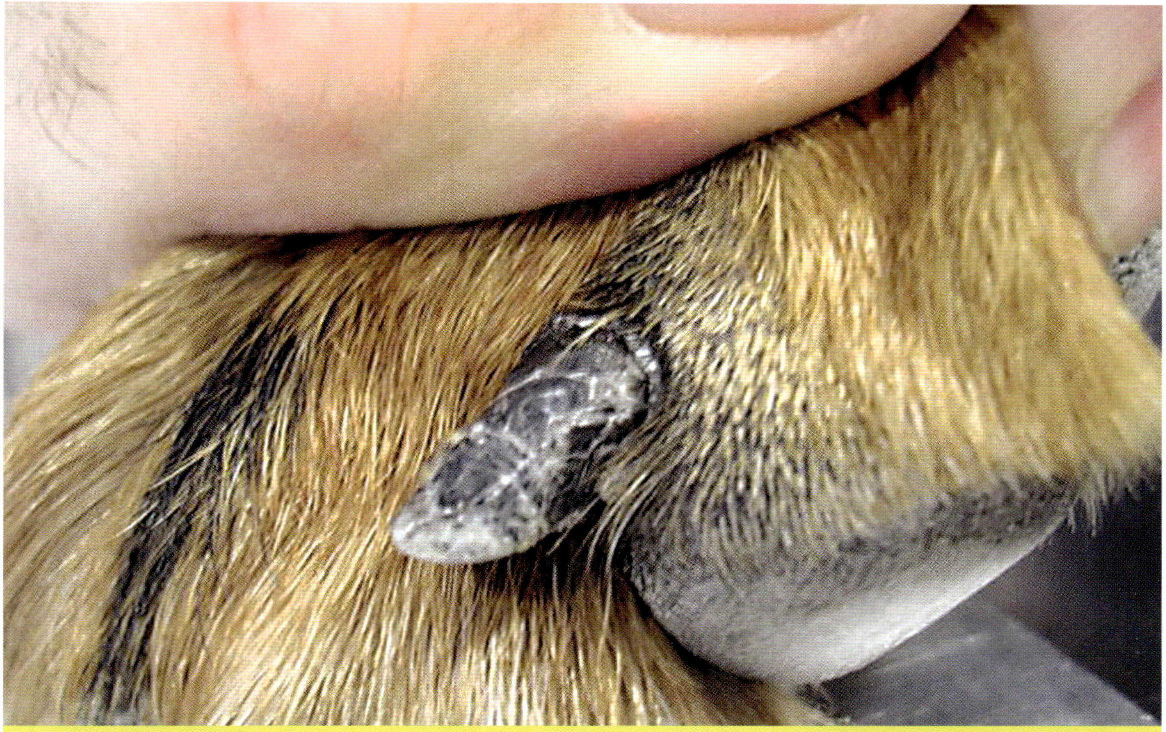

26 Brittle nail at onset of lupoid onychodystrophy. Image courtesy of Xulio Rodríguez Lorenzo.

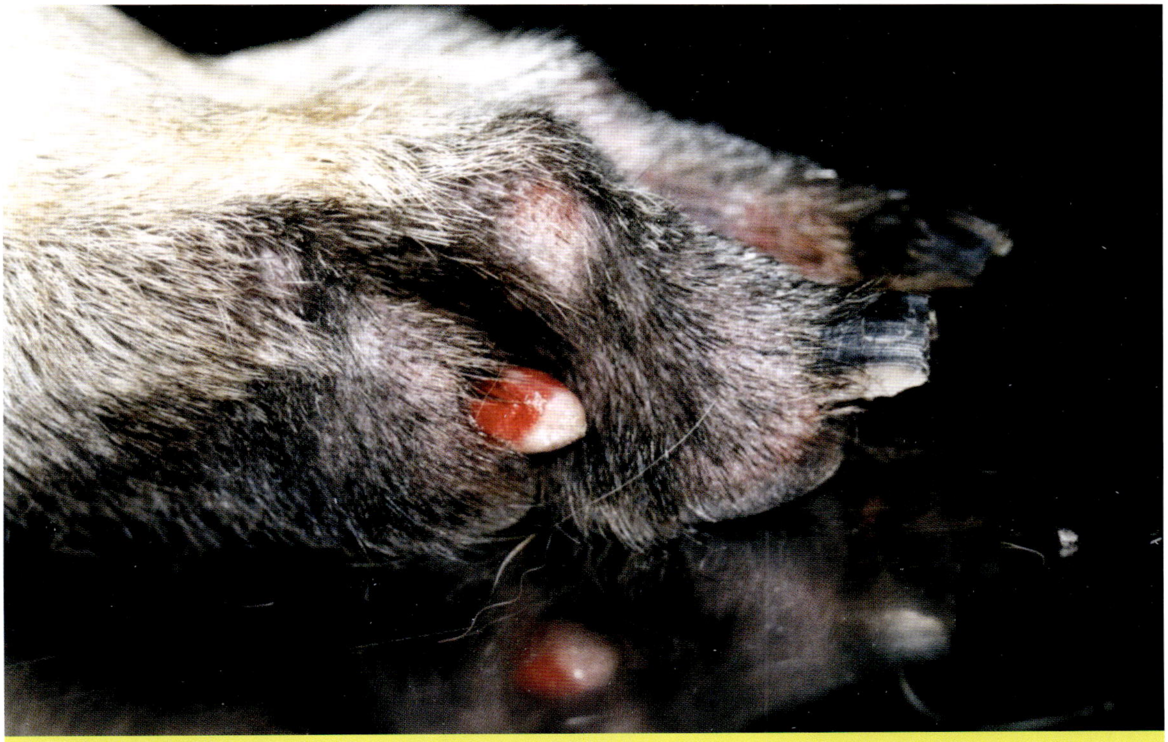

27 Detached nail and broken nail in a case of lupoid onychodystrophy.

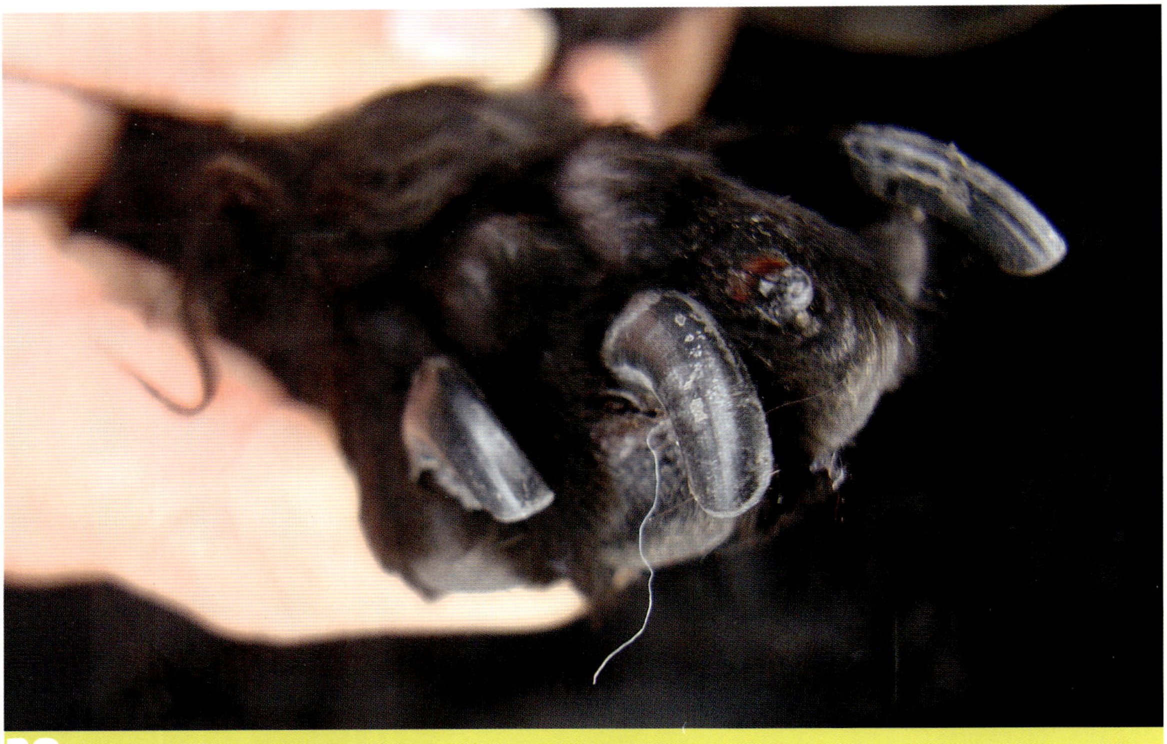

28 Deformed nail and exposed nail matrix in a dog with lupoid onychodystrophy.

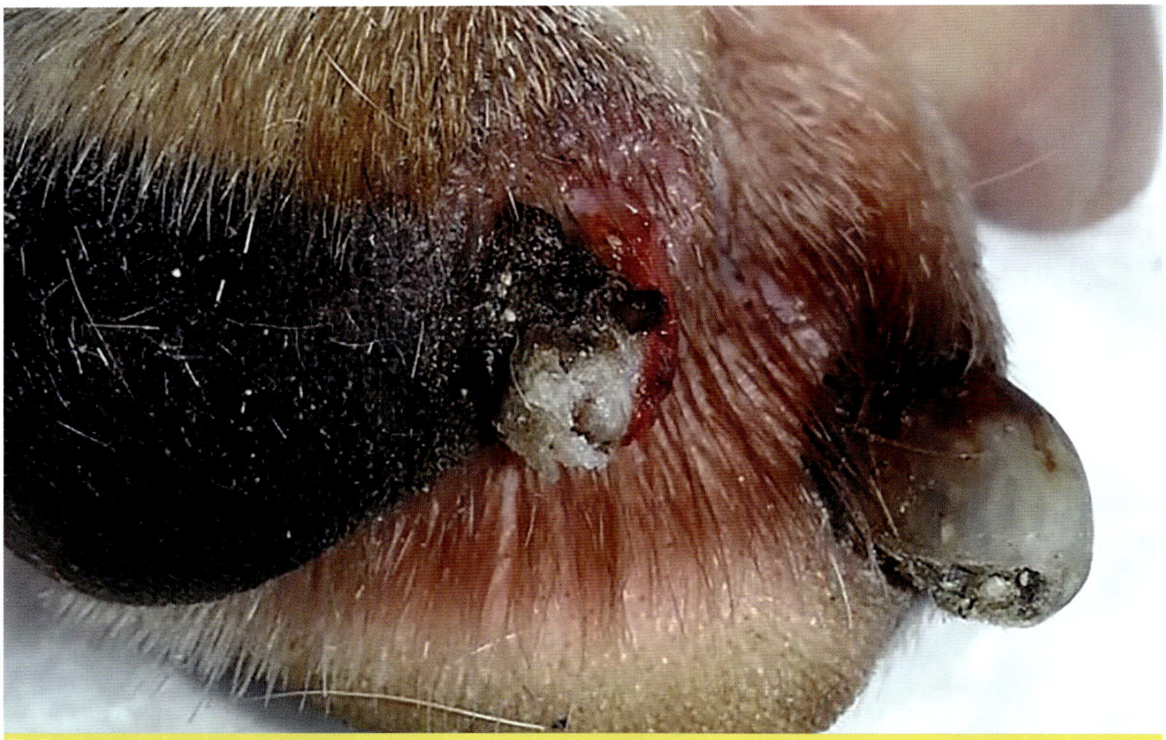

29 Onychomalacia in a dog with lupoid onychodystrophy. Note the consistency of the nail.

# Sterile nodular panniculitis

## Lesion aetiology/pathogenesis and clinical picture

This is an immune reaction of unclear aetiology and pathogenesis that affects the adipose tissue of the hypodermis in dogs and cats. It can affect animals of any age, breed, and sex, although it is more commonly reported in Dachshunds and Poodles.

In some cases, pancreatitis and pancreatic tumours can underlie this clinical presentation. Drug reaction is another suspected cause in some cases.

Lesions consist of solitary or grouped nodules. Clinical signs include prostration and the presence of fluctuating nodular lesions that fistulise to the exterior, discharging haemorrhagic fatty fluid. These nodules are more frequent on the trunk.

## Diagnostic method

Diagnosis is based on a clinical picture consisting of moveable nodules beneath the skin and cytology compatible with adipose tissue and pyogranulomatous inflammation. Biopsy is the ideal method.

The presence of pancreatic alterations increases the likelihood of a diagnosis of sterile nodular panniculitis.

## Main differential diagnoses

- Tumours
- Cysts
- Granulomas

## Treatment

Surgery is one treatment option and often provides good results. In cases of multiple nodules, treatment with glucocorticoids at immunosuppressive doses can be attempted. Some cases may respond to vitamin E, doxycycline-nicotinamide, and cyclosporine.

If the lesions are due to pancreatic alterations, resolution of the latter can resolve the skin lesions.

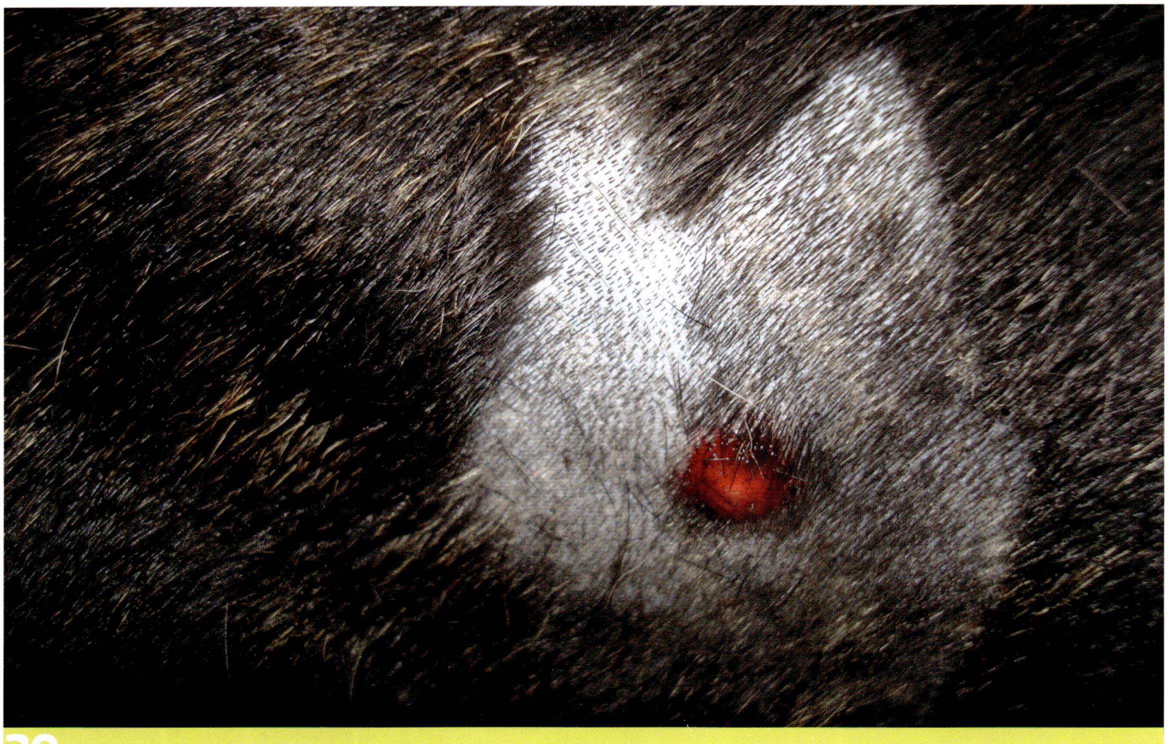

30 Fistulised nodule in a case of sterile nodular panniculitis.

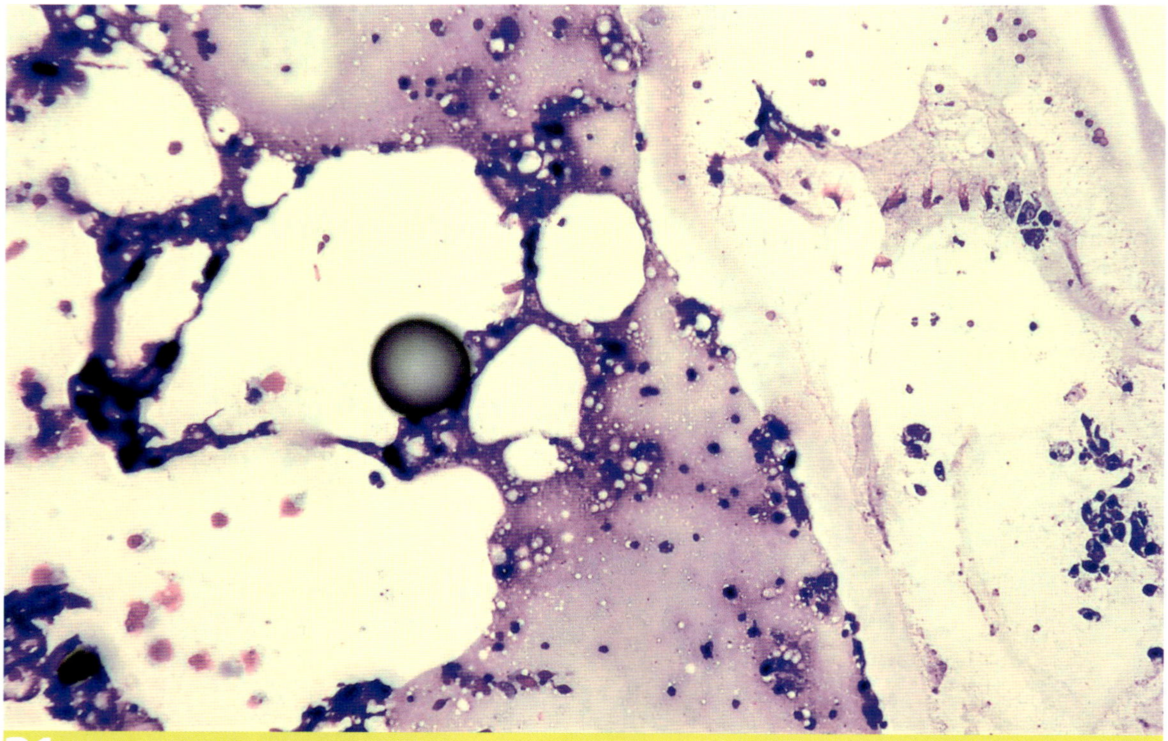

31 Cytology of sterile nodular panniculitis.

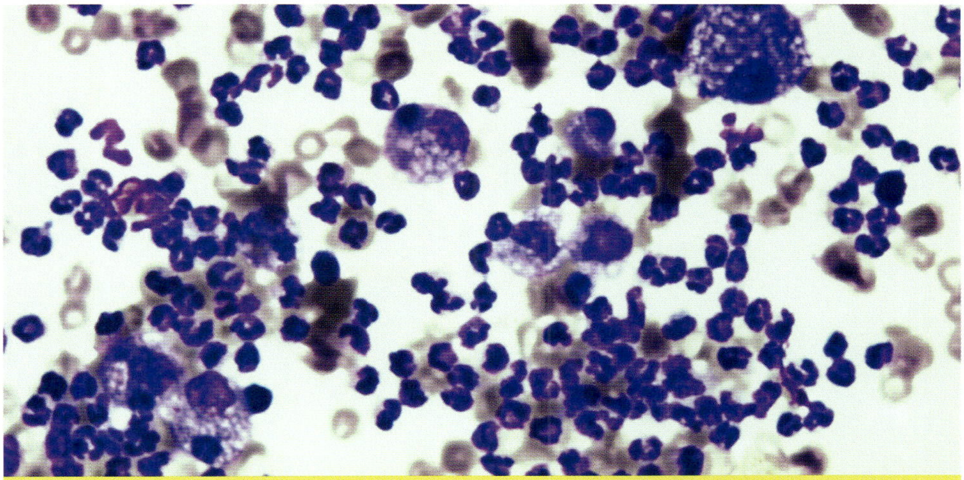

32 Cytology of sterile nodular panniculitis. Note the "foamy" macrophages phagocytosing lipid content.

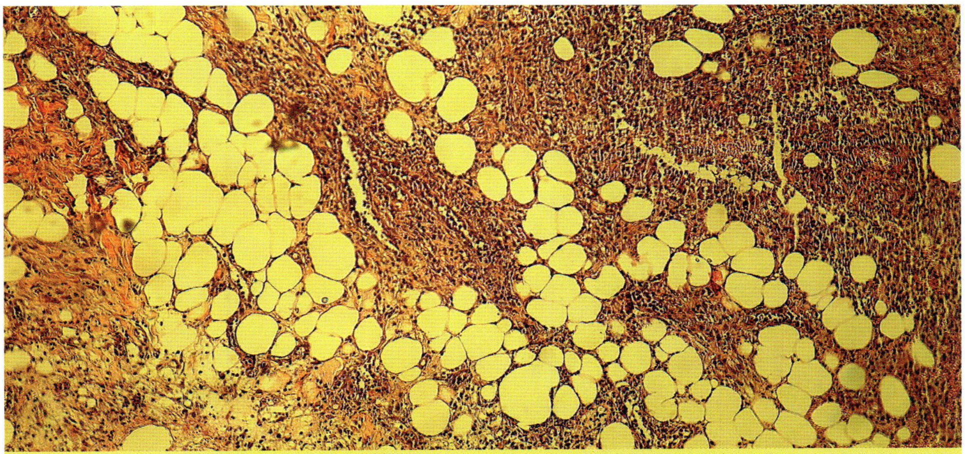

33 Histopathology of sterile nodular panniculitis: the inflammatory infiltrate in the subcutaneous adipose tissue is clearly appreciated.

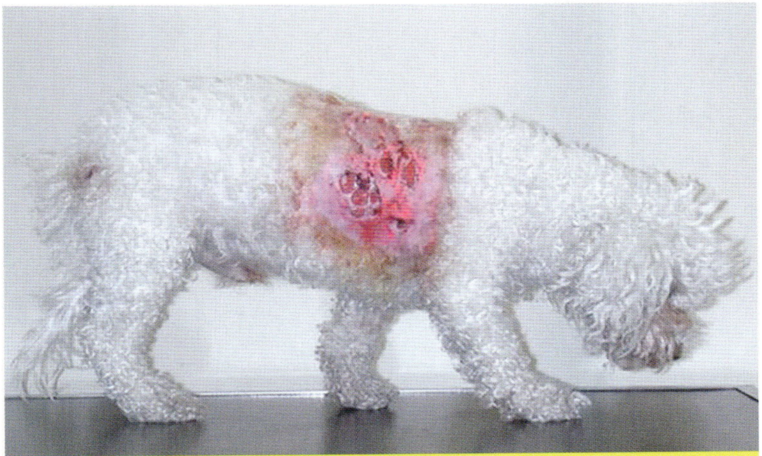

34 Dog affected by sterile nodular panniculitis. Image courtesy of Didier Carlotti (RIP).

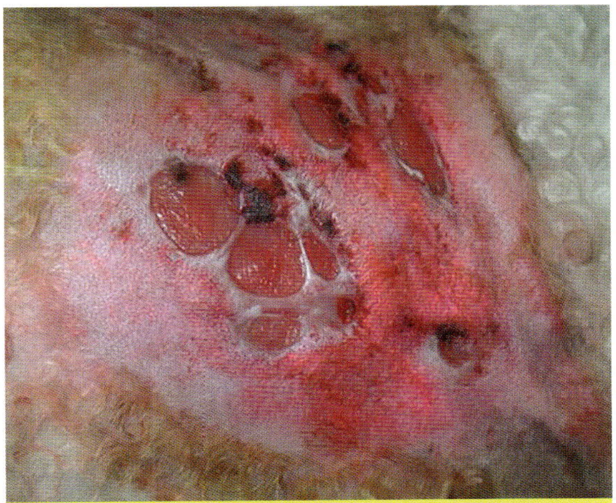

35 Closer view of the dog from the previous image. Image courtesy of Didier Carlotti (RIP).

# Sterile granuloma-pyogranuloma syndrome

## Lesion aetiology/pathogenesis and clinical picture

These skin lesions, which consist of plaques or nodules, are uncommon in dogs and very rare in cats.

The underlying aetiology has not been clearly established, although it may be linked to immune system disorders caused by the presence of bacterial or other antigens that cannot be detected.

## Diagnostic method

Diagnosis is based on cytology showing an absence of microorganisms and on the patient's medical history (see also Figure 2 in Chapter 12).

## Main differential diagnoses

- Other causes of pyogranuloma
- Tumours
- Panniculitis
- Histocytic processes

## Treatment

One option is the use of doxycycline with niacinamide, although this may not be advisable given the possible presence of resistant staphylococci. Glucocorticoids, cyclosporine, azathioprine, or chlorambucil can also be used.

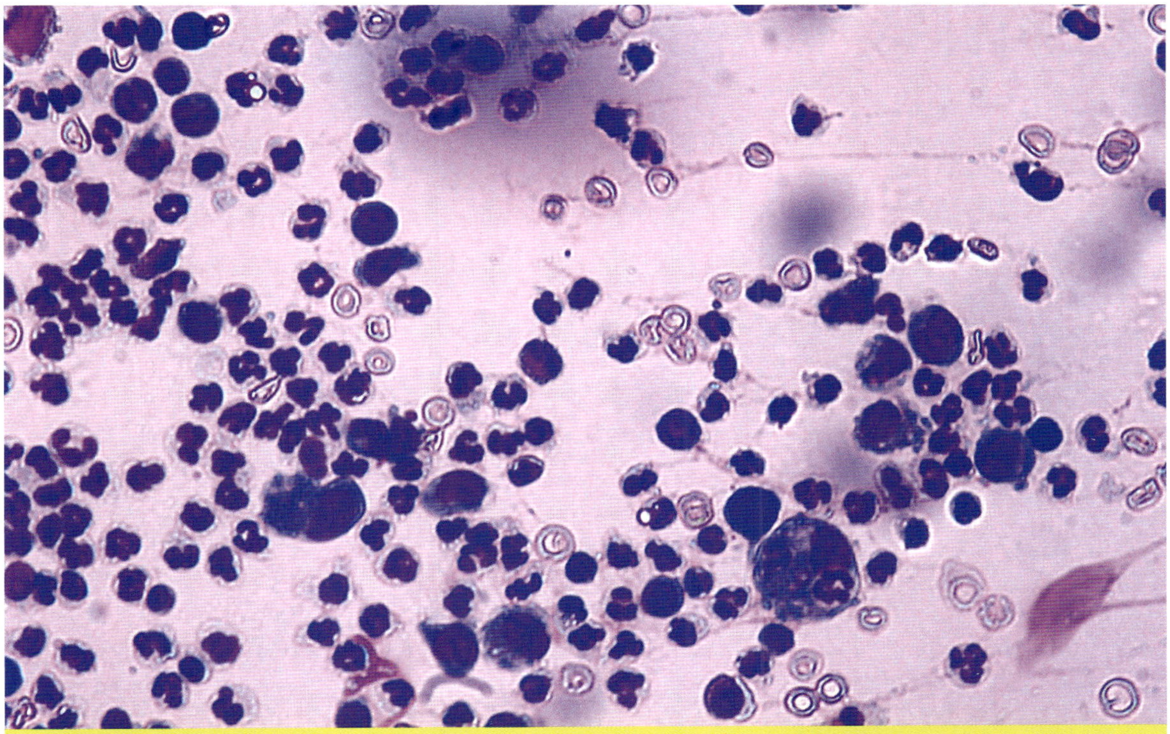

36 Sterile pyogranuloma cytology with active macrophages phagocytosing neutrophils.

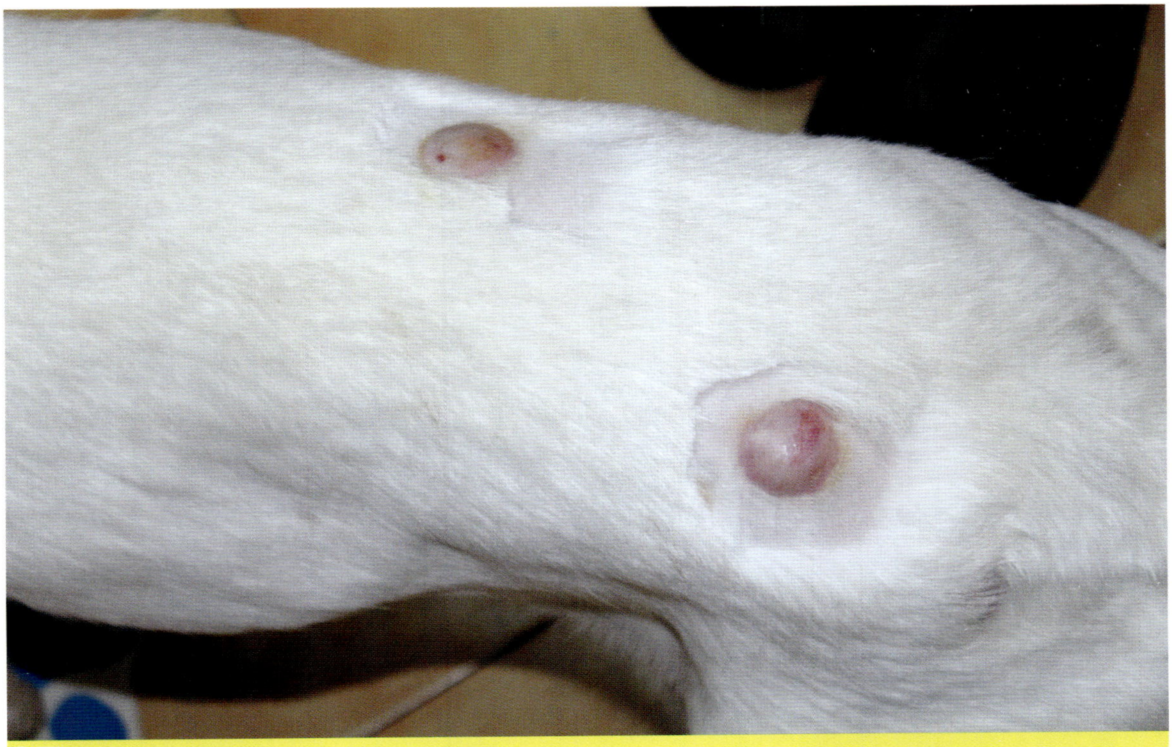

37 Nodules in a dog with pyogranuloma syndrome.

# Sebaceous adenitis

## Lesion aetiology/pathogenesis and clinical picture

This is an autoimmune disease in which the sebaceous glands are attacked. A clear predisposition is described in the Akita Inu, Samoyed, Poodle, and Vizsla. Cats can also be affected by this autoimmune reaction, although it is often associated with another type of systemic disease.

This condition can be idiopathic or associated with either leishmaniasis or hypersensitivity reactions.

The clinical picture appears gradually with diffuse alopecia and a dull, poor quality hair coat. Abundant scaling and follicular casts are observed. In cats, areas of scaling tend to coalesce mainly on the face.

## Diagnostic method

Together with the clinical picture, the affected breed, and a lack of response to conventional treatments, a biopsy will establish the diagnosis. In early stages, it is often difficult to diagnose this disease histologically. It can be confused with other entities. As it progresses, periglandular sebaceous infiltration and subsequent disappearance of these glands becomes much more evident.

## Main differential diagnoses

- Keratinisation disorders
- Endocrinopathies
- Leishmaniasis
- Dermatophytosis
- Follicular dysplasias
- Bacterial folliculitis

## Treatment

It is important to try to stop or delay the disappearance of the sebaceous glands. Moisturising shampoos containing phytosphingosines, ophytrium, glycerin, urea, D-panthenol, liposomes, zinc gluconate, epilobium, etc., are used, as well as propylene glycol lotions. Immunosuppressive drugs are also important and in some cases synthetic retinoids such as acitretin and isotretinoin may be required.

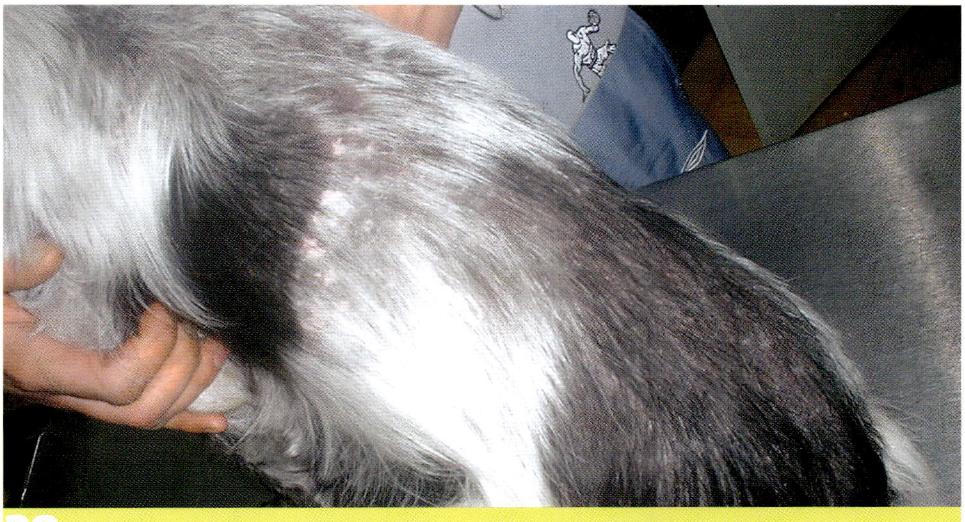

38 Appearance of the coat in a mixed-breed dog with sebaceous adenitis.

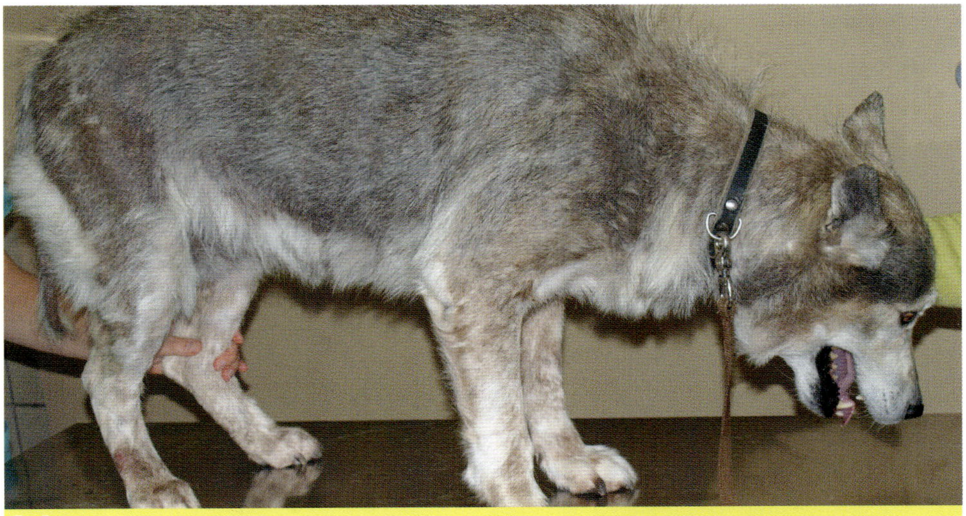

39 Sebaceous adenitis in a mixed-breed dog. Image courtesy of Jose Luis González Arribas.

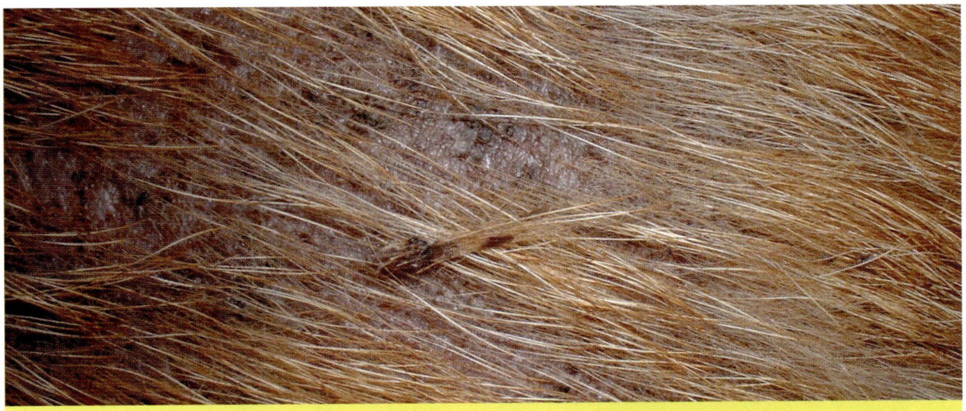

40 Detachment of follicles in casts in a case of sebaceous adenitis.

# Ischaemic dermatopathies

## Lesion aetiology/pathogenesis and clinical picture

Blood vessels can become inflamed by the accumulation of immune complexes, or due to the action of leukocytes or microorganisms. Clear examples of this aetiology are seen in diseases such as erlichiosis, babesiosis, leishmaniasis, and systemic lupus, as well as drug reaction. On many occasions it can be difficult to determine the cause and in some cases the condition is considered idiopathic (e.g. in Jack Russell Terriers, in which the disease is considered breed-specific).

In peripheral areas, such as the edges of the pinnae and the extremities of the limbs and tail, vasculopathy may occur due to vasoconstriction of the capillaries (e.g. due to cold) and in some cases due to hypersensitivity caused by repeated insect bites. The latter is quite frequent in the German Shepherd and its crosses due to the bites of insects on the ears. Idiopathic vasculopathy of the ear margins has also been described. This is a very rare disease and has been reported in Dachshunds and other breeds.

Dermatomyositis is another hereditary immune-mediated vasculopathy described in the Collie and Shetland Sheepdog. The lesions consist of initial scaling, pallor, erosions, ulcers, and gradual necrosis with marked scarring, subsequently progressing to muscular involvement.

## Diagnostic method

Diagnosis is established based on the clinical picture and histological examination. Leishmaniasis must always be ruled out. Histopathology usually enables a definitive diagnosis.

## Main differential diagnoses

- Other forms of vasculitis
- Keratinisation disorders
- Leishmaniasis
- Drug reactions

## Treatment

Avoid the cause in cases of infections or insects. In localised cases of idiopathic origin, treatment with pentoxifylline, fibrinolytic creams, and topical tacrolimus may be effective. In cases of disseminated disease, immunosuppressants and pentoxifylline are typically used. Other options include vitamin E and tetracycline-niacinamide.

The combination of pentoxifylline and oclacitinib is a novel therapeutic strategy that can be very effective.

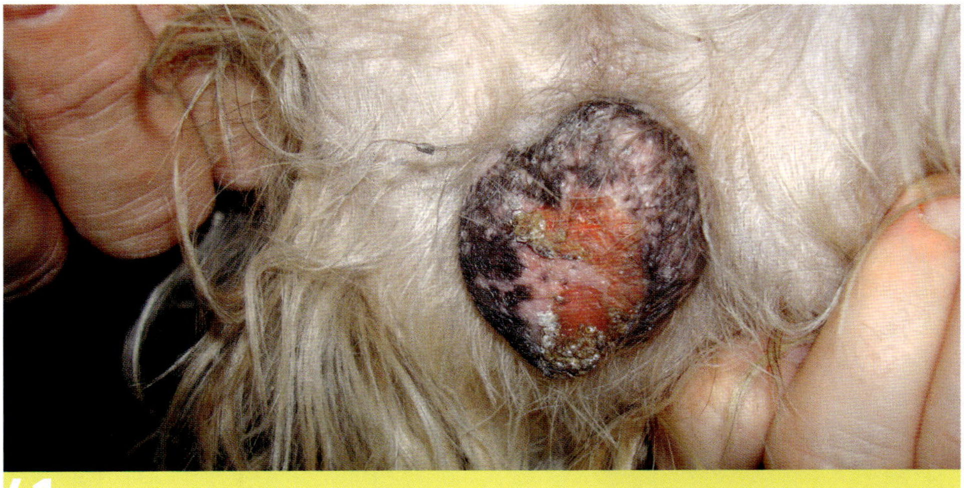

41 Scrotal vasculitis in a lupus-affected Yorkshire Terrier.

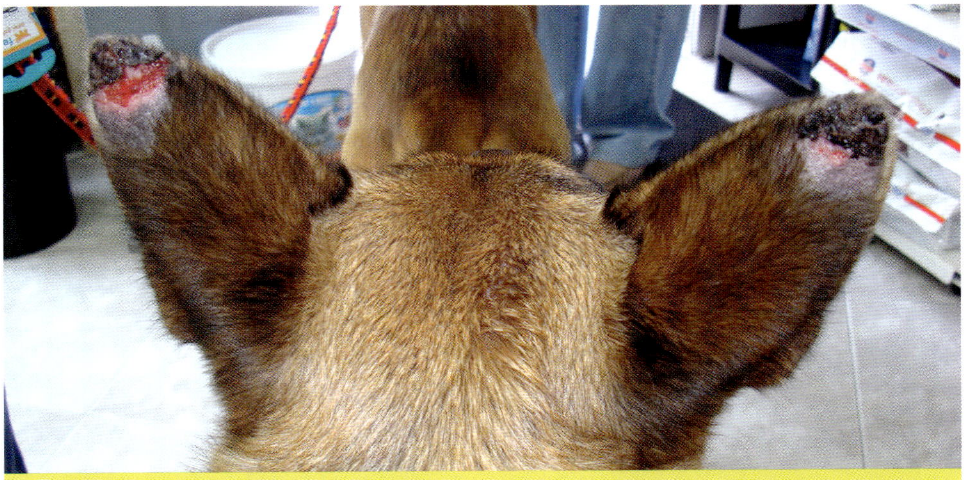

42 Vasculitis of the ear tips and onset of necrosis due to insect bites.

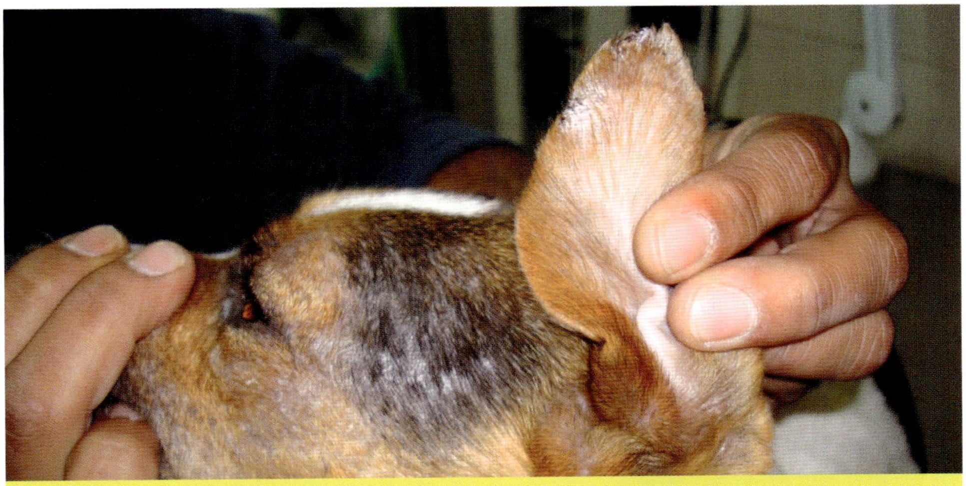

43 Vasculitis of Jack Russell Terriers. Note the ear and facial involvement.

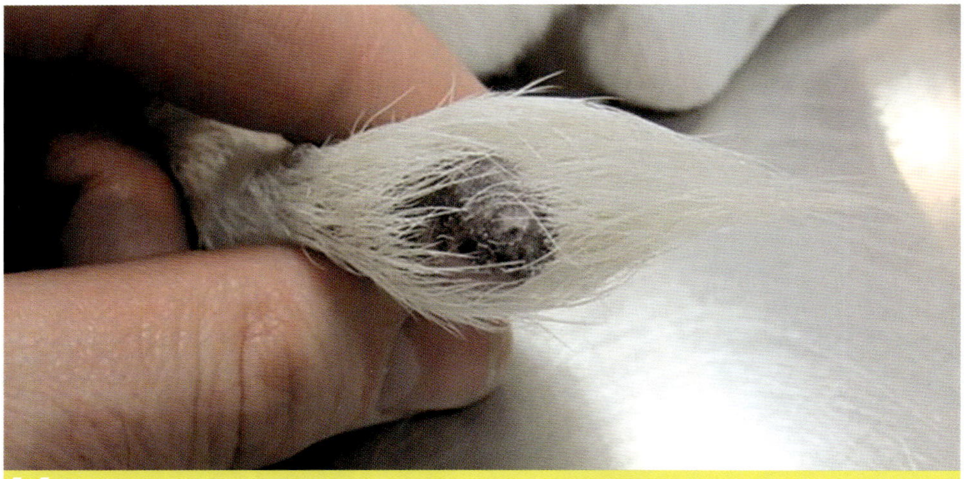

44 Tip of the tail of the dog from the previous image.

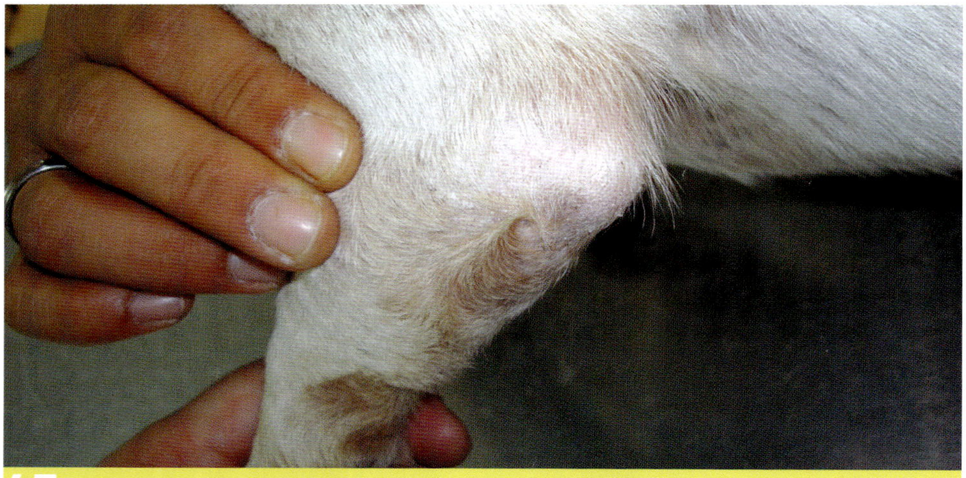

45 Involvement in the bony prominences in a Jack Russell Terrier with vasculitis.

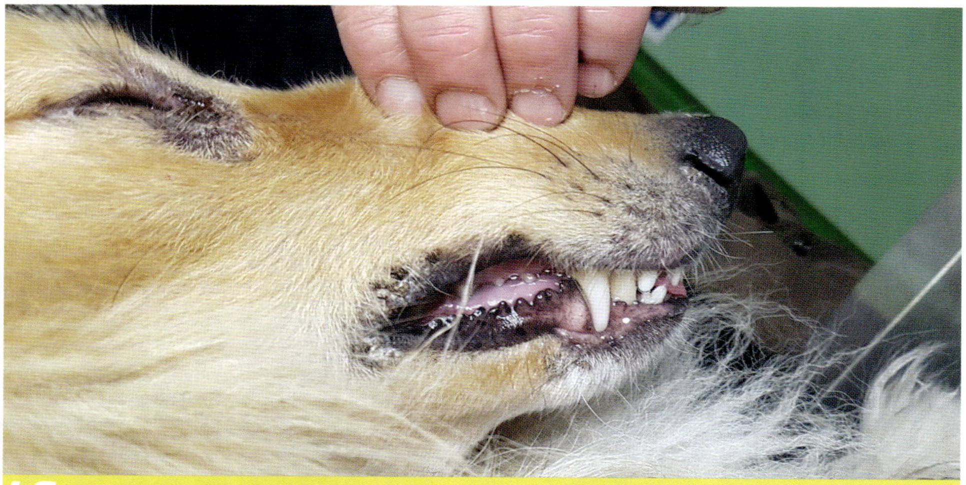

46 Dermatomyositis in a Collie: inolvement of the mucocutaneous junctions of the eyelids and mouth.

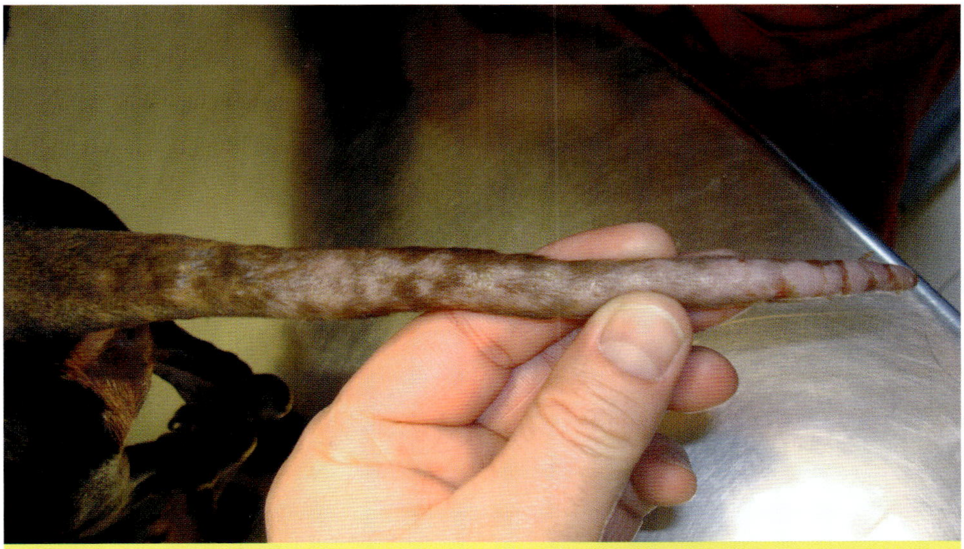

47 Tail of a Dachshund with severe idiopathic vascular disease.

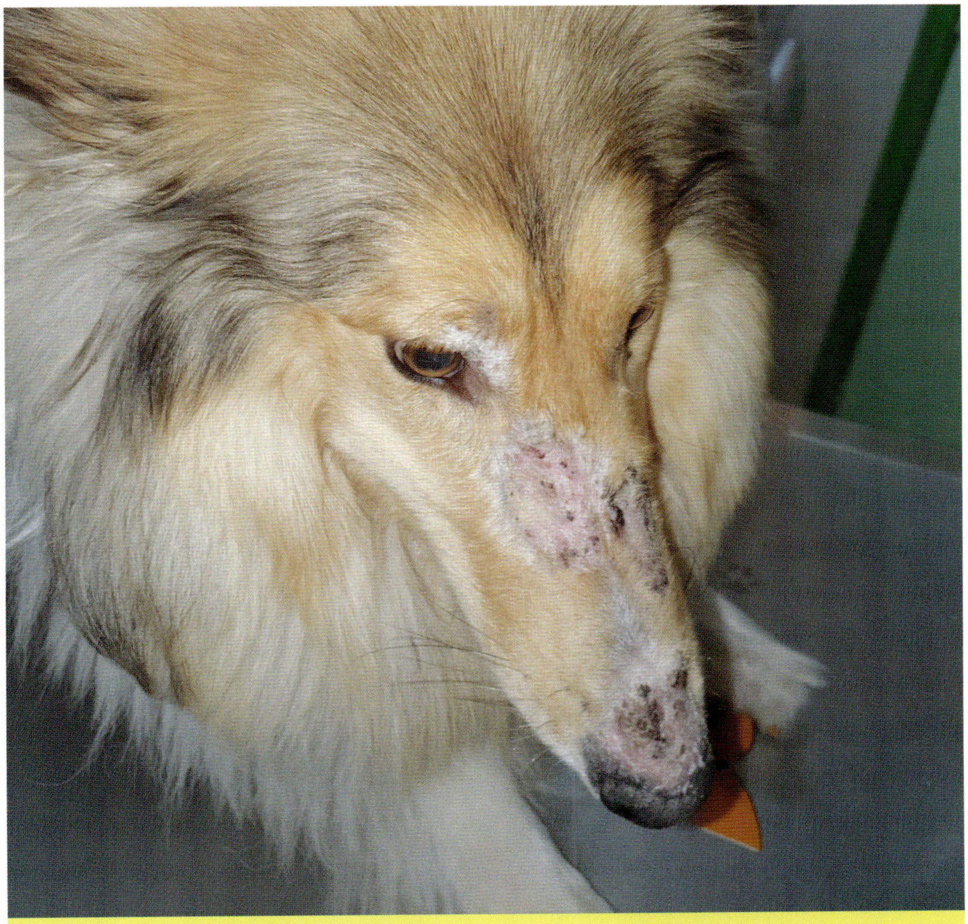

48 Dermatomyositis in a Collie: facial involvement.

# Uveodermatologic syndrome

## Lesion aetiology/pathogenesis and clinical picture

This is a rare disease of dogs consisting of dermatitis combined with depigmentation and uveitis. Autoantibodies are produced against different cellular antigens, mainly melanin (including that of the iris and choroid) and related proteins. Onset usually occurs in young adults. Facial leukoderma occurs with concomitant leukotrichia and uveitis.

## Diagnostic method

Diagnosis is mainly established based on the clinical picture and biopsy.

## Main differential diagnoses

- Vitiligo
- Other autoimmune diseases
- Epitheliotropic lymphoma
- Mucocutaneous pyoderma with depigmentation

## Treatment

Treatment consists of topical and systemic corticosteroids, and in other cases azathioprine or cyclosporine. Treatment response is good, although recurrence is common. It is very important to begin treatment early and to closely monitor the eyes to avoid severe uveitis.

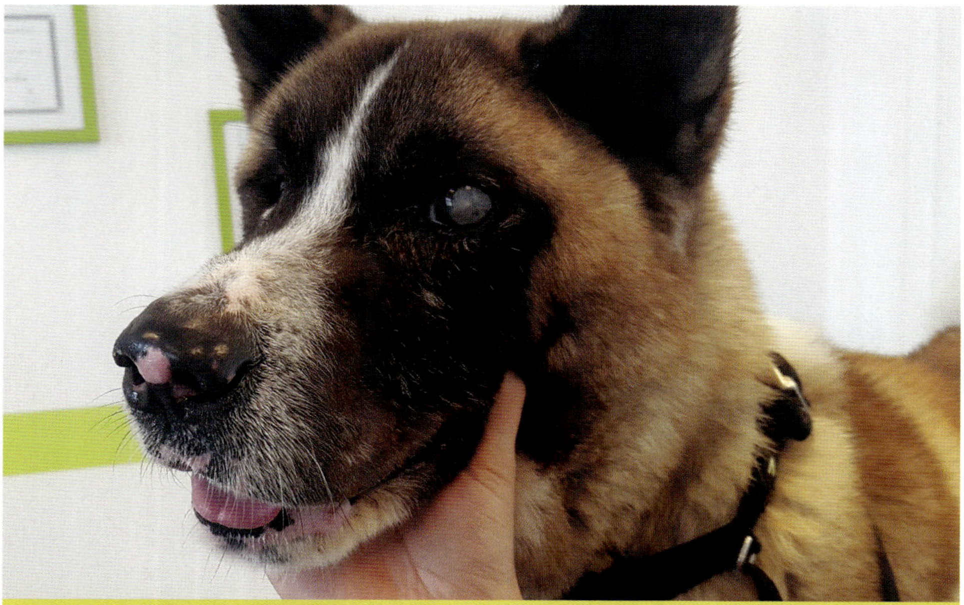

49 Face of an Akita Inu dog with uveodermatological syndrome. Note the eye involvement and the depigmentation of the muzzle and lower lip.

# Fistulas

## Perianal fistulas

### Lesion aetiology/pathogenesis and clinical picture

This disease affects the anal area, rectum, and base of the tail, with the presence of fistulas, concurrent infection, and in many cases colitis. It is thought to be immune-mediated, as it can be resolved or controlled with immunosuppressive drugs and control of colitis can result in resolution of the fistulas.

It is much more common in the German Shepherd, although other breeds can be affected.

### Diagnostic method

Diagnosis is established based on the clinical picture and the response to treatment.

### Main differential diagnoses

- Anal sac fistula
- German Shepherd cellulitis
- Tumours

### Treatment

The combination of cyclosporine, topical tacrolimus, and diets high in omega-3 fatty acids is a commonly used treatment.

In refractory cases, other options include: azathioprine, chlorambucil, salazopyrin, metronidazole and hydrolyzed diets. Recent publications have also described the use of systemic tacrolimus. Successful outcomes have also been recently reported following autologous stem cell implantation into fistulas. Fluorescent light energy (FLE) therapy can also be effective.

In terms of surgical options, laser or cryosurgery can be very effective.

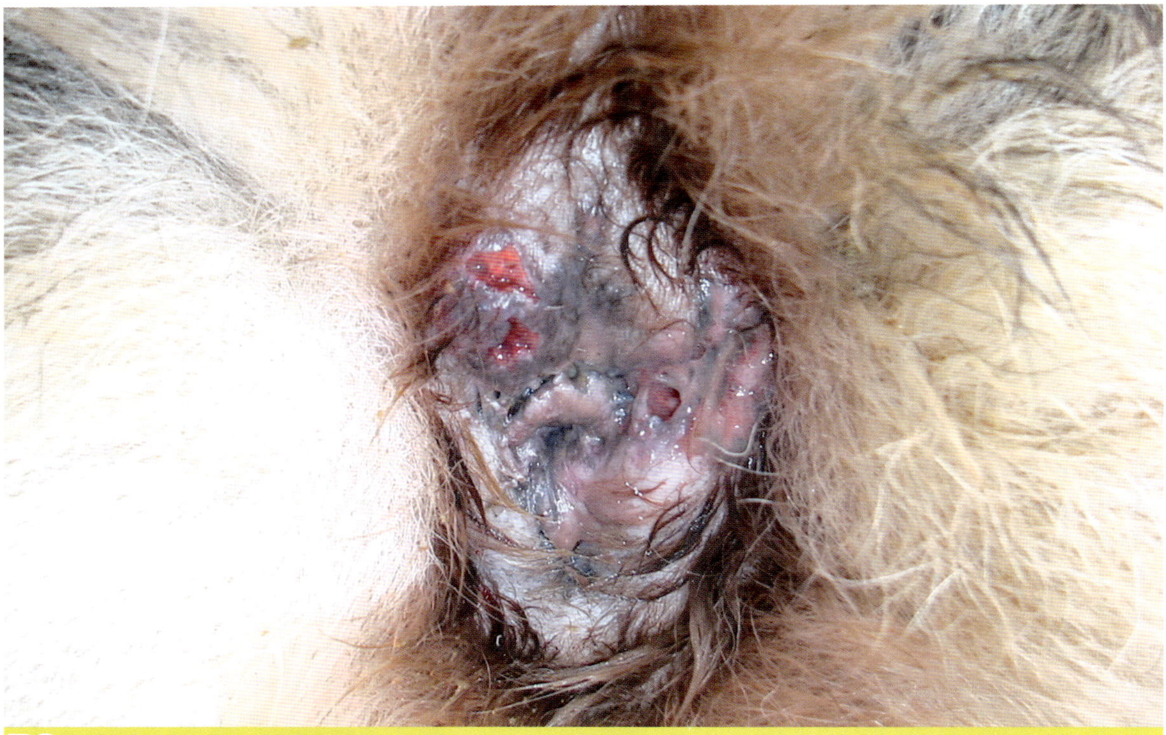

50 Anal fistulisation at the 4 and 10 o'clock position.

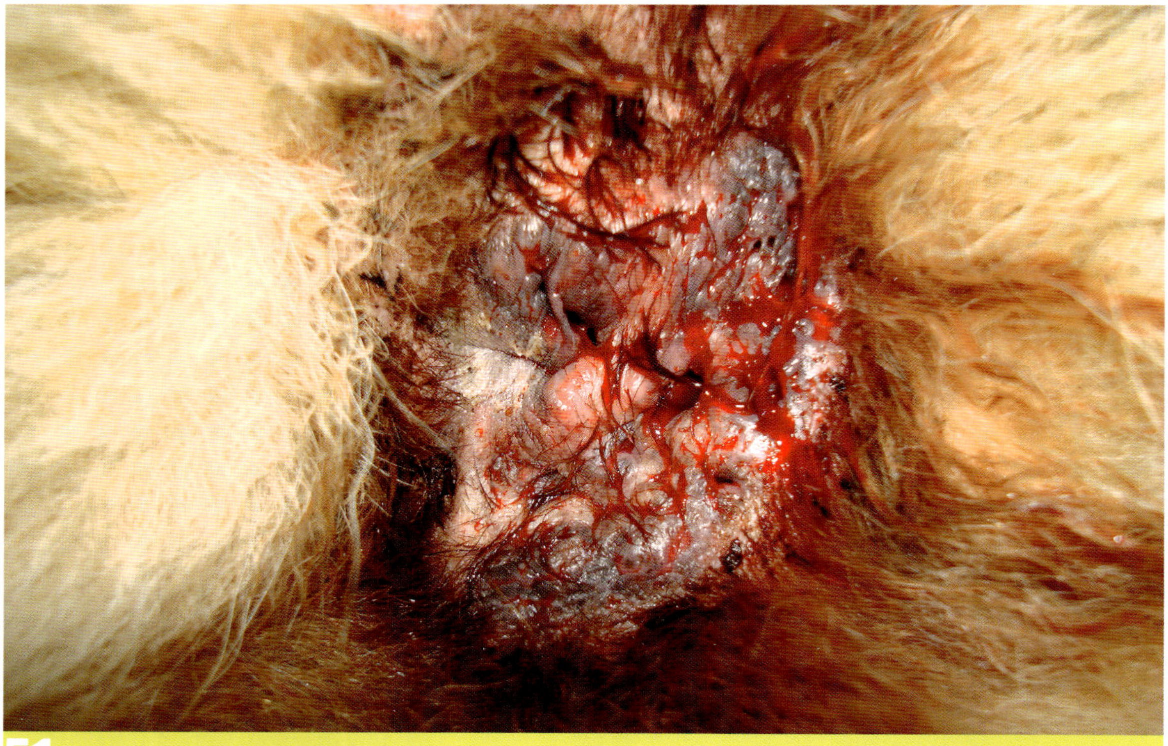

51 Small anal fistulas in a 360° orientation.

# Metatarsal or metacarpal fistulas

## Lesion aetiology/pathogenesis and clinical picture

This infrequent form of sterile dermal or subdermal pyogranuloma may be of immune-mediated origin, and is mainly reported in German Shepherd dogs and their crosses. It almost always affects the palmar or plantar metacarpal or metatarsal area, proximal to the central pad. Fistulas develop, producing seropurulent discharge. These lesions are usually painful, resulting in lameness and licking of the affected area.

In some situations, these fistulas can develop in atypical areas of the metacarpal or metatarsal region.

## Diagnostic method

Diagnosis is established based on the clinical picture, cytology compatible with a pyogranuloma and compatible biopsy findings.

## Main differential diagnoses

- Traumatic ulcers
- Localised pyodermas
- Abscesses

## Treatment

Topical tacrolimus, tetracycline-nicotinamide, glucocorticoids and, in some cases, cyclosporine can be used.

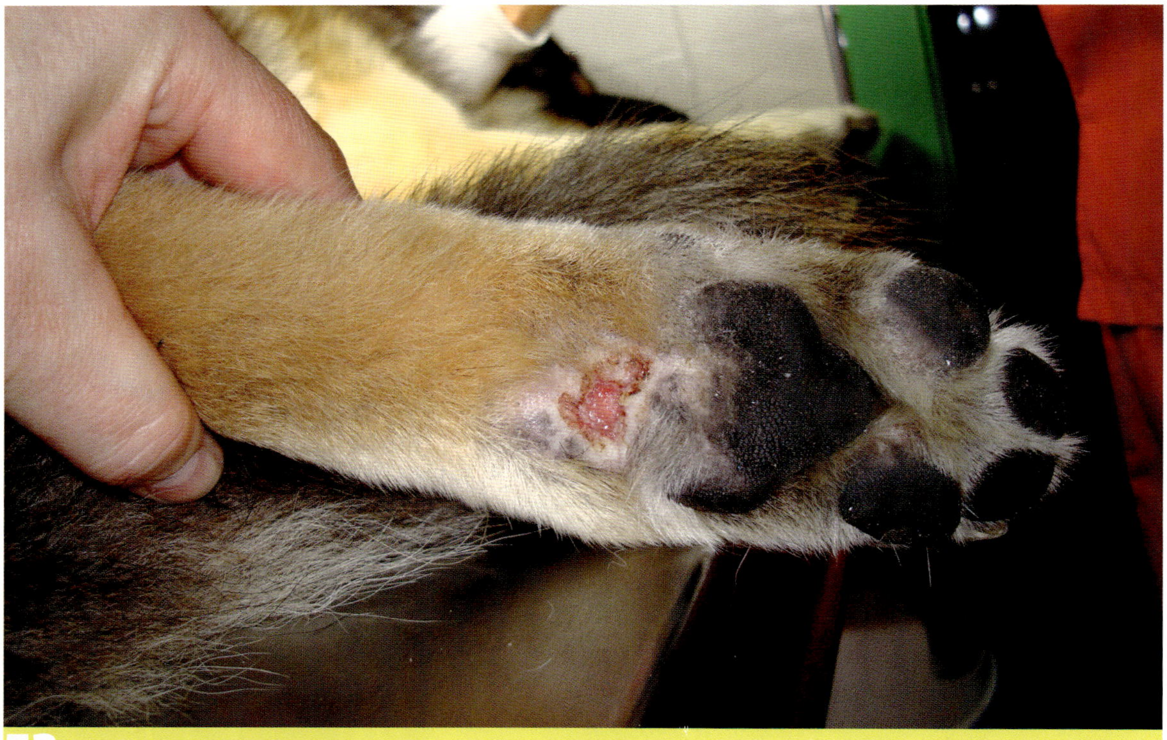

52 Metatarsal fistula in a typical location.

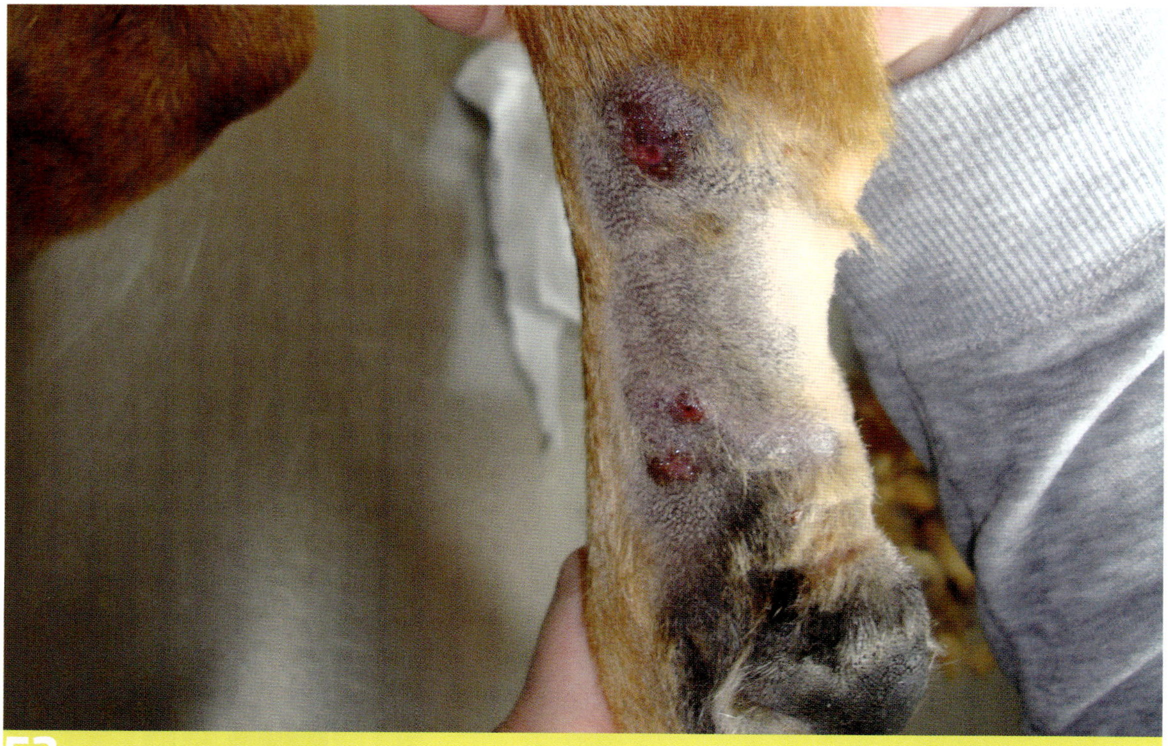

53 Metatarsal fistulas in an atypical location.

# Plasma cell pododermatitis

## Lesion aetiology/pathogenesis and clinical picture

This is a rare, immune-mediated disease that affects the paw pads of cats. It can occur at any age. No breed- or sex-related predisposition is described. Incidence in dogs is extremely low. In cats this condition may be associated with feline immunodeficiency virus.

It consists primarily of gradual inflammation of the central pads, although the other pads can also be affected. The affected pads appear to be filled with fluid and have a soft consistency. It can progress to ulceration and formation of granulomatous tissue. In some cases the skin of the pad does not break and appears deflated and wrinkled.

## Diagnostic method

The clinical picture is obvious. The presence of lymphocytes and plasma cells on cytology and histopathology confirms the diagnosis.

## Main differential diagnoses

- Wounds
- Tumours
- Bacterial or fungal granuloma
- Pemphigus complex

## Treatment

Doxycycline at 10 mg/kg once per day, for 15 days to 1 month, is quite effective.

Treatments with glucocorticoids, cyclosporine, changes in the litter, and topical tacrolimus have been described, with mixed results.

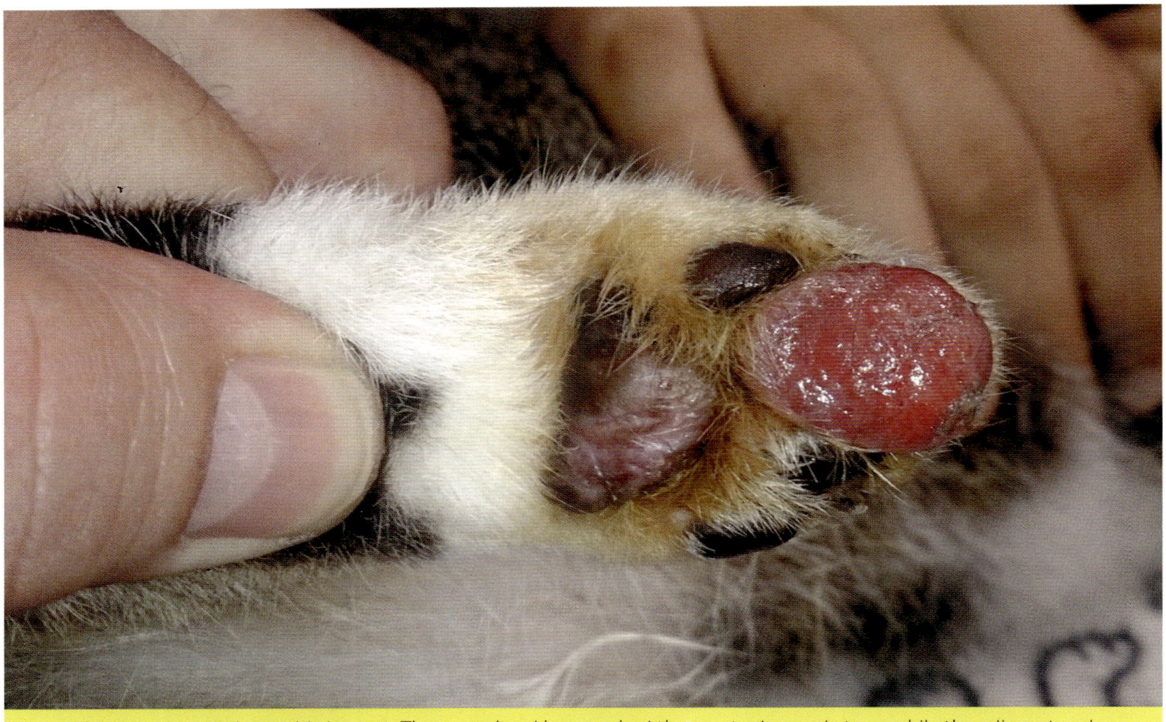

54 Plasmacytic pododermatitis in a cat. The central pad has reached the most advanced stage, while the adjacent pad remains in the most acute phase.

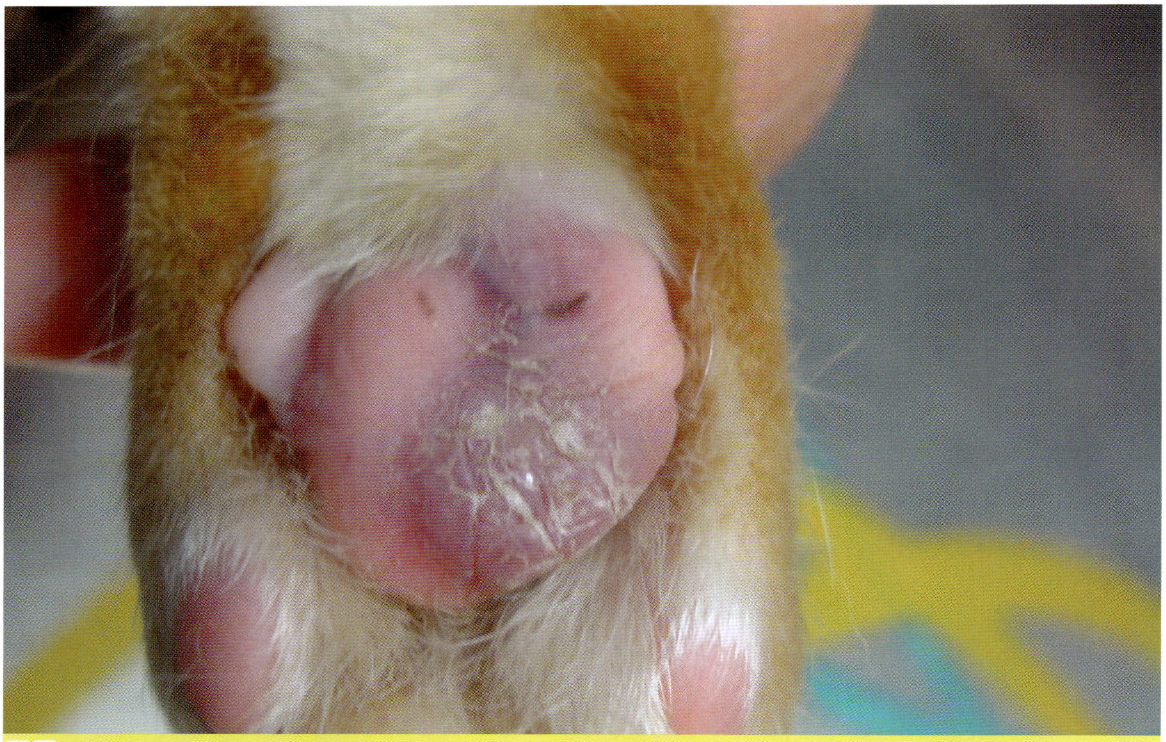

55 Plasma cell pododermatitis: incipient involvement.

# 09

# Dermatosis due to keratoseborrhoeic and pigmentary alterations

# Introduction

This chapter describes the following conditions:

- Primary seborrhoea
- Impaction and fistulas of the anal sacs
- Zinc-responsive dermatosis
- Lichenoid keratosis and lichenoid psoriasiform dermatosis
- Tail gland hyperplasia
- Acne
- Facial dermatosis of Persian and Himalayan cats
- Ulcerative nasal dermatitis of Bengal cats
- Split paw pad disease
- Vitiligo (can also be considered autoimmune)
- Lentigo

Keratoseborrhoeic disorders are a group of dermatoses characterised by an alteration in the production of keratin or products of the specific glands of the skin.

Primary pigmentary alterations consisting of either a lack or the accumulation of pigmentation have been included in this chapter.

# Primary seborrhoea

## Lesion aetiology/pathogenesis and clinical picture

This is a group of skin conditions characterised by excessive scaling and/or sebum production, without an apparent primary cause (and in some cases congenital). Included in this group are senile hyperkeratosis (muzzle and paw pads), vitamin A-responsive dermatosis (American Cocker Spaniel), Miniature Schnauzer comedo syndrome, ear margin seborrhoea (Dachshund) and ichthyosis (Golden Retriever, West Highland White Terrier, etc.).

Cutaneous horns are formed by localised production of compact keratin in cases of hyperplasia of the epidermis or tumours such as squamous carcinomas.

Keratoseborrhoeic disorders in cats are very rare and are usually associated with parasitic infestations, dermatophytosis or metabolic disorders. Bengal cats can develop a congenital form of keratosis of the nasal planum.

## Diagnostic method

Having ruled out external, metabolic, autoimmune, and neoplastic causes, diagnosis is established based on the clinical picture, and often the affected breed.

## Main differential diagnoses

Secondary seborrhoea.

## Treatment

Topical and systemic therapy depending on severity. Frequent therapy with keratolytic, keratoplastic, and keratomodulating and moisturising shampoos, depending on the case, is essential to control the clinical picture. Notable treatments include vitamin A and retinoids, both administered orally, phytosphingosine, derived from the root of *Ophiopogon japonicus*, some seaweed extracts and lipid complexes.

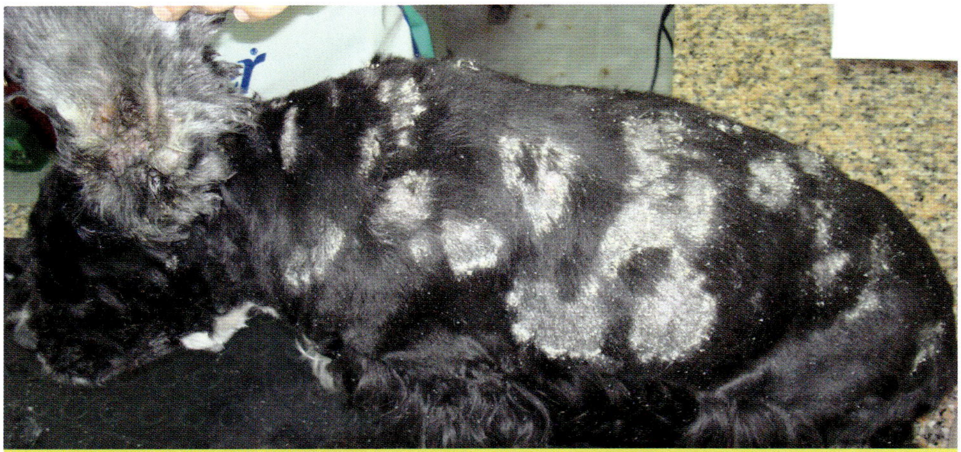

01 Vitamin A-responsive seborrhoea in an American Cocker Spaniel. Note the keratoseborrhoeic plaques and ear involvement.

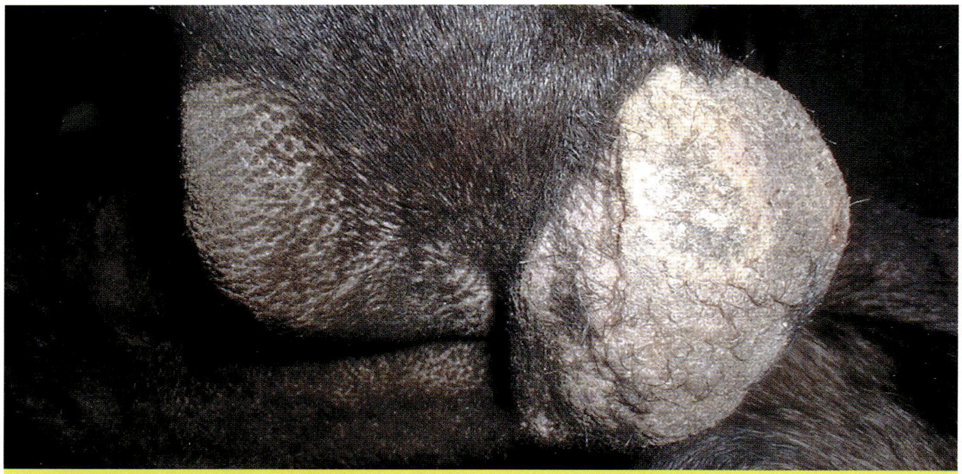

02 Senile hyperkeratosis on the tarsus of a 14-year-old dog.

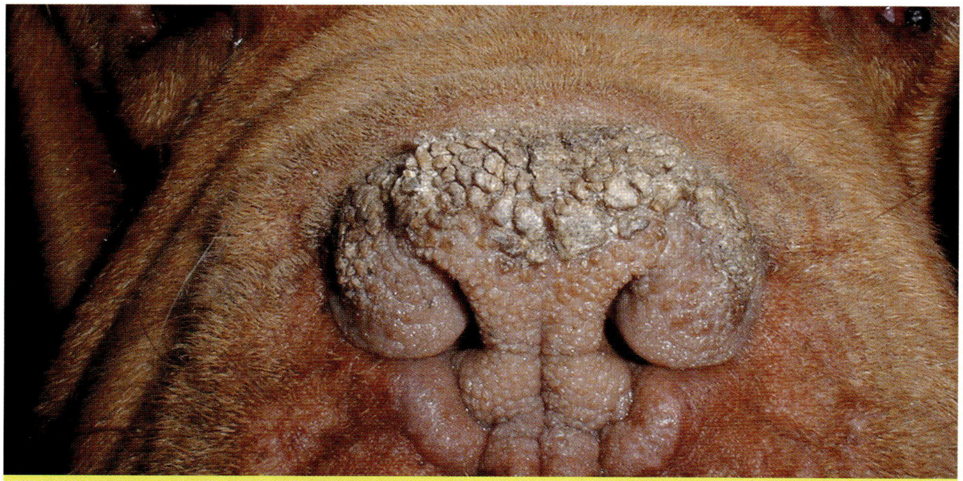

03 Hyperkeratosis on the muzzle of a Dogue de Bordeaux.

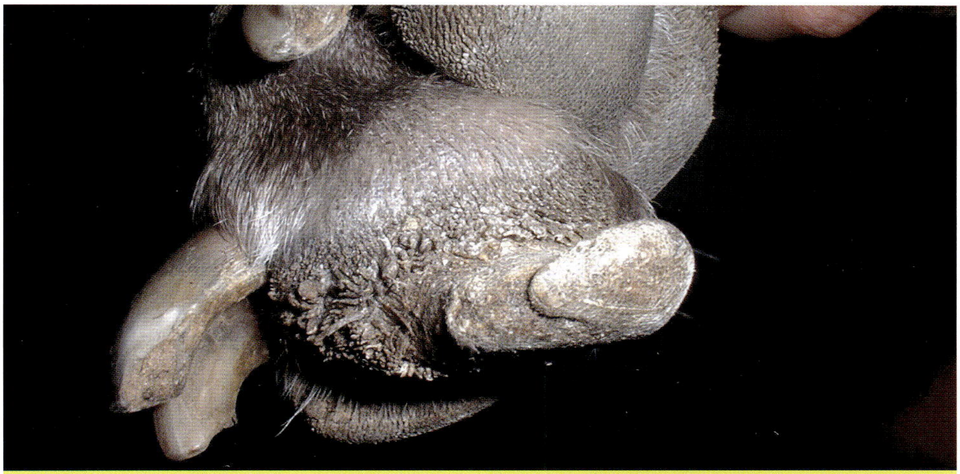

04 Cutaneous horn caused by hyperkeratosis on the paw pad of a Great Dane.

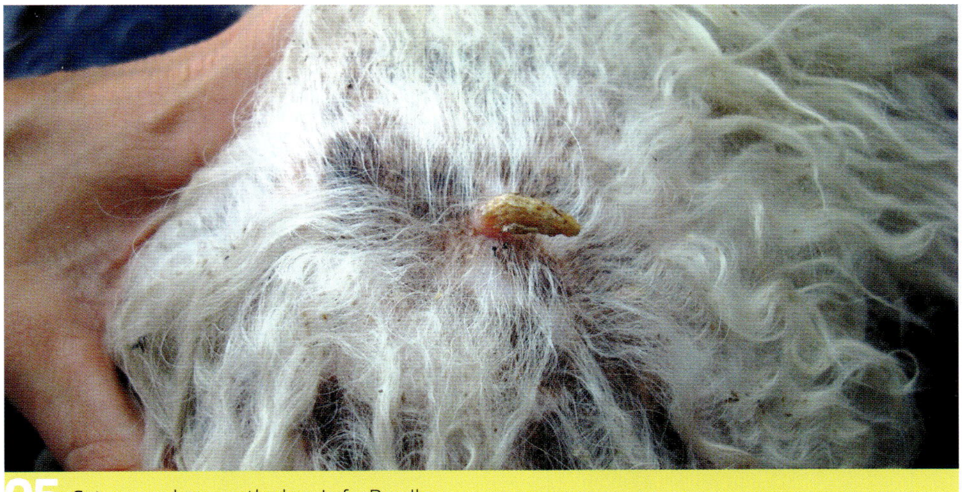

05 Cutaneous horn on the head of a Poodle.

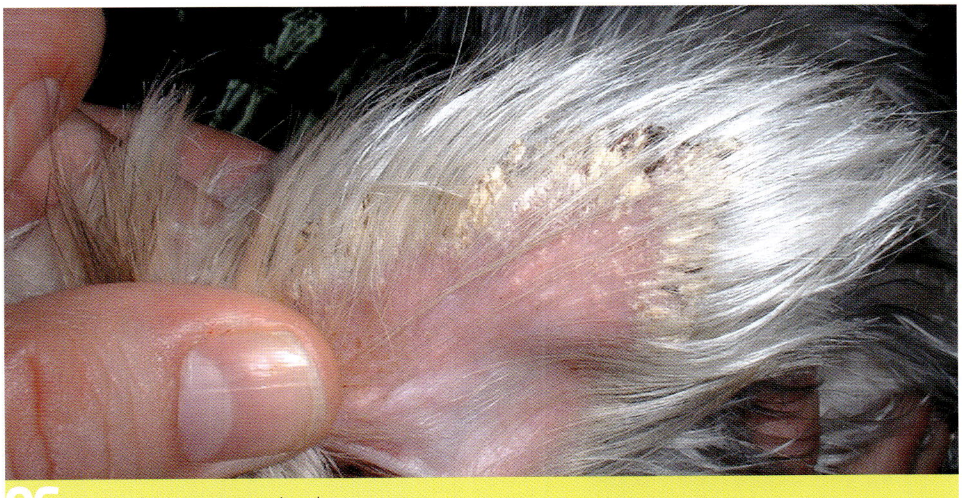

06 Dog with ear margin seborrhoea.

# Impaction and fistulas of the anal sacs

## Lesion aetiology/pathogenesis and clinical description

The anal sacs produce a serous to fatty content containing cellular debris, the consistency of which can change due to inflammatory, infectious, or endocrine alterations. This causes accumulation of the content, resulting in marked inflammation or, in many cases, drainage and the formation of fistulas, which generally coincide with the location of the sacs (4 and 8 o'clock, relative to the anus). Deformation of the area or fistulisation is accompanied by pain due to tenesmus. Affected dogs lick the area constantly and the unpleasant odour released is characteristic.

This condition is rare in cats and is often associated with injuries.

Long-lasting diarrhoea can hinder compression of the sacs, causing the contents to accumulate.

## Diagnostic method

Tenesmus and the clinical picture are characteristic.

## Main differential diagnoses

- Immune-mediated perianal fistulas
- Abscesses
- Wounds
- Tumours

## Treatment

Attempts should be made to identify and correct the cause of the altered production of fluid in the anal sacs.

Specific ointments based on antibiotics and corticosteroids are usually used. Diet should also be modified to favour well-formed stools that compress the sacs. Fibre-based dietary supplements can promote compression of the sacs by the faeces.

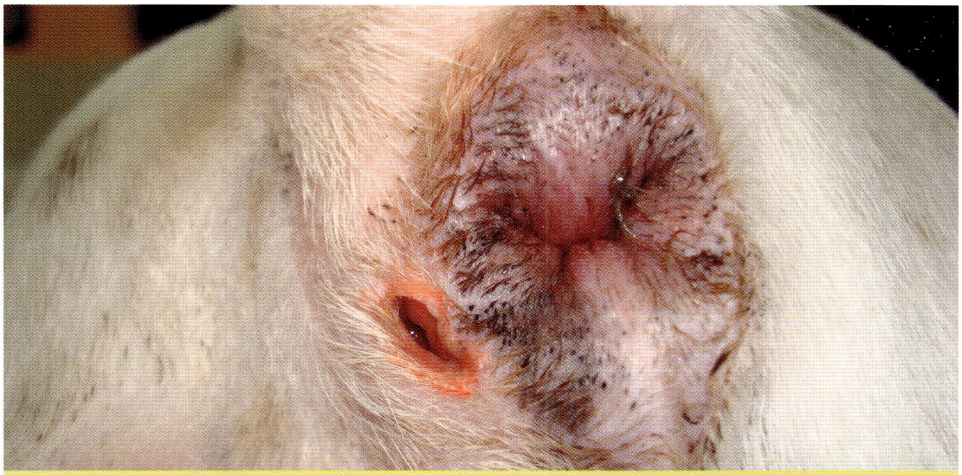

07 Fistulisation of the left anal sac.

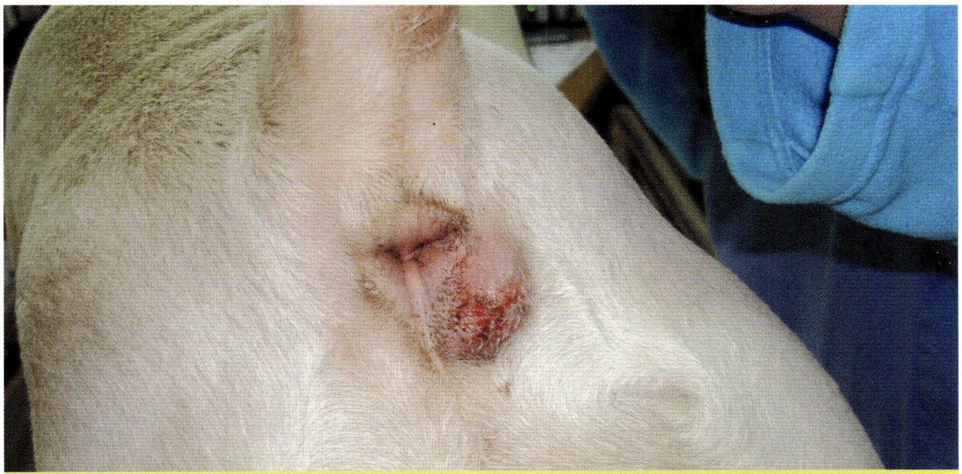

08 Impaction of the right anal sac.

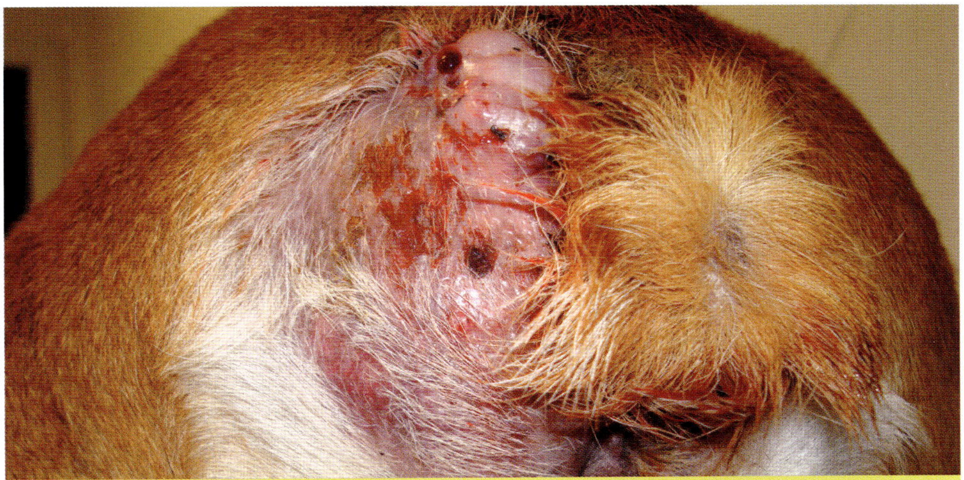

09 Perianal cellulitis caused by rupture of the left anal sac due to infection.

# Zinc-responsive dermatosis

## Lesion aetiology/pathogenesis and clinical description

This is a defect caused by a nutritional deficiency (currently very rare) or impaired capacity to absorb and/or metabolise zinc. It is usually related to genetic defects. A severe form is described in the Bull Terrier (lethal acrodermatitis), while more benign forms typically affect the Siberian Husky and Alaskan Malamute.

Zinc deficiency results in keratinisation and immunodeficiency problems.

The clinical picture of lethal acrodermatitis is characterised by erythema, excoriations, and exfoliation on the face, extremities, and trunk. Abnormal nail formation is another feature.

Diffuse alopecia, whitish exfoliation, and paw pad hyperkeratosis are observed in Nordic breeds. Lesions usually appear on the face, abdomen, and the skin covering bony prominences.

## Diagnostic method

Diagnosis is based on the clinical appearance and the breed of the affected animal. Histology reveals evident parakeratosis. The response to treatment is conclusive.

## Main differential diagnoses

- Other keratinisation disorders
- Malnutrition
- Autoimmune diseases

## Treatment

The prognosis for lethal acrodermatitis is very poor. Palliative treatment options include nutritional supplements, pain relievers, antibiotics, and topical therapy. The more benign forms of dermatosis, such as those that affect Nordic dogs, usually respond to zinc supplementation.

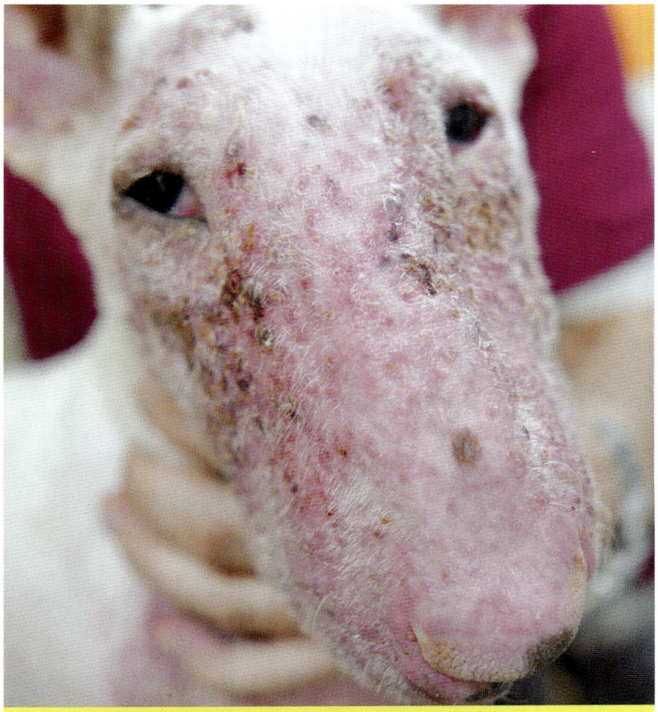

10 Bull Terrier with lethal acrodermatitis. Note the exfoliation and erythema, and the expression suggestive of general malaise.

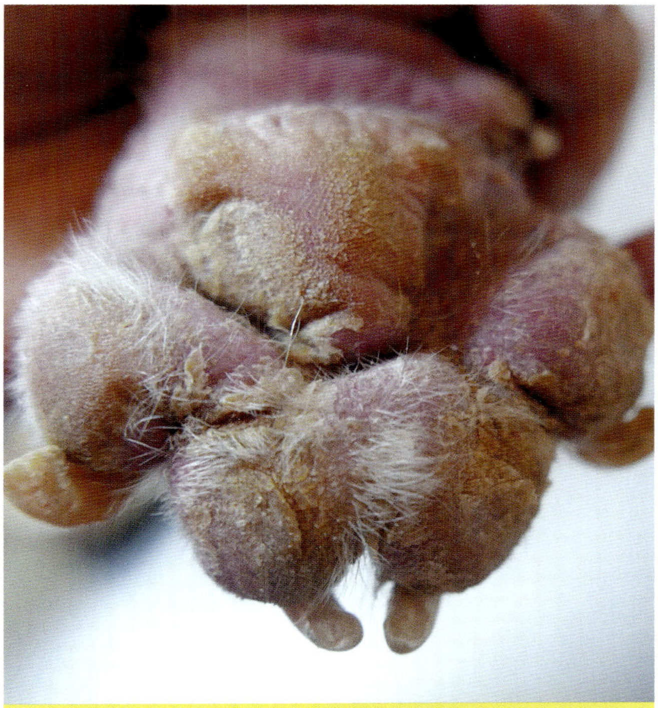

11 Paw pad hyperkeratosis in a Bull Terrier with lethal acrodermatitis.

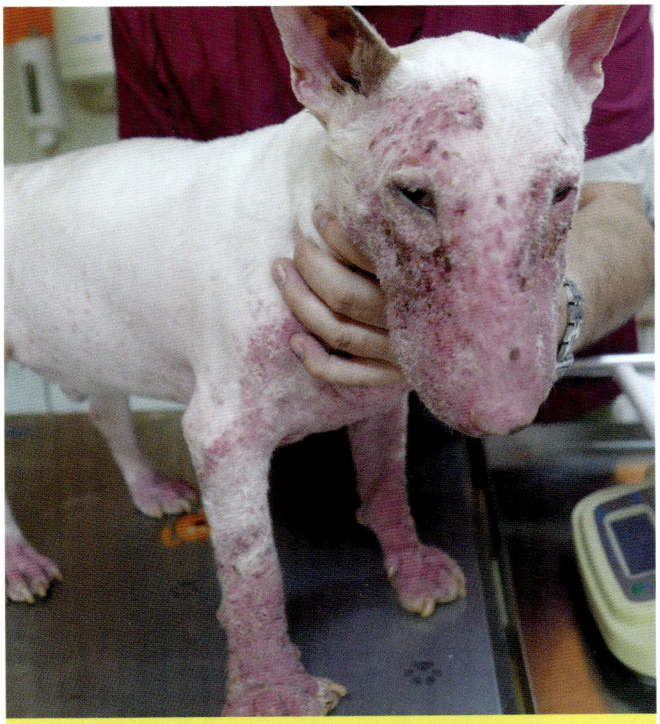

12 Bull Terrier with lethal acrodermatitis: full body appearance. Note the involvement of the limbs.

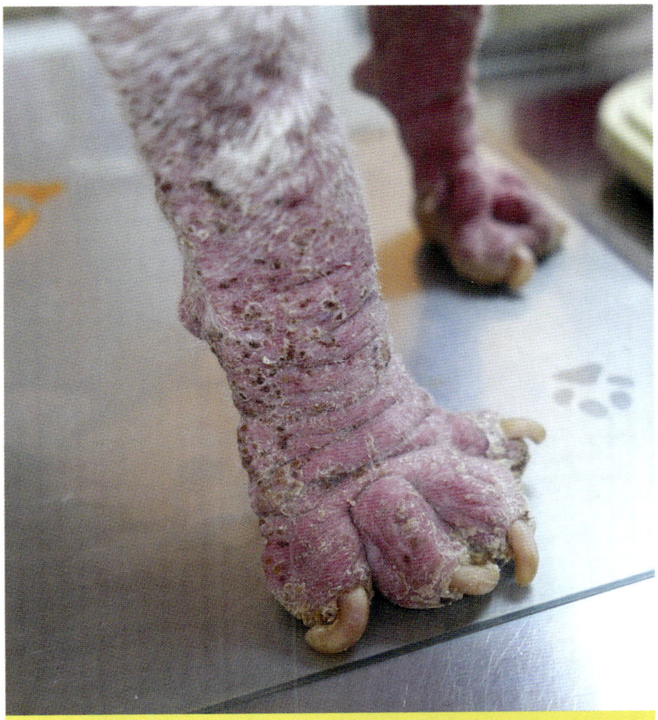

13 Bull Terrier with lethal acrodermatitis. Close-up image of the forelimb showing severe onychodystrophy.

# Lichenoid keratosis and lichenoid psoriasiform dermatosis

## Lesion aetiology/pathogenesis and clinical description

Lichenoid keratosis is a rare skin reaction described in dogs, in which well-circumscribed and adherent keratin plaques or projections occur. Its cause is unknown, although some biopsy findings have indicated an association with skin infections and have implicated immune-mediated mechanisms.

Lichenoid psoriasiform dermatosis is another rare reaction that can occur in the Springer Spaniel, usually on the inner surface of the pinnae. In this case, lesions consist of the accumulation of crusted papules and erythematous plaques. The aetiology is unknown.

## Diagnostic method

Diagnosis is established based on the clinical appearance and histopathology findings.

## Main differential diagnoses

- Lichenoid psoriasiform dermatosis or lichenoid keratosis, depending on the case
- Actinic keratosis
- Viral warts

## Treatment

Treatment consists of topical keratolytic and moisturising treatments. In some cases, retinoids, antibiotics, tacrolimus, and corticosteroids can be administered. Spontaneous remission can occur.

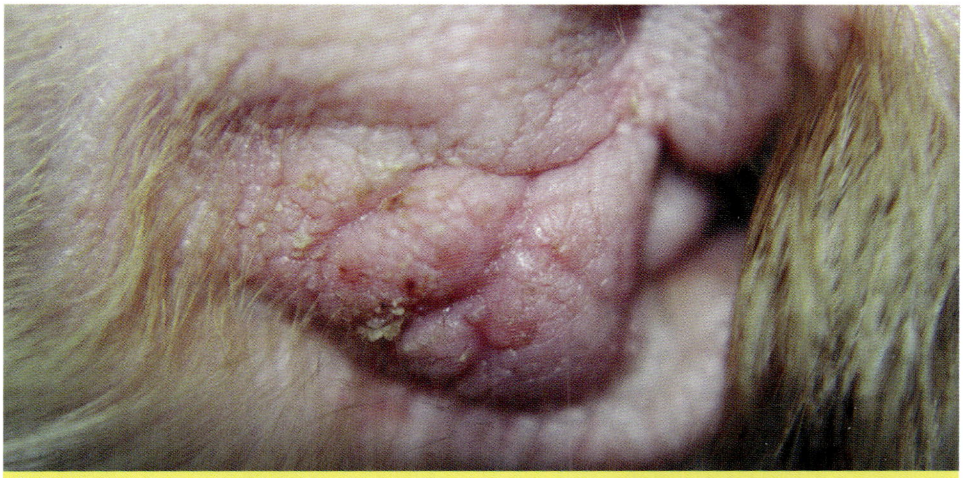

14 Lichenoid psoriasiform dermatosis on the pinna of a Springer Spaniel.

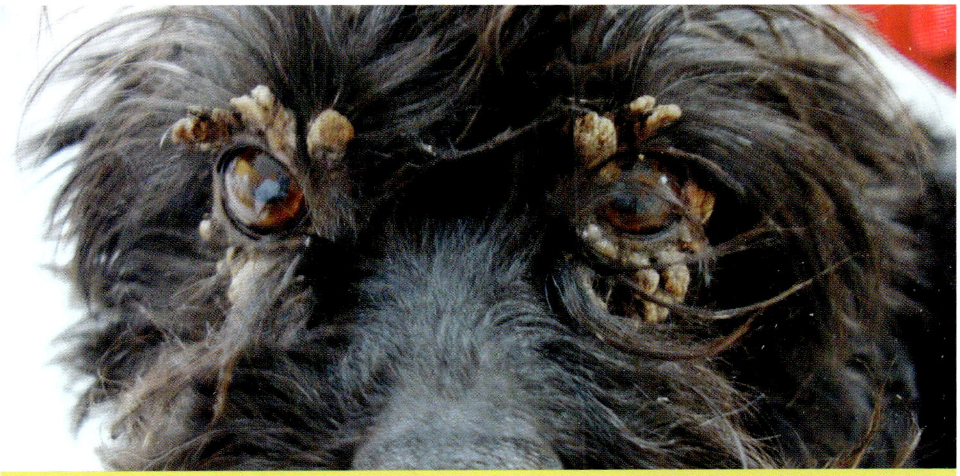

15 Lichenoid keratosis on the eyelids of a Miniature Schnauzer.

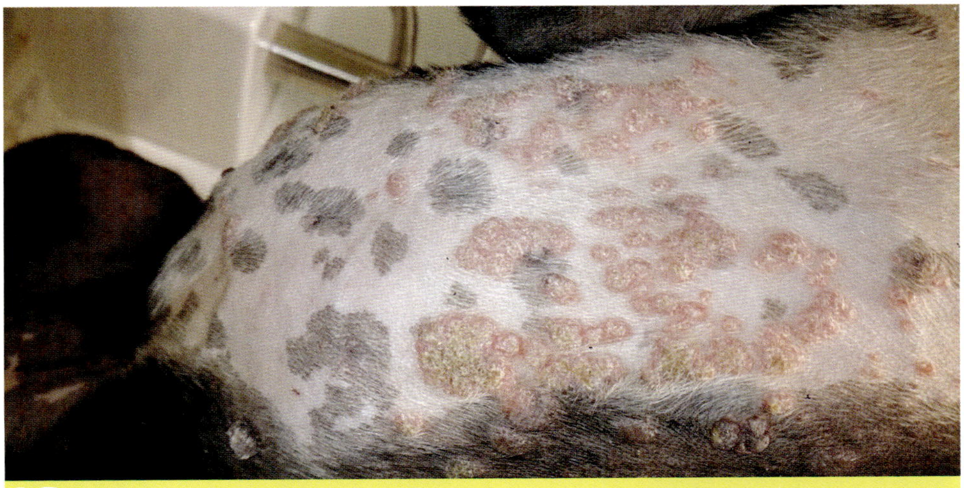

16 Lichenoid reaction on the chest of a dog.

# Tail gland hyperplasia

## Lesion aetiology/pathogenesis and clinical description

In cats, mainly non-neutered males, sebaceous gland hyperplasia can occur on the dorsal aspect of the tail, causing hypersecretion, which usually results in an area of unkempt looking, greasy, clumped hairs.

In dogs with hyperandrogenism, which may or may not be associated with testicular tumours, hyperplasia can also occur in the same area, resulting in the formation of a characteristic plaque of alopecia. In this species, hyperplasia can affect both the sebaceous and hepatoid glands.

Hyperplasia of a single type of gland can also occur in dogs: hyperplasia affecting only the sebaceous glands tends to be more frequent in females.

## Diagnostic method

The clinical picture is quite characteristic.

## Main differential diagnoses

- In cats the clinical picture is highly characteristic
- In dogs it can be confused with various forms of alopecia

## Treatment

Control is usually achieved using topical keratolytics and antiseborrhoeic agents. Neutering does not always guarantee cure.

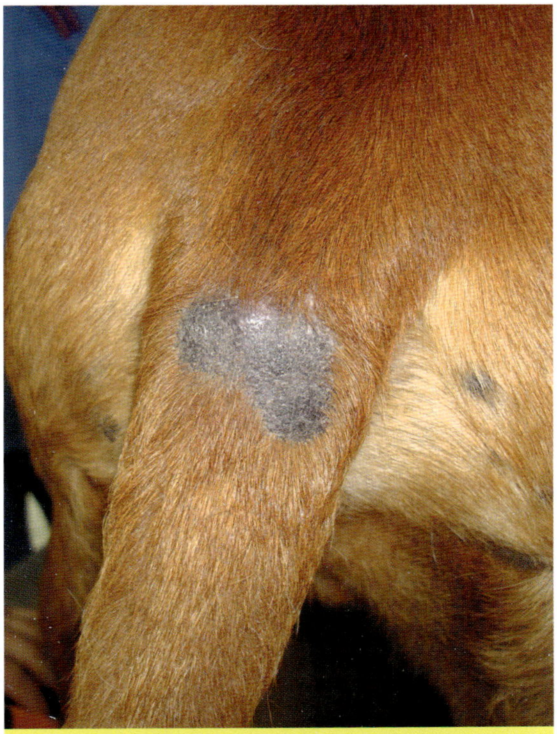

17 Hyperplasia of the supracaudal gland in a dog.

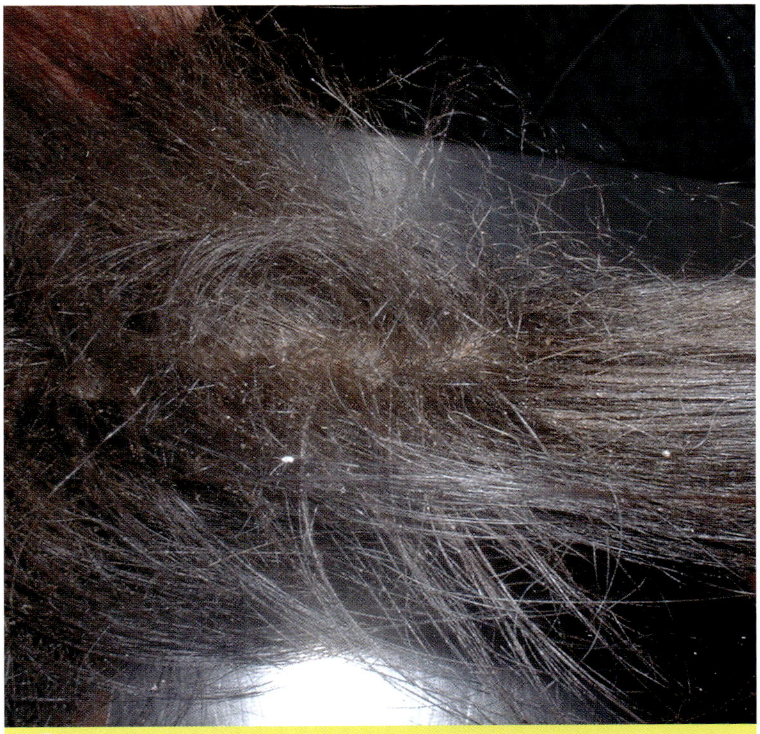

18 Tail gland hyperplasia in a Persian cat.

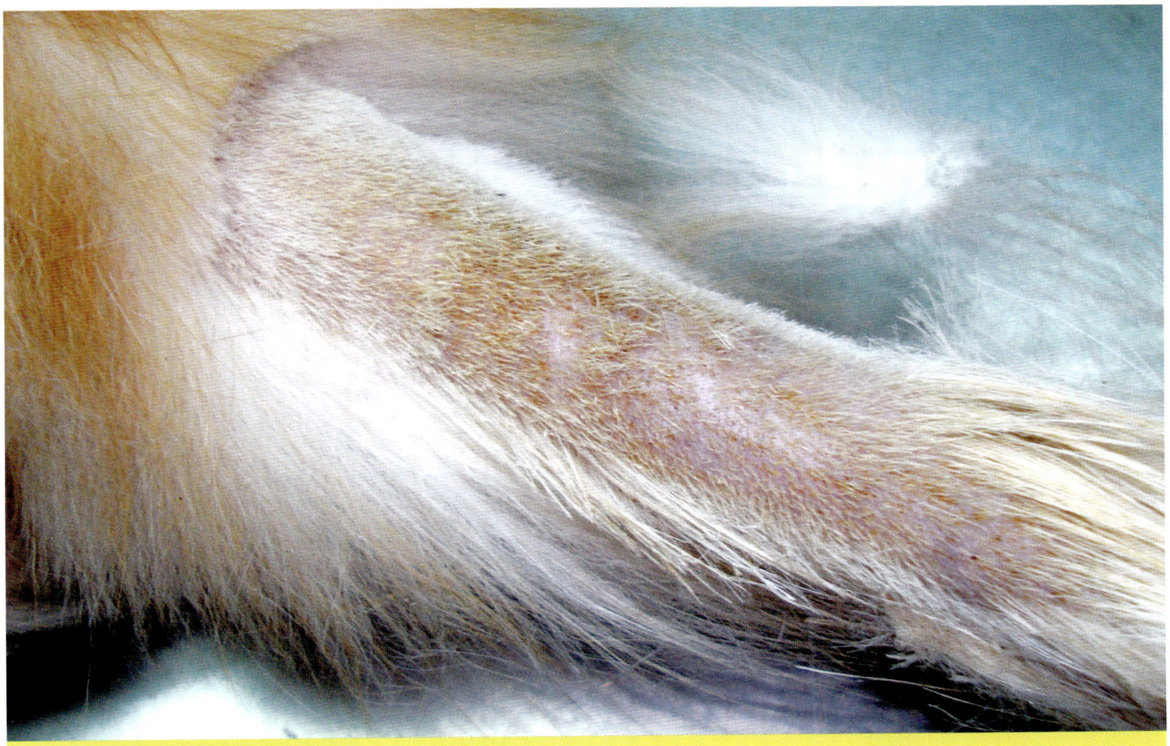

19 Appearance of tail gland hyperplasia in a cat after shaving.

# Acne

## Lesion aetiology/pathogenesis and clinical description

Depending on the underlying aetiology, acne can be classified as a component of several conditions, including infectious, fungal and parasitic diseases, and keratinisation disorders. Regardless of the origin, a common feature is follicular changes with the accumulation of sebum and keratin, due to altered production, plugging, superinfection, parasitic infestation or trauma.

Acne consists of folliculitis and furunculosis that affects the chin region and sometimes the adjacent lips.

However, the origin of this condition frequently differs between dogs and cats. In dogs, mainly short-haired breeds, the incidence of acne is usually higher in younger animals and, although it can be associated with *Demodex* infestation or a dermatophyte kerion, the main cause is thought to be trauma, caused by voracious eating or rubbing of the muzzle during play or scratching. In cats acne is not related to self-trauma: it is purely a follicular keratinisation disorder.

## Diagnostic method

The root cause can be determined based on the characteristic presentation, cytology, scrapings, and trichogram.

## Main differential diagnoses

- Dermatophytosis
- Demodicosis
- Primary keratinisation disorders

## Treatment

In dogs, if parasites, yeasts, and bacteria are controlled, therapeutic management should seek to avoid trauma (e.g. using antivoracity feeders with protrusions or projections in the food area). Benzoyl peroxide can also be very useful owing to its keratolytic effect, while antiseptics can prevent infections. It is important to clean the area thoroughly after dogs play with a ball or with each other. In some cases topical retinoic acid, corticosteroids, or oclacitinib may also be indicated to control furunculosis and itching.

In cats, treatment ranges from the use of topical antiseptics, keratolytics, systemic antibiotics, corticosteroids, and, in some cases, cyclosporine. Oral isotretinoin can be used in very severe cases.

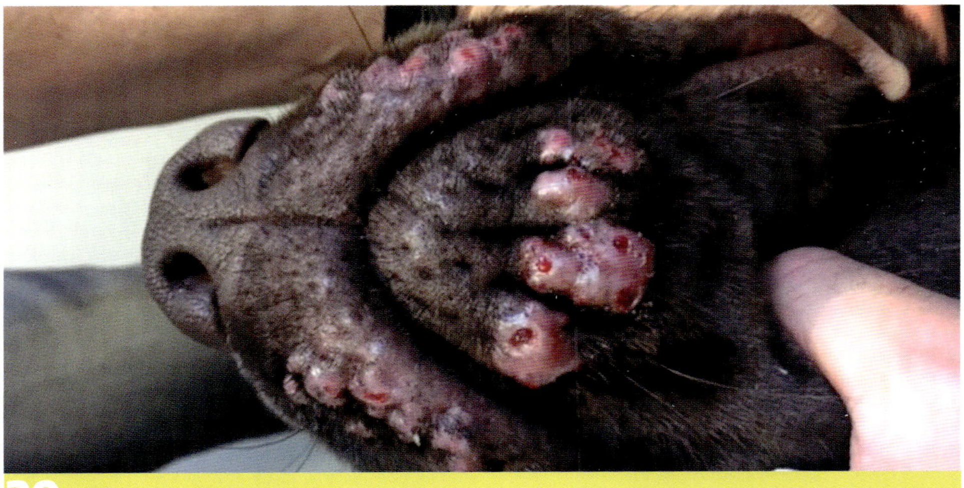

20 Acne with marked furunculosis in a young dog.

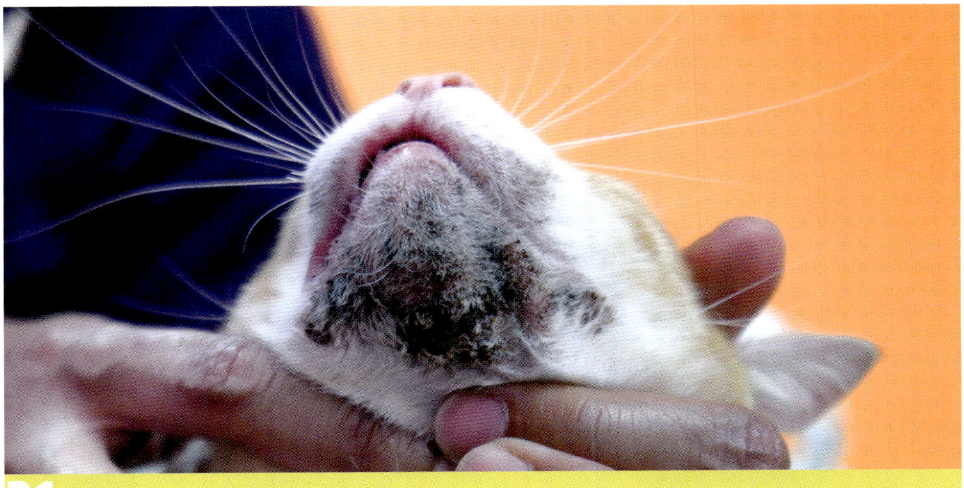

21 Feline acne caused exclusively by a keratinisation disorder.

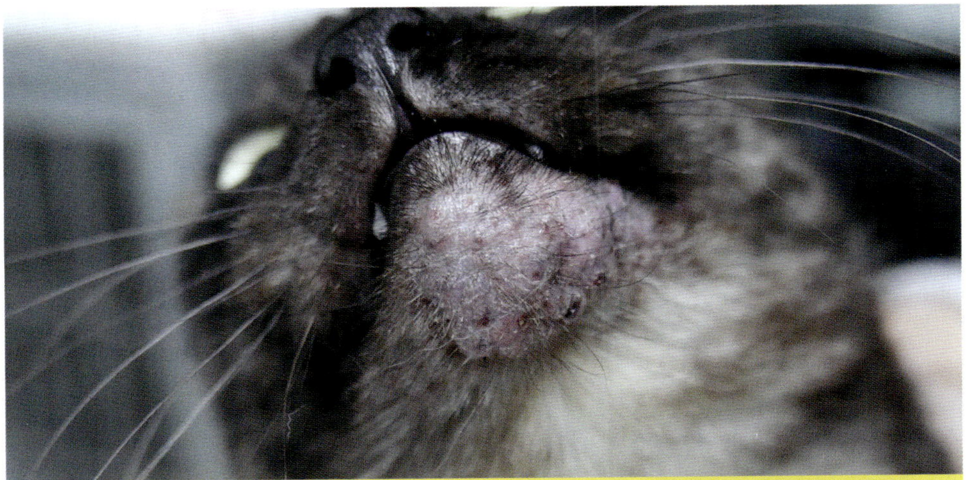

22 Cat with acne with furunculosis due to a dermatophyte kerion.

# Facial dermatosis of Persian and Himalayan cats

## Lesion aetiology/pathogenesis and clinical description

This condition is characterised by the accumulation of dark debris in the skinfolds of the face, mainly around the eyes and on the chin. Moreover, the seborrhoeic discharge can favour the overgrowth of yeast and bacteria. Owing to the characteristic clinical appearance it is also known as "dirty face syndrome".

The origin of this disease is not known, although it should be distinguished from primary causes that produce a similar clinical picture. Brachycephalic characteristics favour this clinical picture.

## Diagnostic method

Diagnosis is established based on the clinical appearance and breed, after ruling out other potential diseases.

## Main differential diagnoses

- Demodicosis
- Feline acne
- Reactive facial pattern due to hypersensitivity or behavioural disorders

## Treatment

Treatment can be very time-consuming and frustrating. Topical chlorhexidine, benzoyl peroxide gels, phytosphingosines, antibiotics, and antifungals can be applied. Systemic antibiotics, corticosteroids, and cyclosporine are other common therapies, as well as elimination diets. Oclacitinib is another potential therapeutic option.

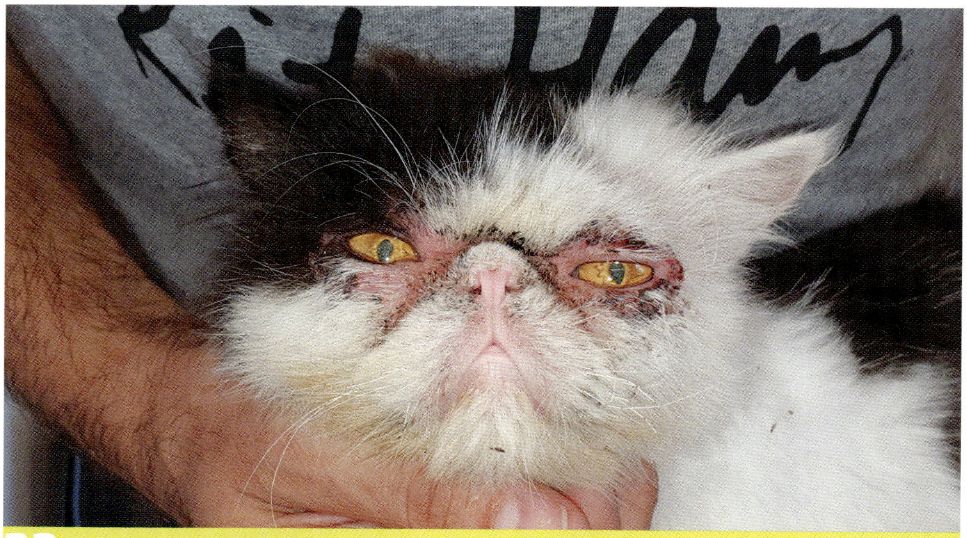

23 Persian cat with dirty face syndrome.

# Ulcerative nasal dermatitis of the Bengal cat

## Lesion aetiology/pathogenesis and clinical description

This is a dermatitis that exclusively affects the muzzle and the skin above it in Bengal cats. Over time the nose becomes hyperkeratotic, leading to the formation of crusts and, sometimes, fissures.

## Diagnostic method

The clinical presentation is quite characteristic.

## Main differential diagnoses

- Pemphigus complex
- Facial herpesvirus
- Squamous cell carcinoma

## Treatment

Topical administration of moisturisers, tacrolimus, or corticosteroids is usually quite effective. In some cases oral prednisolone treatment may be necessary.

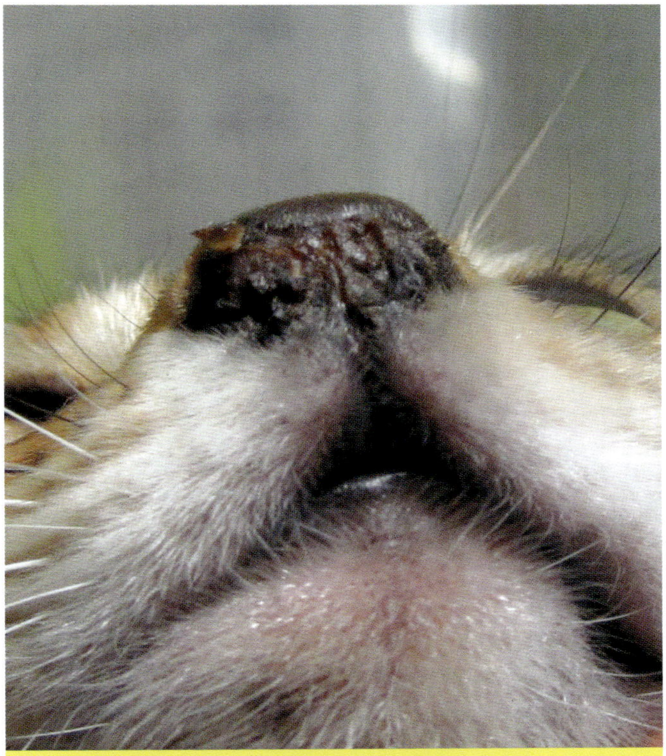

24 Ulcerative nasal dermatitis. Note the nasal hyperkeratosis.

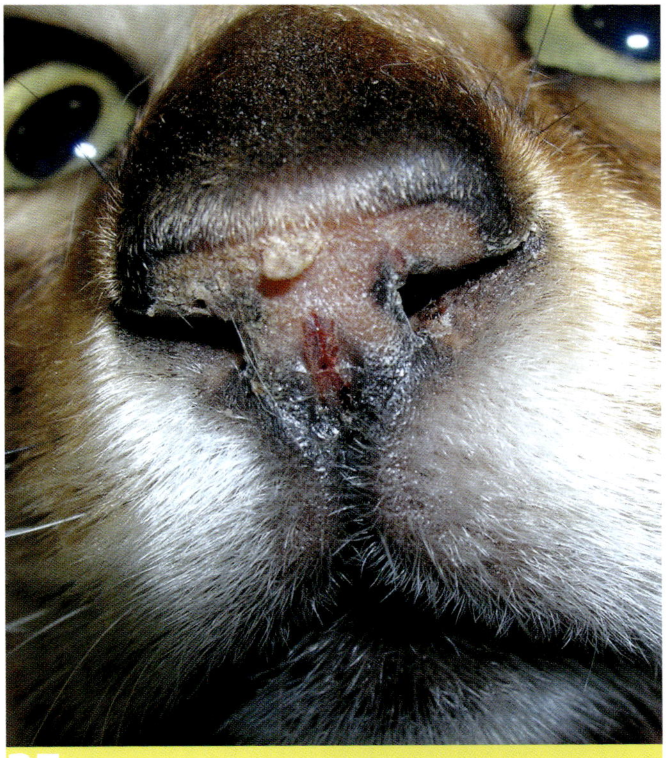

25 Ulcerative nasal dermatitis. Note the fissure in the centre.

# Split paw pad disease

## Lesion aetiology/pathogenesis and clinical description

This is a very rare syndrome of unknown aetiology caused by a possible defect in cornification of the paw pads. Episodes can occur between long periods of normalcy. Licking to relieve the pain often causes concomitant interdigital pyoderma.

Certain animals can be affected by idiopathic defects in paw pad formation, related to foci of hyperkeratosis that detach or repeated trauma. Likewise, irritative reactions caused by contact with wet concrete floors and the use of antiseptic or cleaning substances can favour detachment.

## Diagnostic method

Diagnosis is based on the clinical appearance and biopsy findings.

## Main differential diagnoses

- Split paw pad due to caustic burns
- Contact dermatitis
- Autoimmune bullous diseases
- Adverse food reaction (some dogs respond to elimination diets)
- Keratinisation disorders
- Interdigital pyoderma

## Treatment

As the aetiology of this syndrome is unknown, there is no specific treatment. Creams, analgesics, and antibiotics can provide relief. It is important to ensure that the surface on which the animal walks is comfortable and does not exacerbate the problem.

Picric acid is often used in animals with idiopathic paw pad defects, although it can sometimes cause irritation. Continuous contact with wet surfaces should be avoided and, in the case of partial detachment of the periphery of the paw pad, it is advisable to trim the flap of the detached pad to prevent further progression. In some cases, the use of rubber booties may be recommended.

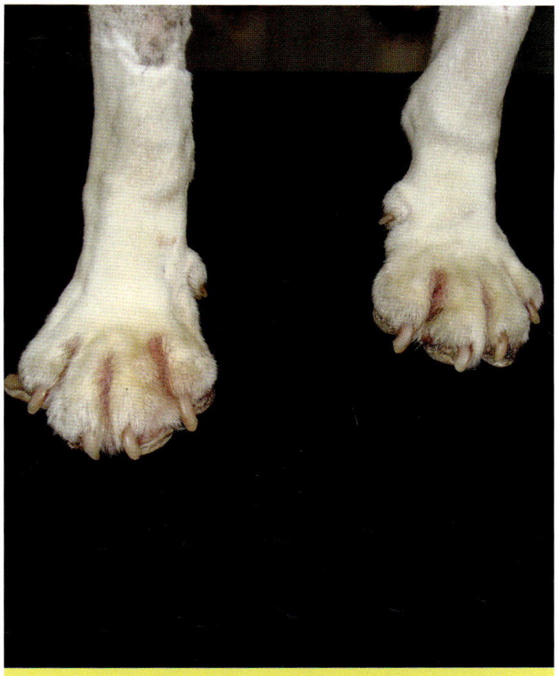

**26** Marked splitting of the paw pads in a 2-year-old Boxer.

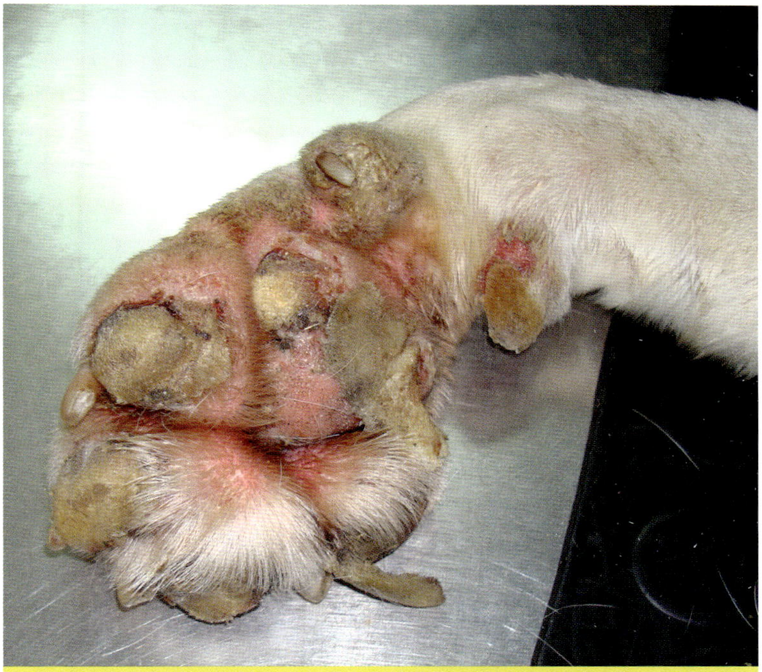

**27** Appearance of the split paw pads in the dog from the previous image.

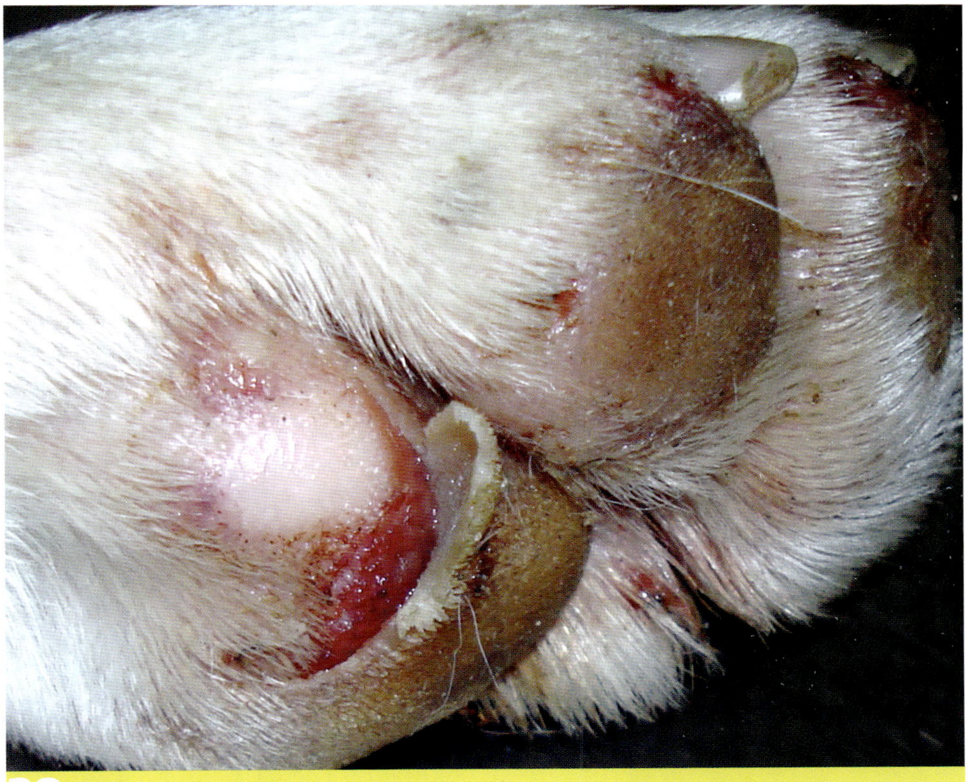

**28** Split paw pad in a dog with idiopathic paw pad defects.

# Vitiligo

## Lesion aetiology/pathogenesis and clinical description

This is an acquired disorder characterised by melanocytopenia and hypomelanosis, which leads to leukoderma and leukotrichia. Onset generally occurs from the first year of life, starting on the nose, lips, and the areas around the eyes and paw pads.

It is more common in dogs, in particular certain breeds such as the Rottweiler and Doberman Pinscher, and much less so in cats, although it can occur in Siamese cats.

The aetiology is poorly understood, but may involve a combination of a lack of pigment production and the production of autoantibodies against melanocytes.

## Diagnostic method

The clinical presentation and evolution are usually characteristic. In some circumstances this condition has been associated with hypoadrenocortisism and diabetes mellitus in dogs.

## Main differential diagnoses

- Lupus
- Uveodermatologic syndrome
- Epitheliotropic lymphoma
- Dermatomyositis
- Mucocutaneous pyoderma
- Piebaldism

## Treatment

To date, there is no effective treatment for large affected areas, although in cases affecting small areas of skin it may be possible to control the process with topical tacrolimus. It is important to avoid UVA damage using sunscreen.

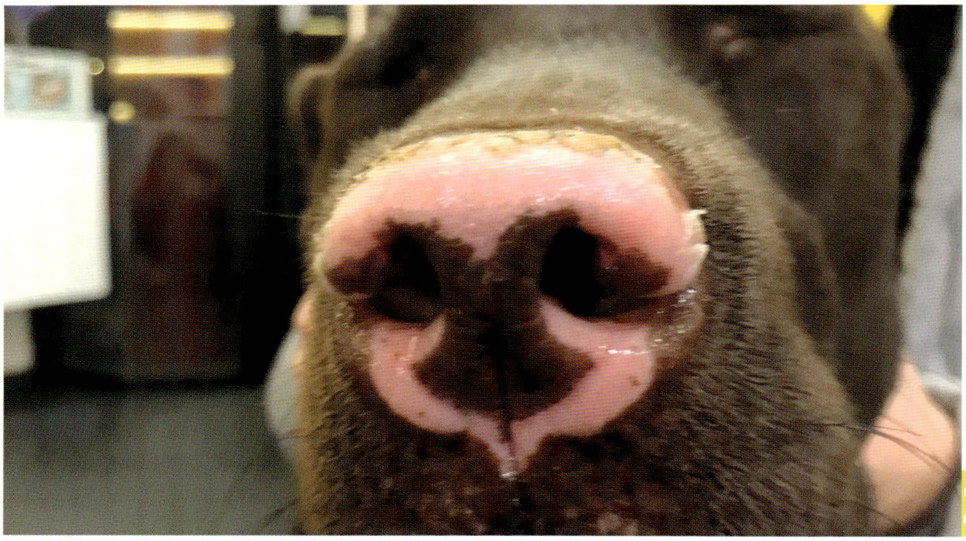

29 Onset of vitiligo on the nose and lips of a Labrador.

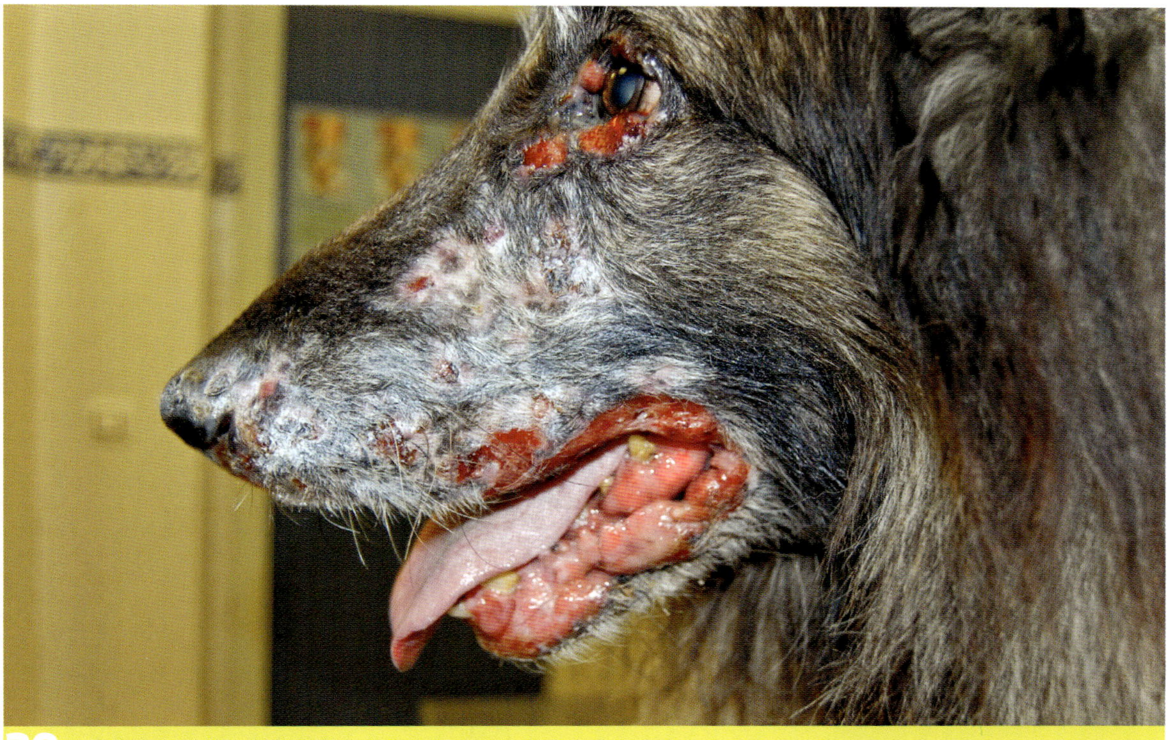

30 Depigmentation of skin and hair in a Belgian Tervuren with epitheliotropic cutaneous lymphoma.

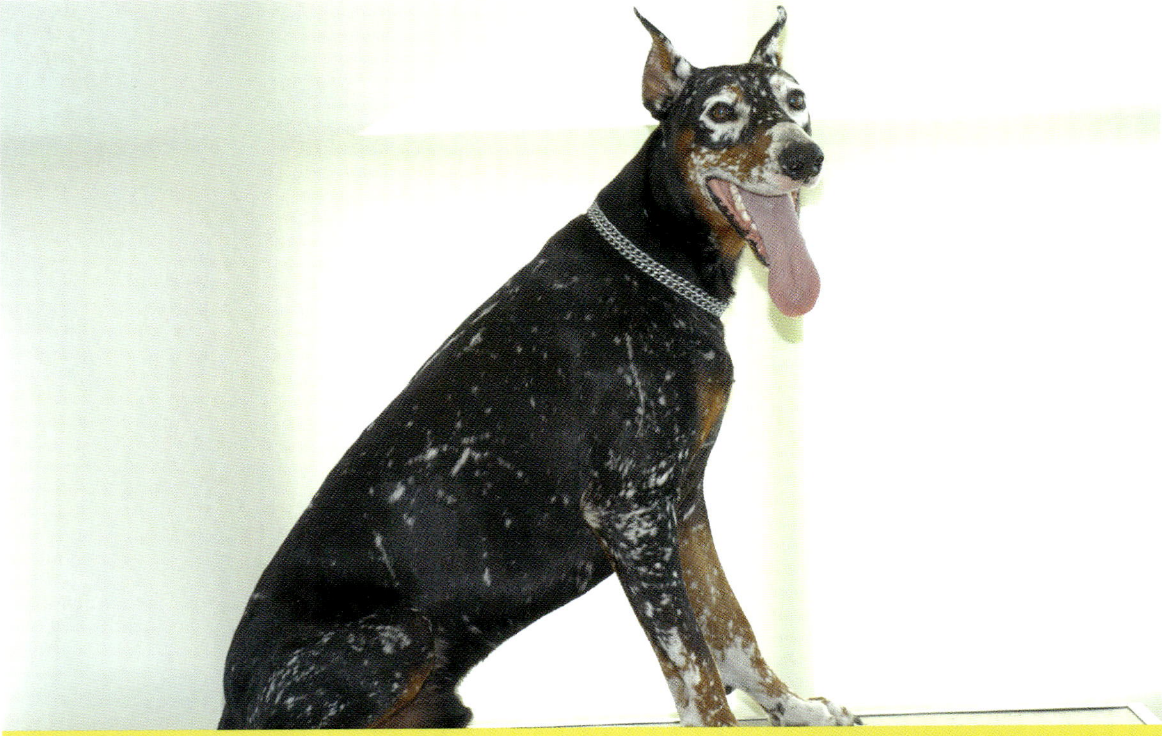

31 Generalised vitiligo in a Doberman. Image courtesy of Didier Carlotti (RIP) and Debora Trenti.

# Lentigo

## Lesion aetiology/pathogenesis and clinical description

This condition consists of focal hyperpigmentation in the form of dark brown to black macules or small spots.

The underlying aetiology is unknown, although it has been associated with papillomavirus in dogs. There is a generalised form known as canine lentiginosis profusa.

It is quite common on the muzzle and lips of calico and orange cats. It is an exclusively aesthetic issue, with no implications for the animal's health.

## Diagnostic method

Diagnosis is established based on the clinical presentation and progression.

## Main differential diagnoses

- Pyoderma
- Demodicosis
- Tumours and pseudotumours

## Treatment

As this is exclusively a cosmetic issue, no treatment is required.

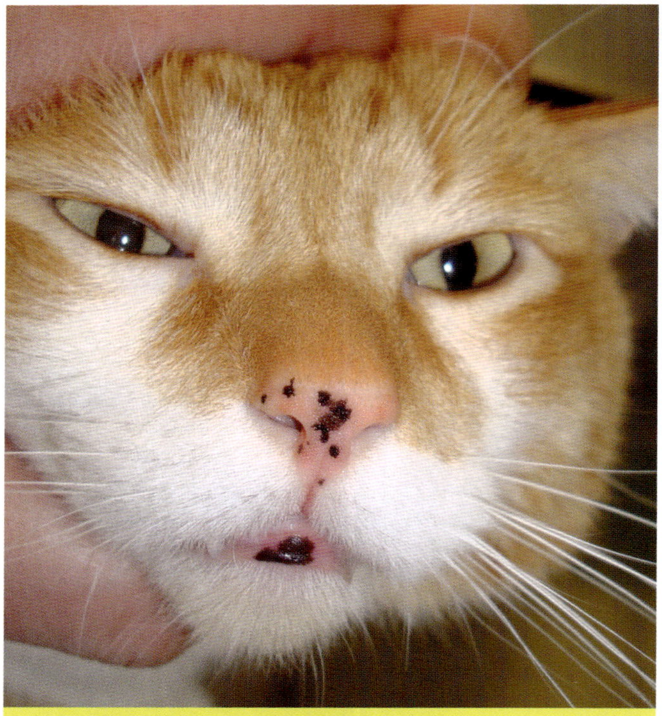

32 Classic lentigo affecting the nose and lip in an orange cat.

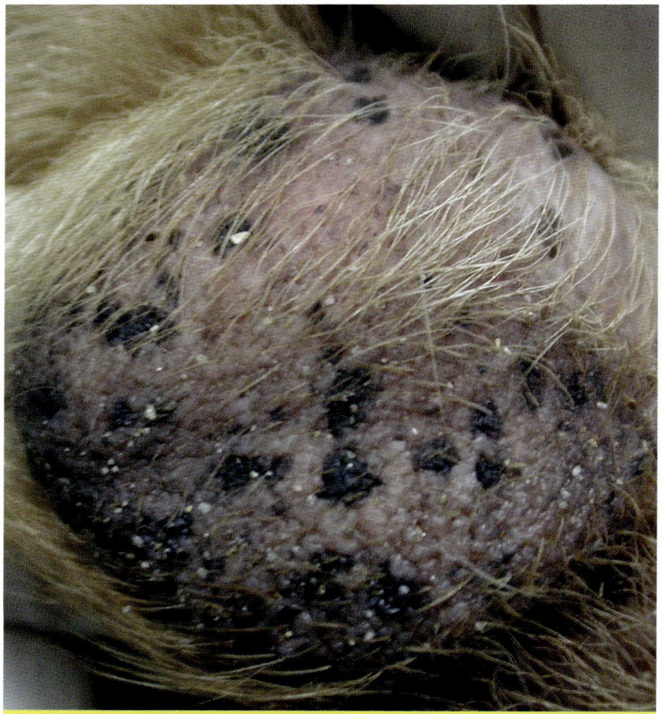

33 Scrotal lentigo. Image courtesy of the Somaza Pérez Veterinary Clinic (Spain).

# 10 Most frequent tumours

# Introduction

Tumours are the result of abnormal, irreversible cell proliferation that is not coordinated with the surrounding tissues. They are caused by an inheritable change in gene expression in the cells of origin.

There are certain exceptions to the irreversibility of cell proliferation (e.g. histiocytoma and papilloma). Moreover, in exceptional circumstances (e.g. transmissible venereal tumour), the immune response can result in tumour resolution.

The tumours that most frequently affect dogs and cats are:

- Lipoma and liposarcoma
- Mast cell tumour
- Histiocytoma
- Reactive histiocytosis
- Histiocytic sarcoma
- Epitheliotropic T-cell lymphoma
- Cutaneous plasmacytoma
- Basal cell tumours
- Feline paraneoplastic alopecia
- Adenoma and carcinoma of the hepatoid glands
- Papillomas
- Soft tissue sarcomas
- Squamous cell carcinoma
- Actinic keratosis
- Cutaneous metastasis of mammary adenocarcinoma
- Melanoma
- Transmissible venereal tumour

In oncology, photo atlases can be of limited value as the appearance of tumours can vary greatly. In this chapter we will present some examples, although the most important aspects are the cytological and histopathological features, based on which diagnosis can be established.

# Lipoma and liposarcoma

## Lesion aetiology/pathogenesis and clinical picture

These are tumours of mesenchymal origin formed by adipocytes that are located in the dermis and hypodermis, and in some cases infiltrate the muscle. The benign form (lipoma) tends to be much more frequent, particularly in older and somewhat overweight animals, and can include both encapsulated and infiltrative lipoma.

## Diagnostic method

Tumour shape can be highly variable. In some cases the tumour may be mobile beneath the skin, while in others it is highly infiltrated and immobile. Cytology provides information on the cell type, and biopsy confirms the degree of malignancy. Cytology can provide information on the degree of malignancy if the cellular characteristics are taken into account.

## Main differential diagnoses

- Various tumours
- Cysts

## Treatment

Resection is not always easy, especially in the case of infiltrative lipomas. Intratumoural administration of depot corticosteroids such as triamcinolone acetonide can reduce tumour size, thereby facilitating resection.

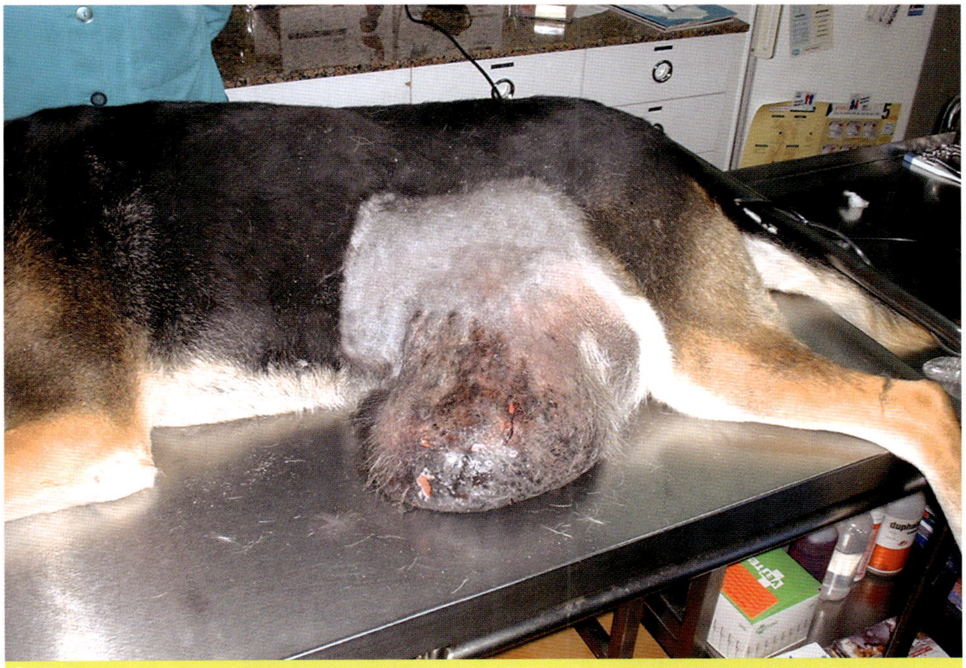

01 Infiltrative lipoma that appeared 1 year earlier.

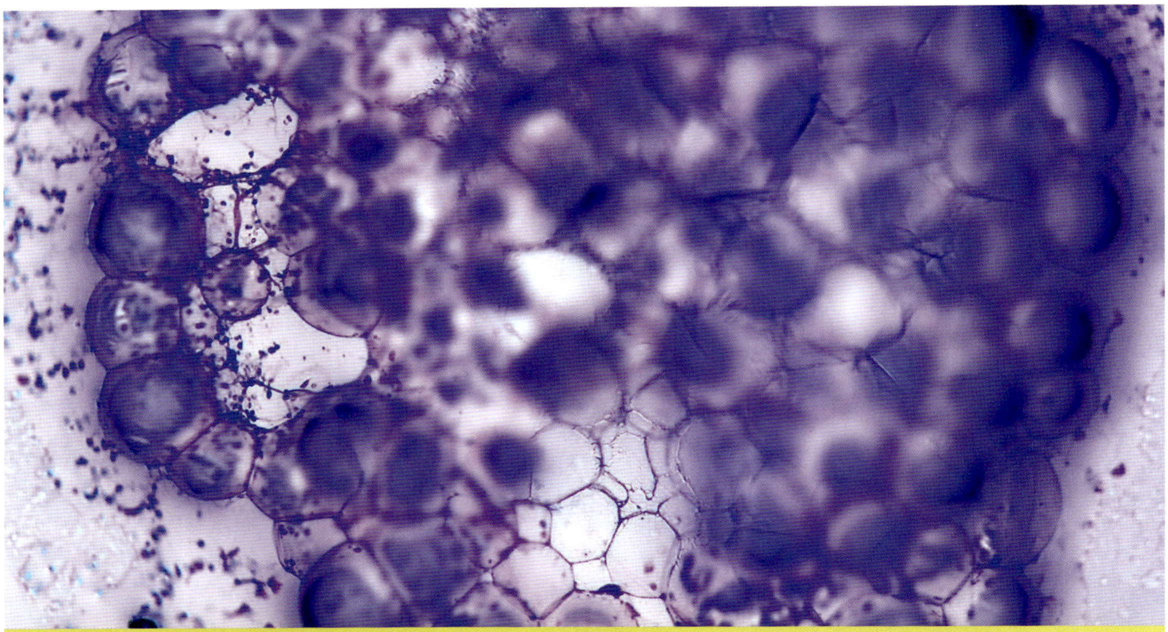

02 Lipoma cytology.

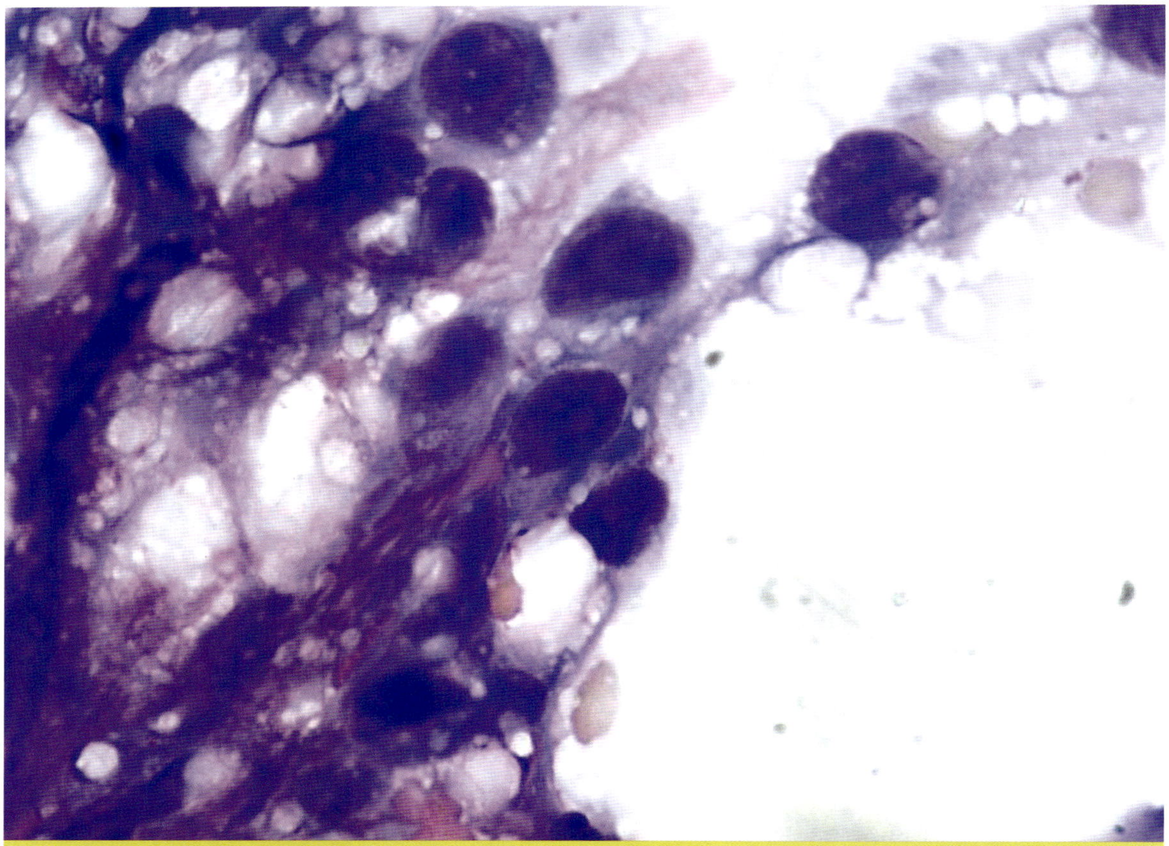

03 Liposarcoma cytology.

# Mast cell tumour

## Lesion aetiology/pathogenesis and clinical picture

These are tumours formed by round mast cells that can proliferate uncontrollably. They are more common in dogs than cats. In dogs the degree of malignancy can vary greatly. In cats these tumours are usually benign. Young cats can develop a differentiated form of cutaneous mast cell tumour (histiocytic mast cell tumour), in which cytology shows clusters of larger epithelioid cells.

A certain predisposition to cutaneous mast cell tumour is described in dog breeds such as the Boxer, Staffordshire Bull Terrier, Labrador, Boston Terrier, and Bull Terrier. The clinical presentation is so variable that it is impossible to provide a specific description.

## Diagnostic method

While the clinical appearance is never diagnostic, sudden changes in size and the itching caused by the release of inflammatory mediators, known as Darier's sign, can be. Cytology is an essential tool in almost all cases to determine the type of cells involved and the degree of differentiation. It is very important to try to determine the stage once the grade has been determined.

In some cases there is no direct relationship between the degree of differentiation and biological behaviour. For example, Shar Peis can have a low-grade tumour that nonetheless displays highly malignant behaviour.

## Main differential diagnoses

- Various tumours
- Abscesses
- Cysts

## Treatment

Whenever possible, radical surgery is usually the best approach. Depending on the grade and stage of the tumour, oncotherapy using agents such as lomustine, tyrosine kinase inhibitors, corticosteroids, and vinblastine can be indicated.

A product containing tigilanol tigliate for intratumoural application can be an excellent tool in the case of nonmetastatic mast cell tumours in dogs to avoid anaesthetic risk during surgery, and in cases of tumours located in areas unsuited to surgical intervention, such as the distal limbs or the face.

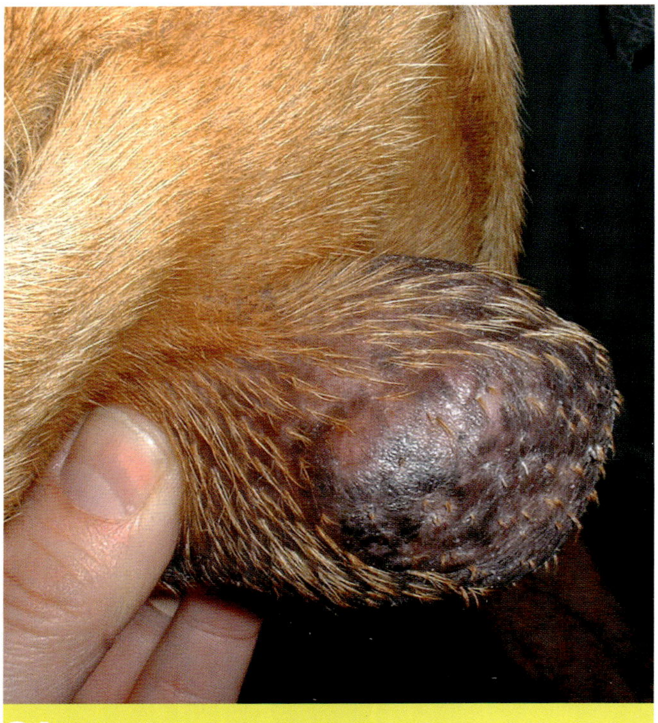

04 Scrotal mast cell tumour: quite frequent in Boxers.

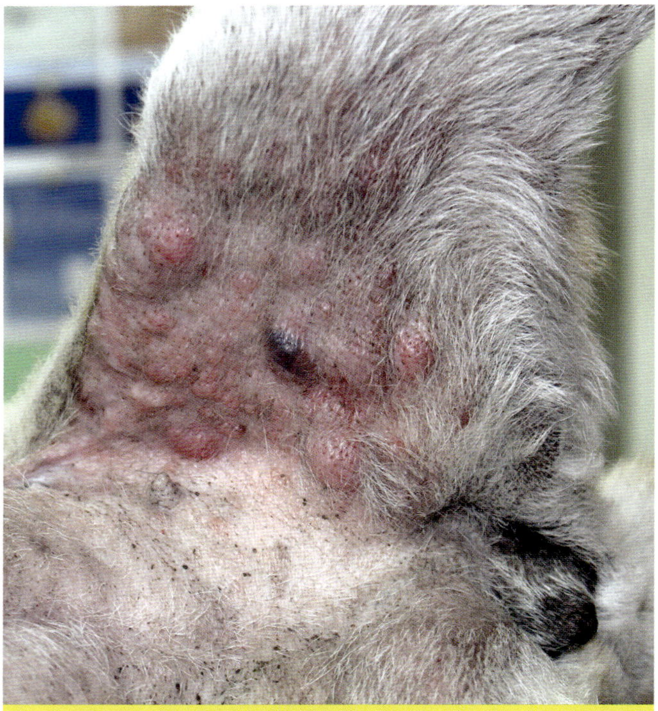

05 Mast cell tumour with disseminated satellite nodules in a Shar Pei. Poor biological behaviour.

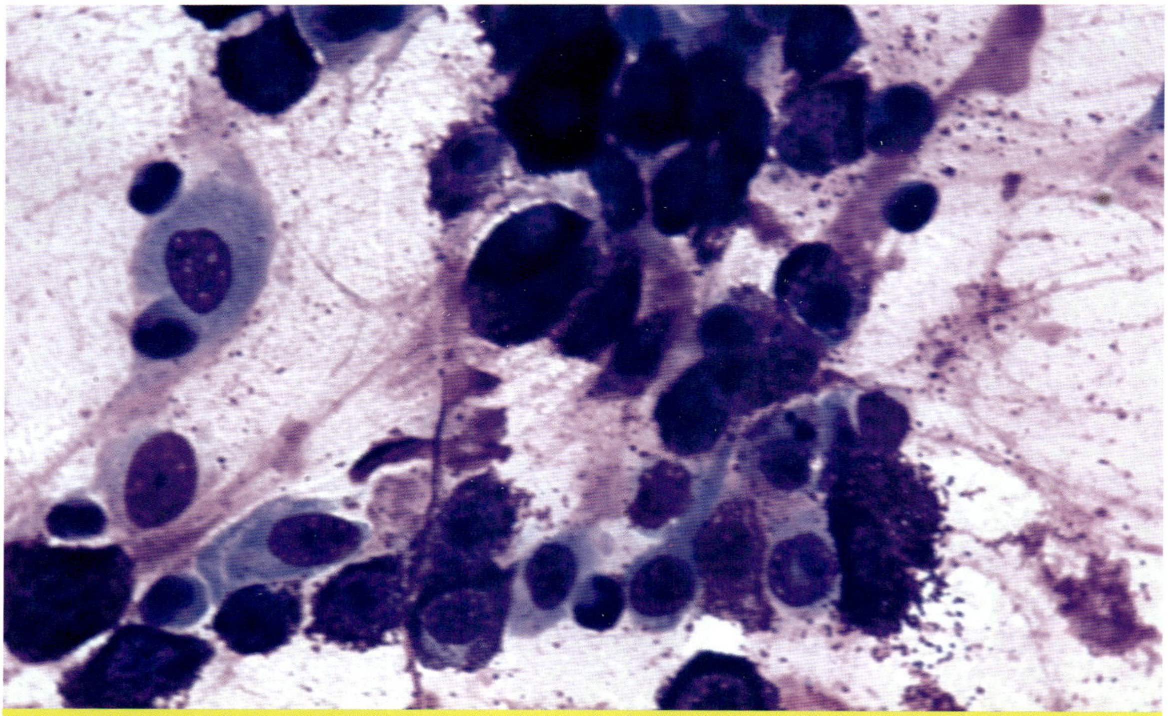

06 Cytology of a low-grade mast cell tumour. Note the granule-containing mast cells and mesenchymal cells, which provide structure to the tumour.

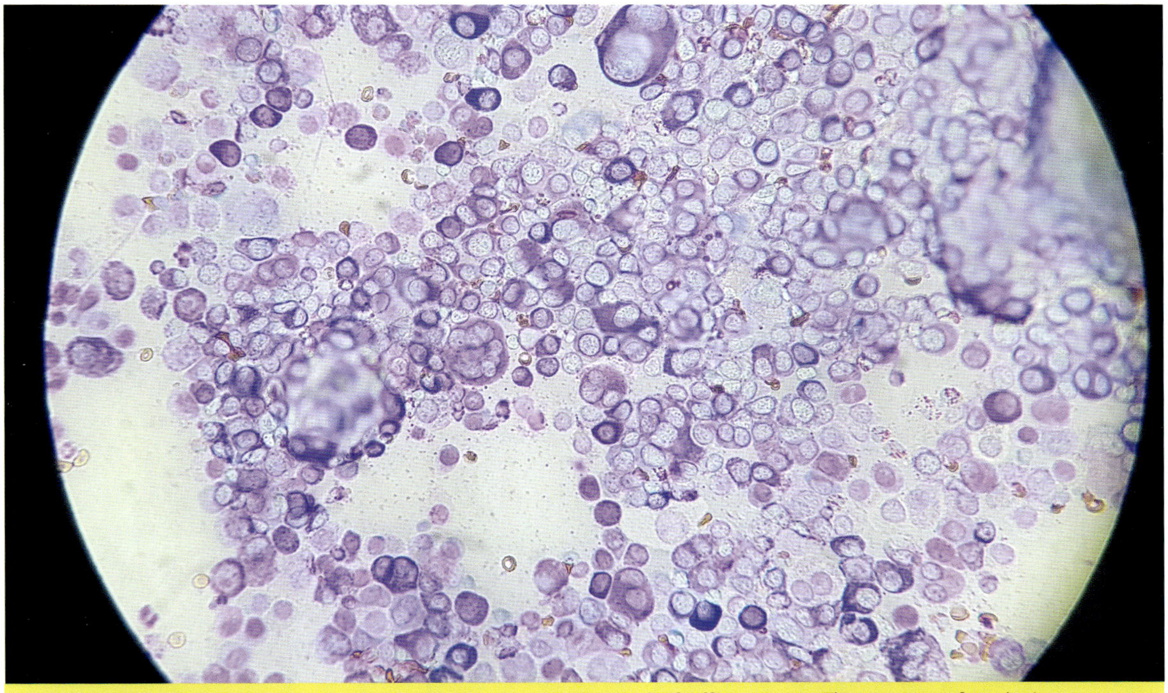

07 Cytology of a high-grade mast cell tumour showing a marked lack of differentiation. The presence of marked anisocytosis and unpaired mitoses indicate a high degree of malignancy. Immunocytochemistry may be required to establish diagnosis in these cases.

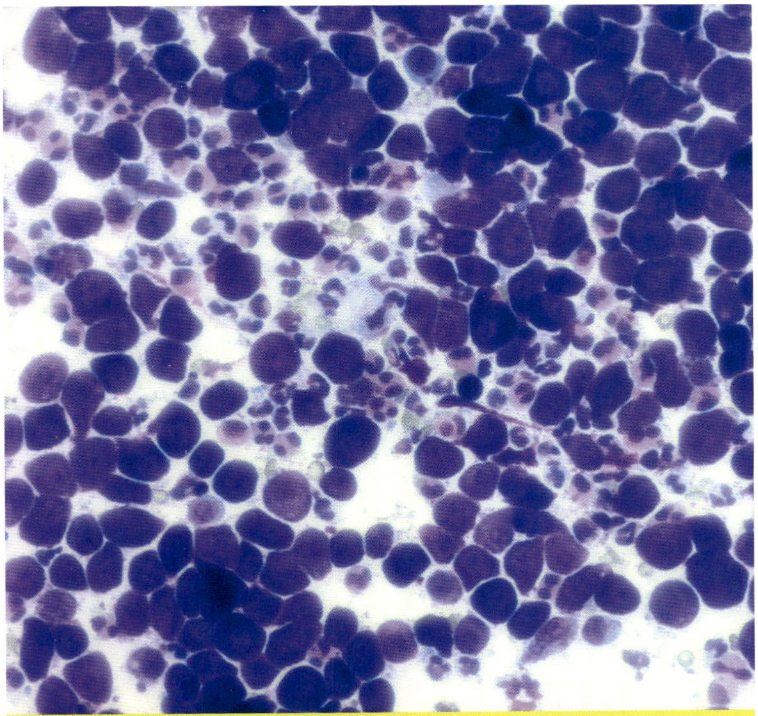

08 Cytology of a histiocytic mast cell tumour in a 3-year-old cat. Note the clustered large cells.

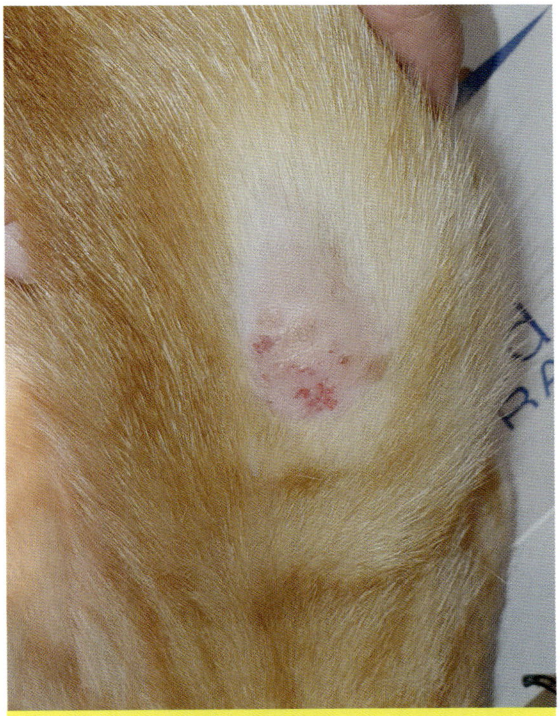

09 Appearance of a histiocytic mast cell tumour in a cat.

# Histiocytoma

## Lesion aetiology/pathogenesis and clinical picture

This is a generally benign, round cell tumour caused by the proliferation of Langerhans cells. It usually occurs in young animals (up to 2 years of age), mainly in the Shar Pei, Boxer, and French Bulldog breeds. It is very rare in cats.

It is characterised by a protruding, erythematous, and often eroded nodule of about 1 cm in diameter. It is typically located on the muzzle, extremities, and ears, where a more aggressive form of tumour can develop.

These tumours usually resolve on their own within a few weeks or months. However, in some individuals they may behave somewhat erratically and recur frequently.

## Diagnostic method

Diagnosis is established based on the clinical picture and cytological and histopathological findings. The presence of lymphocytes on cytology may be indicative of impending resolution.

## Main differential diagnoses

- Dermatophyte kerion
- Other tumours
- Nodular form of demodicosis
- Acral lick dermatitis

## Treatment

This tumour usually self resolves within a few months. In some cases surgery may be necessary.

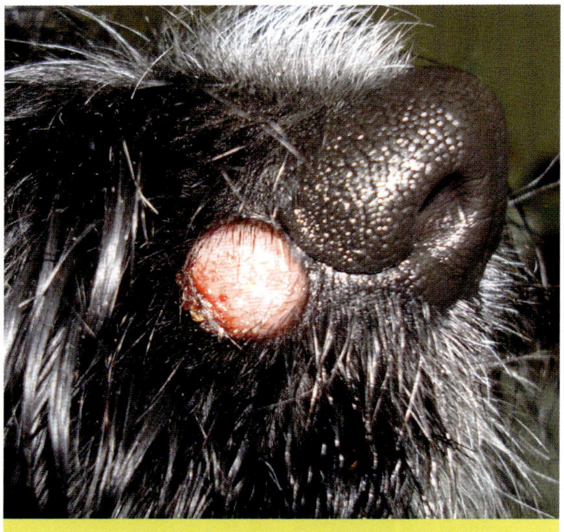

10 Histiocytoma on the muzzle of a mixed-breed puppy.

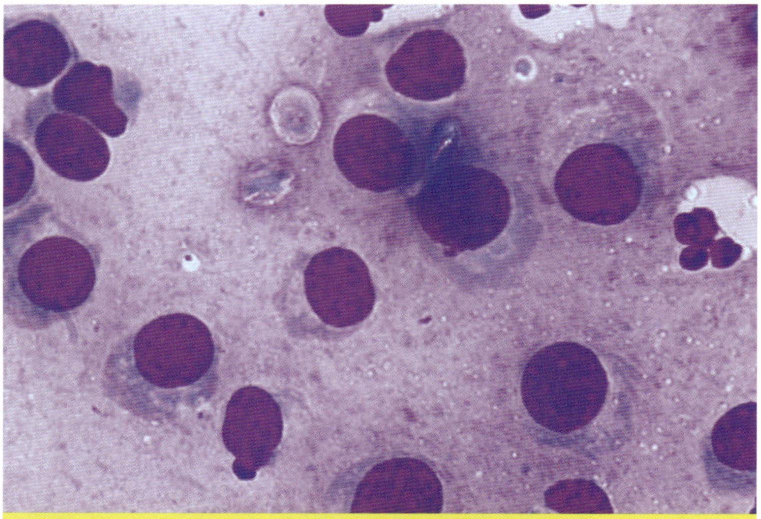

11 Histiocytoma cytology. Note the characteristic chromatin nuclei of histiocytic cells.

# Reactive histiocytosis

## Lesion aetiology/pathogenesis and clinical picture

Reactive histiocytosis is the uncontrolled proliferation of histiocytes in the skin and sometimes in internal organs.

The aetiology is unknown, but does involve immune system alterations.

It presents as multiple nodules (approximately 1 cm in diameter) that may ulcerate, located on the face, ears, trunk, and extremities.

## Diagnostic method

Diagnosis is established based on the clinical picture, cytology, and histopathology. In many cases immunohistochemistry is confirmatory.

Cytology reveals benign-appearing histiocytes, often accompanied by multinucleated giant cells.

## Main differential diagnoses

- Other tumours
- Infectious granulomas

## Treatment

Surgery can be effective in isolated cases, although the prognosis is usually guarded, given the unpredictability of the treatment result. Treatments used to date include corticosteroids and cyclosporine, tetracycline or doxycycline/niacinamide, vitamin E, and essential fatty acids. Spontaneous resolution is also described.

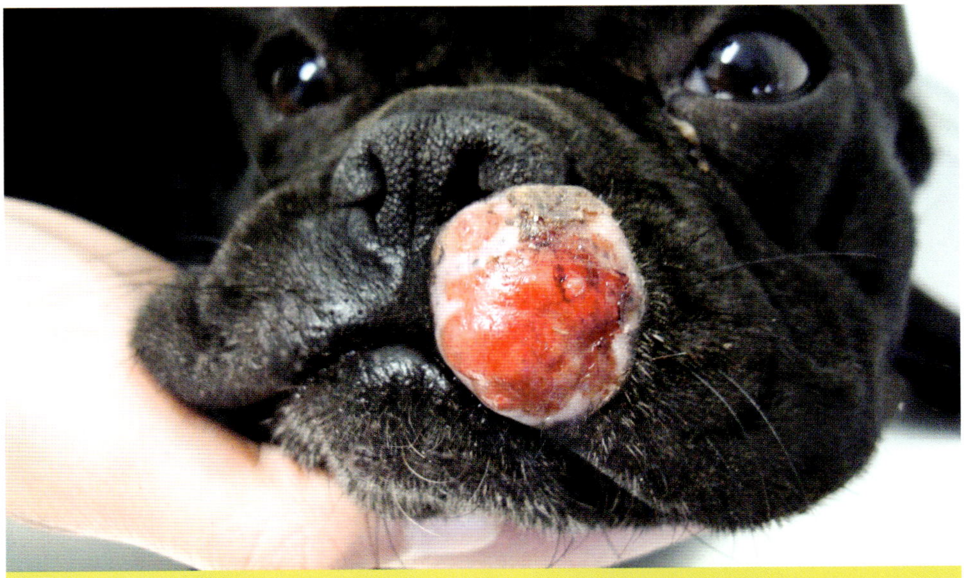

12 Ulcerated nodule in a 6-year-old French Bulldog with refractory reactive histiocytosis.

# Histiocytic sarcoma

## Lesion aetiology/pathogenesis and clinical picture

This is another variant of histiocytic proliferative disorders (which involve dendritic cells or macrophages).

Histiocytic sarcoma is a tumour that can be either localised or disseminated, and disproportionately affects the Golden Retriever, Bernese Mountain Dog, and Rottweiler. It mainly affects the limbs, appearing as a soft, localised, and rapidly growing tumour. The disseminated form can affect several internal organs.

## Diagnostic method

This tumour is derived from dendritic cells, and features marked anisocytosis and anisokaryosis. Mitosis and erythrophagocytosis may be observed.

## Main differential diagnoses

- Other tumours
- Inflammatory granulomas

## Treatment

Generally, the prognosis is poor. Early surgery, in localised cases, may be the only option. Chemotherapy has not shown effective results: the response to this treatment is poor.

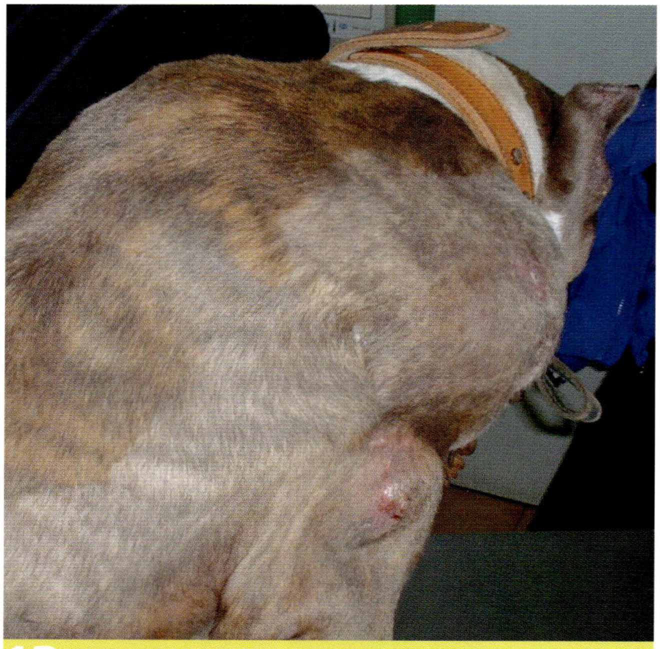

13 Histiocytic sarcoma in the shoulder and elbow area of a dog.

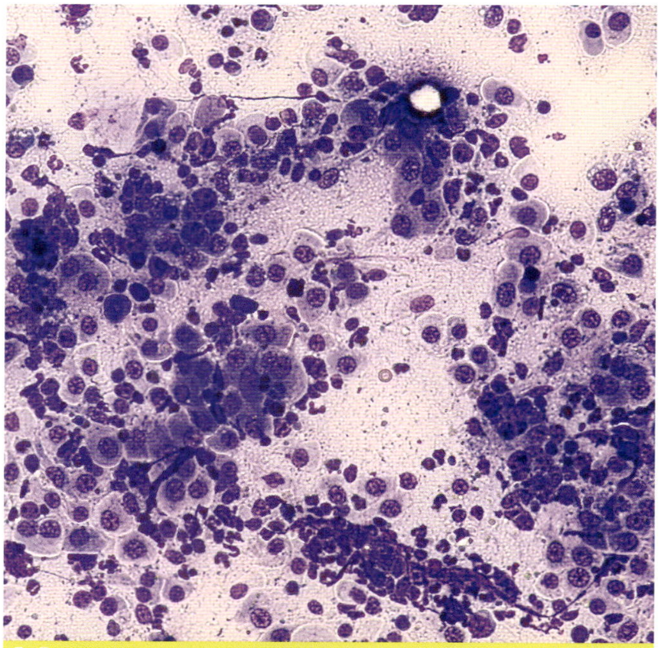

14 Cytology of a highly undifferentiated histiocytic sarcoma.

# Epitheliotropic T-cell lymphoma

## Lesion aetiology/pathogenesis and clinical picture

This tumour is the result of the proliferation of neoplastic T cells in the epidermis, also known as mycosis fungoides. Affected animals are usually no younger than 8 years of age and, according to retrospective studies, it is more frequent in animals that have experienced chronic inflammation of the skin (atopic). In cats it is a much less frequent disease.

It can present in different stages, starting as a leukoderma, progressing to erythroderma and scaling, and later giving rise to ulcerated nodules and plaques. It can affect the mucocutaneous junctions and facial region at first, subsequently spreading throughout the body.

Itching is usually present in affected dogs.

## Diagnostic method

Diagnosis is based on the clinical appearance, cytology, and histopathology. The clinical appearance can be highly variable, making initial diagnosis difficult.

## Main differential diagnoses

- Vitiligo
- Other tumours
- Keratinisation disorders
- Inflammatory erythroderma
- Non-neoplastic lymphocytosis

## Treatment

The general prognosis is guarded to poor, with a maximum survival of 2 years. Oncotherapy is based on the administration of lomustine, tyrosine kinase inhibitors, and corticosteroids. In refractory cases the protocol for multicentric lymphoma can be used. Systemic retinoids have shown efficacy in some cases.

Pruritus can be controlled with lokivetmab, since mutated T cells can produce IL-31.

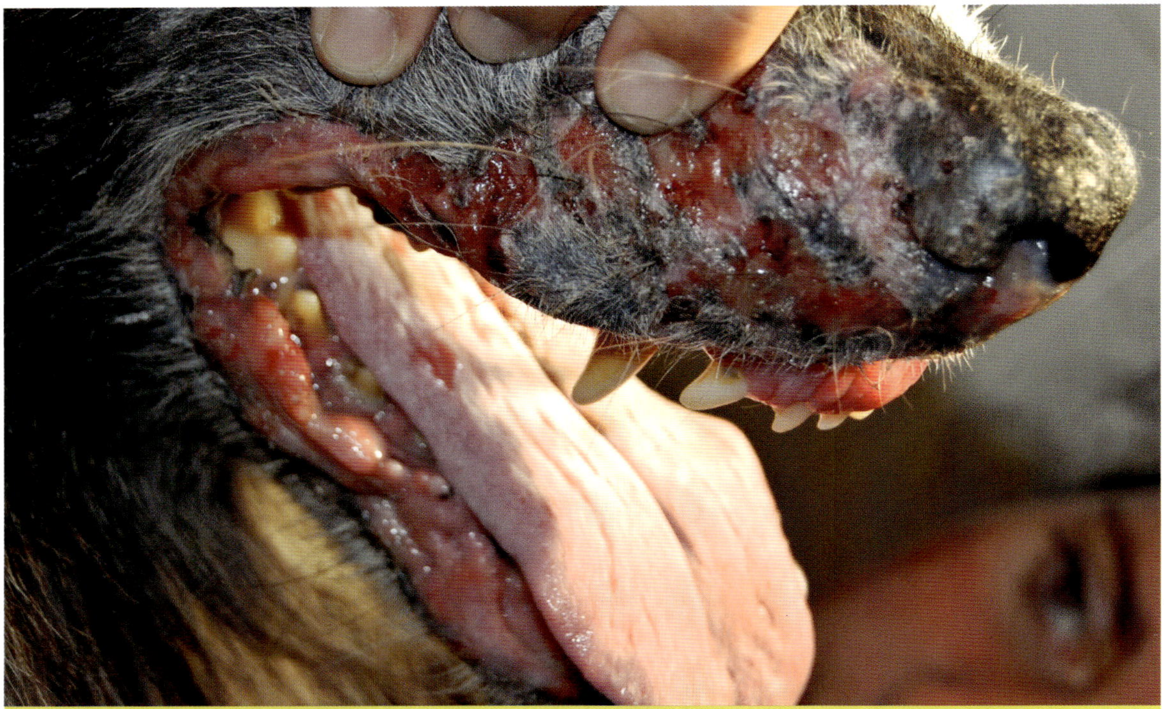

**15** Epitheliotropic lymphoma in a 12-year-old Belgian Tervuren. Lesions are observed on the tongue and inside the mouth, as well as on the mucocutaneous junctions. See also Image 30 in Chapter 9.

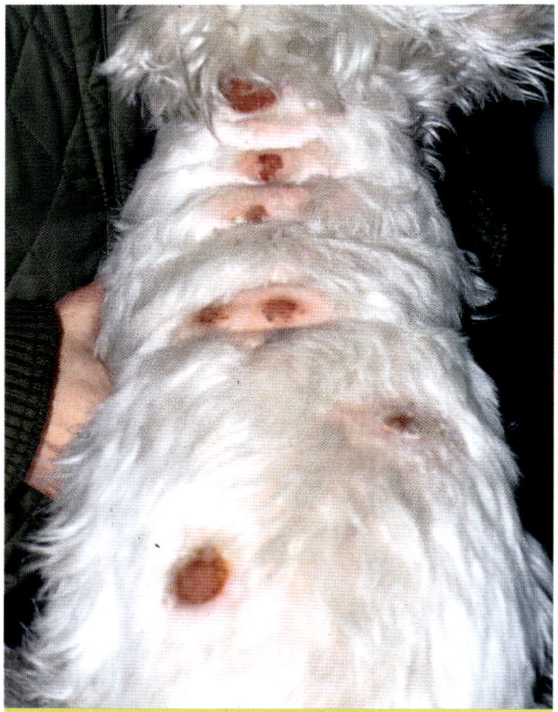

**16** Nodules and plaques in a dog with epitheliotropic lymphoma. Image courtesy of José Luis González Arribas.

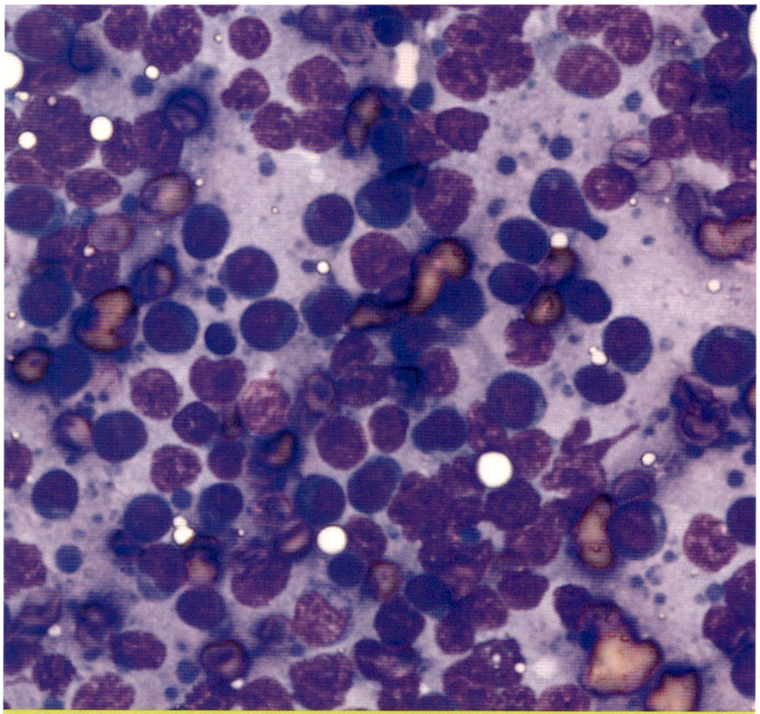

**17** Cytology of an epitheliotropic lymphoma. Note the tennis racket-shaped lymphocytes, which are compatible with T cells.

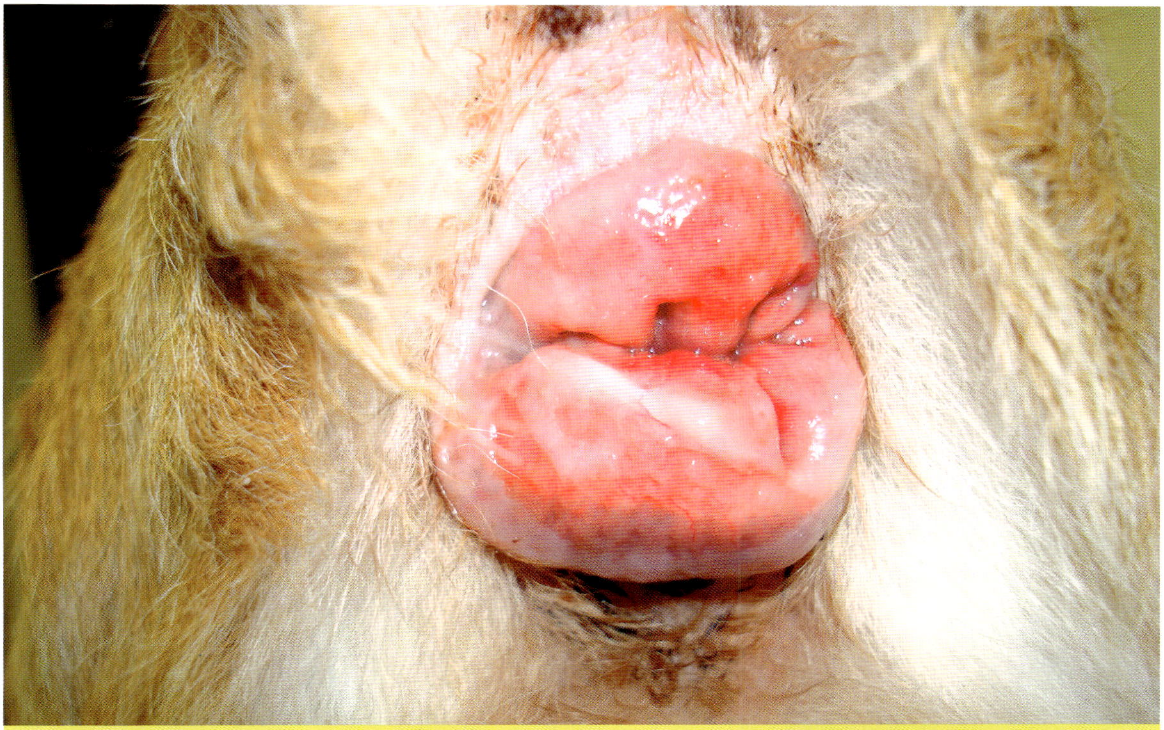

18 Anal mucocutaneous involvement in a dog with epitheliotropic lymphoma.

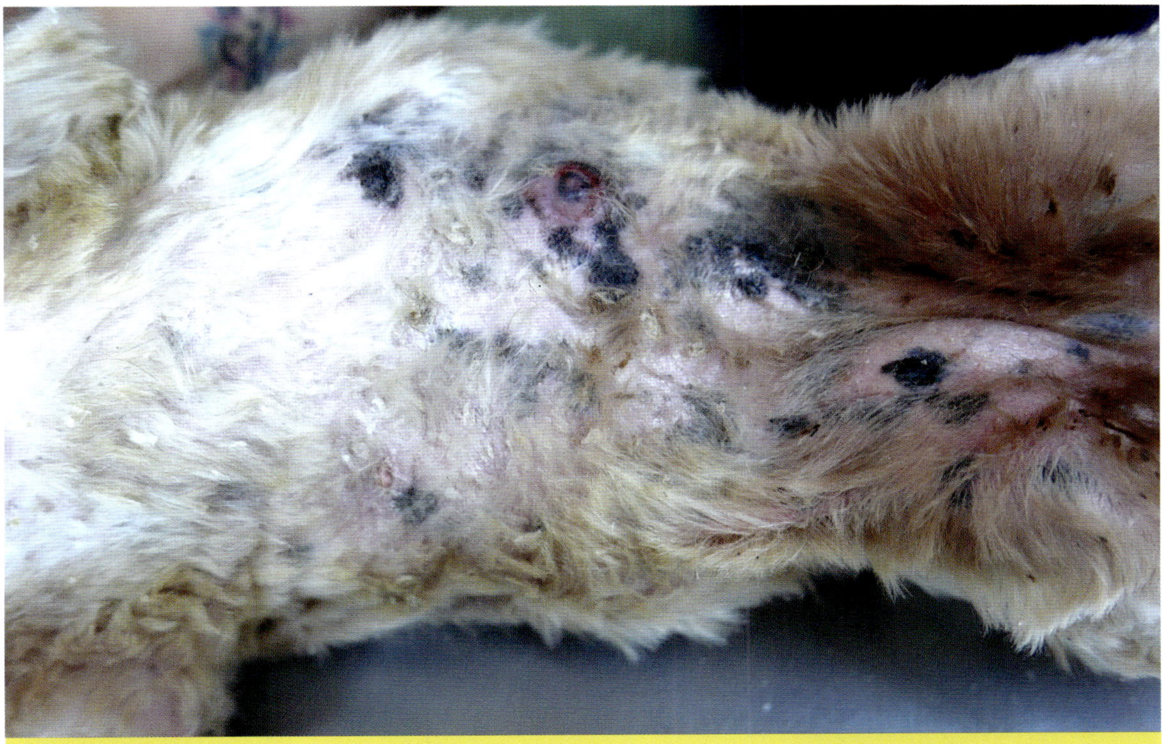

19 Ulcerated and crusted lesions highly indicative of epitheliotropic lymphoma.

# Cutaneous plasmacytoma

## Lesion aetiology/pathogenesis and clinical picture

This tumour is common in dogs and rare in cats. It consists of a round cell tumour derived from extramedullary plasma cells, although in some cases it may be associated with multiple myeloma. It usually appears in older dogs, mainly on the trunk and limbs. This tumour tends to be solitary and can affect the mucocutaneous junctions.

## Diagnostic method

Cytology and histology are the appropriate techniques to establish diagnosis and the degree of differentiation.

## Main differential diagnoses

Other tumours.

## Treatment

Surgery, if feasible, is usually effective. Radiation therapy and, in some situations, chemotherapy can be used.

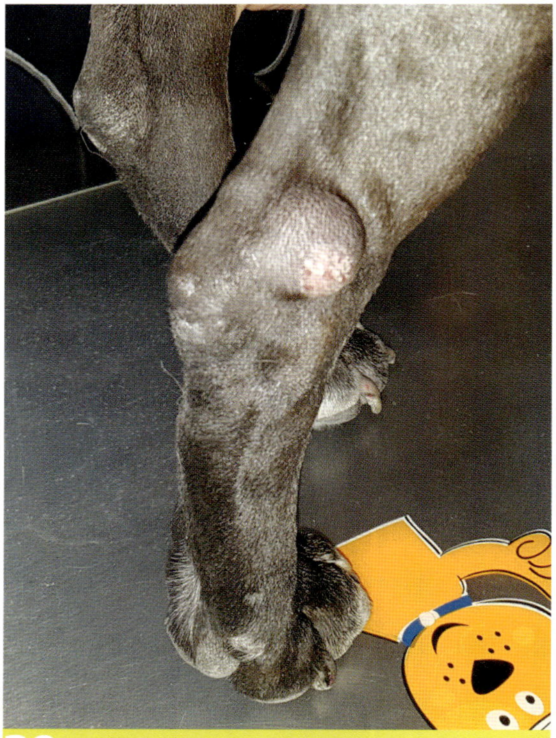

20 Plasmacytoma on the limb of a dog.

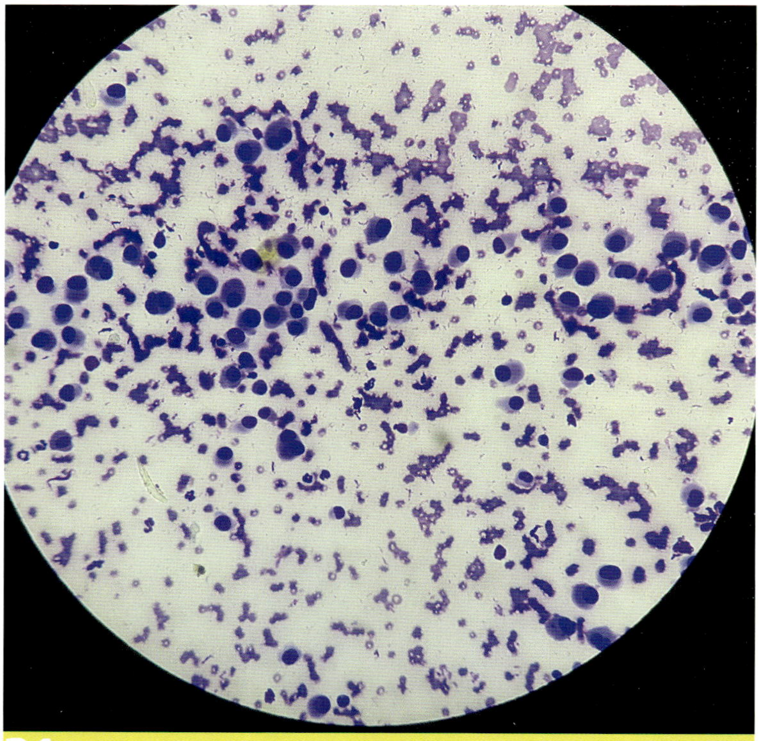

21 Plasmacytoma cytology.

# Basal cell tumours

## Lesion aetiology/pathogenesis and clinical picture

These are usually benign tumours and are much more frequent in cats. They arise from the basal cells of the epidermis and, in contrast to the human form, do not appear to be actin-induced.

They are usually solitary tumours and occur most frequently on the head, neck, limbs, and back. They are usually firm, rounded, and encapsulated.

The malignant presentation is much less frequent.

## Diagnostic method

Histopathology shows a highly homogeneous circumscribed proliferation of basaloid cells.

## Main differential diagnoses

- Other tumour types
- Granulomas
- Cysts

## Treatment

Surgery if necessary.

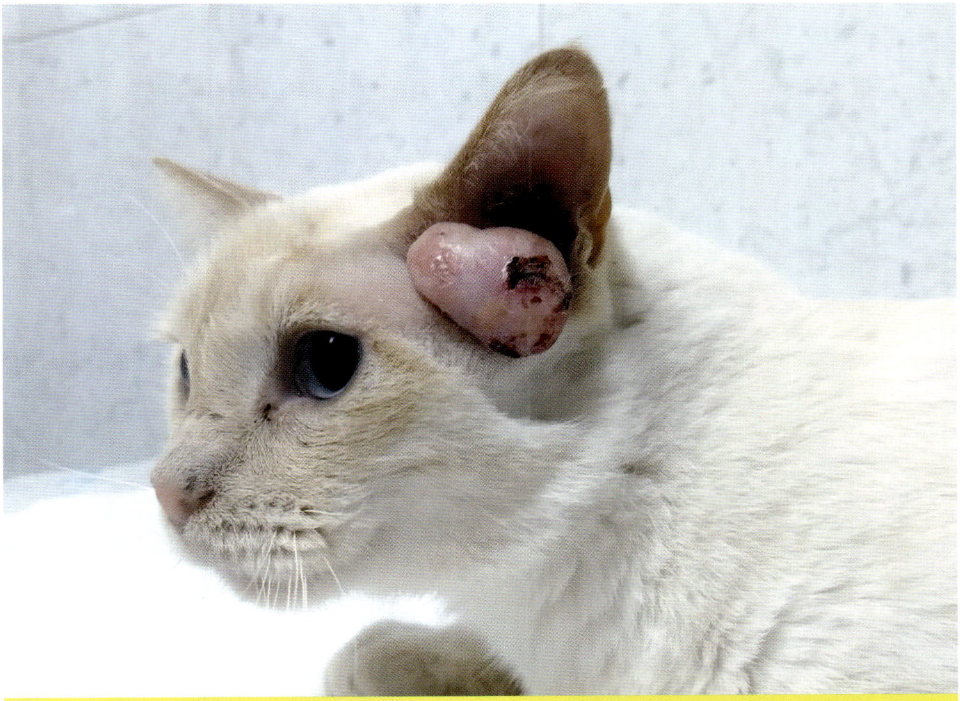

22 Basal cell carcinoma next to a cat's ear.

# Feline paraneoplastic alopecia

## Lesion aetiology/pathogenesis and clinical picture

This dermatosis occurs specifically in cats and is characterised by the absence of hair, which is easily shed, and by atrophic and very shiny skin in ventral areas. It is associated with pancreatic tumours, although the pathogenesis is unknown. *Malassezia* overgrowth may occur.

## Diagnostic method

Diagnosis is established based on the clinical appearance, histopathology, and ultrasound confirmation of the tumour.

## Main differential diagnoses

- Dermatophytosis
- Drug reaction
- Other cachexia-inducing tumours

## Treatment

The prognosis is bad. Treatment is only possible if the tumour is operable.

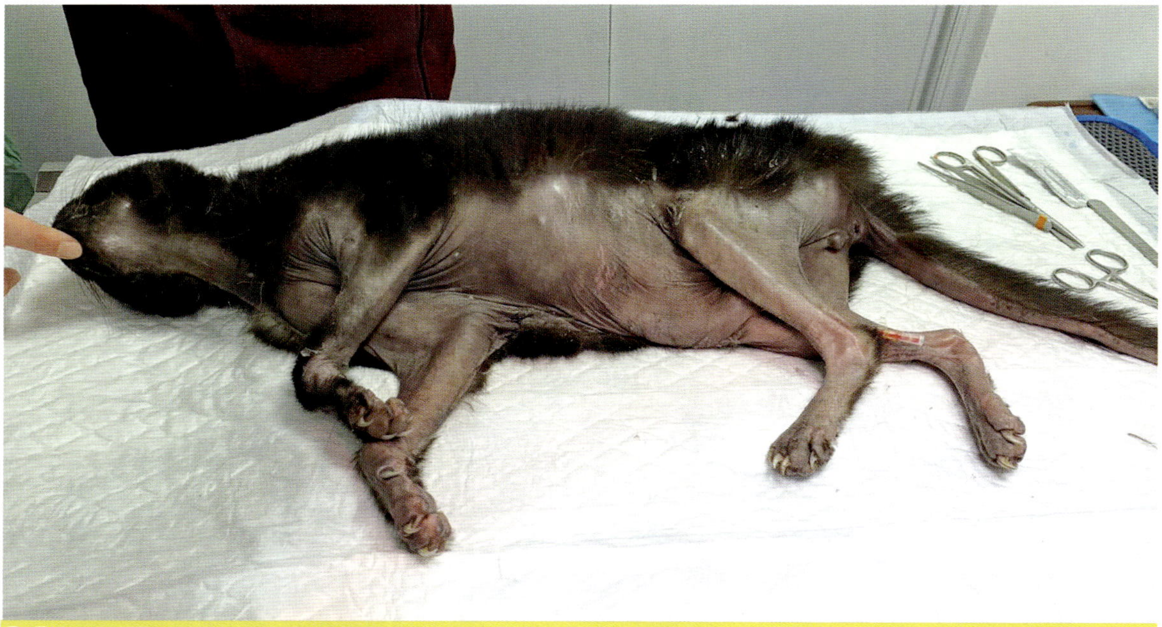

**23** General appearance of a cat with paraneoplastic alopecia.

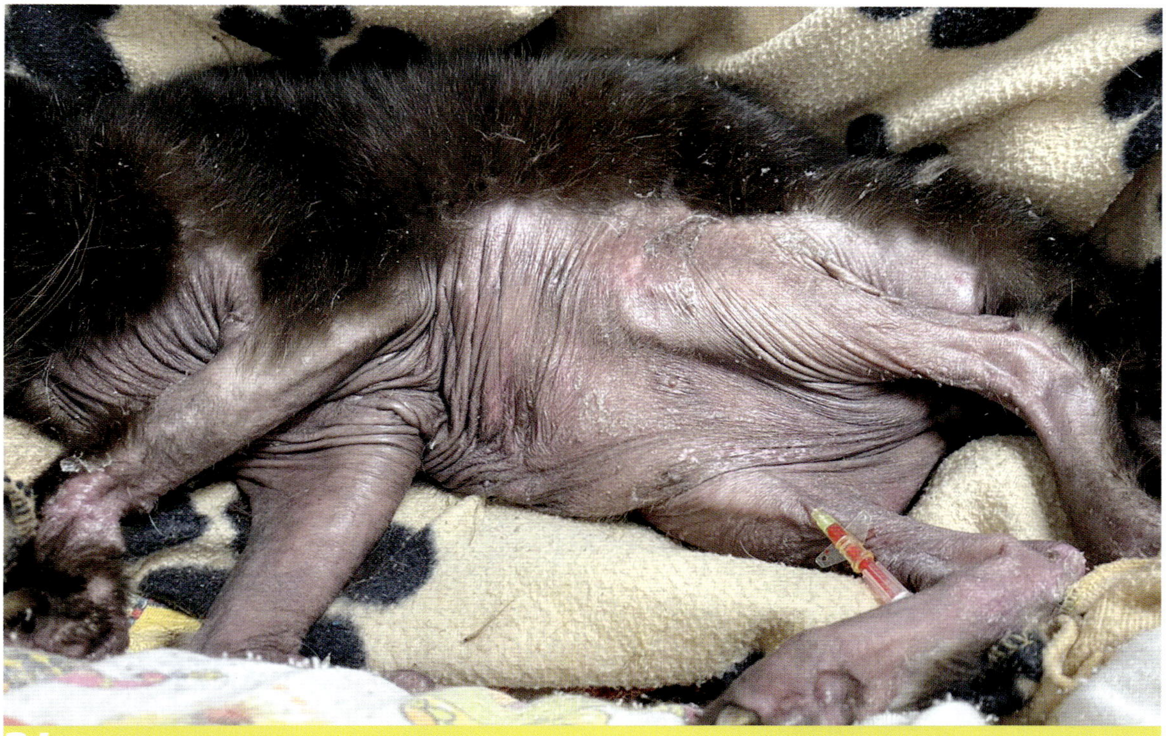

24 View of the abdomen of the cat from the previous image.

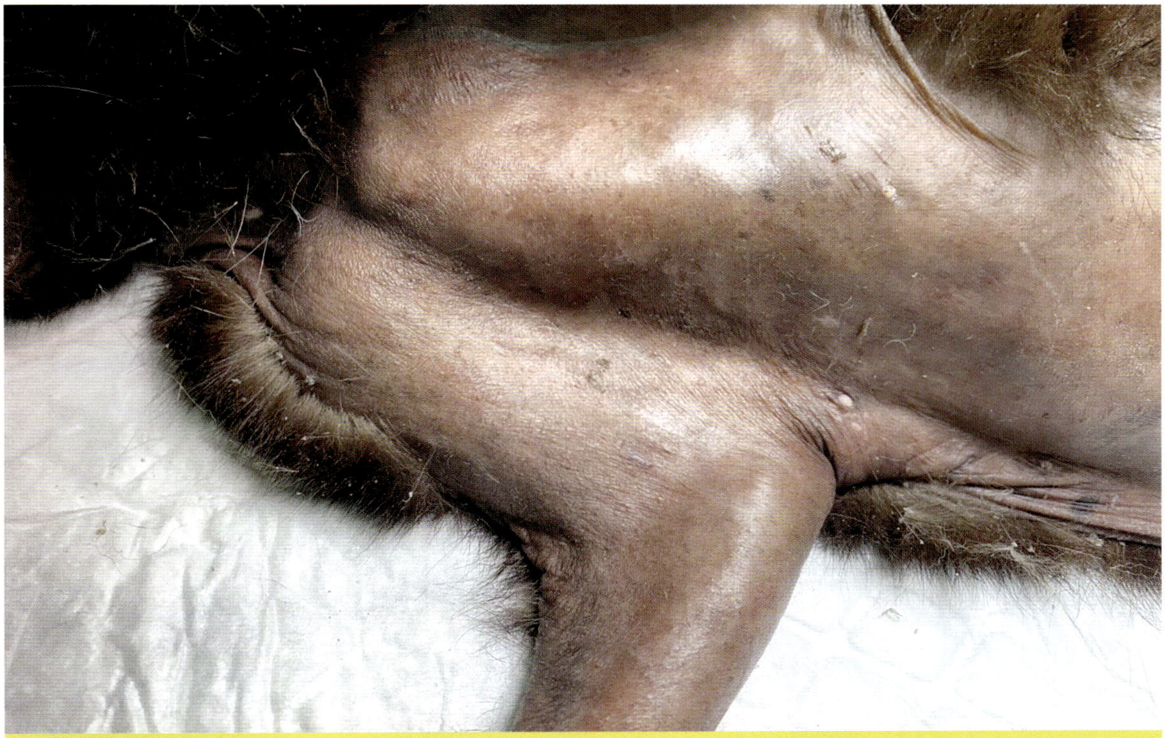

25 Close-up image of the skin in the axillary area.

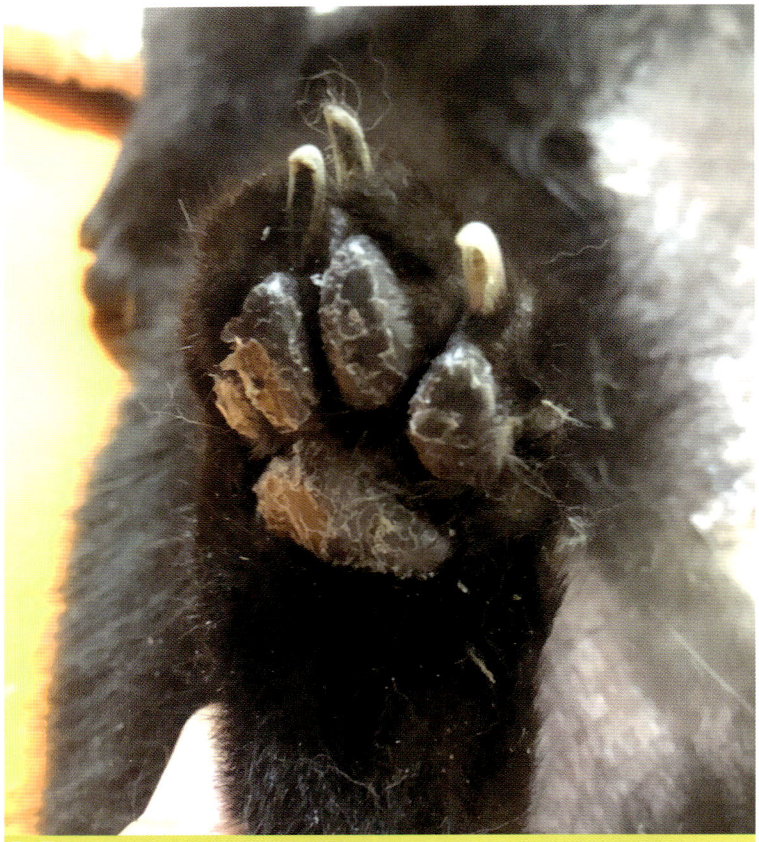

26 Paw pad of a cat with paraneoplastic alopecia displaying onychodystrophy.

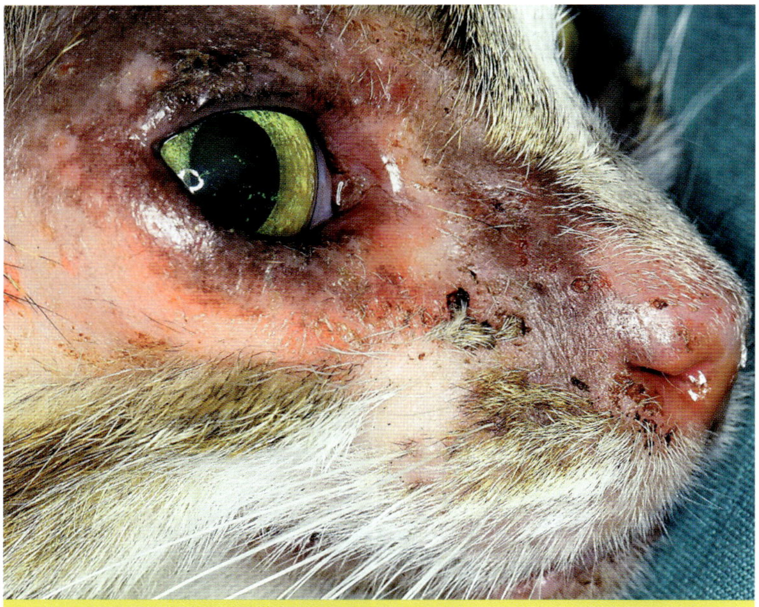

27 Facial appearance of a cat with paraneoplastic alopecia. Image courtesy of Didier Carlotti (RIP).

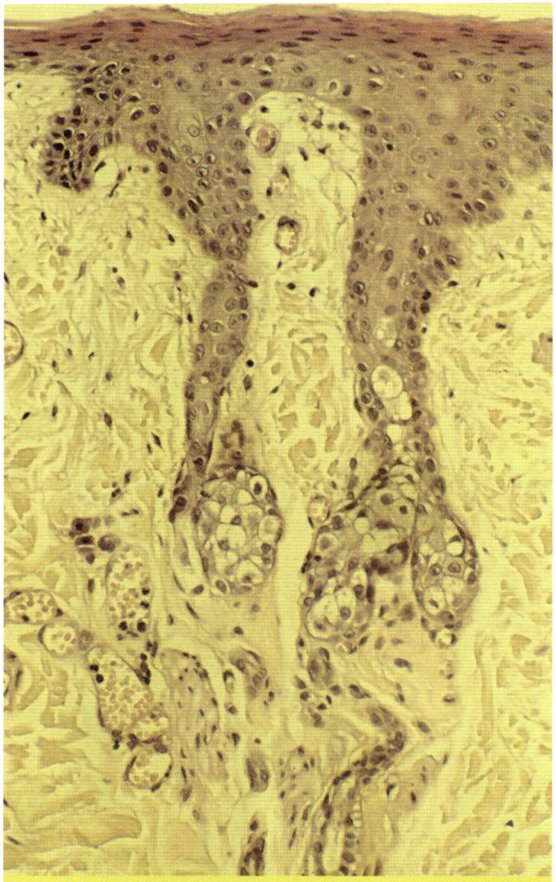

28 Histopathology of the patient from the previous image showing hyperplasia of the epidermis, absence of the corneal layer, and follicular atrophy. Image courtesy of Didier Carlotti (RIP).

# Adenoma and carcinoma of the hepatoid glands

## Lesion aetiology/pathogenesis and clinical picture

These are tumours of the perianal or hepatoid glands that typically affect dogs over 8 years of age. Most are usually benign adenomas, with a strong androgenic influence. Adenocarcinomas are clinically very similar, making them macroscopically indistinguishable from benign adenomas. Generally, the tumours are irregular in shape and usually occur in the perianal or perigenital area, or at the base of the tail.

## Diagnostic method

Diagnosis is established based on the clinical appearance, cytology, and biopsy.

Cytology is a reliable technique to identify the cell type, but does not always enable distinction of adenomas from adenocarcinomas.

## Main differential diagnoses

- Other tumours
- Anal sac diseases
- Perianal fistulas

## Treatment

In cases of adenoma, resolution can usually be achieved by neutering or, if surgical intervention is not feasible, the use of antiandrogens such as deslorelin implants. In adenocarcinoma the prognosis is worse and patients must undergo early surgical intervention to achieve cure.

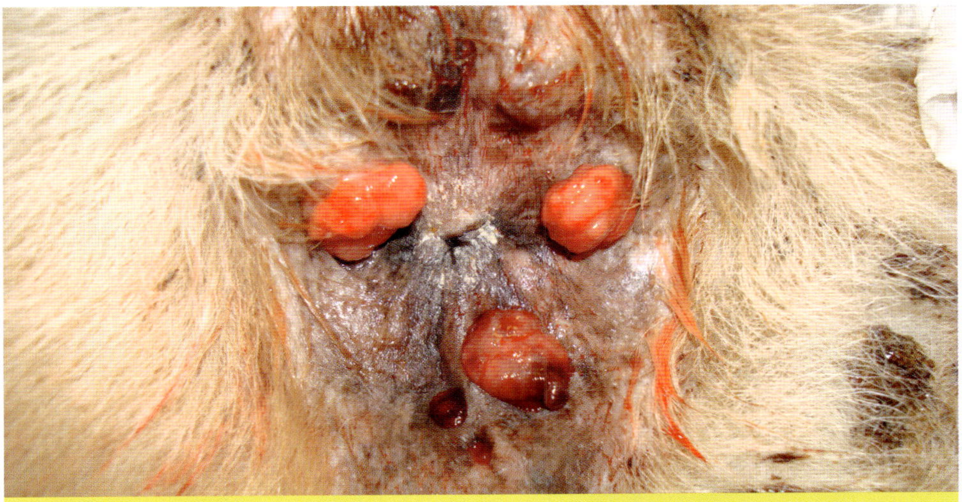

29 Hepatoid gland adenomas.

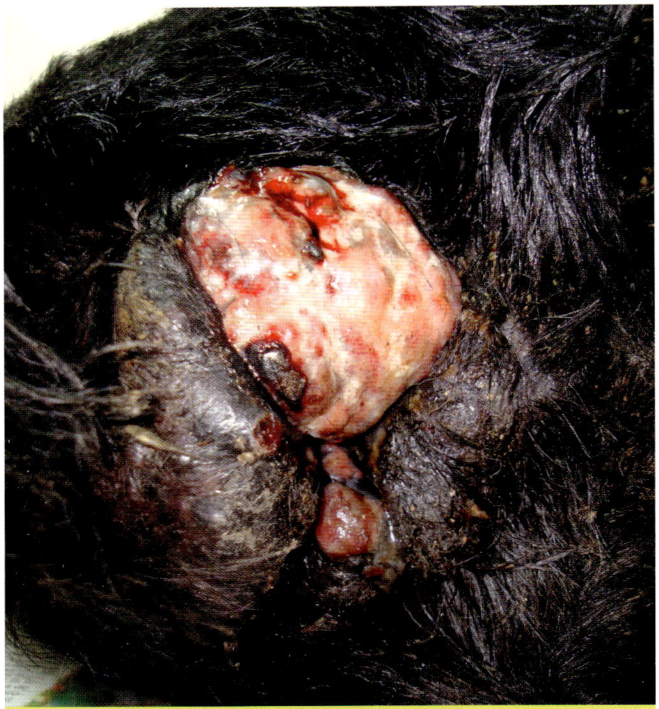

30 Irregular, slow growing hepatoid gland adenoma in a 9-year-old Giant Schnauzer.

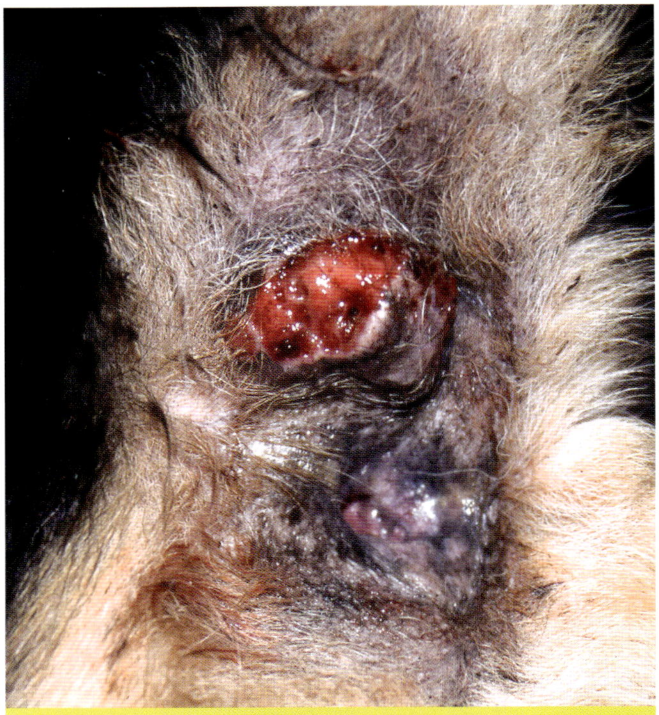

31 Adenocarcinoma of the hepatoid glands in a 10-year-old German Shepherd.

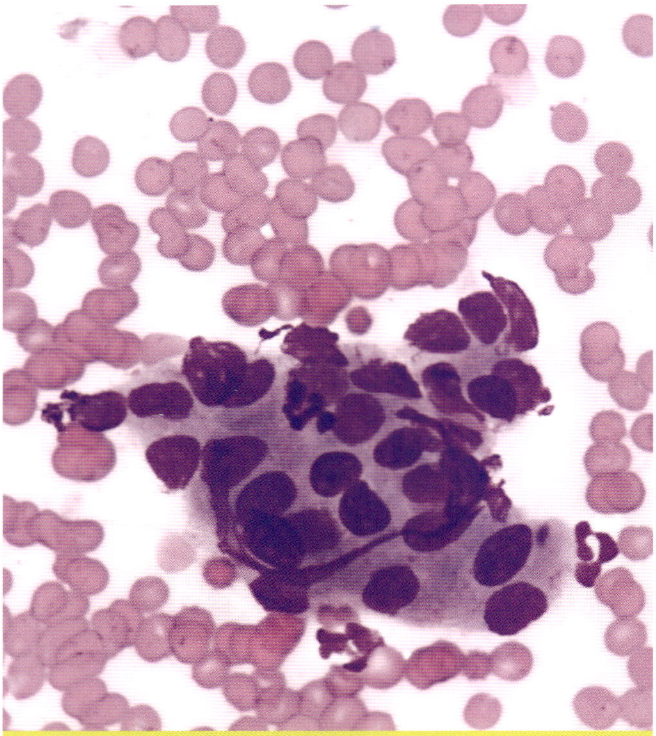

32 Cytology of a hepatoid gland adenoma showing epithelial cells.

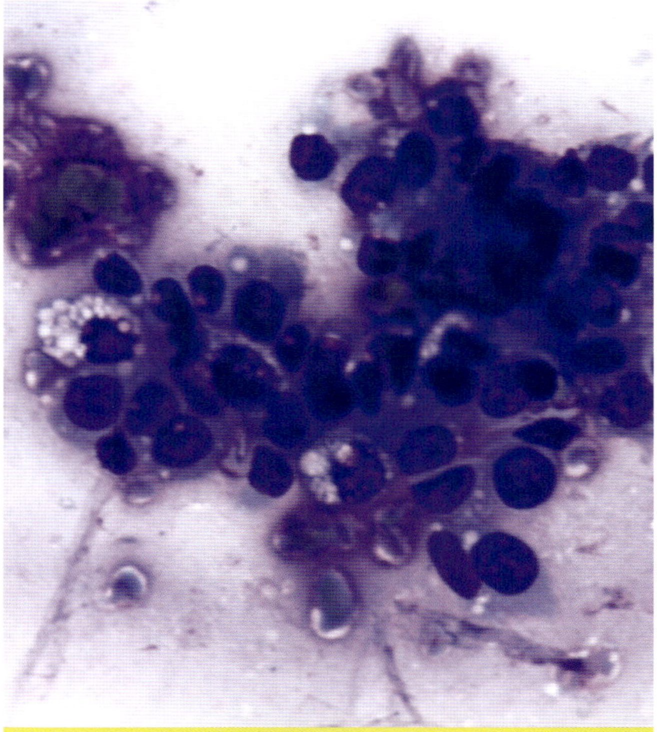

33 Cytology of hepatoid gland adenocarcinoma.

# Papillomas

## Lesion aetiology/pathogenesis and clinical picture

Papilloma is the result of thickening of the epidermis supported by projections from the dermis, often forming peduncles. Many are viral in origin (discussed in Chapter 5), while others are squamous papillomas.

## Diagnostic method

Diagnosis is established based on the clinical appearance and histopathology. Cytology is important to rule out other types of tumours. Viral forms are more common in young or immunosuppressed animals. Nonviral forms are more common in adult and senior dogs.

## Main differential diagnoses

- Other tumours
- Pseudotumours
- Cysts

## Treatment

Surgery.

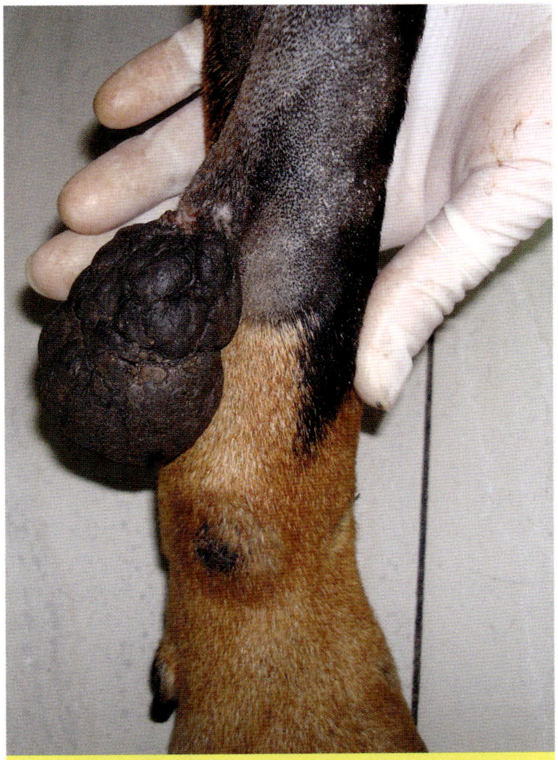

34 Nonviral papilloma on the forelimb of a Doberman.

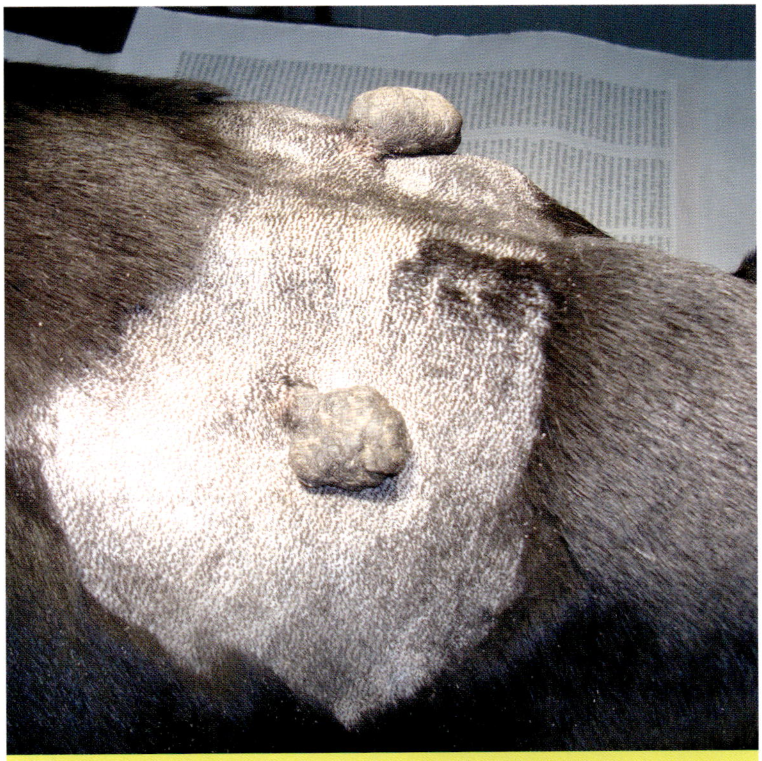

35 Papillomas on the back of a 12-year-old mixed-breed dog.

# Soft tissue sarcoma

## Lesion aetiology/pathogenesis and clinical picture

This type of tumour is derived from mesenchymal cells, and includes various tumours with similar biological behaviour. They are often collectively referred to as fibromas and fibrosarcomas, but can involve muscle, vascular, nerve, and other cells.

They can affect both dogs and cats. The malignant forms are usually highly recurrent, with little metastatic potential.

There is a variant of this tumour induced by the injection of different substances. This is mainly described in cats at the injection site.

Another variant is solar-induced cutaneous haemangiosarcoma.

## Diagnostic method

Compatible cytology and biopsy.

## Main differential diagnoses

Other tumours.

## Treatment

Radical surgery, preferably compartmental. In some cases radiation therapy may be applied. Intratumoural administration of tigilanol tiglate is currently being studied.

In cases of injection-induced variants in cats (feline injection-site sarcoma, FISS), very radical surgery is required and radiation therapy can be attempted. Intratumoural recombinant IL-2 may also be useful.

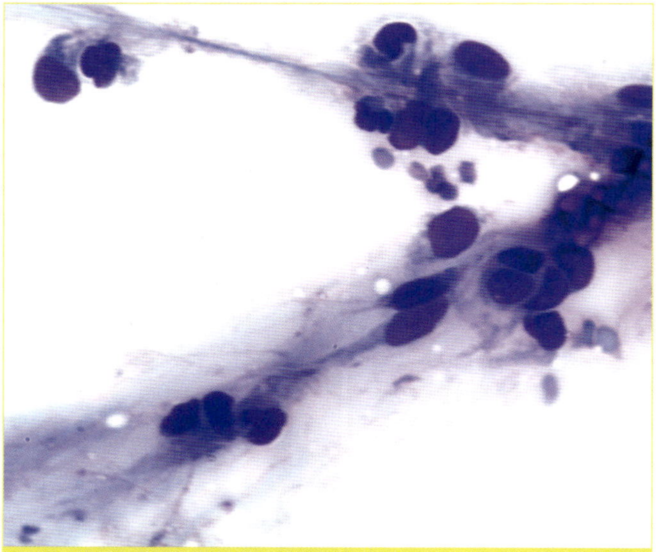

36 Cytology of a feline postvaccination fibrosarcoma.

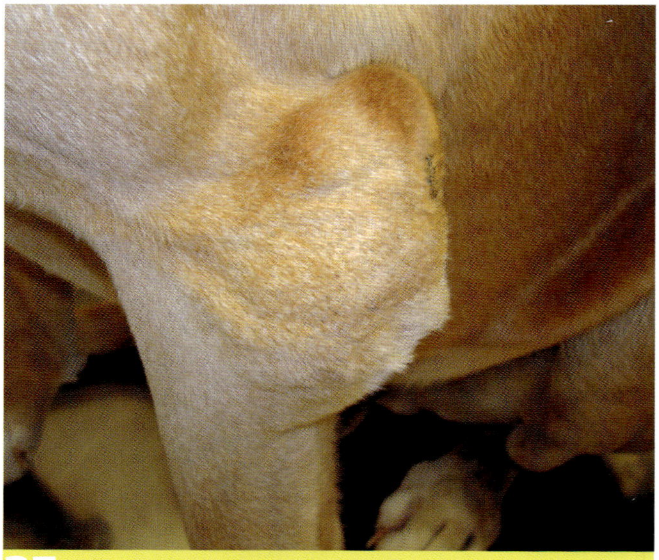

37 Haemangiopericytoma on the elbow of a 9-year-old Boxer.

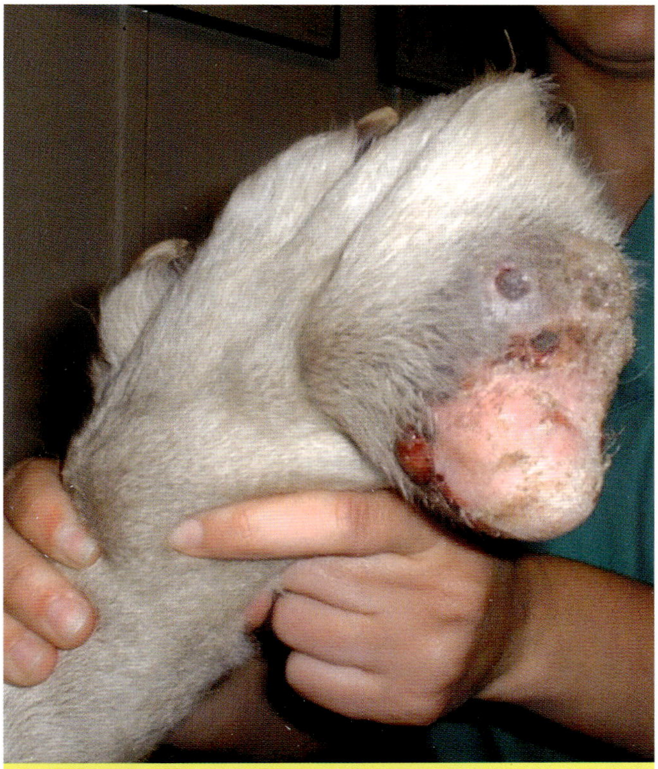

38 Schwannoma on the digit of a 9-year-old Mastiff.

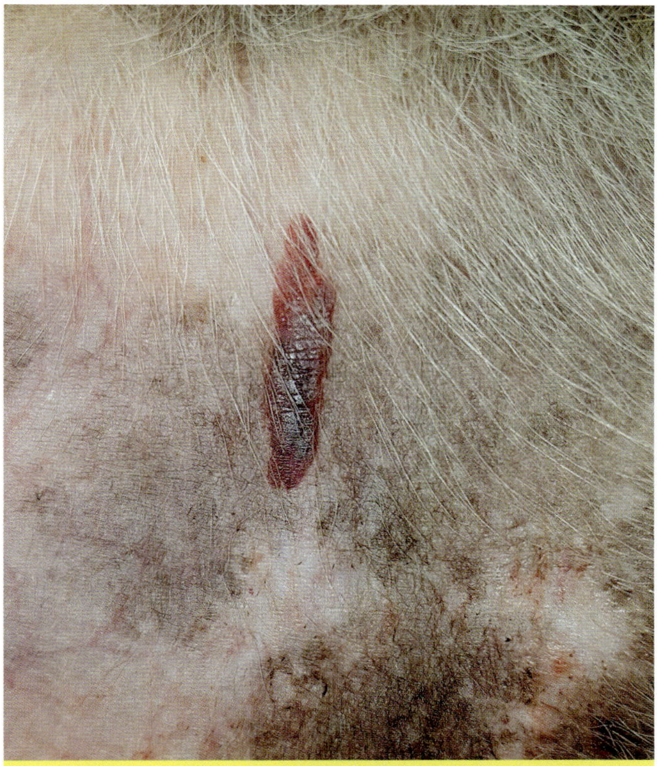

39 Cutaneous haemangiosarcoma.

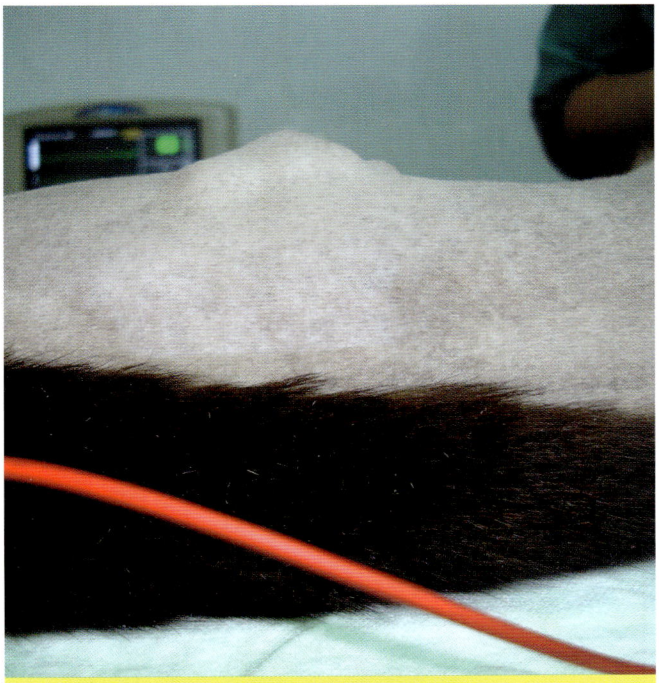

40 Injection-site sarcoma in a cat. Note the tumour in the area prepared for excision.

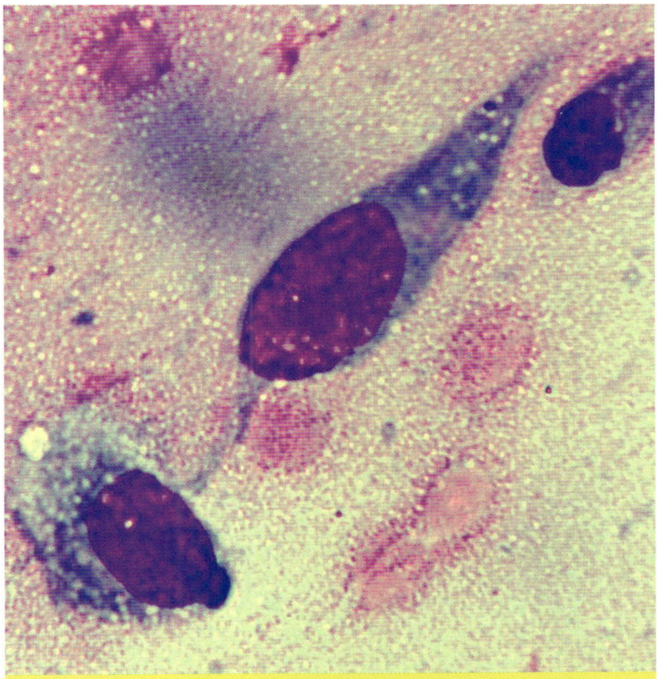

41 High magnification image of malignant mesenchymal cells. Vacuoles are visible in the cytoplasm and nucleus.

# Squamous cell carcinoma

## Lesion aetiology/pathogenesis and clinical picture

This tumour of keratinocytes more commonly affects animals with white coats and mainly appears in areas with less hair. A very aggressive variant affects the nail matrix of the digits and appears more frequently in large, black coat breeds such as the Giant Schnauzer.

In dogs it can manifest as a tumorous or ulcerated and scaling form, mainly in animals with a high degree of sun exposure. In cats, mainly those with white coats, it can also affect the areas most exposed to the sun, such as the tips of the ears and the nose.

## Diagnostic method

Diagnosis is based on the clinical appearance and cytology and biopsy findings. Cytology does not enable easy differentiation of precancerous stages (e.g. actinic keratosis) from squamous cell carcinoma (SCC).

## Main differential diagnoses

- Actinic keratosis
- Other forms of carcinosis

## Treatment

Radical surgery, cryotherapy, imiquimod are options in very early stages. Given the receptors expressed in this tumour, tyrosine kinase inhibitors may be useful.

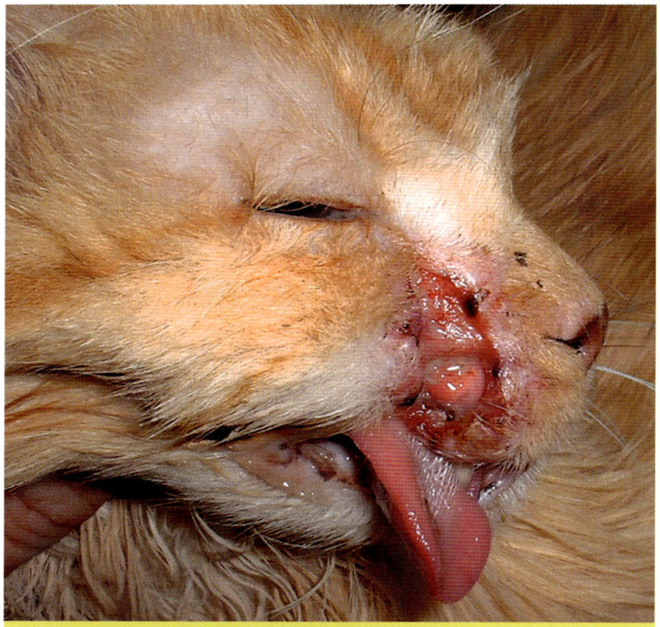

42 Squamous cell carcinoma on the face of a 9-year-old cat.

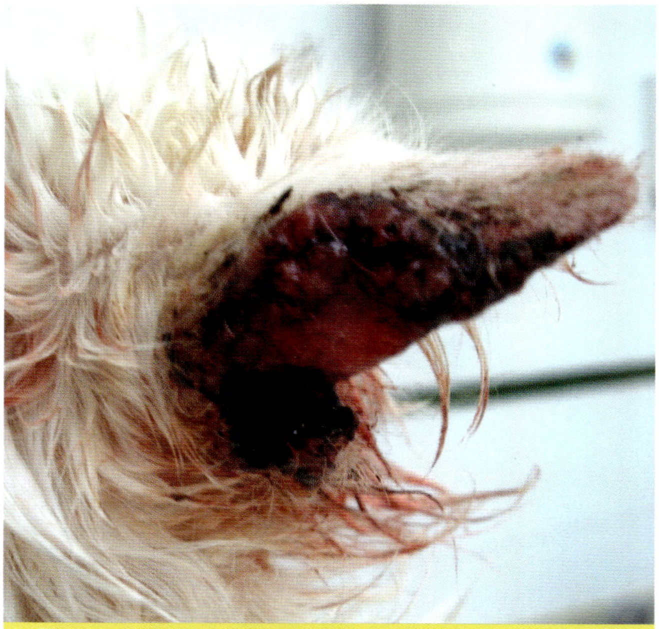

43 Squamous cell carcinoma on the ear of a white cat.

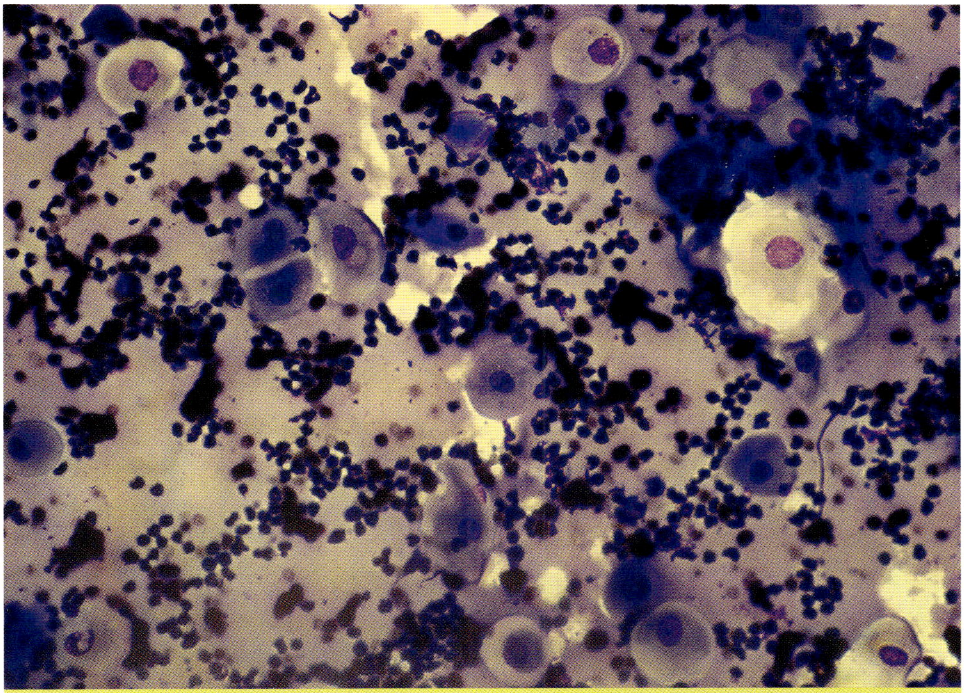

44 Squamous cell carcinoma cytology.

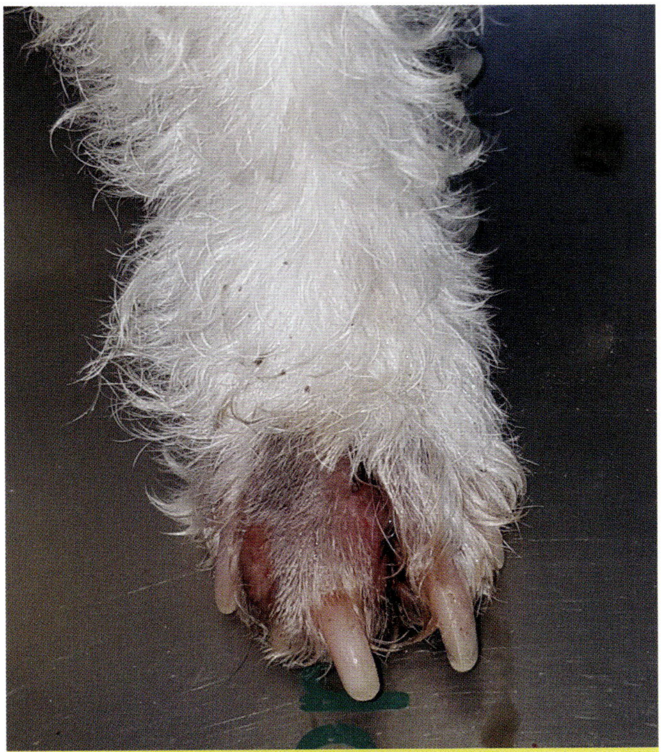

45 Carcinoma of the nail matrix. Note the thickening of the affected digit.

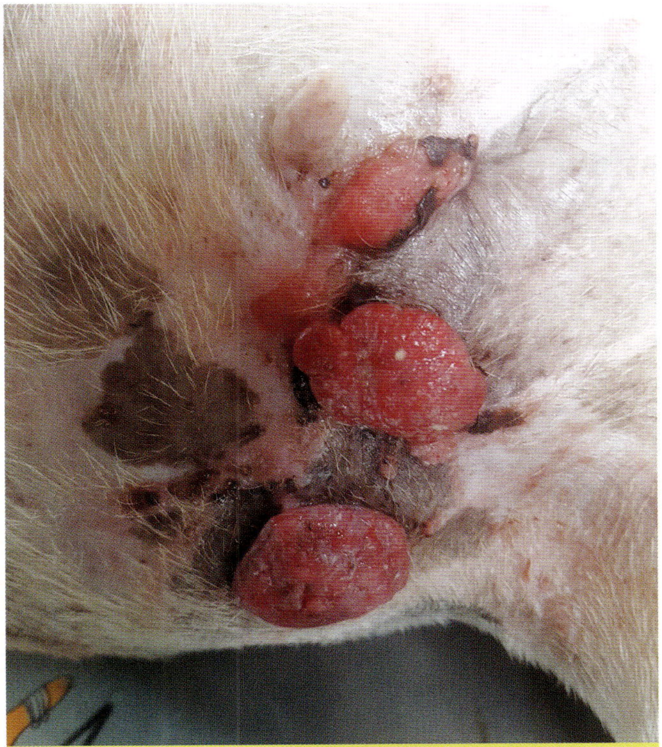

46 Solar-induced squamous cell carcinoma nodules on the abdomen of a Bull Terrier.

# Actinic keratosis

## Lesion aetiology/pathogenesis and clinical picture

Ultraviolet radiation-induced epidermal dysplasia. This occurs mainly in glabrous areas of skin in dogs and cats with high levels of exposure to the sun. It presents as erythematous areas with shiny, scaly, crusted skin, and diffuse alopecia. In some cases exfoliation and even ulceration may be observed. This may be indicative of malignant squamous cell carcinoma.

## Diagnostic method

Diagnosis is based on the clinical appearance and histopathology. Cytology can be indicative but not definitive. UVA radiation can also alter mesenchymal cells and elastin fibres.

## Main differential diagnoses

- Squamous cell carcinoma
- Alopecia with erythema due to other causes

## Treatment

Avoidance of the sun, use of sunscreen, tattooing, retinoids, imiquimod, liposome-encapsulated photolyase (DNA repairsomes), and cryotherapy can be effective.

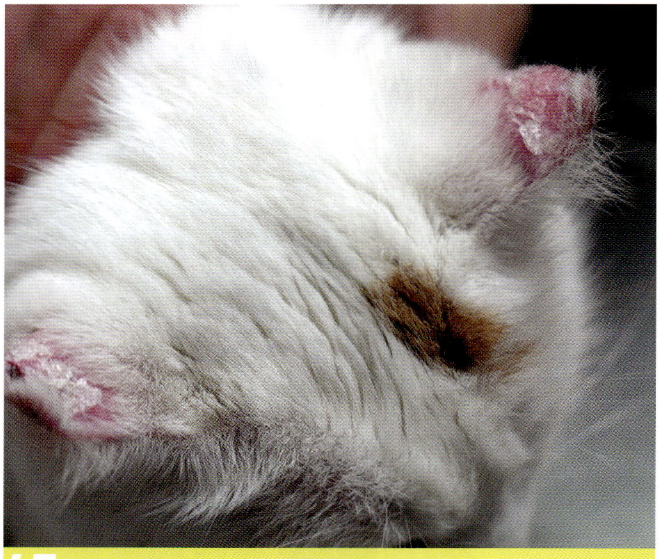

47 Actinic keratosis on both ears of a white cat.

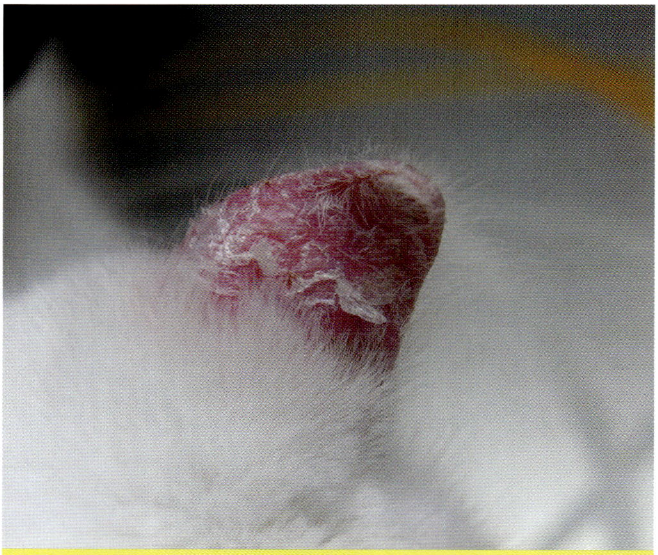

48 Actinic keratosis: close-up image.

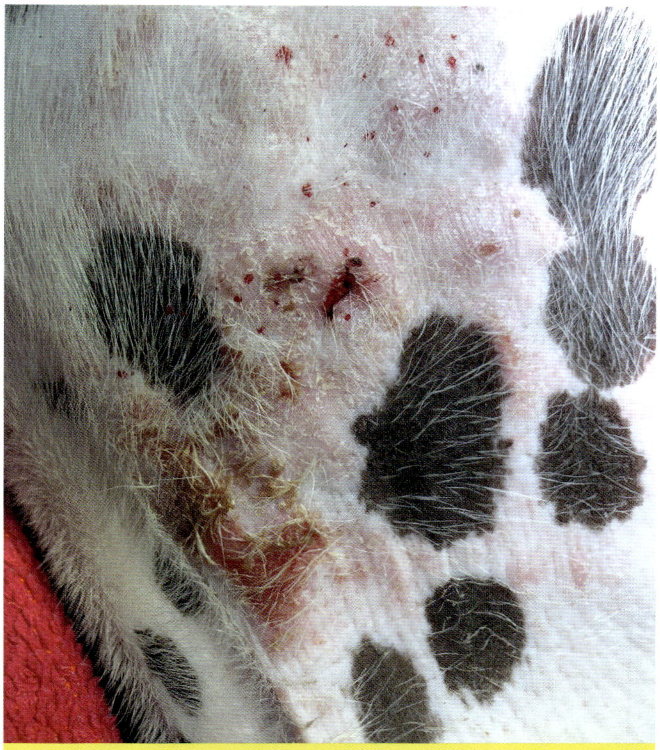

49 Actinic keratosis and furunculosis on the abdomen of an 8-year-old Dogo Argentino.

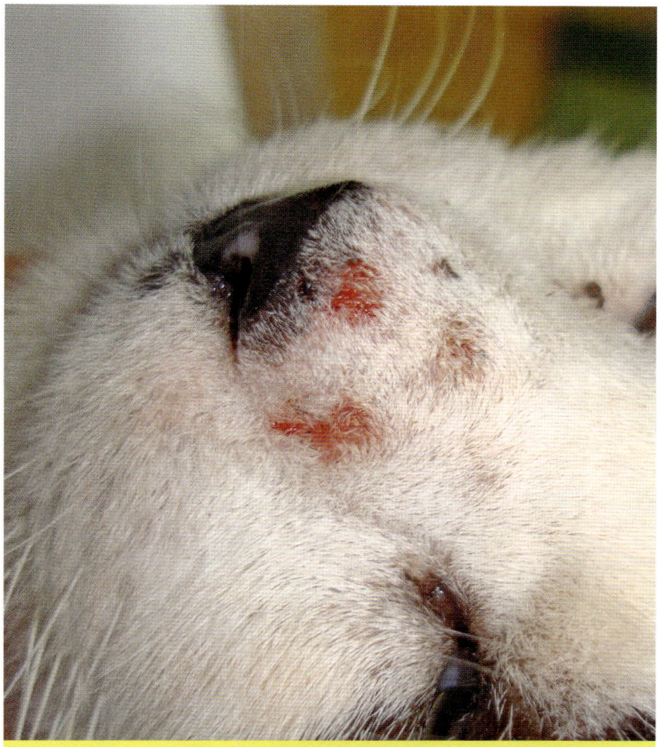

50 Onset of actinic keratosis on the nasal bridge of a cat.

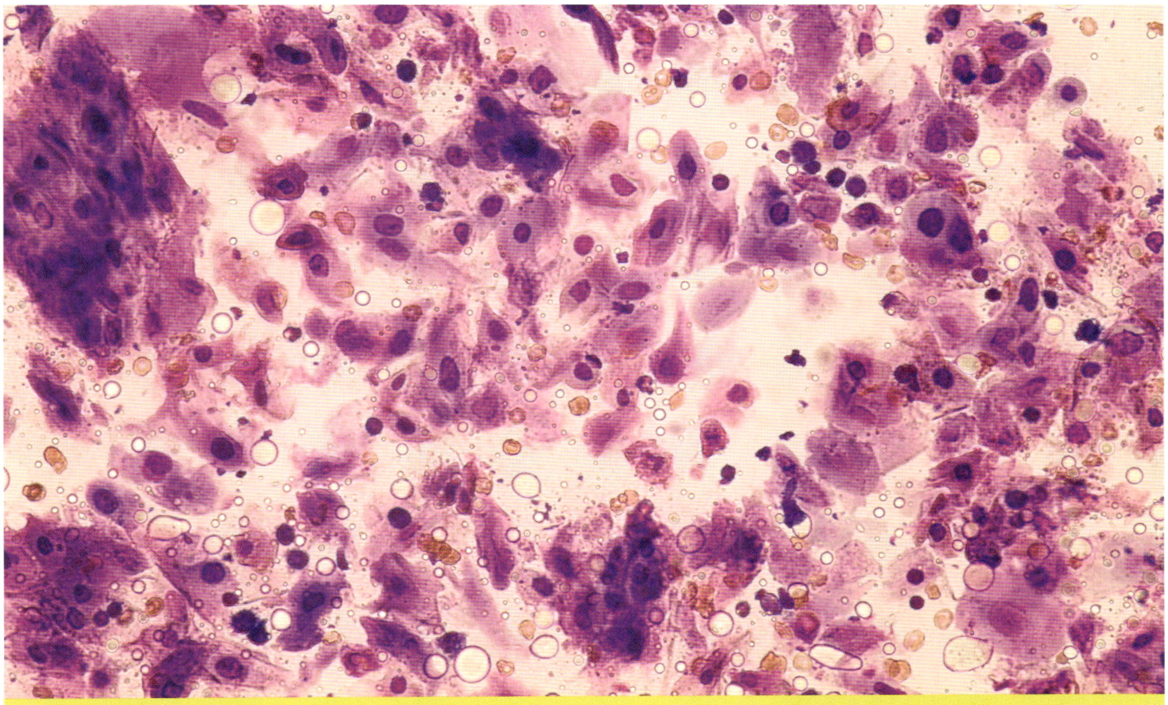

51 Cytology showing solar-induced dysplasia of epithelial and mesenchymal cells.

# Cutaneous metastasis of mammary adenocarcinoma

## Lesion aetiology/pathogenesis and clinical picture

In areas of skin adjacent to breast tumours, and sometimes further afield, adenocarcinoma can spread via the bloodstream to the skin, giving rise to what is known as carcinomatosis or inflammatory carcinoma. This usually manifests with erythema, crusting, and ulceration, and generally represents a terminal stage.

## Diagnostic method

Diagnosis is based on the clinical appearance and cytology findings compatible with adenocarcinoma.

## Main differential diagnoses

- Other carcinomas
- Deep pyodermas
- Actinic keratosis

## Treatment

Cutaneous metastasis of mammary adenocarcinoma has a very poor prognosis. Radical surgery and chemotherapy can be attempted.

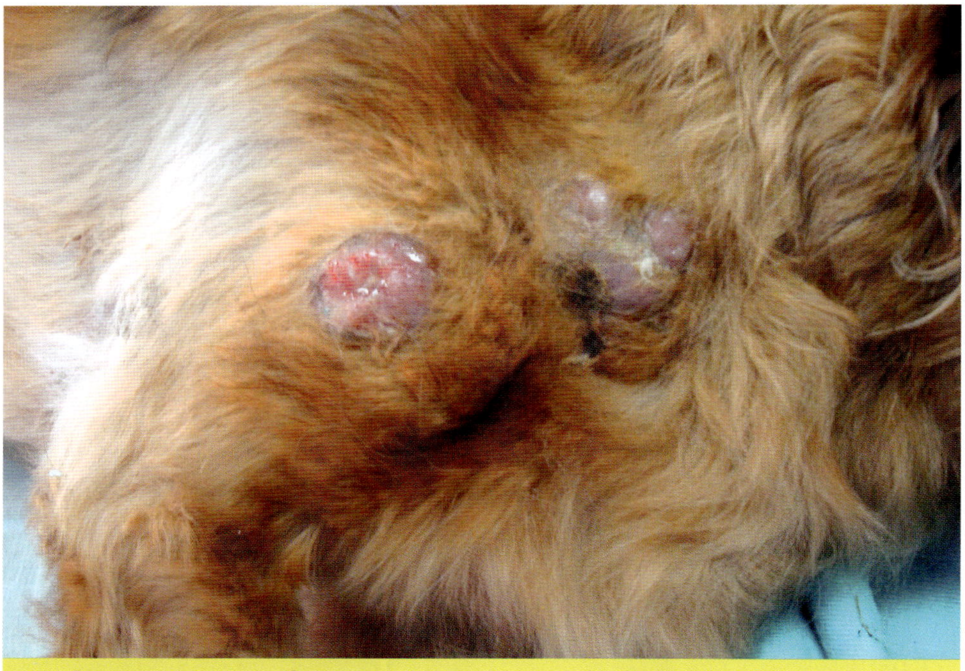

52 Cutaneous metastasis of mammary adenocarcinoma on the shoulder skin of a 14-year-old female dog.

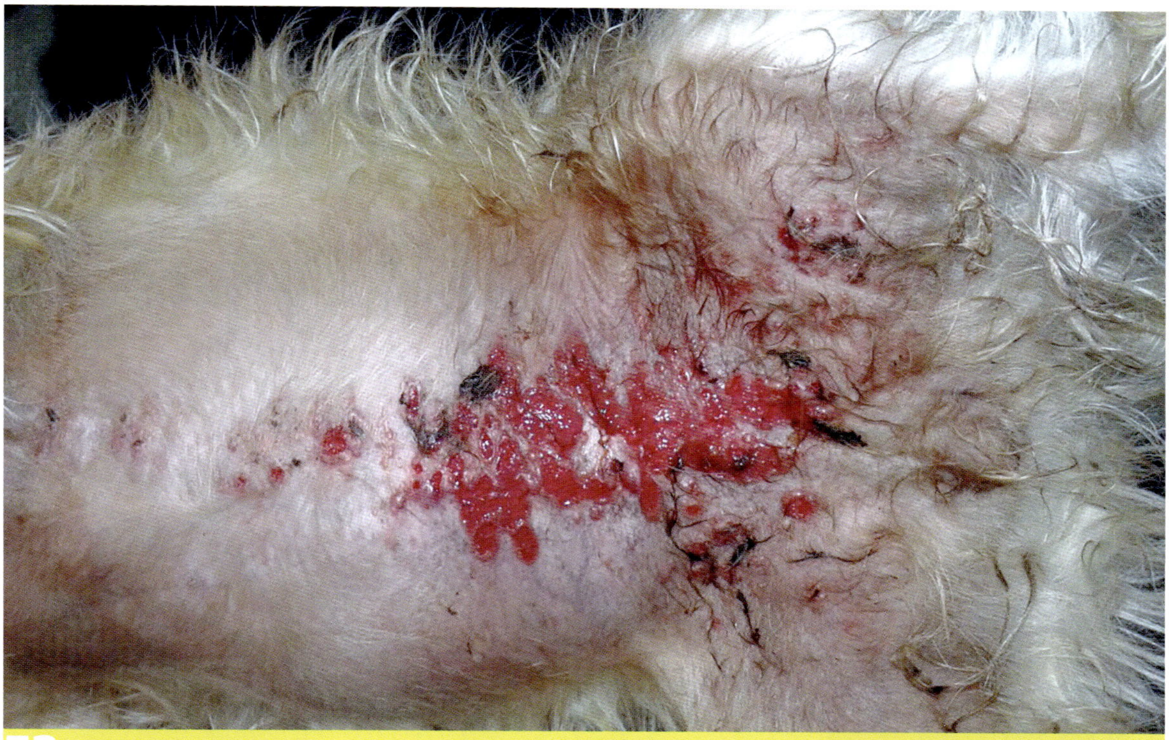

53 Mammary carcinomatosis on the skin of a female dog 1 month after surgery.

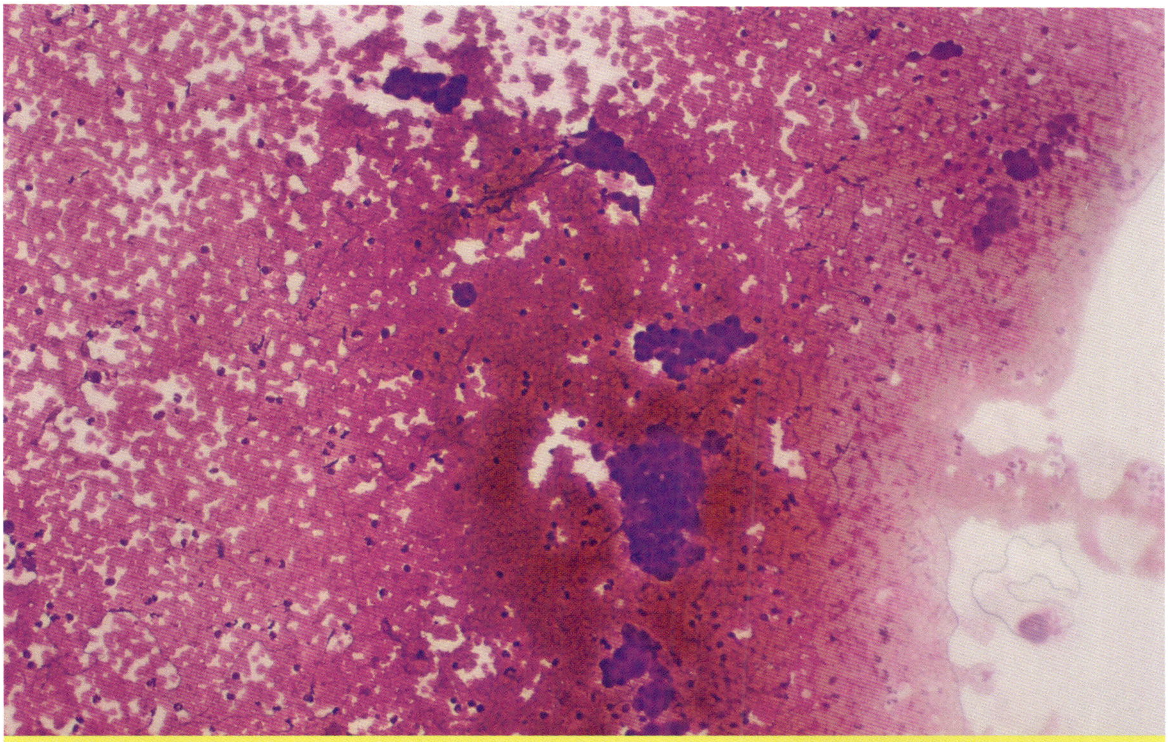

54 Cytology of cutaneous carcinomatosis due to breast adenocarcinoma. Note the groups of tumour cells.

# Melanoma

## Lesion aetiology/pathogenesis and clinical picture

These are melanocytic tumours with varying degrees of malignancy. They are described using various different terms, from melanocytoma for benign forms to melanosarcoma for malignant forms. They can manifest as irregular tumours, spots, or simple macules, which should be monitored closely. The prevalence of malignant tumours tends to be higher in cats. In dogs, tumours in certain locations (e.g. the digits, lips, eyelids, or gums) can increase the risk of malignancy.

## Diagnostic method

Diagnosis is established based on the tumour evolution and appearance, as well as cytology and biopsy findings.

## Main differential diagnoses

- Mast cell tumour
- Lentigo
- Melanocytic nevus or hamartoma

## Treatment

A vaccine is available for oral forms and is used to try to increase cellular immunity against tumour cells. Radical and early surgery is the best therapeutic option. Selective cyclooxygenase-2 inhibitors and carboplatin can be used as chemotherapeutic agents.

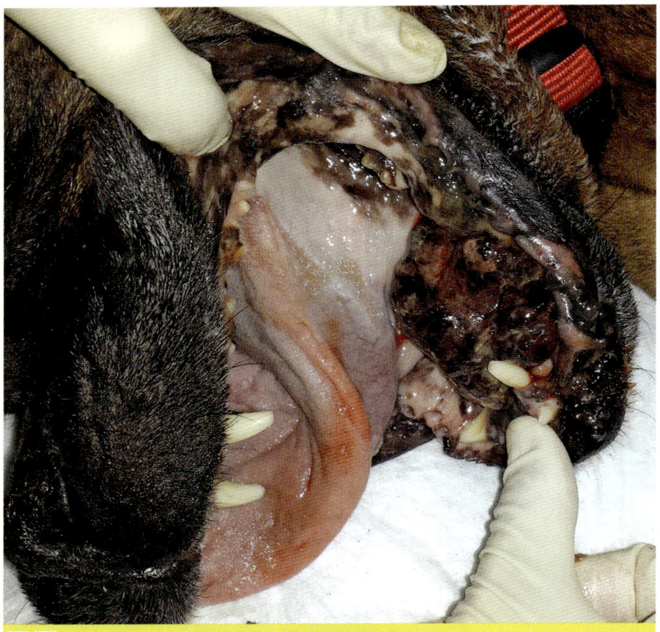

55 Invasive melanoma in the mouth of a Boxer.

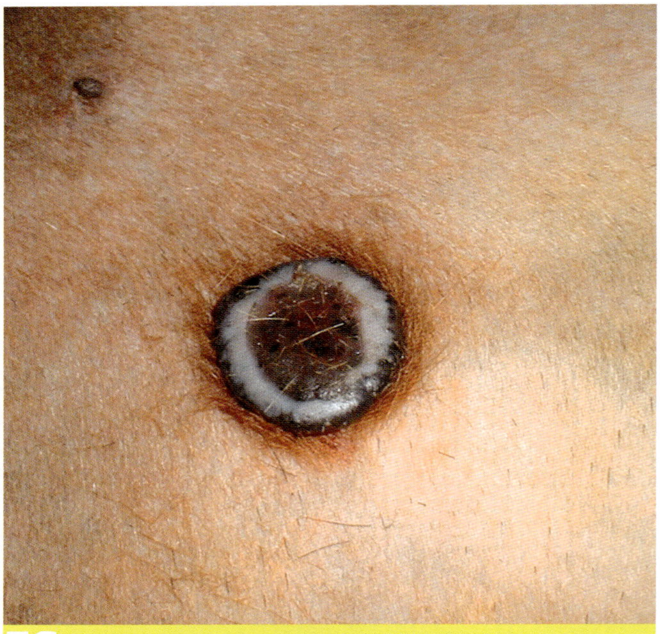

56 High-grade melanoma on the abdomen of a 9-year-old Boxer.

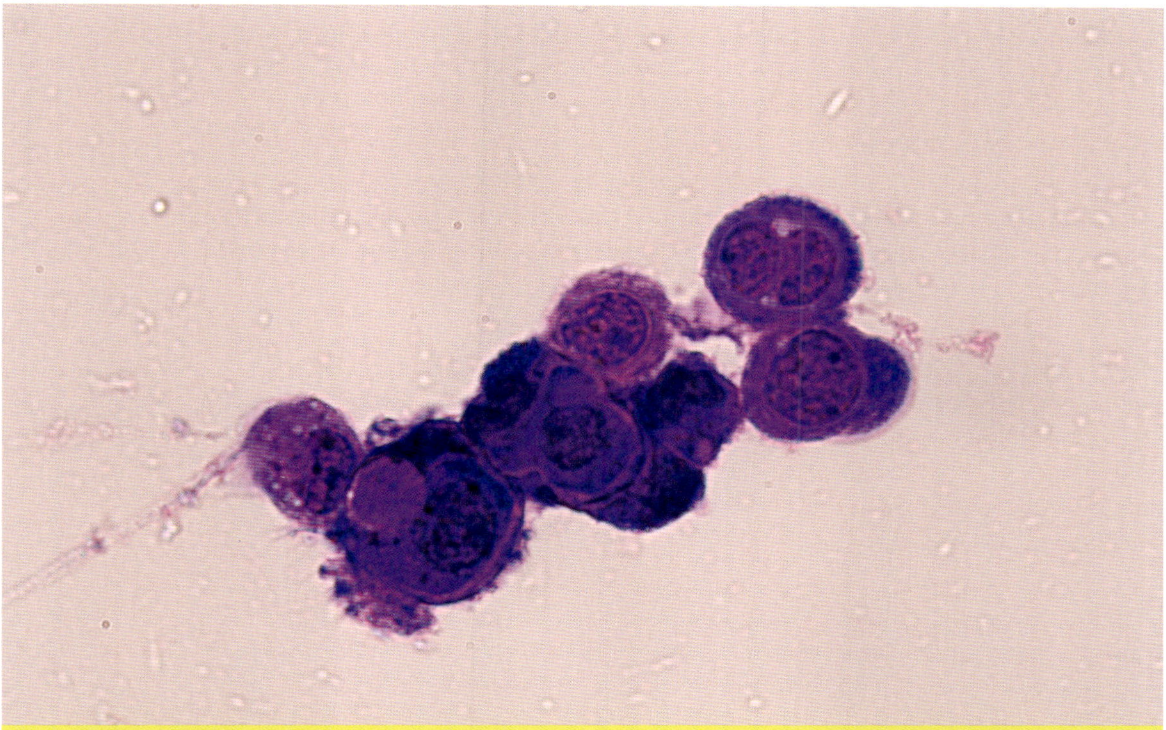

57 Melanocytes exhibiting multiple signs of malignancy.

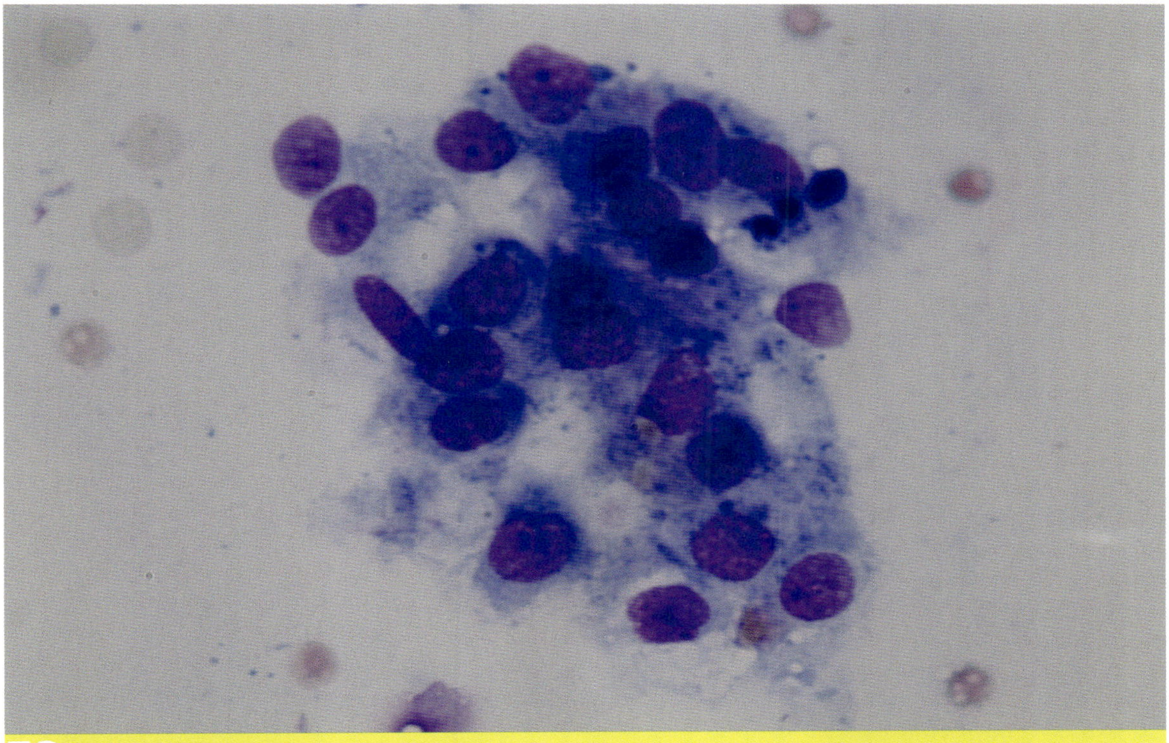

58 Melanoma cytology. Pigment granules are evident.

# Transmissible venereal tumour

## Lesion aetiology/pathogenesis and clinical picture

This tumour type is relatively frequent in certain (mainly tropical) countries. Its origin is unknown, although it is known to be contagious. It is transmitted by sexual contact, licking, and biting. It has a very irregular appearance and develops in the genital and perigenital areas and on the face. In cases of postmicturition occult bleeding, care should be taken to investigate the presence of a tumour in inconspicuous areas.

## Diagnostic method

Diagnosis is established based on the clinical appearance, clinical history, and cytology and biopsy findings.

## Main differential diagnoses

Tumours in perineal, genital, and facial areas.

## Treatment

Cases of spontaneous remission are described. Vincristine treatment tends to produce a good response.

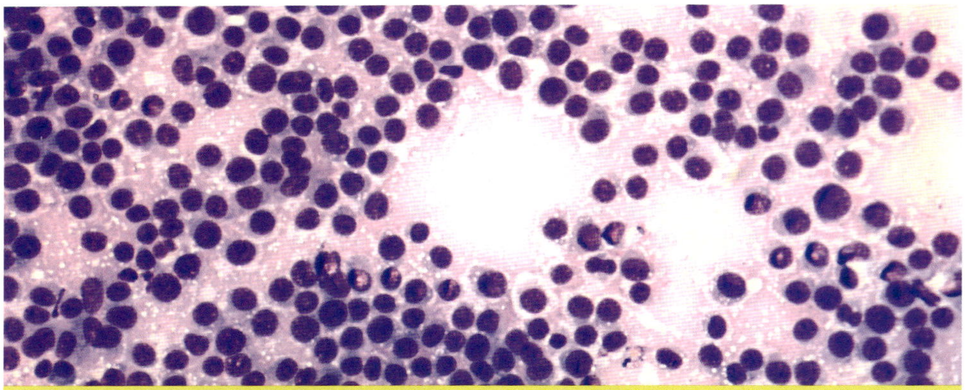

59 Cytology of a transmissible venereal tumour containing typical round cells with well-defined vacuoles.

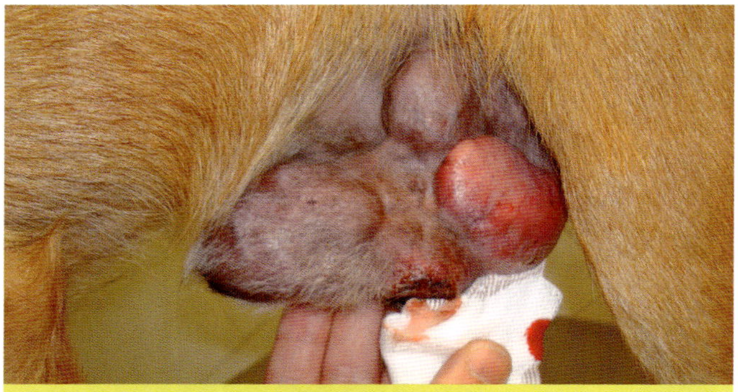

60 Transmissible venereal tumour in the preputial area of a male.

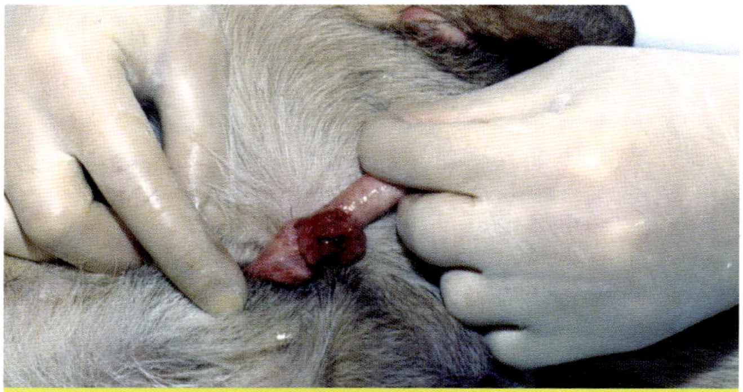

61 Transmissible venereal tumour deep in the preputial mucosa. Cause of haematuria.

# 11 Most frequent pseudotumours

# Introduction

Pseudotumours are disorganised nonmonoclonal tissue masses, usually consisting of growths of normal tissue where it does not belong. In this chapter we will discuss the most common forms:

- Hamartomas
- Cysts
- Cutaneous horns
- Cutaneous outgrowths
- Canine interdigital granulomas
- Keratosis
- Fibropruritic nodules
- Nodular dermatofibrosis
- Cutaneous polyps

# Hamartomas

## Lesion aetiology/pathogenesis and clinical picture

These are stable malformations of hereditary or congenital origin that are restricted to the skin.

They are usually exaggerated growths of normal histological structures. They can occur at any age, but tend to be more frequent in animals of advanced age.

Depending on their location, they can be:

- Collagenous
- Hair follicle-derived
- Melanocytic (benign melanoma)
- Pigmented epidermal
- Sebaceous gland-derived
- Scrotal vascular

## Diagnostic method

Diagnosis is established based on the clinical appearance and the histopathological findings. Cytology findings can be highly variable.

## Main differential diagnoses

The differential diagnosis includes all types of tumours and pseudotumours.

## Treatment

The only effective treatment is surgical resection, which is performed when the tumour begins to bother the patient.

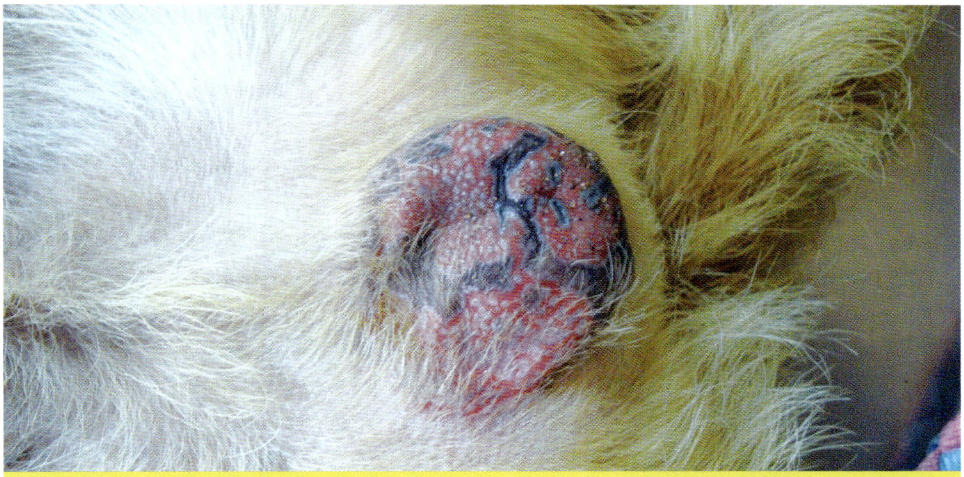

01 Vascular hamartoma.

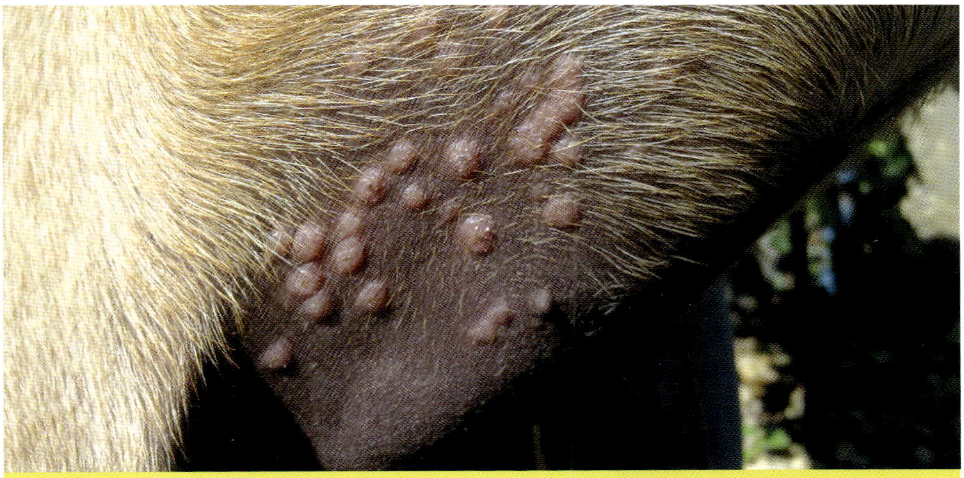

02 Collagenous hamartoma. Image courtesy of María del Mar Bustabad.

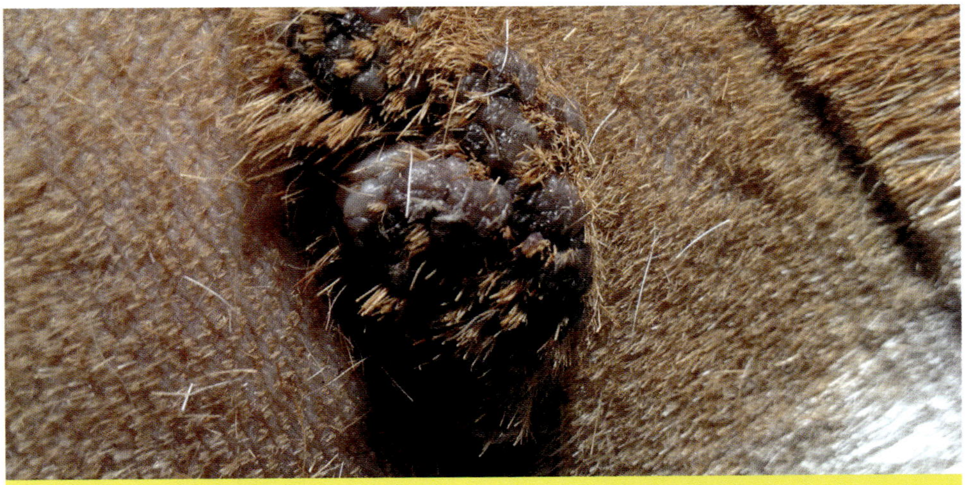

03 Follicular hamartoma.

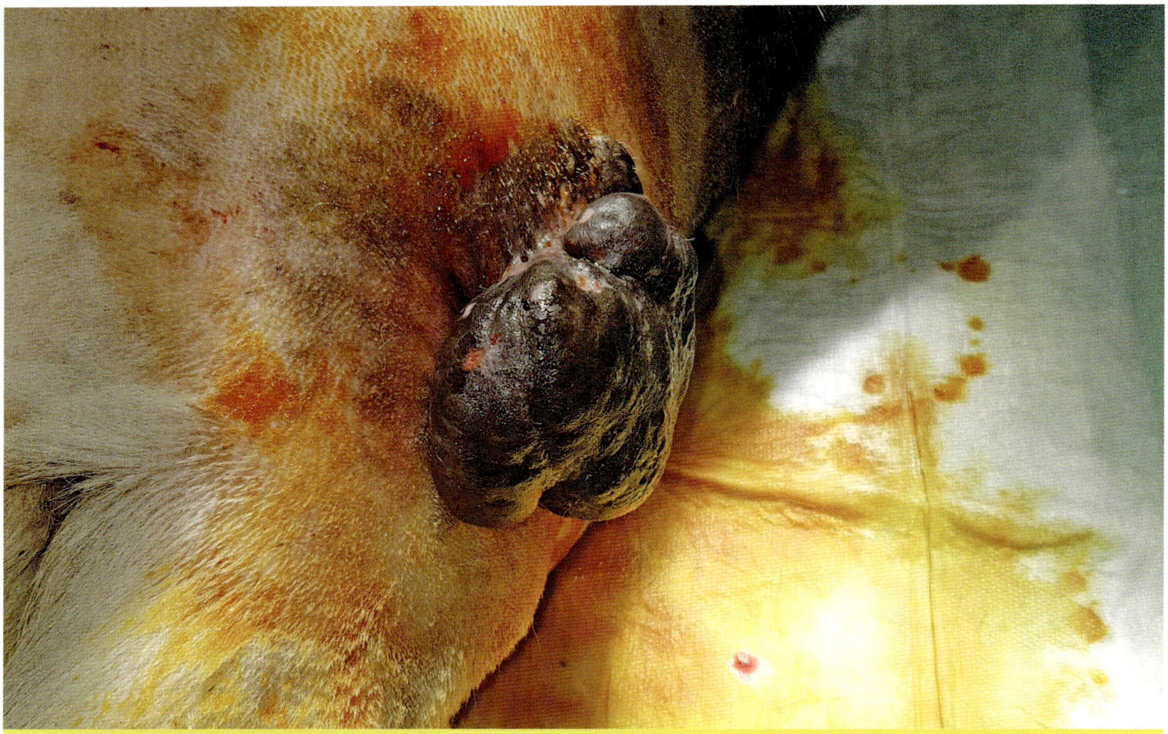

04 Melanocytic hamartoma.

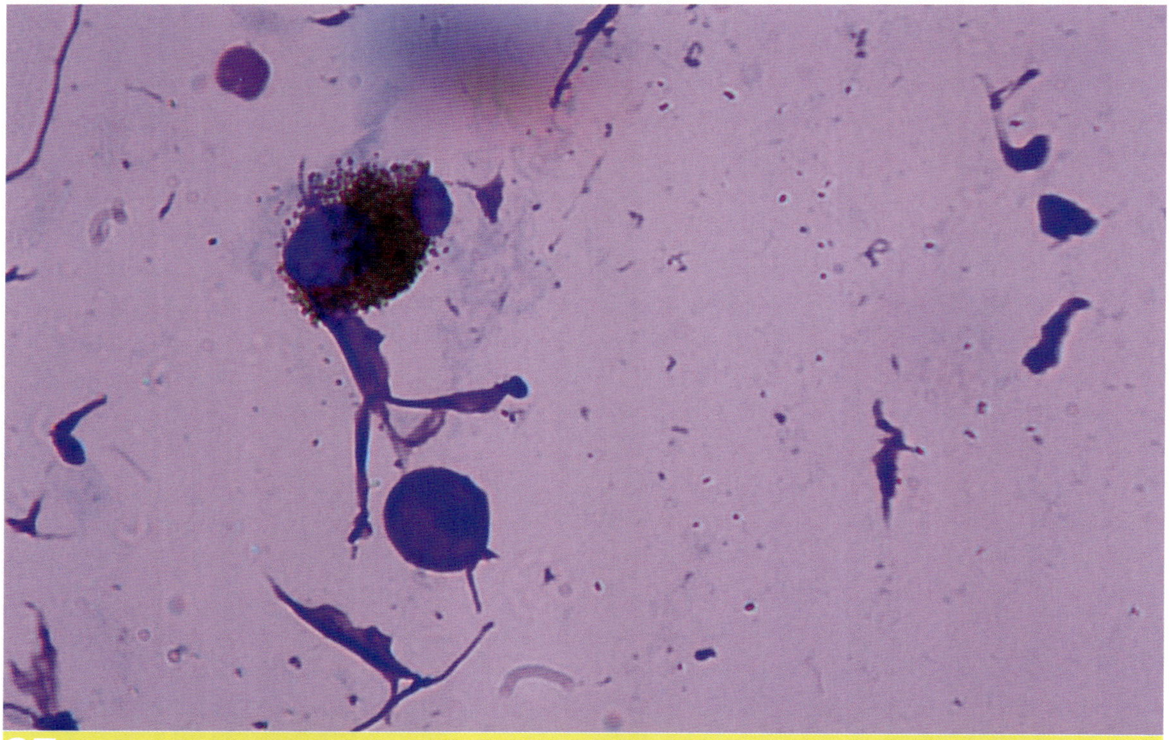

05 Cytology of melanocytic hamartoma. Note the melanin granules in the cell.

# Cysts

## Lesion aetiology/pathogenesis and clinical picture

These are cavities that are filled with liquid or solid material and are usually integrated into different structures:

- Apocrine cyst or apocrine or ceruminous cystomatosis
- Dermoid cysts
- Infundibular cysts

## Diagnostic method

Infundibular cysts are caused by degenerative changes in the hair follicle or in the adjoining glands and their ducts.

However, dermoid cysts constitute complete replication of the skin structure in the dermis or subcutis.

Apocrine cysts or apocrine cystomatosis are cavities filled with glandular fluid. A clear example is that which develops in the ears of some cats, containing content from the ceruminous glands.

## Main differential diagnoses

- Other tumours
- Abscesses
- Bullae

## Treatment

Removal is often indicated owing to the discomfort that they cause in the patient, as well as the consequences of scratching and the subsequent infections that can develop.

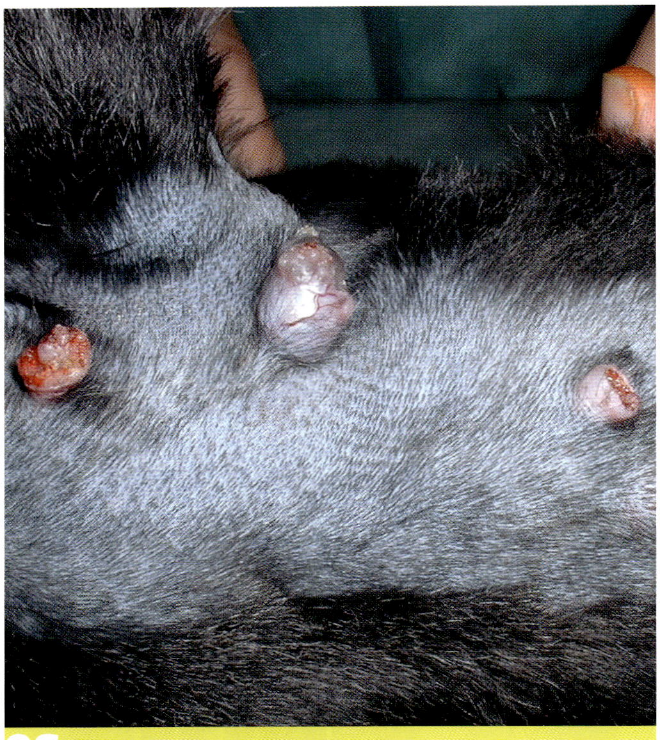

06 Multiple infundibular keratinous cysts.

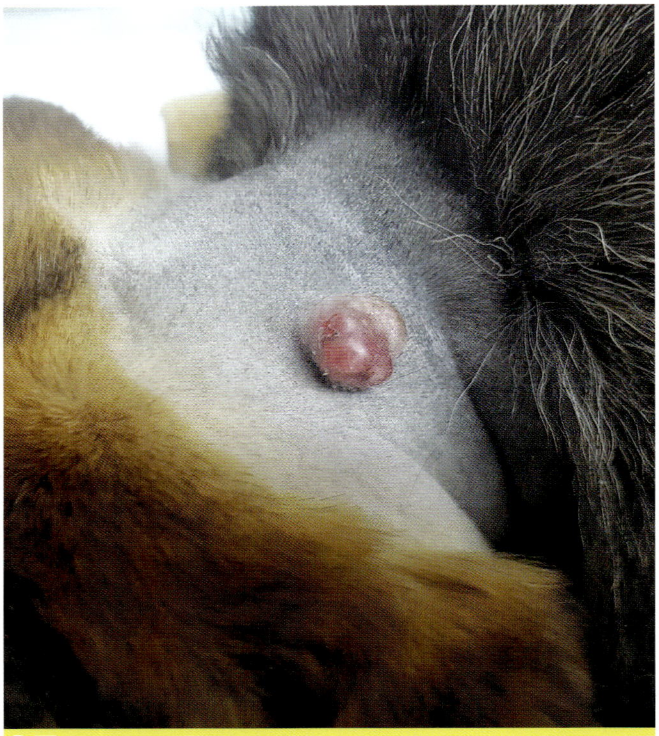

07 Trichilemmal cyst.

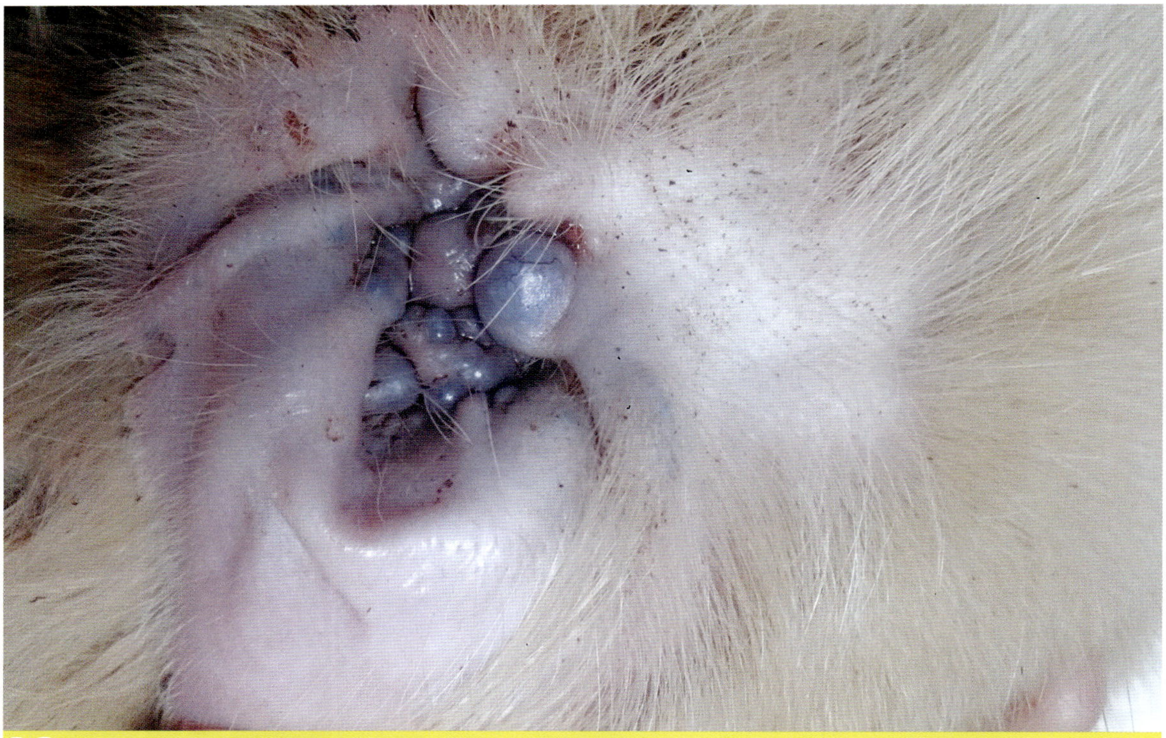

08 Feline cystomatosis. Ceruminous cysts in a cat's ear.

# Cutaneous horns

## Lesion aetiology/pathogenesis and clinical picture

These are rare, conical or cylindrical, very hard keratotic masses. They are usually long (up to 5 cm). They can be idiopathic in origin, or caused by chronic irritation as a consequence of poor stance, papillomas, or actinic keratosis.

## Diagnostic method

Diagnosis is based mainly on the clinical appearance and the clinical history.

## Main differential diagnoses

- Localised hyperkeratosis of other aetiologies
- Keratosis lichenoides
- Keratinous cysts

## Treatment

Resection can be difficult, and therefore softening with caustic solutions is often necessary.

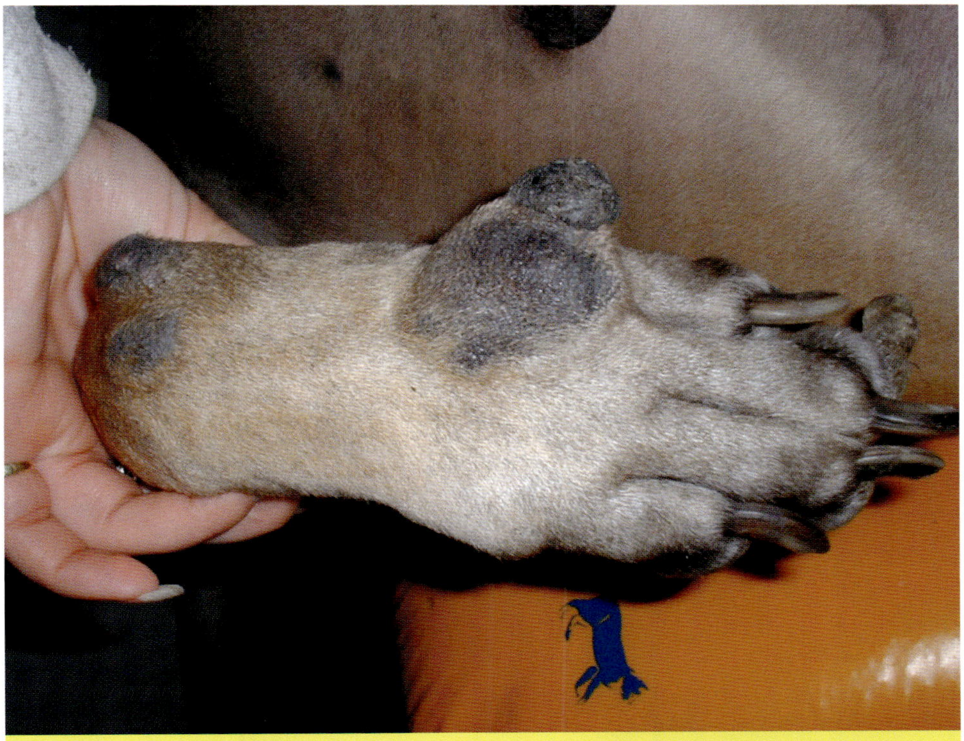

09 Cutaneous horn in a dog.

# Cutaneous outgrowths

## Lesion aetiology/pathogenesis and clinical picture

These are small masses of tissue that form on the surface of the skin. They are generally benign and painless, and do not grow or change. They are produced by an alteration in skin turnover, mainly in senior animals.

## Diagnostic method

Diagnosis is based primarily on appearance and biopsy findings.

## Main differential diagnoses

- Papillomas
- Other forms of verrucous hyperplasia

## Treatment

Removal, if necessary.

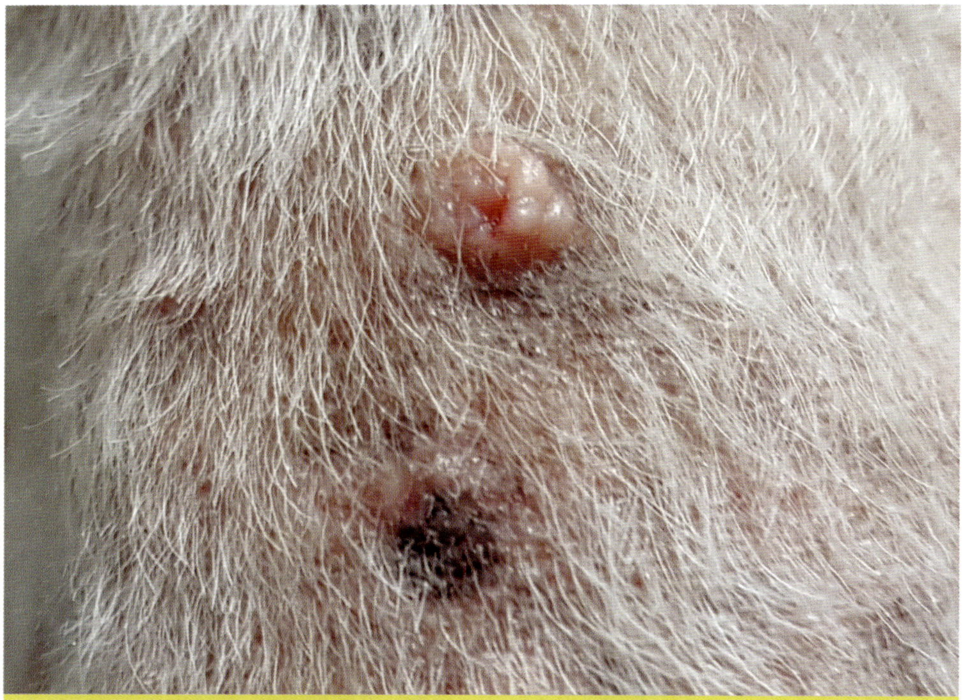

**10** Skin growth on the back of a 15-year-old Poodle.

# Canine interdigital granuloma

## Lesion aetiology/pathogenesis and clinical picture

Excluding foreign bodies, interdigital granulomas or cysts are usually the consequence of follicular rupture and formation of a furuncle around the hair, which acts as a foreign body. This type of lesion can be more common in brachycephalic breeds and dogs with orthopaedic problems.

## Diagnostic method

The clinical presentation is very characteristic.

## Main differential diagnoses

- Cysts
- Tumours

## Treatment

Surgery is not usually necessary. Patients usually respond to topical or systemic corticosteroids. In recurrent cases, systemic cyclosporine and topical tacrolimus can be used. In obese dogs or those with poor stance due to joint pain, the therapeutic objective is to reduce the patient's weight or alleviate pain using analgesics.

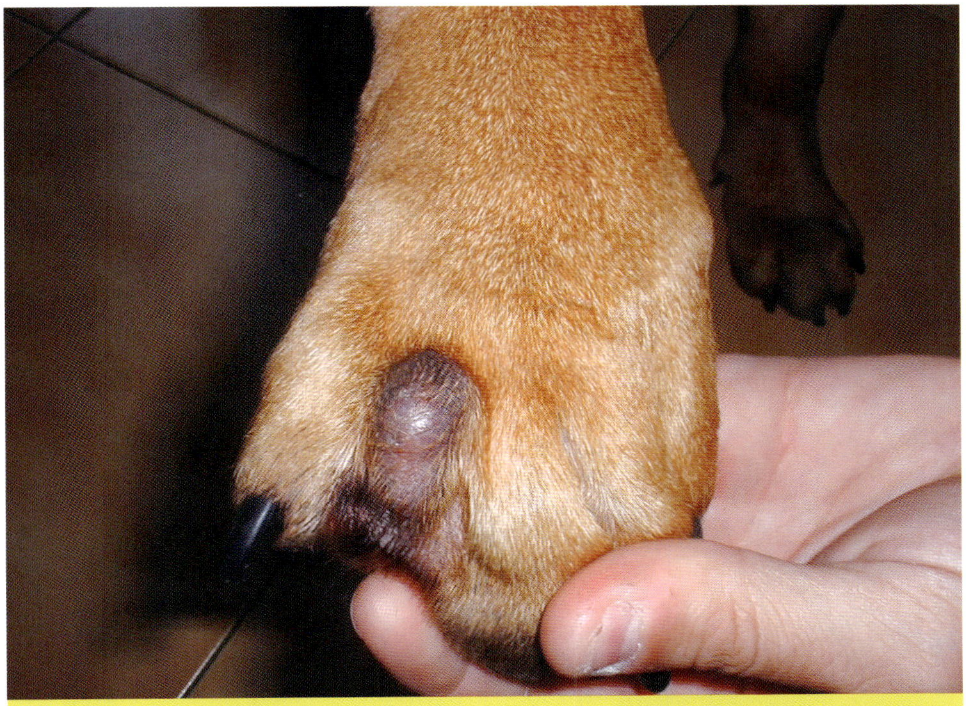

11 Follicular interdigital granuloma in a dog.

# Keratosis

## Lesion aetiology/pathogenesis and clinical picture

Keratosis is a reactive proliferation of keratinocytes that form firm, well-defined plaque-like lesions. Possible forms include:

- Lichenoid (see Chapter 9)
- Actinic (see Chapter 10)
- Seborrhoeic

## Diagnostic method

Biopsy findings allow precise determination of the lesion origin.

## Main differential diagnoses

- Other forms of secondary keratosis
- Epitheliotropic lymphoma

## Treatment

Treatment depends on the lesion aetiology. Sun exposure should be avoided. In other cases, antibiotics and antiseborrhoeic substances should be used.

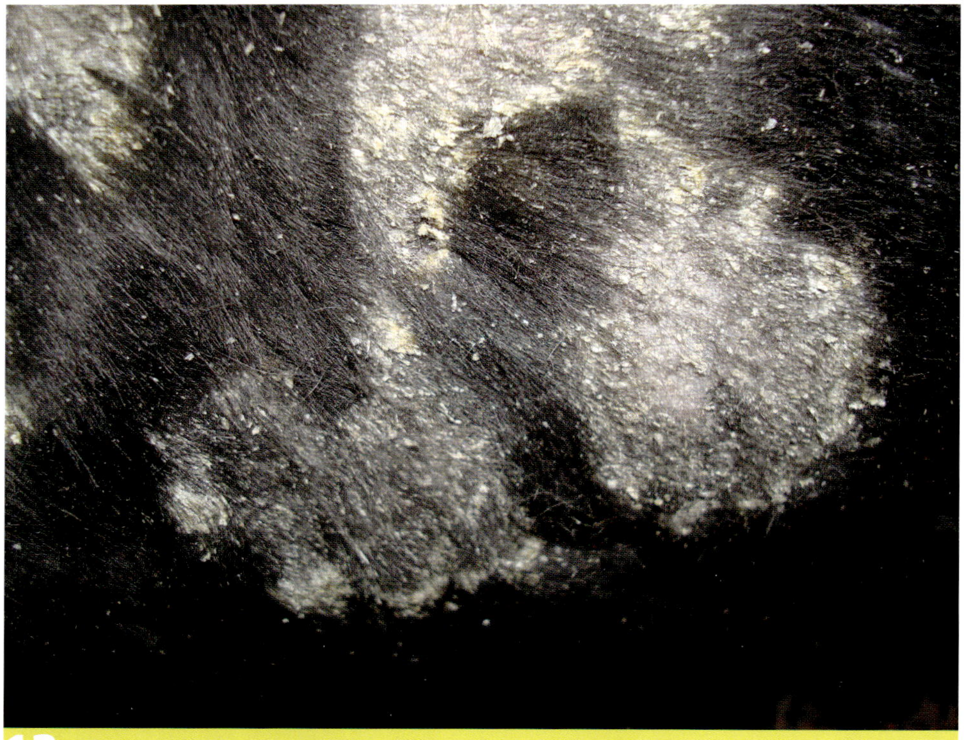

12 Seborrhoeic keratosis plaques in a dog.

# Fibropruritic nodules

## Lesion aetiology/pathogenesis and clinical picture

These are caused by cutaneous hyperplasia as a consequence of chronic inflammation, often due to itching. They can be observed on the lower back of dogs with flea allergy dermatitis.

## Diagnostic method

The clinical appearance and history are usually sufficient to establish diagnosis.

## Main differential diagnoses

- Nodular tumours
- Other pseudotumours

## Treatment

Treatment of the inflammation usually results in remission.

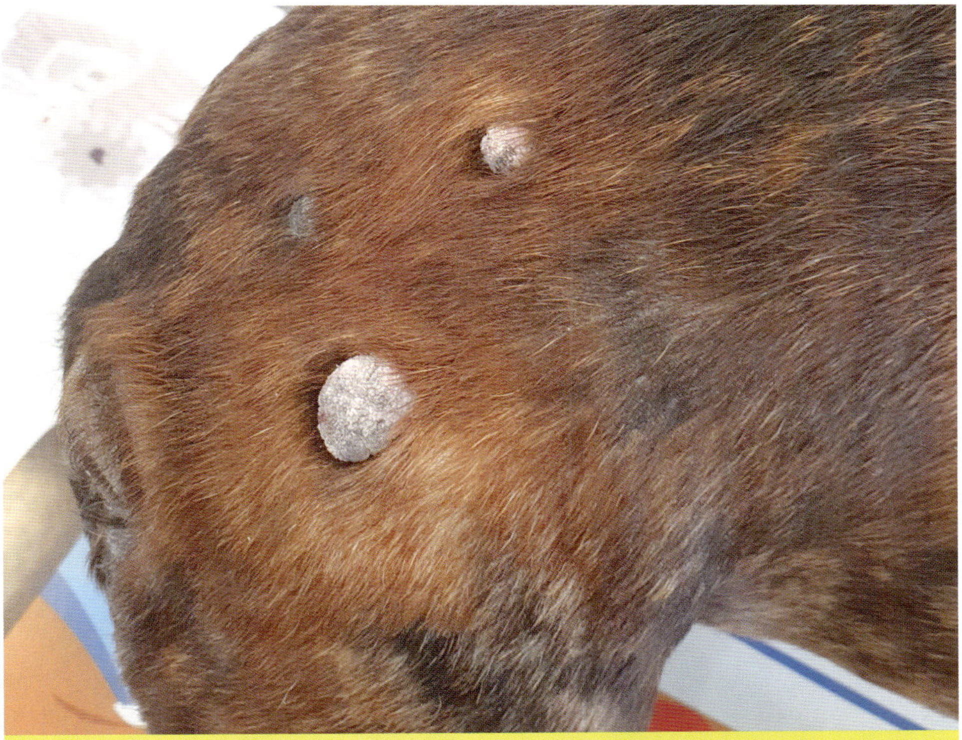

13 Nodules in the lumbar area of a dog with flea allergy dermatitis.

# Nodular dermatofibrosis

## Lesion aetiology/pathogenesis and clinical picture

Dogs with kidney tumours and skin nodules may show overexpression of transforming growth factor beta 1 (TGF-β1), a fibrosis-stimulating cytokine, resulting in a paraneoplastic reaction that gives rise to nodular fibrosis on the limbs.

## Diagnostic method

The appearance of the lesion and the presence of renal problems can help orient the diagnosis.

## Main differential diagnoses

- Primary tumours
- Other pseudotumours

## Treatment

Surgery, if successful, can be curative.

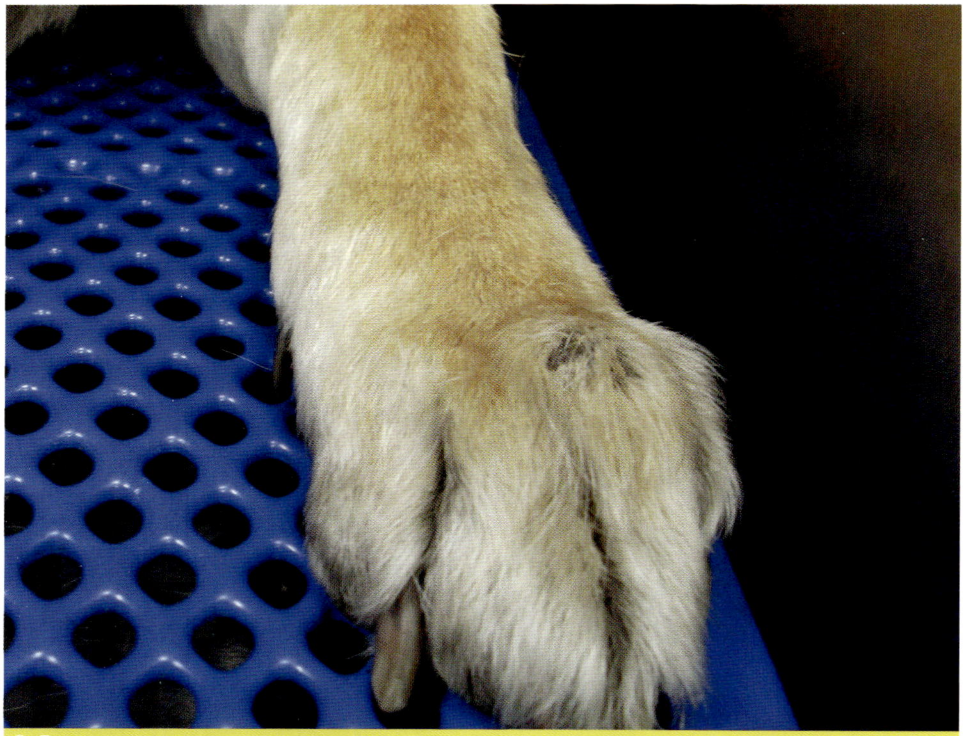

14 Nodular dermatofibrosis on the limb of a German Shepherd. Image courtesy of Mónica Lores.

# Skin polyp

## Lesion aetiology/pathogenesis and clinical picture

Local trauma, irritation, or furunculosis can result in hyperplasia of epidermal and dermal collagen. Skin polyps have a polypoid appearance and form on the trunk or at pressure points in middle-aged or older dogs.

## Diagnostic method

Diagnosis is based on the clinical appearance.

## Main differential diagnoses

- Cutaneous outgrowths
- Collagenous hamartomas
- Tumours

## Treatment

Surgery is the only recommended treatment.

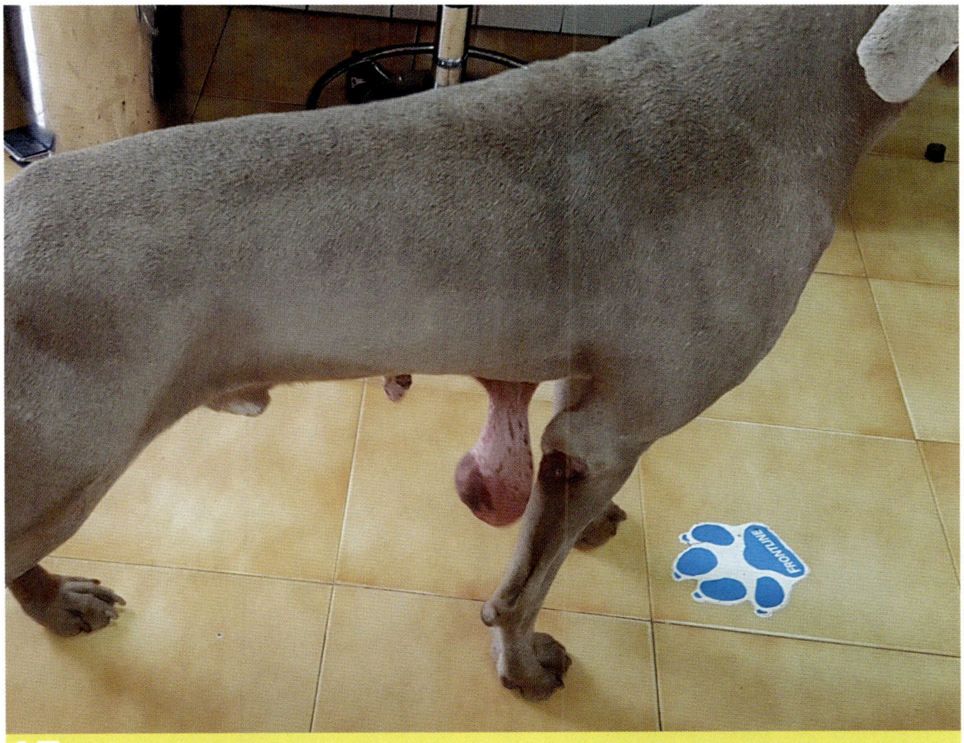

15 Cutaneous polyp.

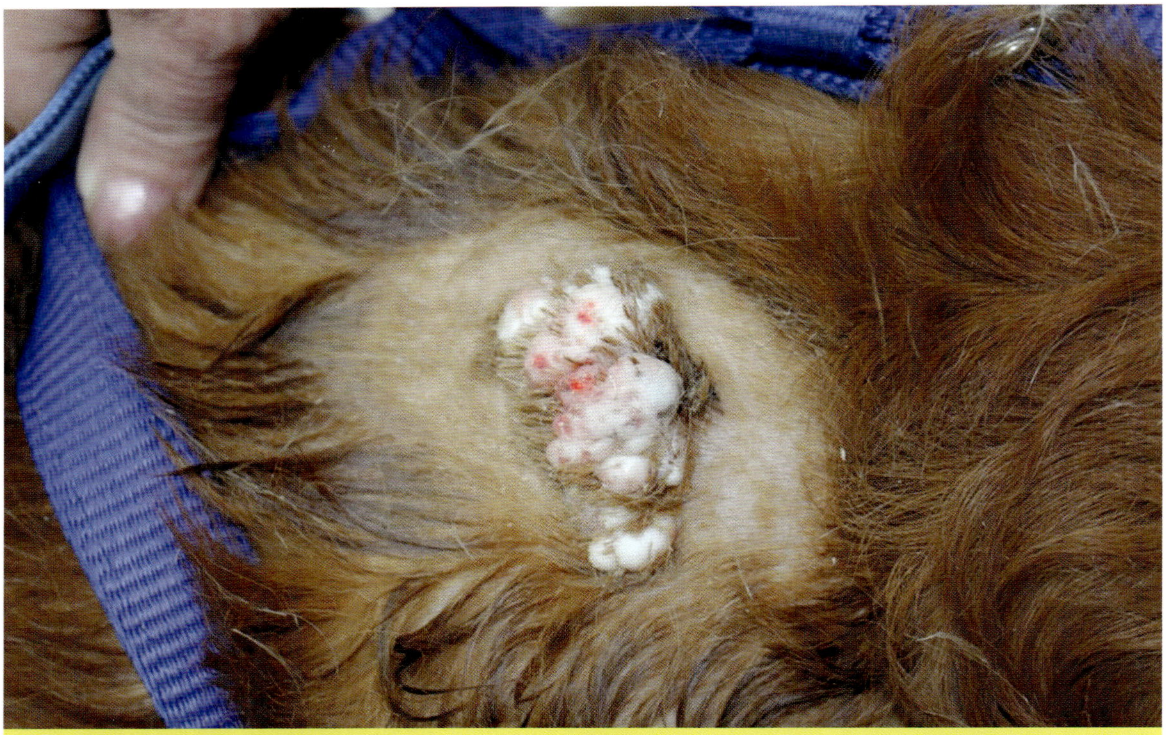

16 Collagenous polyp in a senior dog.

# 12

# Noninflammatory and nonendocrine forms of alopecia

# Introduction

This chapter describes the following types of alopecia:

- Breed-specific alopecia
- Follicular dysplasia
- Pattern alopecia
- Cyclic alopecia of the flanks and nasal bridge
- Anagen and telogen effluvium
- Post-clipping alopecia
- Traction alopecia
- Post-injection alopecia/alopecia due to local application of substances
- Alopecia areata and pseudopelade
- Feline psychogenic alopecia

This chapter discusses forms of alopecia without skin inflammation or systemic hormonal alterations.

The aetiology of alopecia X remains a matter of debate: this form could be included in the present chapter as it may be due to alterations in follicular receptors.

Post-injection alopecia or that caused by topical application of medications can involve inflammation due to vasculitis. Nonetheless, this form of alopecia is caused by externally applied substances and therefore it is included in this chapter.

# Breed-specific alopecia

## Lesion aetiology/pathogenesis and clinical picture

Certain dog and cat breeds have been bred for a complete lack of hair, for aesthetic, hypoallergenic or therapeutic reasons, owing to the heat they emit. Alopecia in these animals is not considered a primary disease. The most well known are the Chinese Crested Dog, the Mexican Naked Dog or Xoloitzcuintle, and the Sphynx cat. Potential concomitant diseases in these animals include xerosis, comedones, retention of dead epidermis (milia), and pyodermas.

These animals usually have miniaturised atrophic follicles.

Interestingly, the majority of allergies caused by pets may be due to allergens contained in the secretions of their sebaceous and salivary glands, and in their excreta. Allergic reactions occur as a consequence of inhalation or contact with skin scales, impregnated hair, urine, saliva, or serum. Thus, hair is not one of the main allergens in these animals.

## Diagnostic method

Small clumps of hair may be observed in some areas of the body. It is very important that the veterinary clinician is familiar with the breed standard.

## Main differential diagnoses

Generalised alopecia of another origin.

## Treatment

Breeders do not expect hair to grow and are only concerned with keeping the skin healthy, hydrated, and free of comedones and milia.

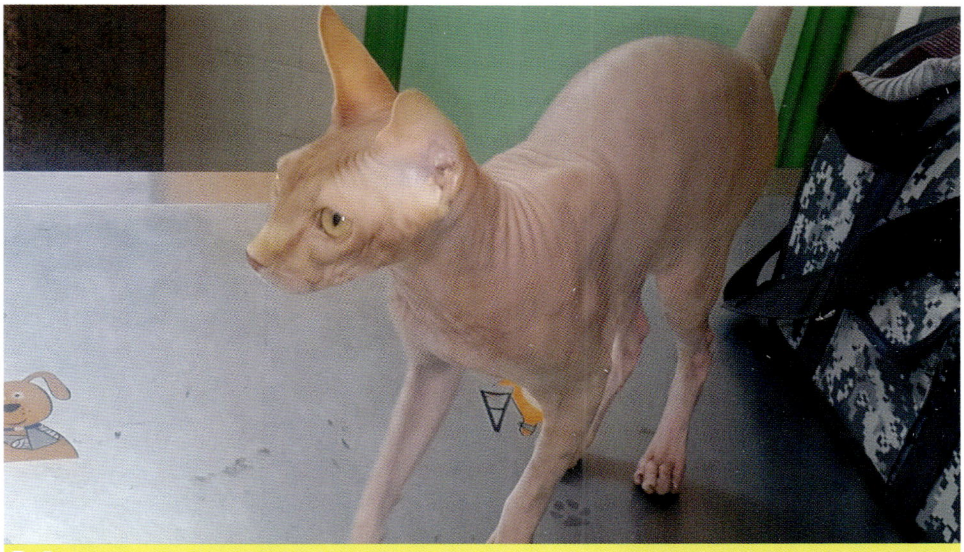

01 Breed-specific alopecia in a Sphynx cat.

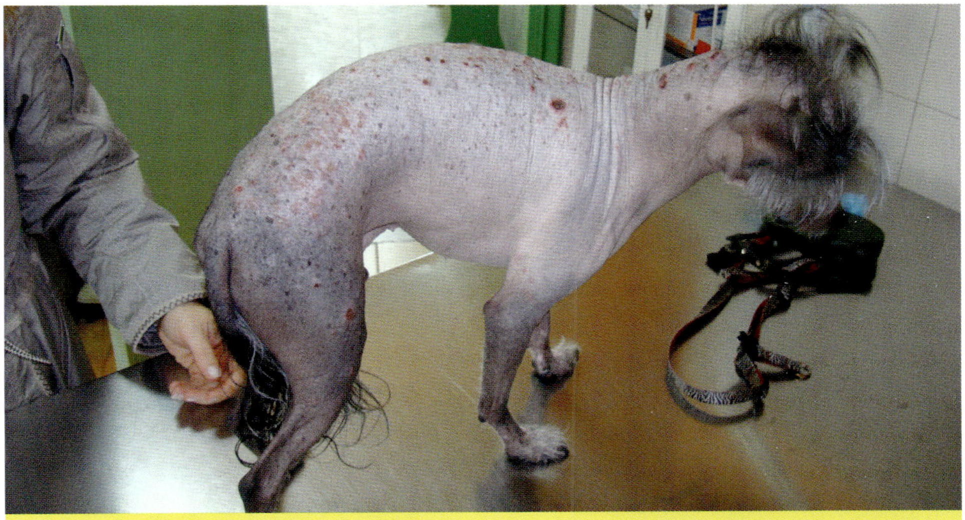

02 Chinese Crested Dog with sterile granuloma syndrome.

# Follicular dysplasia

## Lesion aetiology/pathogenesis and clinical picture

These are congenital forms of alopecia associated with malformed hair follicles. These follicles can produce hairs with altered pigmentation or general development, or may even fail to produce hair. Dogs are more frequently affected. There are three types of dysplasia:

- Colour dilution follicular dysplasia
- Follicular dysplasia of black hair
- Nonseasonal, non-colour-related dysplasia

## Diagnostic method

Diagnosis is established based on the clinical picture, trichogram, and biopsy findings.

It is essential to identify the three layers of the hair and melanin granules in order to confirm the alteration.

## Main differential diagnoses

- Various dysplasias
- Endocrine alopecia
- Dermatophytosis
- Demodicosis
- Effluvium

## Treatment

These are predominantly aesthetic alterations that should be treated to avoid associated problems such as dry skin and pyoderma. Melatonin administration can be helpful in early stages.

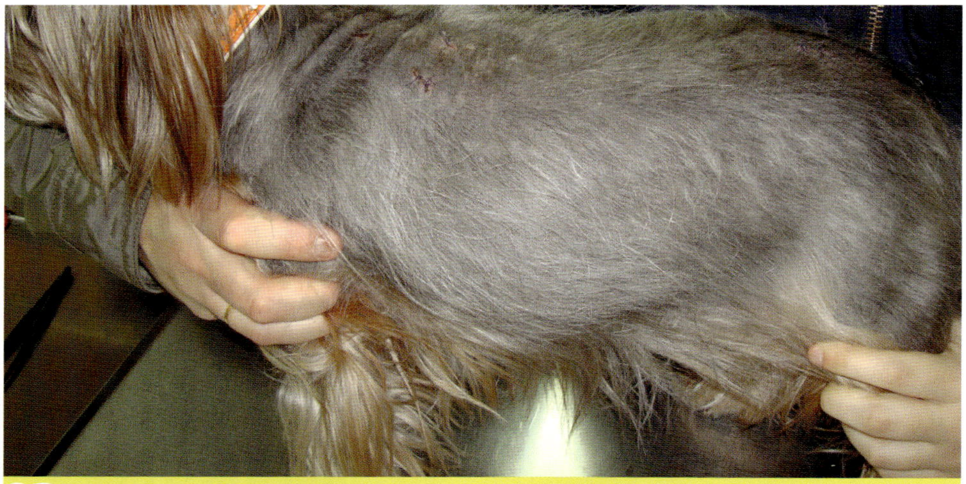

03 Colour dilution follicular dysplasia in a Yorkshire Terrier. Note the alopecia and fragile, grey hair.

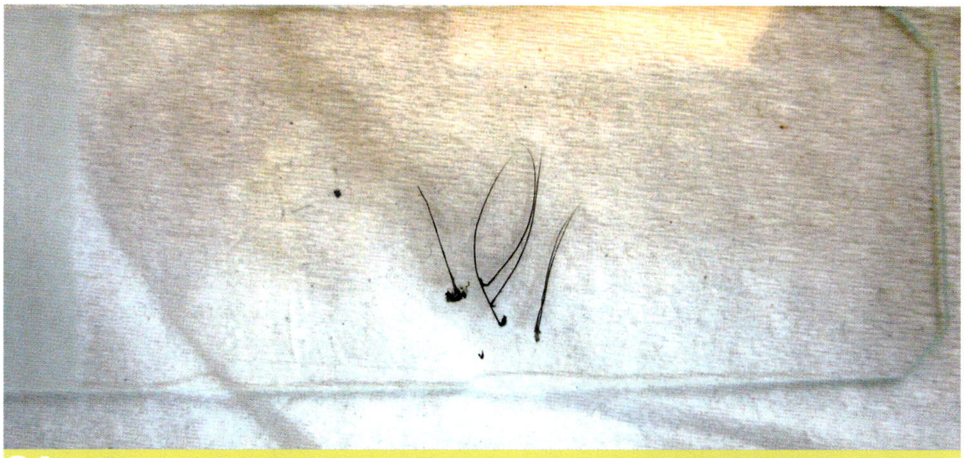

04 Trichogram: macroscopic view of dilated hair roots typical of colour-related follicular dysplasia.

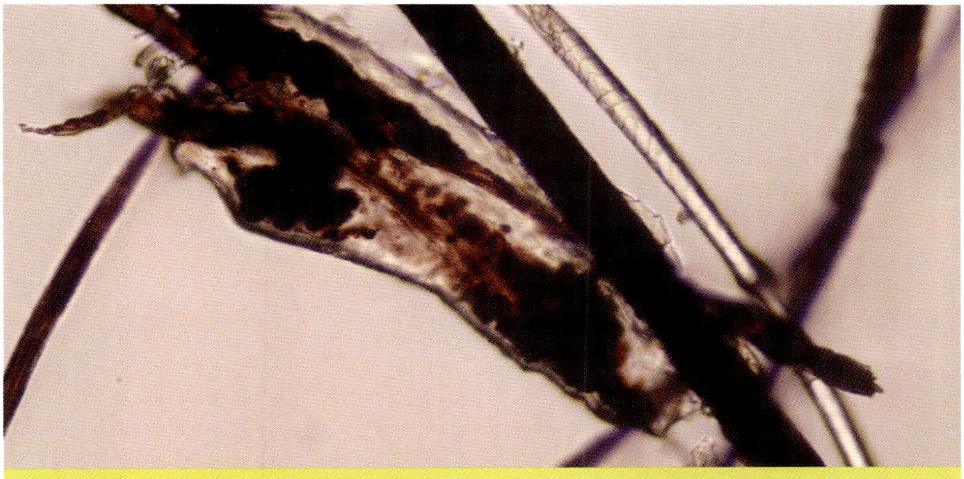

05 Trichogram: capillary defect caused by protrusion of macromelanosomes. Hair breakage is observed.

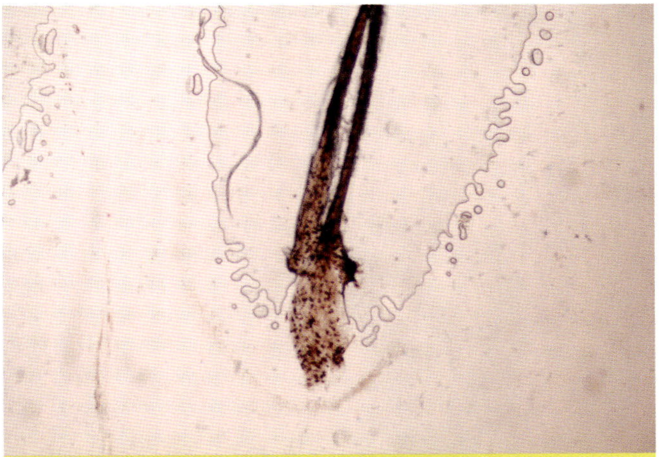

06 Trichogram: typical hair root appearance in a case of follicular dysplasia. Note the scattered melanin granules.

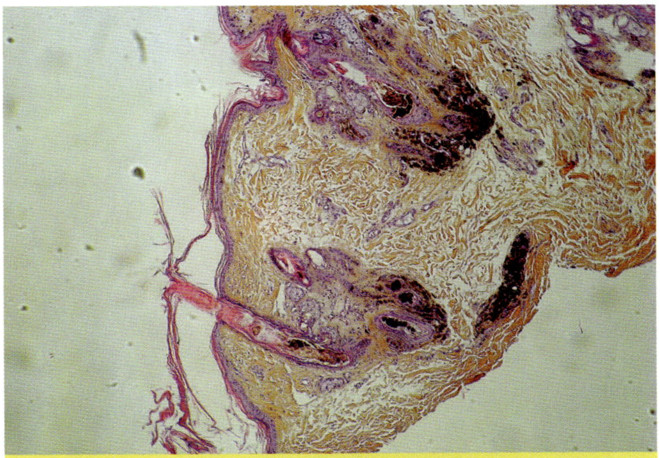

07 Histological image of follicles showing pigmentary incontinence and disorganised formation of altered hairs.

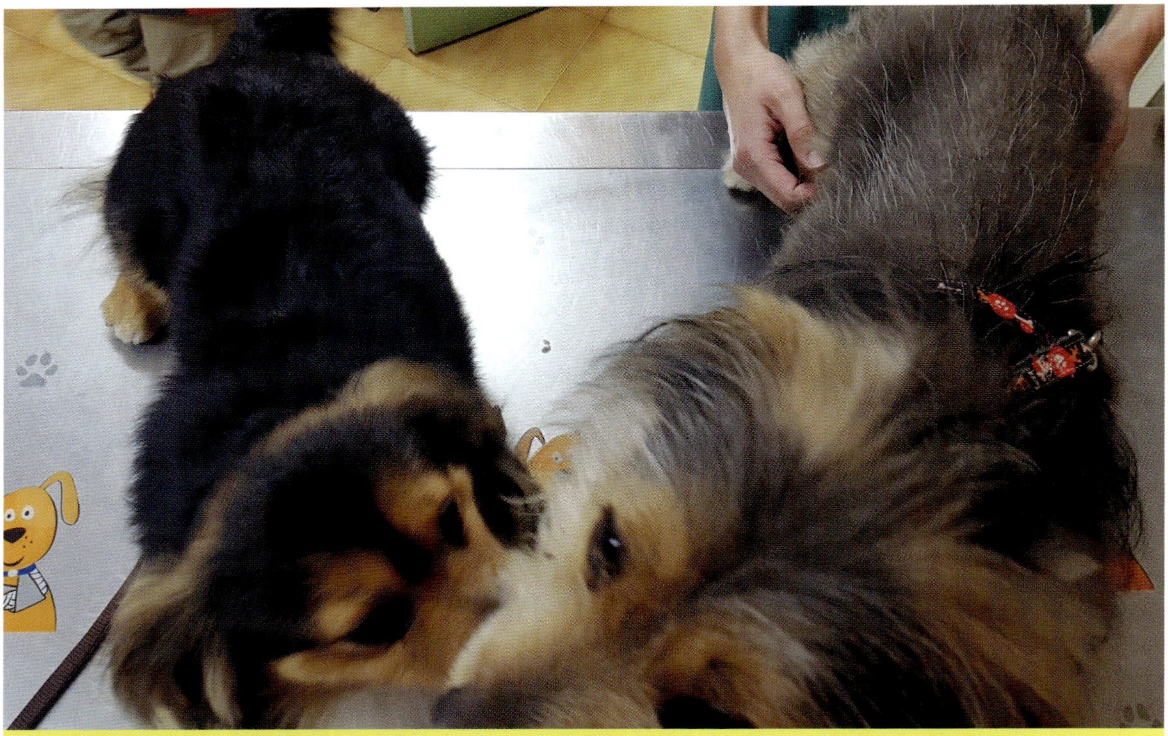

08 Littermates. Note the difference between the healthy hair of one and the dysplastic hair of the other.

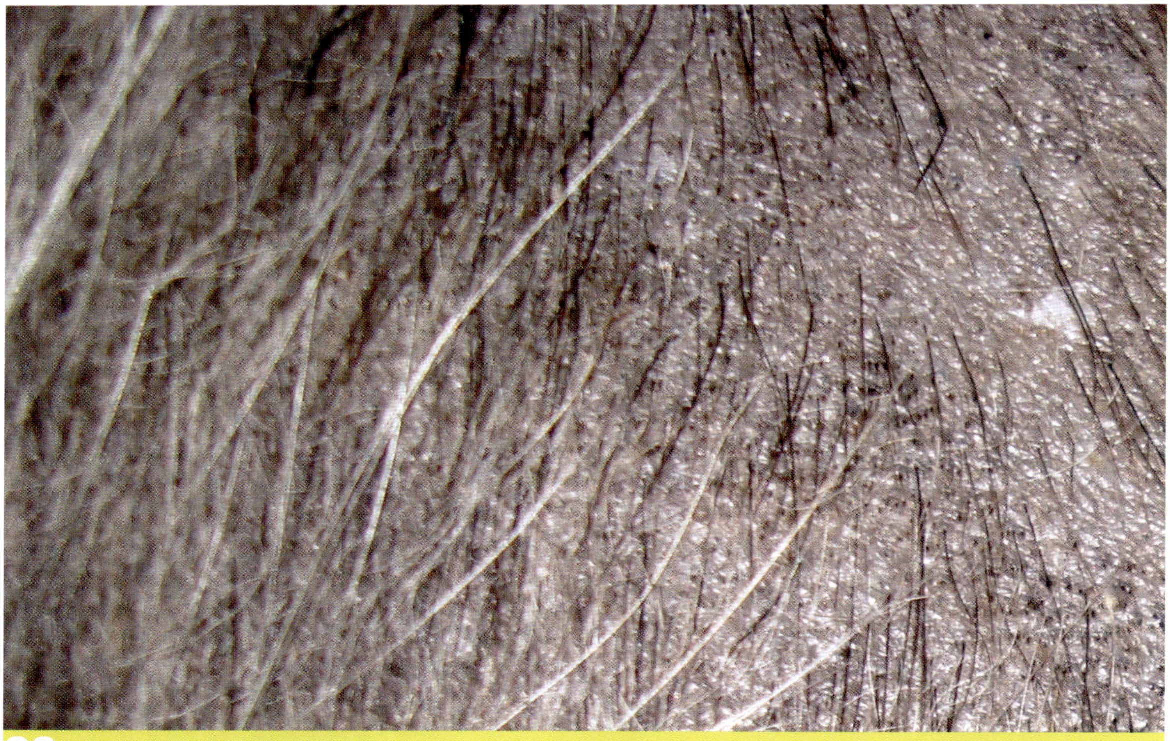

09 Dermoscopic image showing follicular plugging with keratin produced by the dysplastic hair.

# Pattern alopecia

## Lesion aetiology/pathogenesis and clinical picture

This occurs in some dogs and cats of particular breeds. It usually manifests in puberty or early maturity, and is characterised by hair loss in certain areas, including the external surface of the pinnae, preauricular area, buttocks, ventral region of the neck, chest, caudomedial region of the thighs, axillae, and abdomen. The breeds in which it occurs most frequently are the Pinscher, Dachshund, Chihuahua, and Greyhound.

Cats can develop an idiopathic form that affects the preauricular area and sometimes the pinnae.

## Diagnostic method

The clinical appearance and breed enable confirmation of the diagnosis. Histopathology is not usually necessary, but if performed will reveal miniaturisation of the follicles.

## Main differential diagnoses

- Hormonal dermatoses
- Demodicosis
- Dermatophytosis
- Follicular dysplasia

## Treatment

Melatonin can be used to delay hair loss in the affected areas. Topical minoxidil has been used with success in some cases.

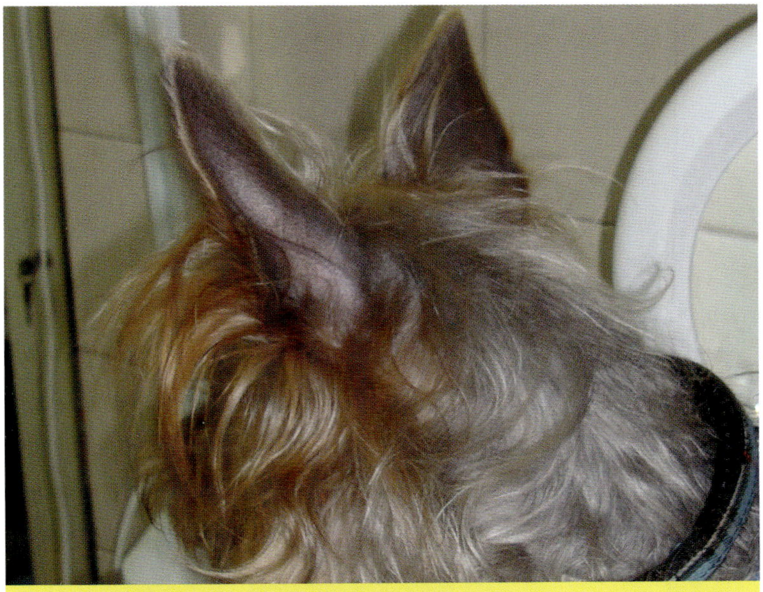

10 Pattern alopecia on the pinnae in a Yorkshire Terrier.

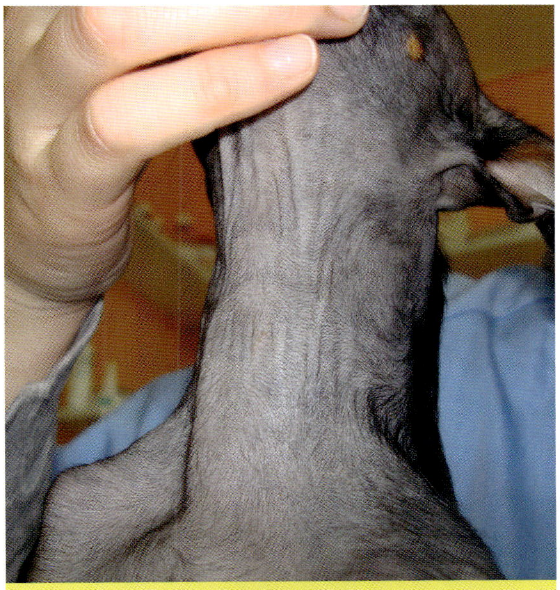

11 Pattern alopecia on the ventral cervical area and chest of a Pinscher.

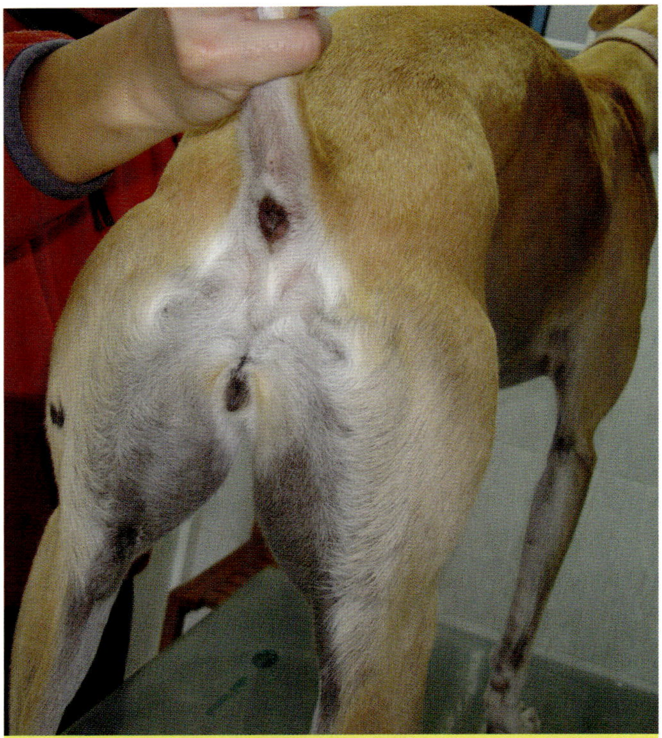

12 Pattern alopecia in the thigh area of a Greyhound.

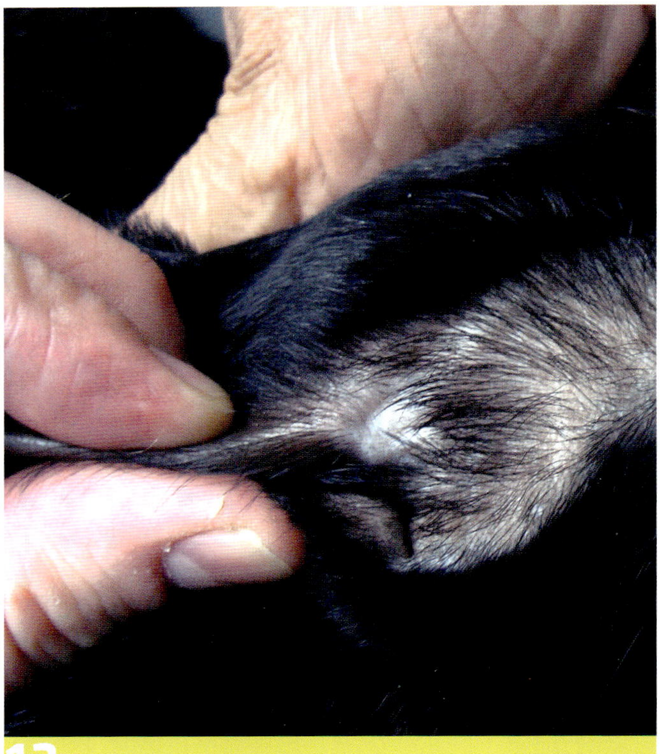

13 Pattern alopecia in the preauricular area in a European Shorthair.

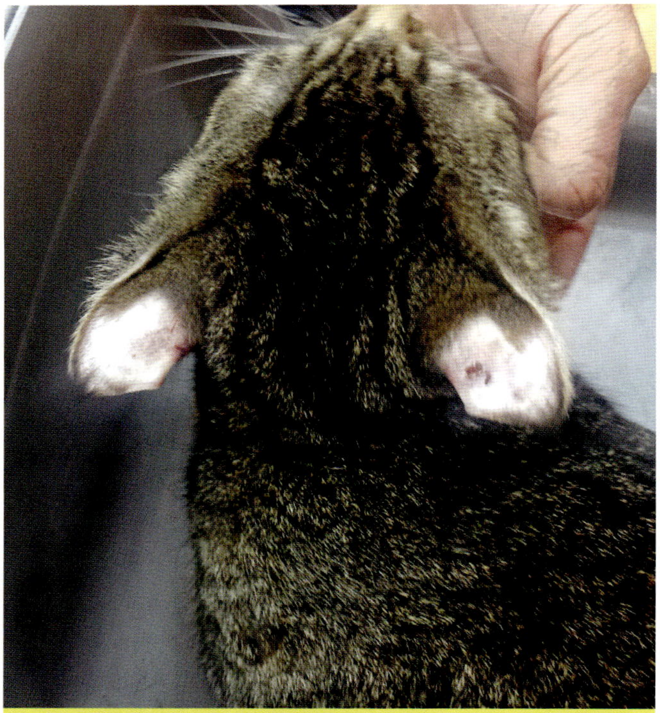

14 Alopecia with no obvious cause on the pinnae of a domestic shorthair cat.

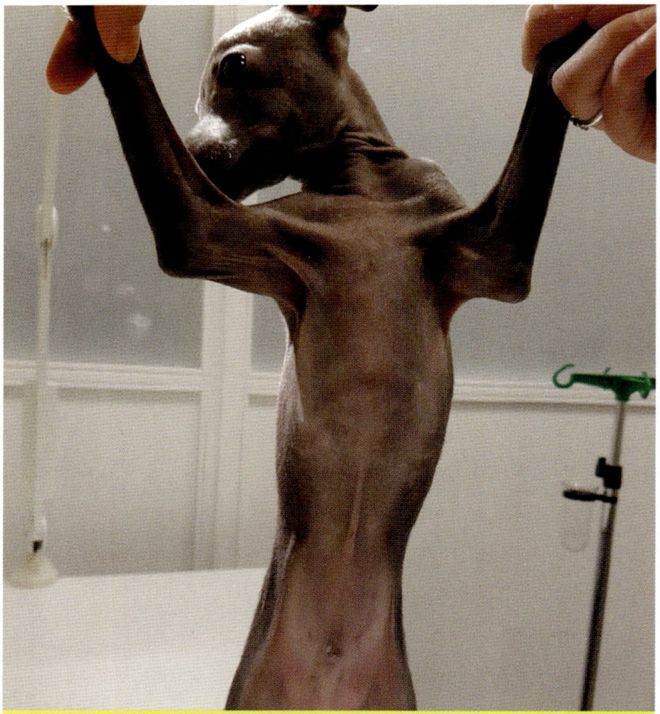

15 Italian Greyhound with generalised alopecia and histopathological findings indicating follicular dysplasia and miniaturisation.

# Cyclic alopecia of the flanks and nasal bridge

## Lesion aetiology/pathogenesis and clinical picture

This form of alopecia occurs in dogs due to cyclical alterations in follicular function that coincide with the darker months of the year. The typical irregular borders, which resemble a geographic map, are quite characteristic. The hair grows back in a few months. Airedale Terriers, Boxers, and English Bulldogs are more commonly affected. Recurrence does not necessarily occur every year. The visible skin is usually hyperpigmented. In some cases the skin of the dorsal area or the rump may be affected.

This same form of alopecia can also occur on the nasal bridge of certain breeds, including the Golden Retriever.

## Diagnostic method

Diagnosis is based on the clinical appearance, history, and biopsy results. The latter is characteristic, revealing a trichilemmal alteration known as "witch's feet", with dilation of the bulb area.

## Main differential diagnoses

- Endocrinopathies
- Dermatophytosis
- Alopecia areata

## Treatment

As this condition self-resolves, often no treatment is selected. It can be prevented by administering melatonin 1 month before the expected onset of recurrence, which is usually in November (northern hemisphere).

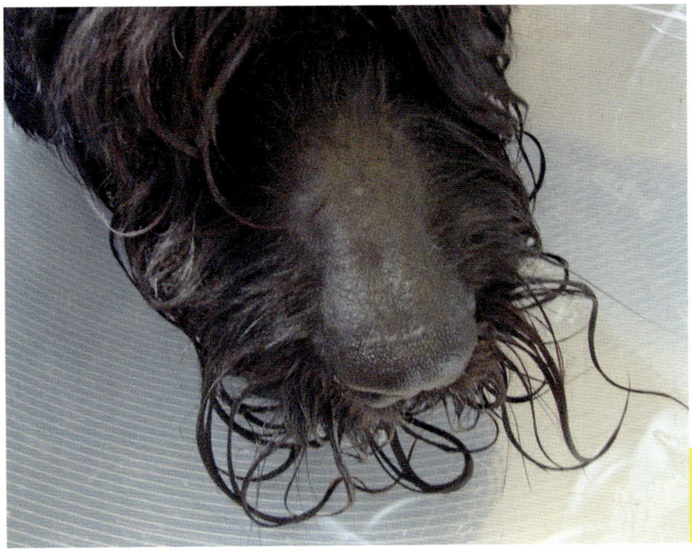

**16** Recurrent alopecia on the nasal bridge of a Giant Schnauzer.

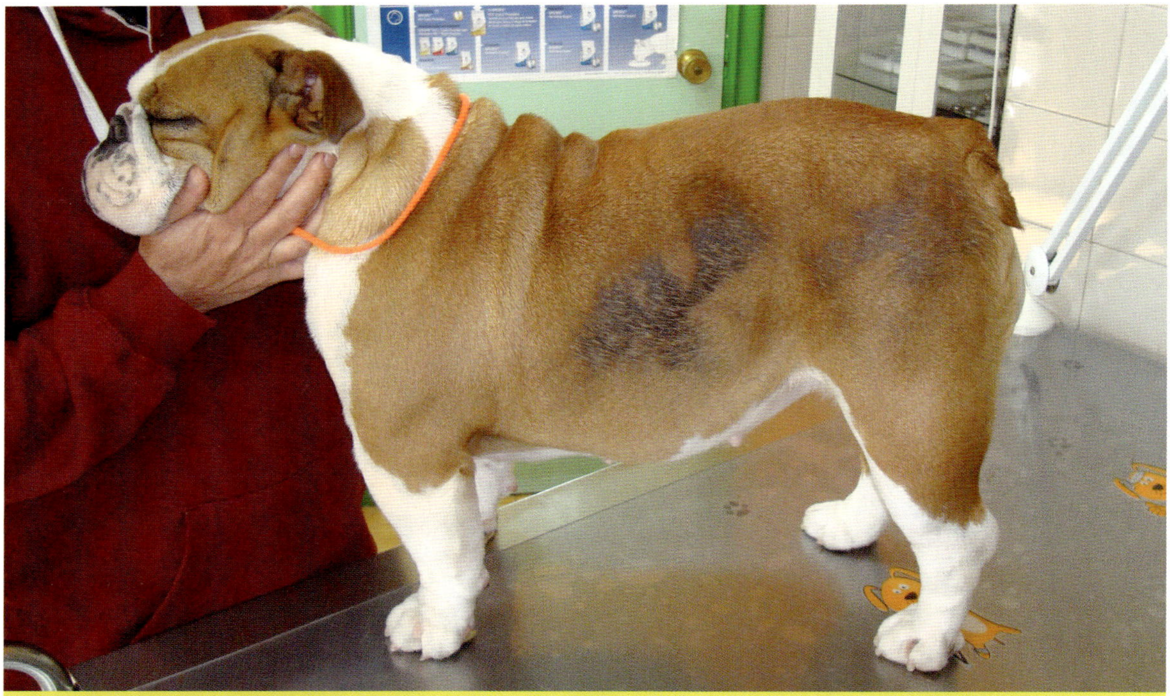

17 Cyclic alopecia of the flanks in a Bulldog. Note the borders of the areas of alopecia and the hyperpigmentation.

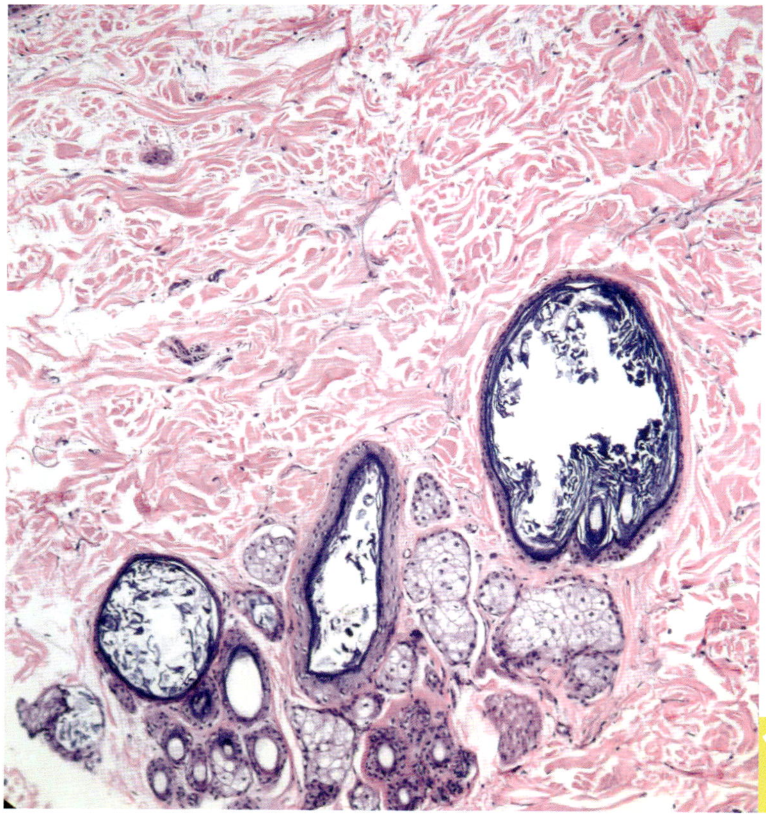

18 Typical histopathology findings in a case of cyclic alopecia with trichilemmal disorder.

# Anagen and telogen effluvium

## Lesion aetiology/pathogenesis and clinical picture

This can occur in both dogs and cats:

- **Anagen effluvium:** due to the action of drugs, infectious diseases, endocrinopathies, or metabolic alterations, the anagen cycle of the hair is affected, resulting in germ cell abnormalities and alterations in hair quality. The hair continues to grow, but in a defective way, and is consequently shed a few days after onset of the problem.
- **Telogen effluvium**: a stressful event, such as pregnancy, serious illness, shock, surgery, or anaesthesia, can cause an abrupt cessation of anagenesis, and sudden synchronisation of abundant hairs in telogen phase (telogen arrest or arrest). After some time (1–3 months), with the next anagen phase, all telogen hairs are eliminated resulting in consequent alopecia.

## Diagnostic method

The clinical history is key to establishing diagnosis.

In cases of anagen effluvium the trichogram reveals anagen characteristics but with dysplasia (cuticular fragility due to defective capillary formation). In the case of telogen effluvium, the trichogram shows hairs with telogen characteristics. Biopsy can also help establish diagnosis.

## Main differential diagnoses

- Dermatophytosis
- Alopecia areata and pseudopelade
- Endocrinopathies
- Other follicular dysplasias

## Treatment

Melatonin treatment can be helpful in these cases, although stopping the root cause will resolve the problem.

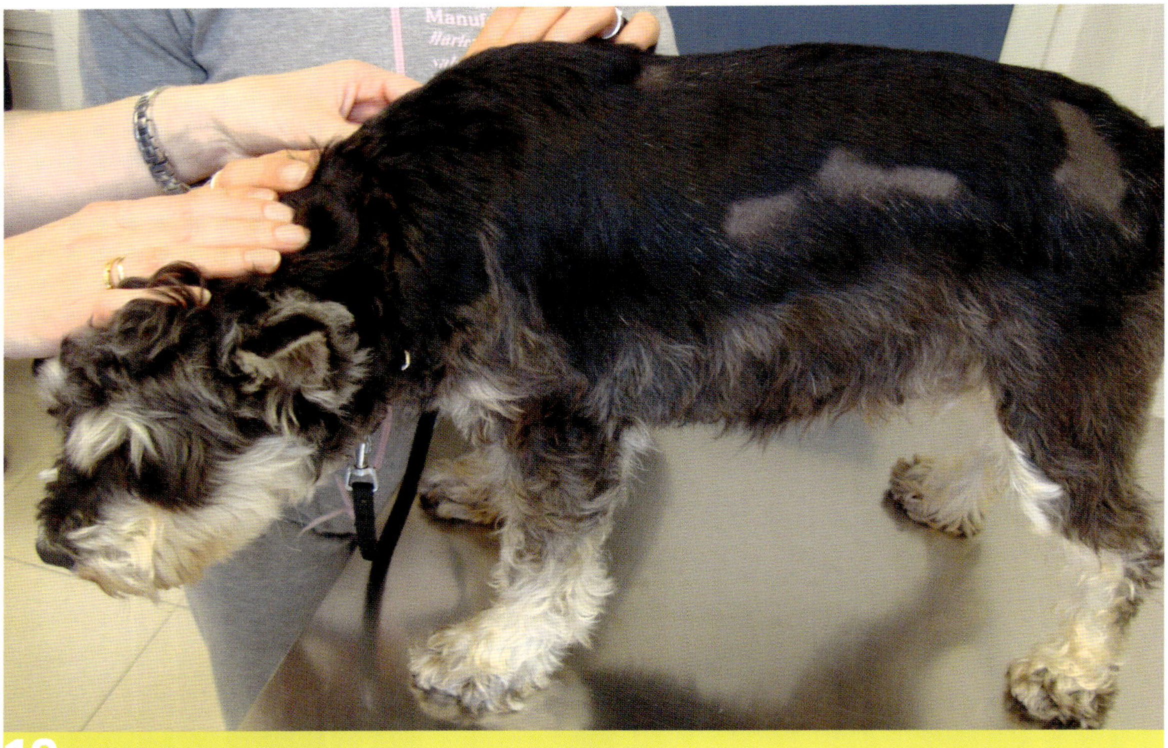

19 Telogen effluvium in a Schnauzer dog 1 month after giving birth.

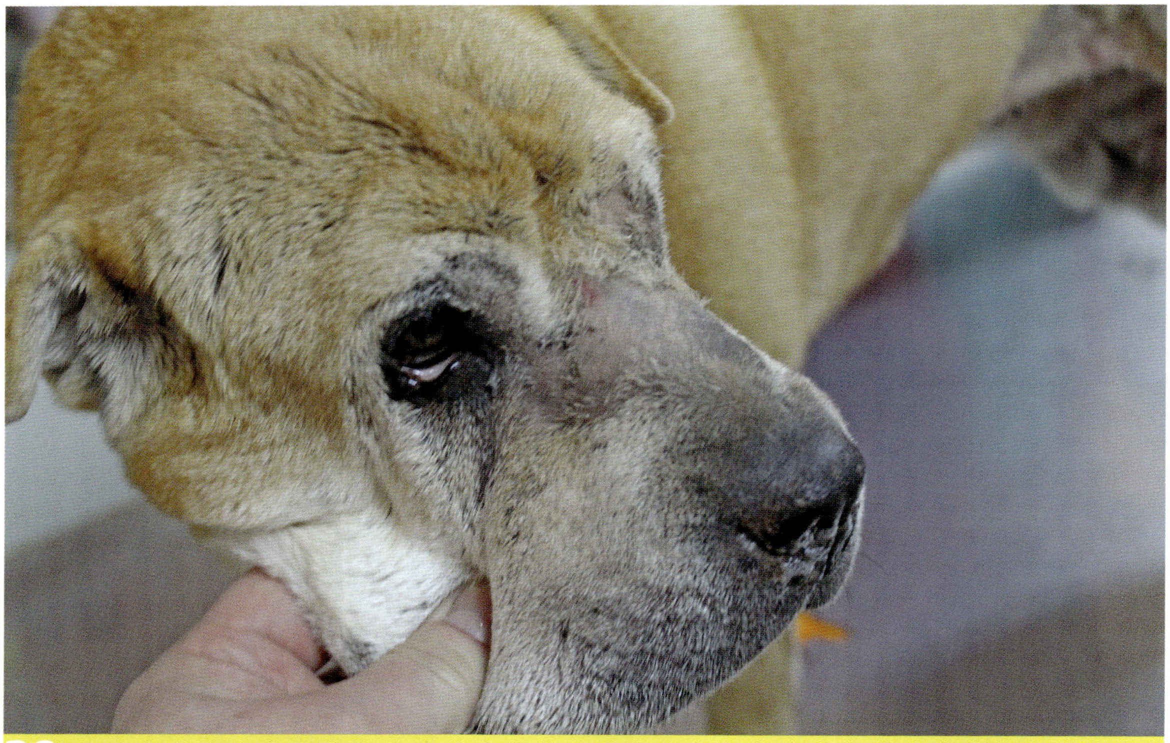

20 Chemotherapy-induced anagen effluvium in a Shar Pei.

# Post-clipping alopecia

## Lesion aetiology/pathogenesis and clinical picture

This is a form of alopecia of unknown origin that occurs after clipping some or all of the dog's hair. It is usually more common in Nordic breeds. Some theories propose that this constitutes an energy saving mechanism in these breeds, whereby follicles remain in telogen phase for long periods. Other theories suggest that alopecia is caused by cooling or direct UVA irradiation of the follicles.

## Diagnostic method

Diagnosis is based on the history and clinical picture.

## Main differential diagnoses

Endocrinopathies.

## Treatment

Hair usually regrows after several months. Follicle reactivation can be attempted using thyroxine and/or pentoxifylline.

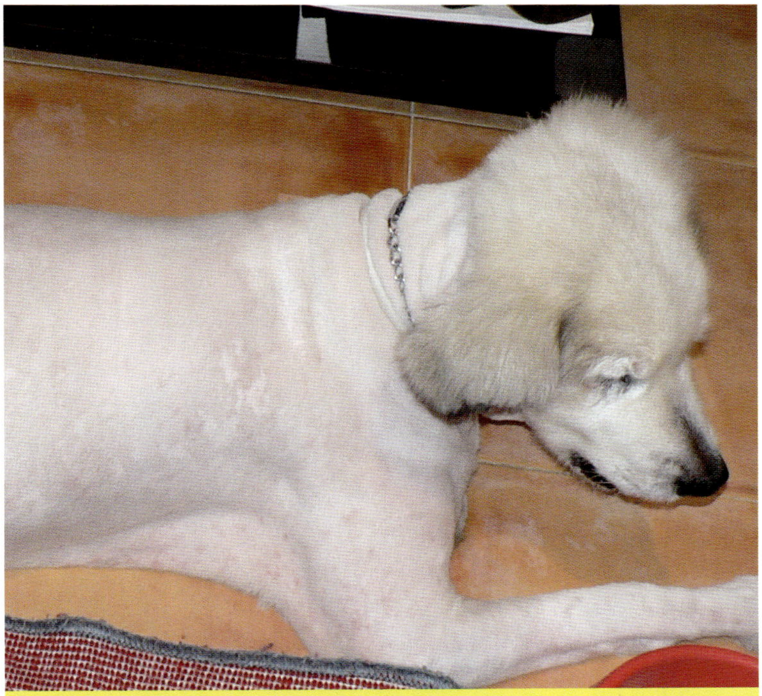

21 Post-clipping alopecia in a Pyrenean Mastiff 6 months after hair clipping.

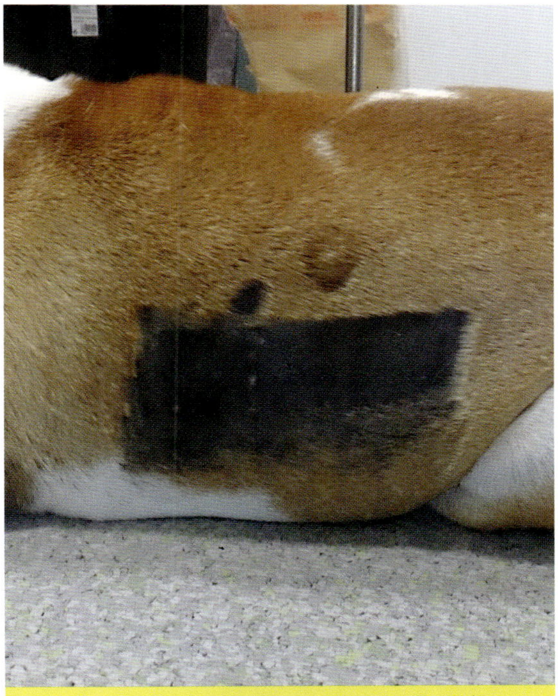

22 Alopecia and hyperpigmentation in an English Bulldog 4 months after clipping for an intradermal allergy test.

# Traction alopecia

## Lesion aetiology/pathogenesis and clinical picture

This is an uncommon disorder that occurs in dogs that experience excessive traction on the hairs of the head due to the use of hairpins or rubber bands. Alopecia, erythema, and in some cases small keratin cysts occur in the centre of the head or on one side, coinciding with the area of the tied up hair. It is more common in breeds such as the Yorkshire Terrier, Shih Tzu, and Poodle.

## Diagnostic method

Diagnosis is based on the history and clinical appearance.

## Main differential diagnoses

- Dermatophytosis
- Alopecia areata
- Demodicosis

## Treatment

Treatment involves correcting the excessive traction applied to the hair before the lesion becomes chronic and irreversible. Pentoxifylline may be helpful in the early stages.

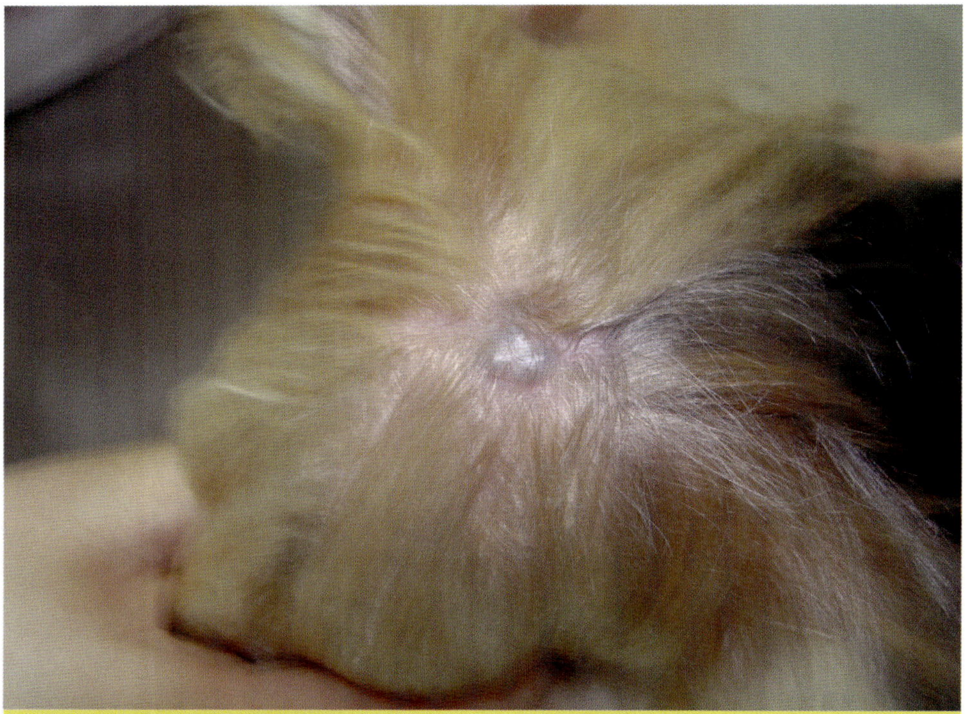

**23** Alopecia in the centre of the head of a Yorkshire Terrier due to excessive traction caused by hair ties. Note the formation of keratin cysts.

# Post-injection alopecia/alopecia due to local application of substances

## Lesion aetiology/pathogenesis and clinical picture

This skin condition of dogs and cats could be classified as a drug reaction, but in this case it refers to specific lesions caused by the application of certain injectable drugs, which cause vasculitis or skin atrophy, or topical medications, which cause scaling, erythema, and sometimes pemphigoid reactions.

The injectable drugs that most commonly cause these reactions are progestogens, corticosteroids, and vaccines. Topical medications include corticosteroids, spot-on parasiticides, and, in some more generalised cases, certain shampoos.

Intramuscular injections can also cause this type of reaction, although less frequently.

In the case of nodule formation after injection, it is essential to ensure that neoplastic fibrosis (injection-site sarcoma, ISS) does not occur. To this end, the 1-2-3 rule should be followed:

1. Growth observed 1 month after injection.
2. Measures more than 2 cm.
3. Does not go away after 3 months.

## Diagnostic method

Diagnosis is based on the medical history, location, and clinical appearance.

## Main differential diagnoses

- Alopecia areata
- Dermatophytosis
- Demodicosis

## Treatment

It is important to act early by slowing down the process, for example using topical tacrolimus, systemic pentoxifylline, or, in some cases, tetracycline-nicotinamide.

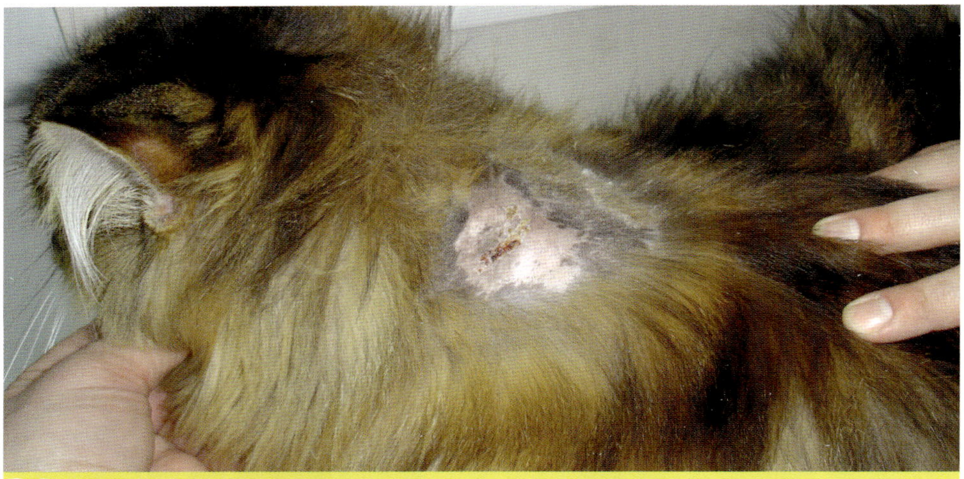

24 Alopecia in the cervical area of a cat following application of spot-on medication.

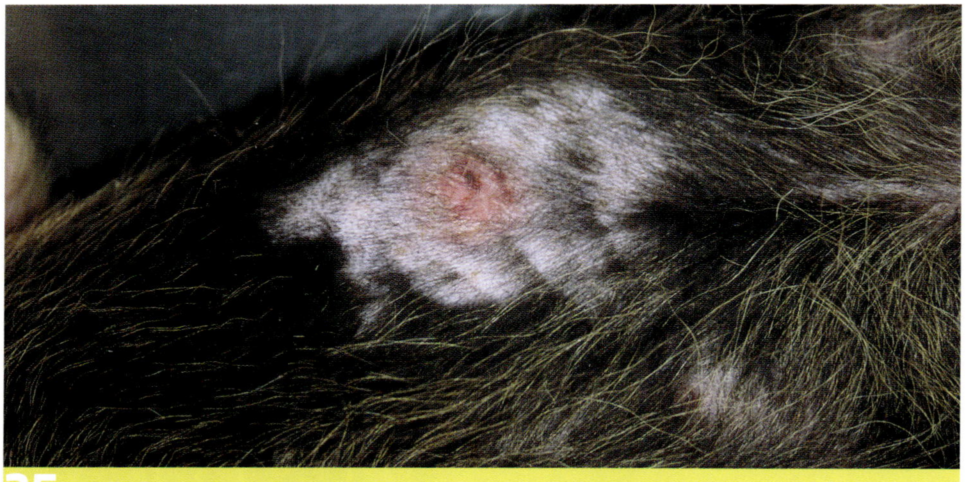

25 Alopecia, erythema, and atrophy following administration of the rabies vaccine.

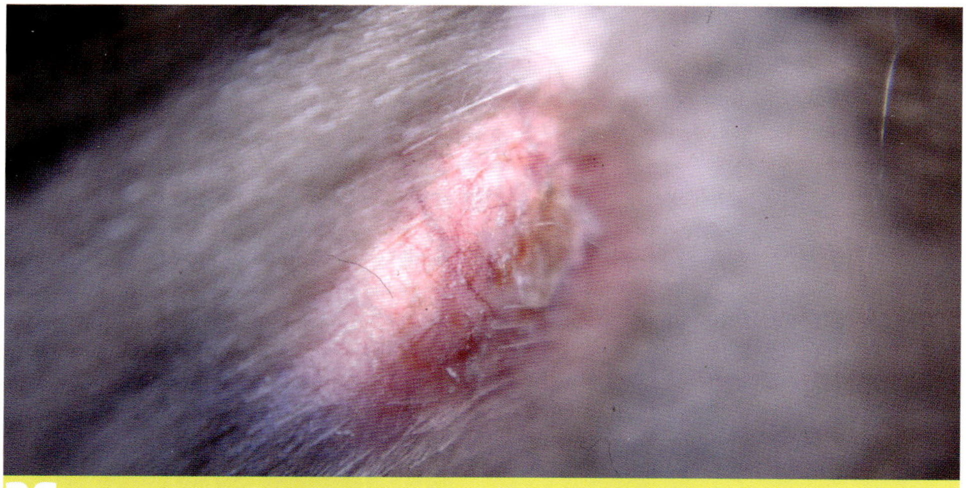

26 Cutaneous atrophy at the site of depot corticosteroid injection.

# Alopecia areata and pseudopelade

## Lesion aetiology/pathogenesis and clinical picture

Alopecia areata is a form of alopecia possibly caused by an immune-mediated/autoimmune reaction against cells of the hair follicles in anagen phase in dogs and cats. The areas of alopecia are well-defined, and can be isolated, multiple, or generalised. The process can begin by affecting melanocytes, resulting in subsequent leukotrichia.

Pseudopelade is a very rare disorder, similar to alopecia areata but targeting the cells of the follicular isthmus.

## Diagnostic method

Diagnosis is based on the history, clinical picture, and biopsy findings. These are primarily noninflammatory conditions, and diagnosis without biopsy is difficult.

In alopecia areata, trichography can be diagnostically useful when it reveals characteristic fracture of the hair shaft (exclamation mark-like appearance).

## Main differential diagnoses

- Dermatophytosis
- Demodicosis
- Vitiligo
- Skin reaction to topical application of substances

## Treatment

There is no specific effective treatment. Spontaneous resolution can occur. Recovery has been reported in cats treated with cyclosporine and dogs treated with corticosteroids and topical minoxidil.

Oclacitinib may be another option in cases of alopecia with immune-mediated mural folliculitis. In this author's experience dealing with pseudopelade, oclacitinib proved highly effective, resulting in hair recovery.

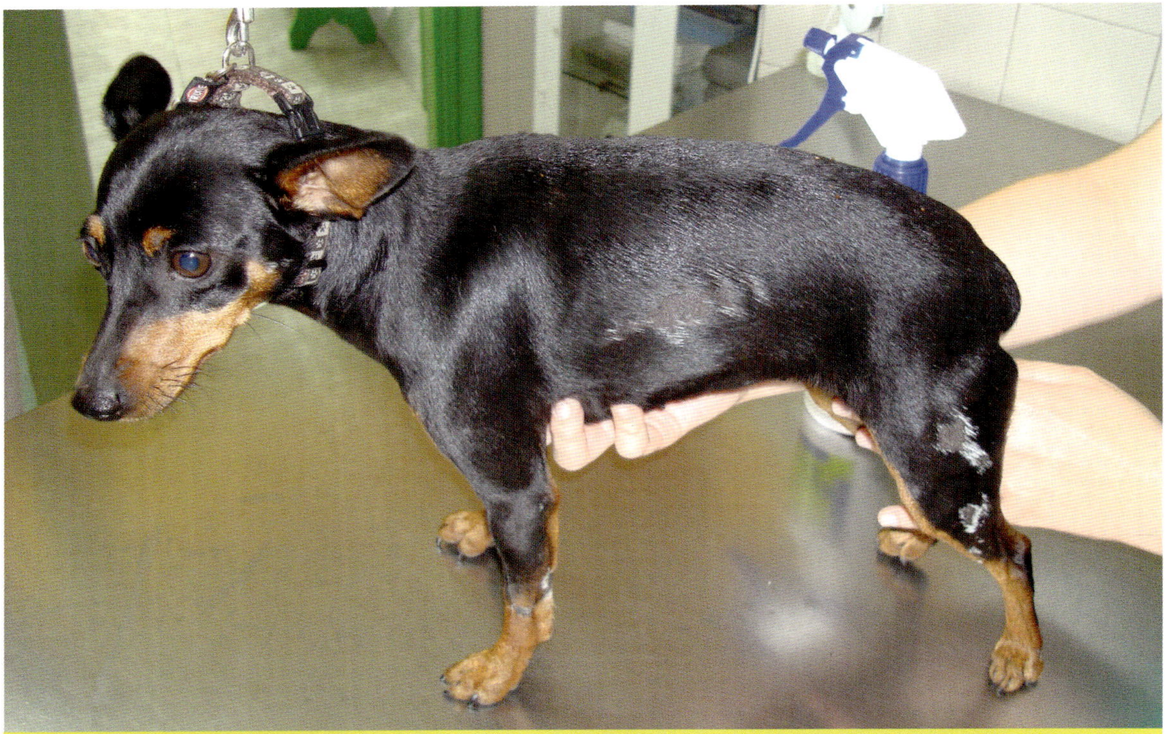

**27** Alopecia areata in a Pinscher. Foci of alopecia surrounded by leukotrichia.

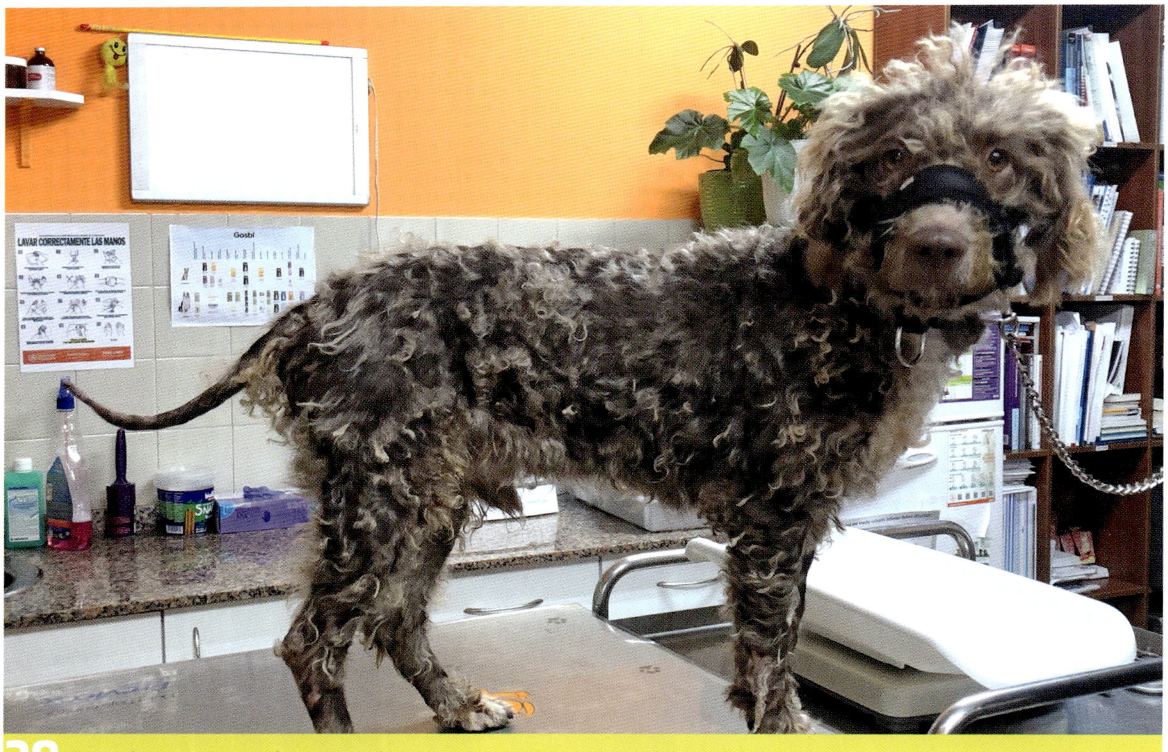


**28** Spanish Water Dog with pseudopelade. Note complete alopecia of the tail and patches all over the body.

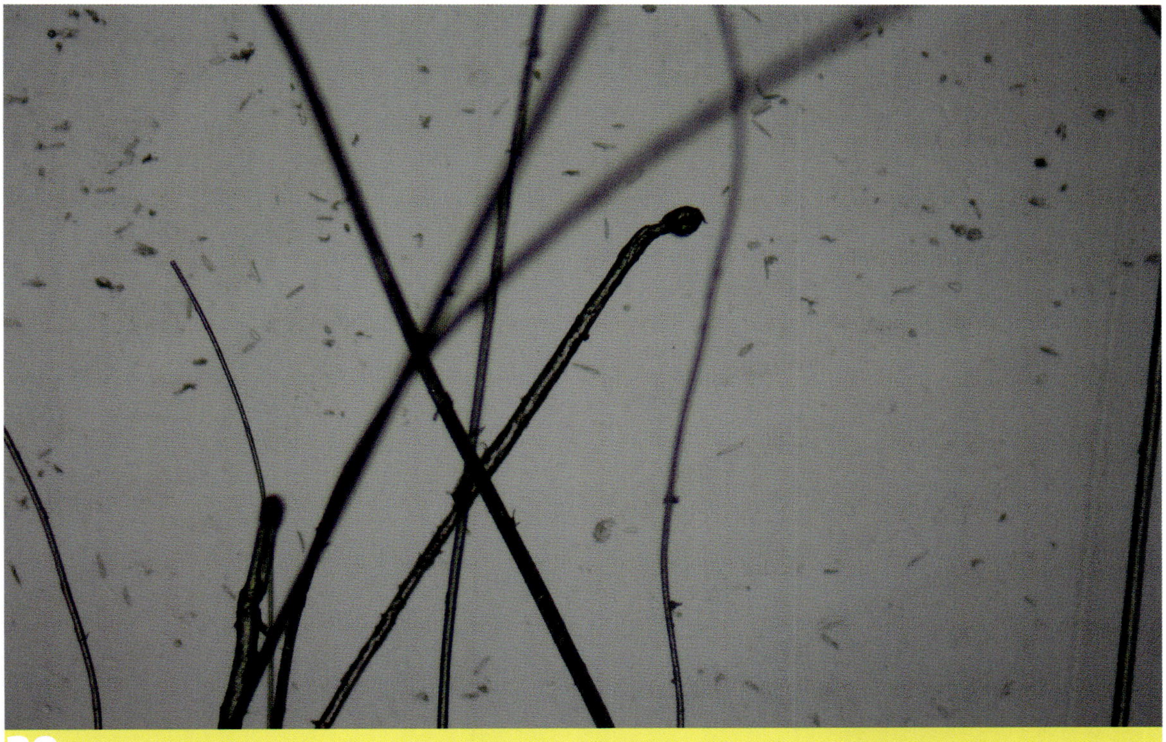

29 Trichography in a case of alopecia areata. Note the exclamation mark-like appearance of the hair root.

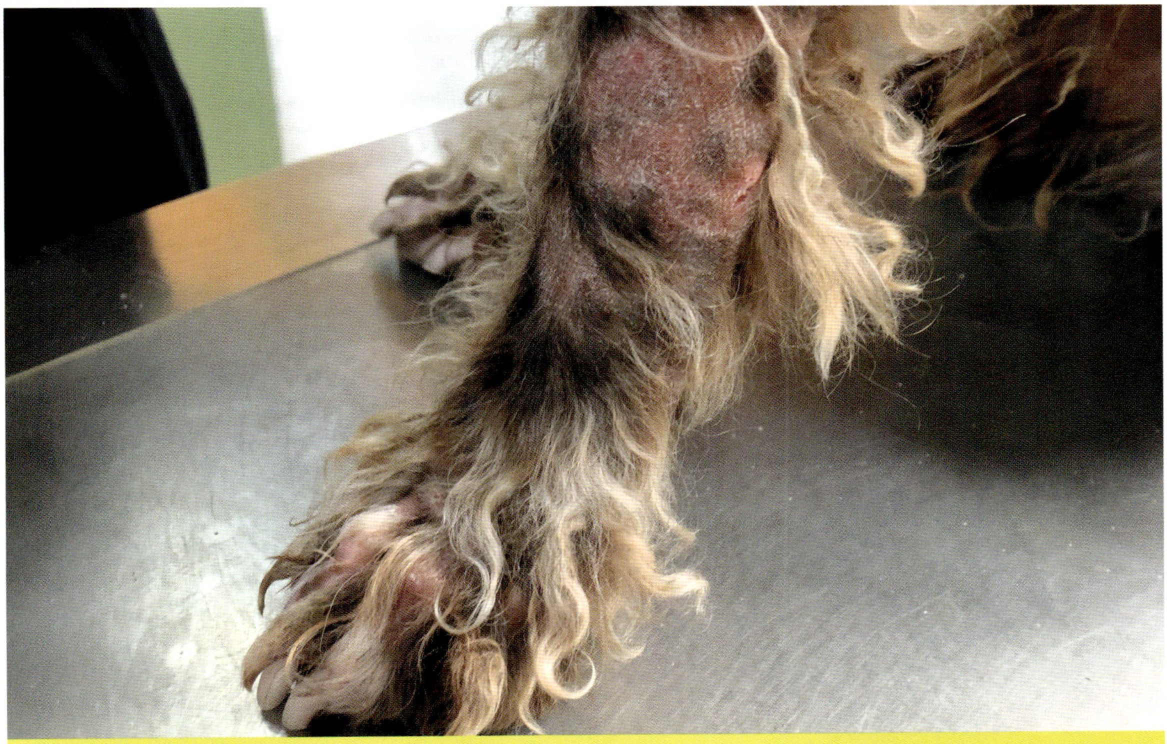

30 Alopecia of the distal forelimb in a case of pseudopelade.

# Feline psychogenic alopecia

## Lesion aetiology/pathogenesis and clinical picture

This is a form of alopecia in cats caused by excessive grooming due to behavioural disorders. It is less common than other forms of self-induced alopecia in cats with hypersensitivity, parasitic conditions, or dermatophytosis. It can also be caused by licking induced by pain in a specific area.

A psychological origin is demonstrated after ruling out any of the other aforementioned aetiologies. It usually occurs in areas that the cat can reach, such as the abdomen, back, legs, or buttocks. This disorder can be triggered by the arrival of a new inhabitant in the house, or a change in the orientation of the furniture.

## Diagnostic method

Diagnosis is based on the clinical history, trichogram findings, and a lack of response to corticosteroids, flea treatments, NSAIDs, and elimination diets. It should be taken into account that stress can sometimes aggravate self-induced alopecia due to hypersensitivity.

## Main differential diagnoses

Inflammatory self-induced alopecia.

## Treatment

It is important to correct any alterations of the environment in which the animal lives, and to energise or enrich the environment. This can be achieved using toys, games, pheromones, creating hiding places, providing more litter trays, etc. In some cases, the administration of psychotropic drugs such as amitriptyline, clomipramine, or fluoxetine may be necessary.

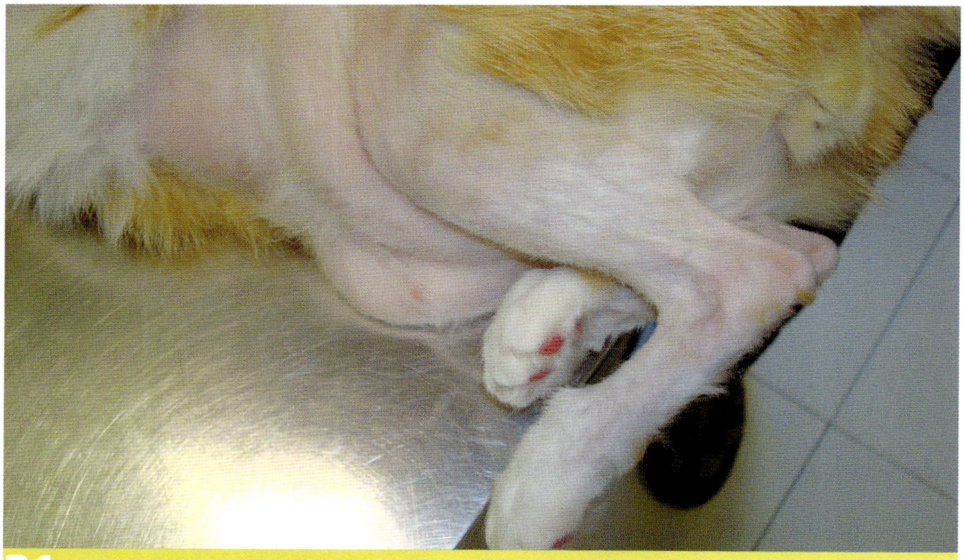

**31** Alopecia of the hindlimbs that does not respond to anti-inflammatory treatment.

# 13 Miscellaneous conditions

# Introduction

This chapter includes clinical pictures and diseases that do not fit easily into the previous chapters, or dermatoses that warrant separate discussion owing to the area they affect or their characteristics. The chapter also includes images that may be useful in daily clinical practice:

- The most common dermatophytoses: microscopic differential diagnosis
- Nail diseases
- Disorders of the paw pads
- Canine facial dermatoses
- Acral mutilation syndrome
- Collagen diseases:
  - Cutaneous asthenia
  - Feline auricular chondritis

# The most common dermatophytoses: microscopic differential diagnosis

Dermatophytosis (see Chapter 3) is a disease caused by keratolytic fungi, which, as discussed previously, can produce highly variable clinical pictures. In general, knowing exactly which dermatophyte is causing a given infection is important because it allows us to determine both the source and the prognosis. For example, fungi of the genus *Trichophyton* may be more stubborn when it comes to treatment.

Observation of macroconidia in colonies grown in DTM (dermatophyte test medium) is the best way to differentiate fungi. The hyphae of *Trichophyton* are also highly characteristic, enabling identification even in the absence of macroconidia.

Images of the most common macroconidia of saprophytic fungi are included to facilitate recognition.

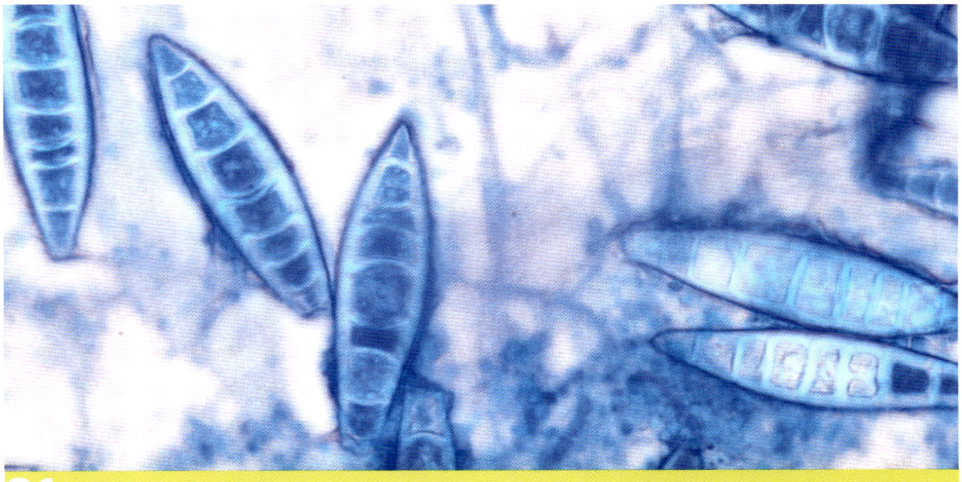

01 Macroconidia of *Microsporum canis* with a characteristic double wall.

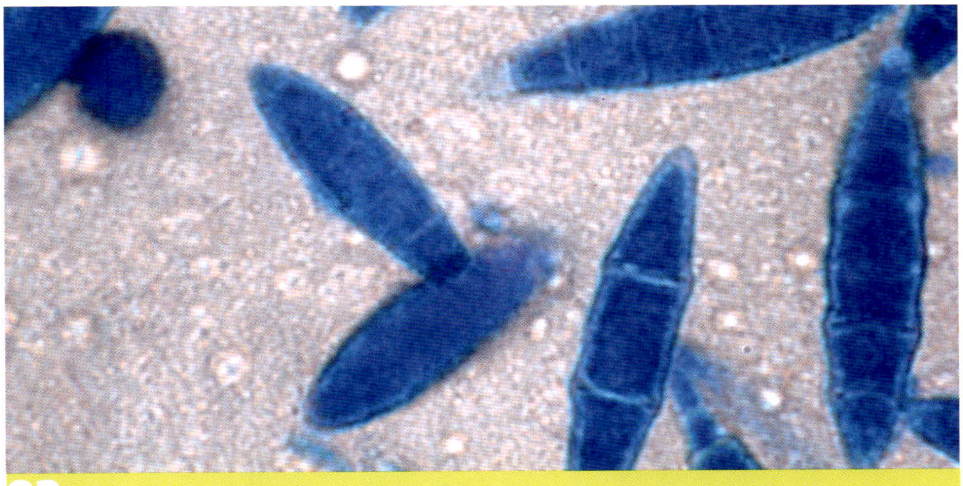

02 Macroconidia of *Microsporum gypseum*, exhibiting a single wall and fewer cells.

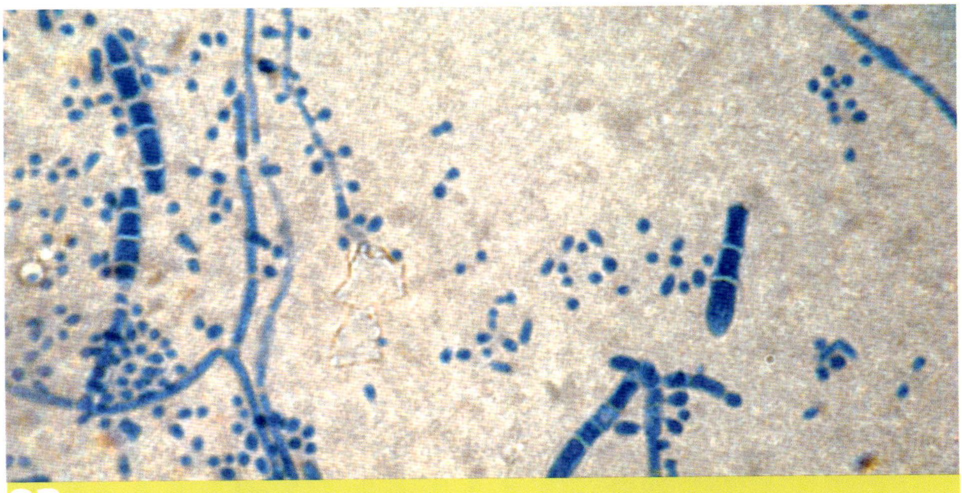

03 Macroconidia of *Microsporum persicolor*.

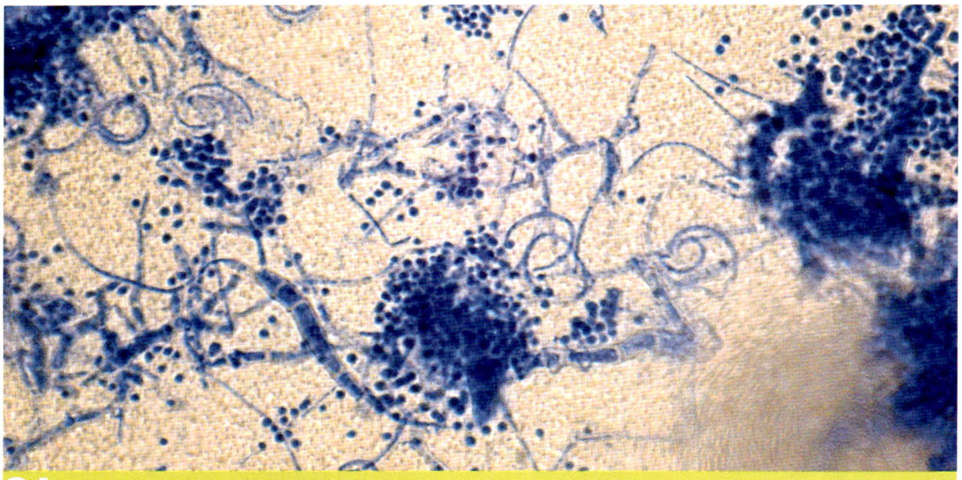

04 Macroconidia and hyphae of *Trichophyton mentagrophytes*. Note the typical spiral hyphae.

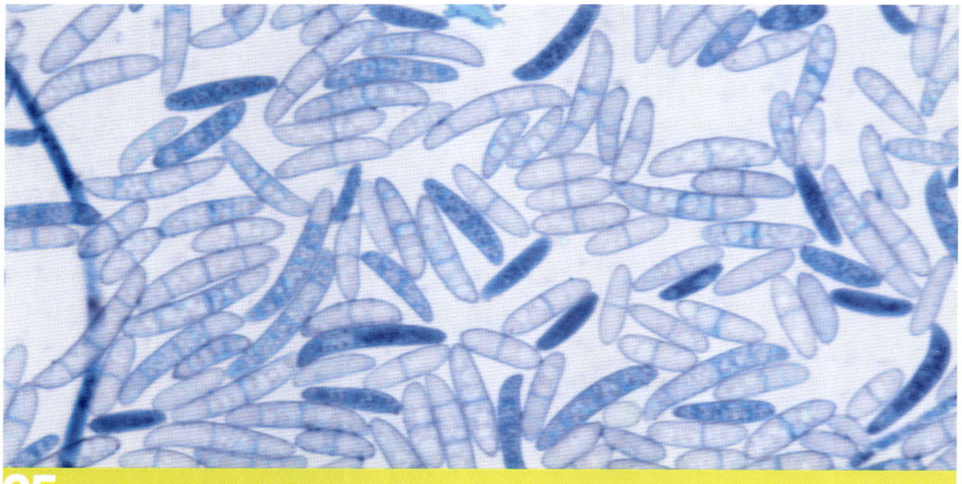

05 Macroconidia of genus *Fusarium*.

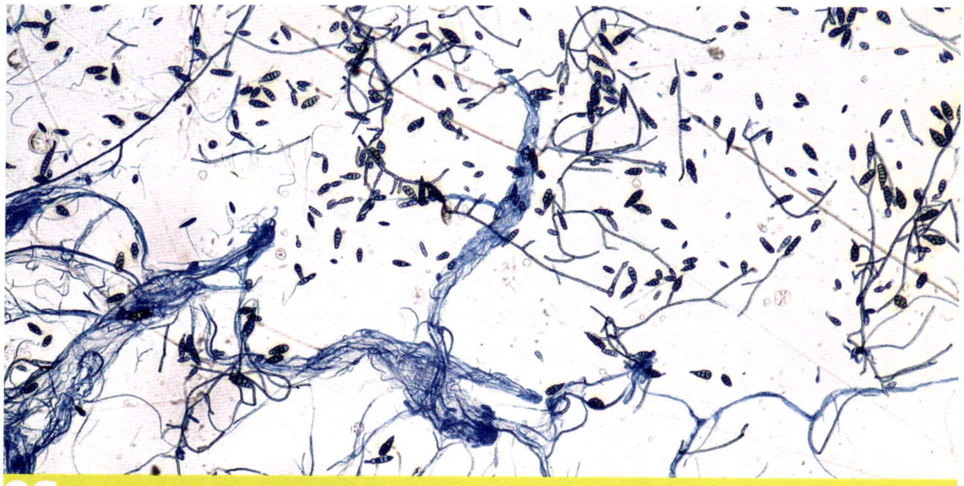

06 Macroconidia of genus *Alternaria*.

# Nail diseases

Nails are specialised skin appendages with a multitude of functions, and can be targeted by many diseases, causing great discomfort in patients.

Specific nomenclature is used to describe the different disorders that can affect the nails, some of which are represented in the following images.

| Nail disorders: nomenclature. | | |
|---|---|---|
| **Name** | **Meaning** | **Example** |
| Onyxis or onychia | Abnormal nail | Any condition that causes altered nail formation |
| Onychoschisis | Splitting of the nail | Trauma |
| Onychorrhexis or onychoclasis | Breakage of nails that are brittle or fragile | Onychomycosis |
| Onychomadesis | Nail shedding | Lupoid onychodystrophy |
| Onychogryphosis | Hypertrophy and abnormal curvature | Leishmaniasis |
| Onychodystrophy | Abnormal formation | Paronychia |
| Onychomalacia | Softening of the nail | Nutritional deficiency |
| Paronychia | Inflammation or infection of nail folds | Bacteria, fungi |

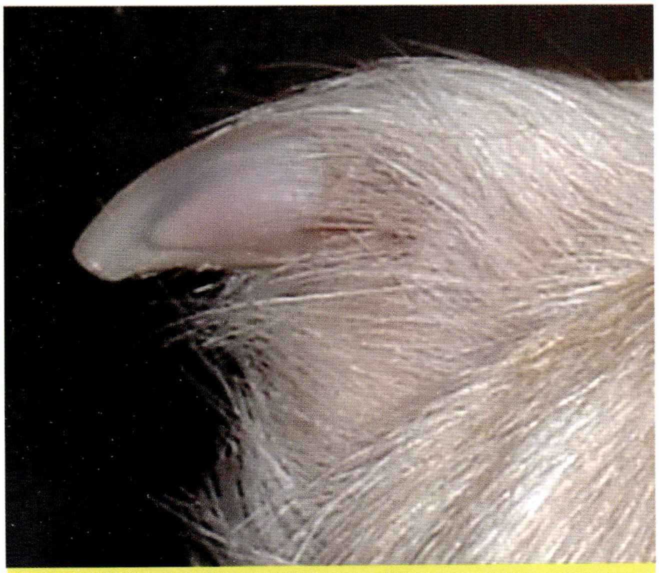

07 Normal nail with visible chorion.

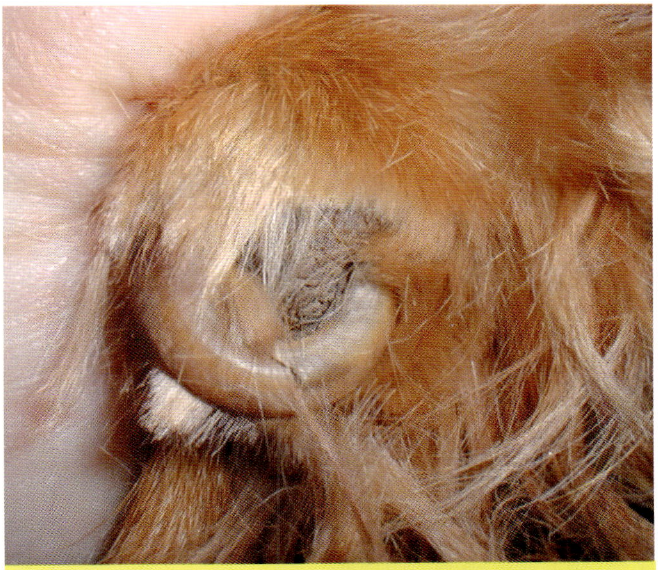

08 Onychoschisis. Nail fracture.

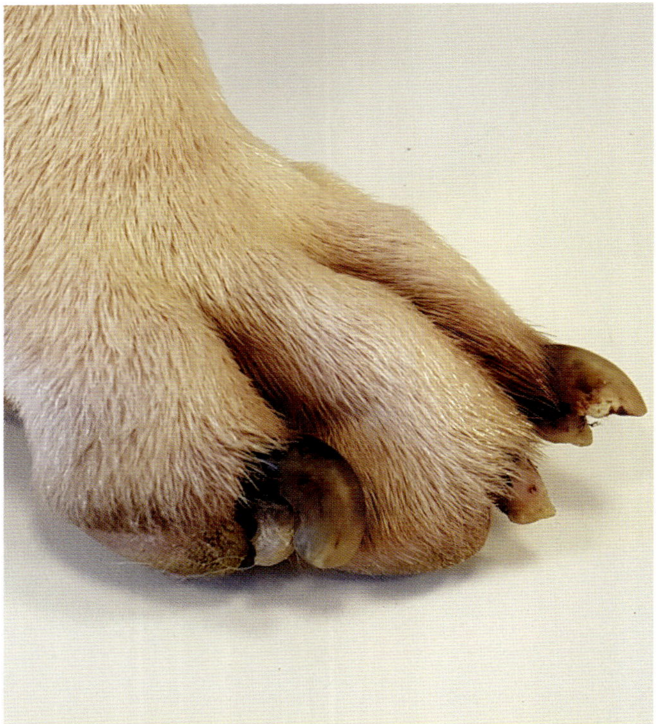

09 Onychorrhexis. Breakage of nails that are brittle or fragile.

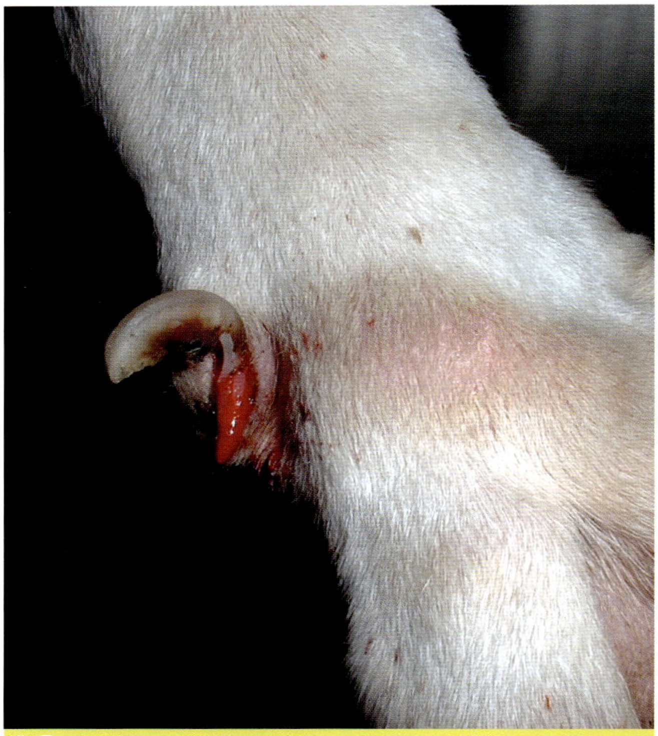

10 Onychomadesis. Nail shedding.

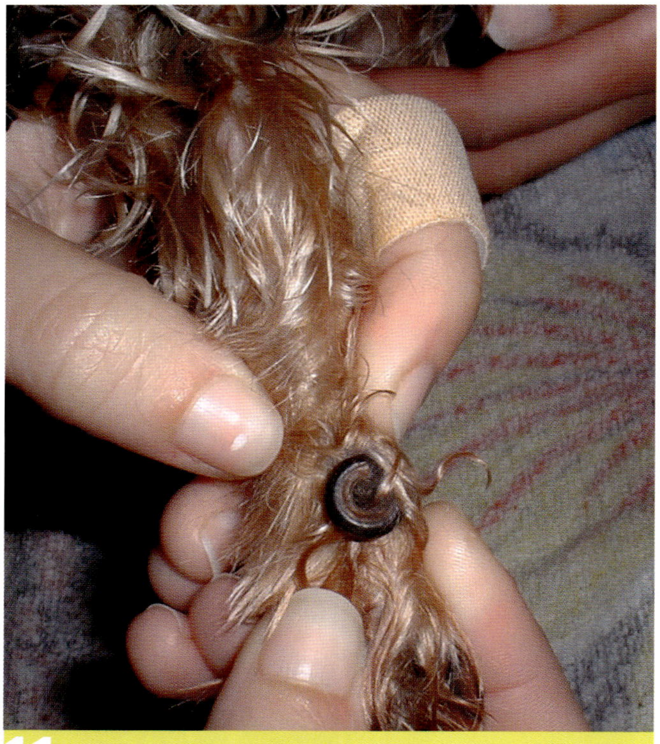

11 Onychogryphosis. Hypertrophy and abnormal curvature.

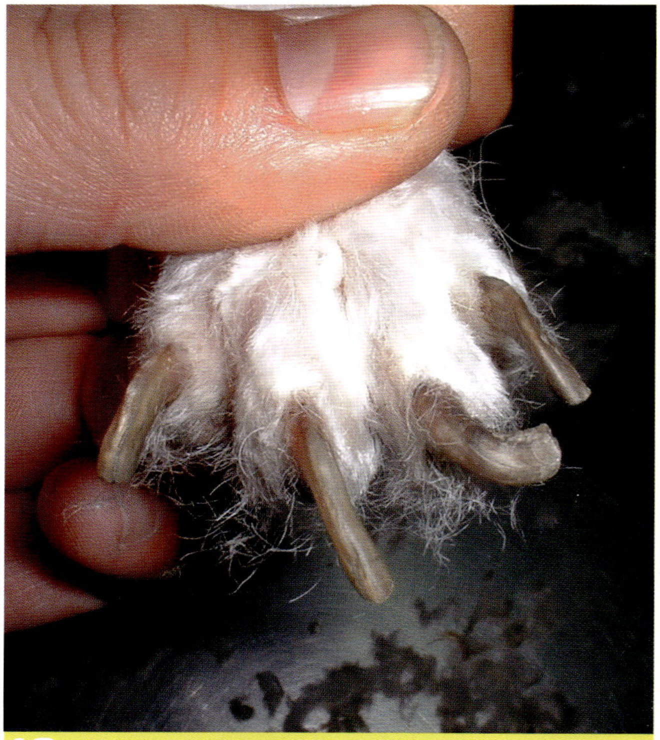

12 Onychodystrophy. Abnormal nail formation.

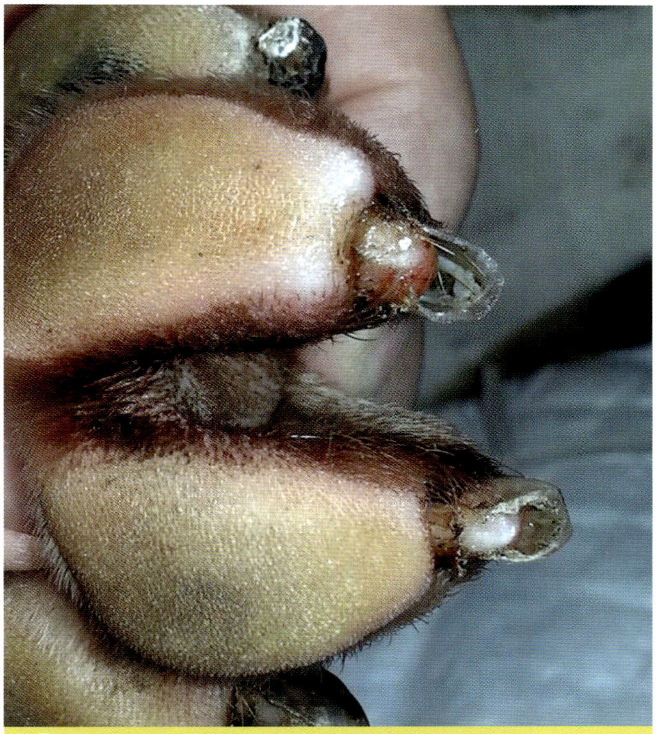

13 Onychomalacia. Softening of the nail.

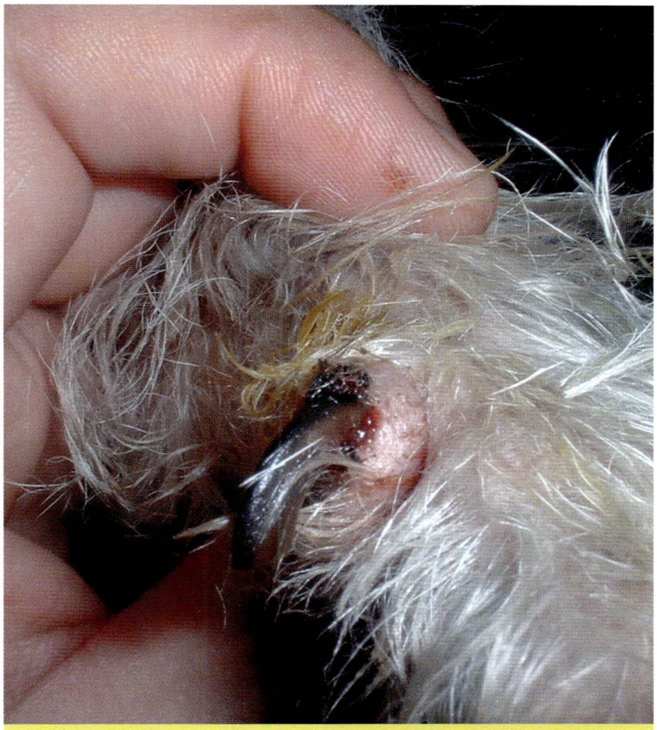

14 Paronychia. Inflammation of the nail folds.

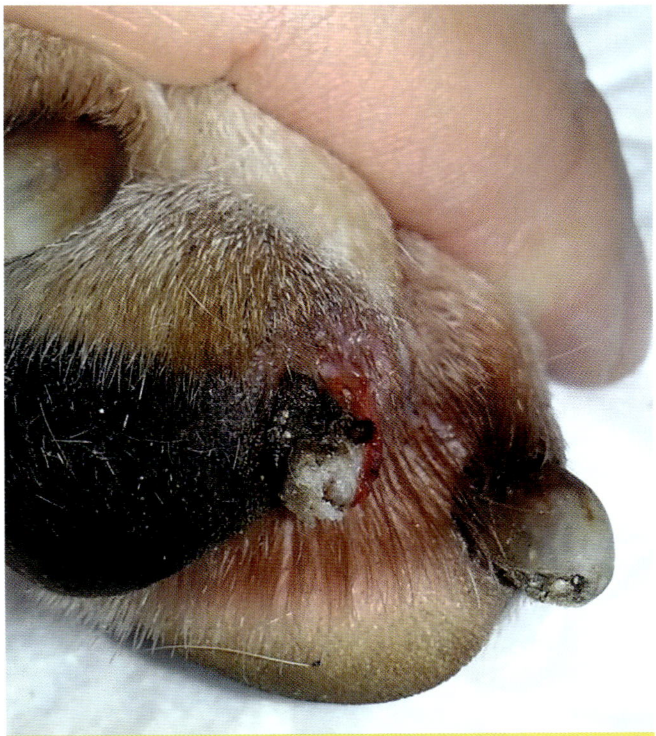

15 Bacterial paronychia. Lupoid onychodystrophy with infection.

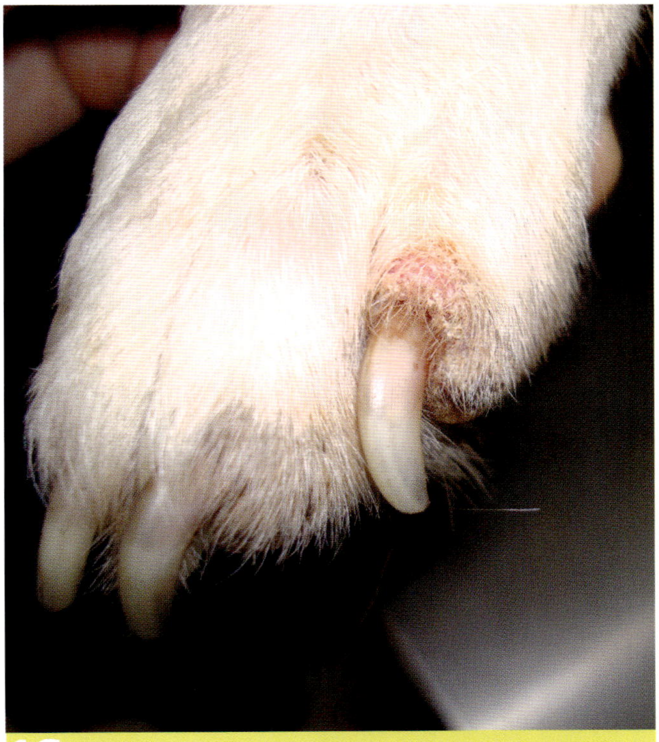

16 Paronychia due to dermatophytes.

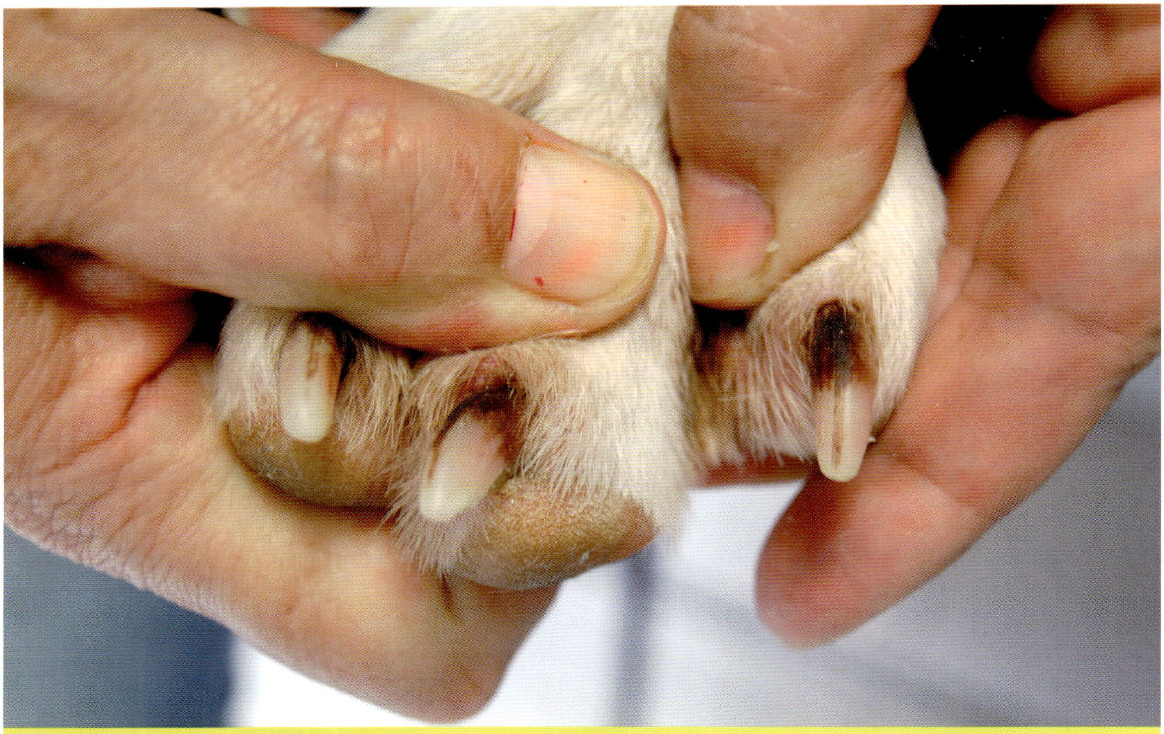

17 Paronychia caused by *Malassezia* with typical discolouration of the nail.

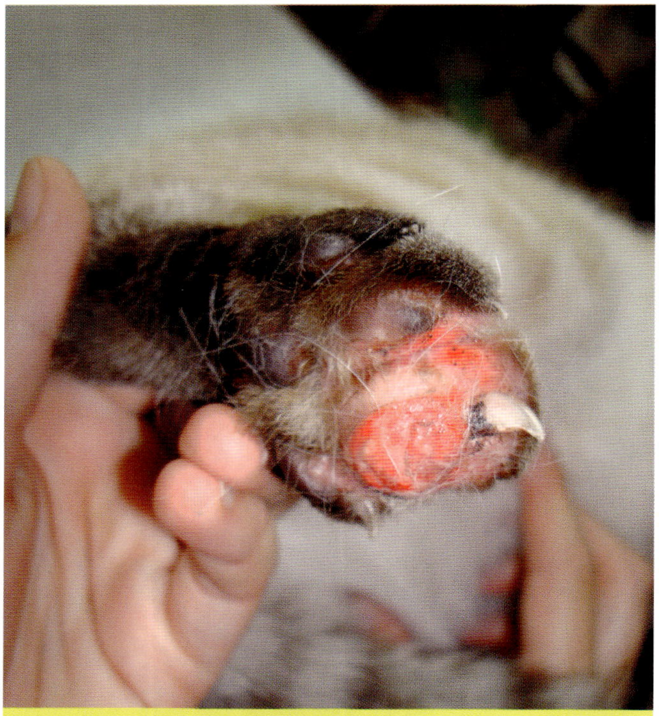

18 Paronychia due to feline eosinophilic granuloma.

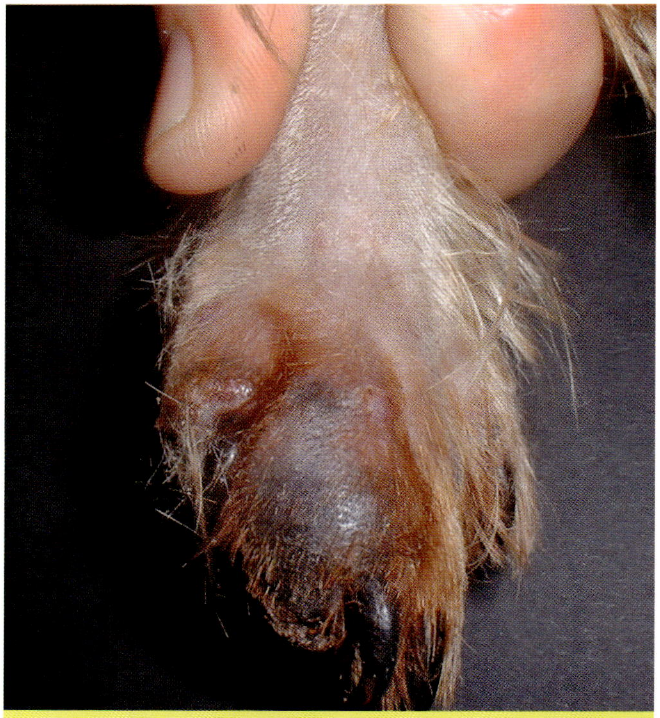

19 Paronychia due to neoplasia. Subungual squamous cell carcinoma.

# Disorders of the paw pads

The paw pads are keratinised formations that contain eccrine glands and lack follicles. They serve as shock absorbers and protect the animal during movement, while also providing grip. They also play a role in pheromonal marking.

Paw pads can be affected by keratinisation disorders (excessive or deficient keratinisation), and by other diseases (mainly vascular, autoimmune, immune-mediated, or traumatic).

The images below show some examples of paw pad involvement in different diseases.

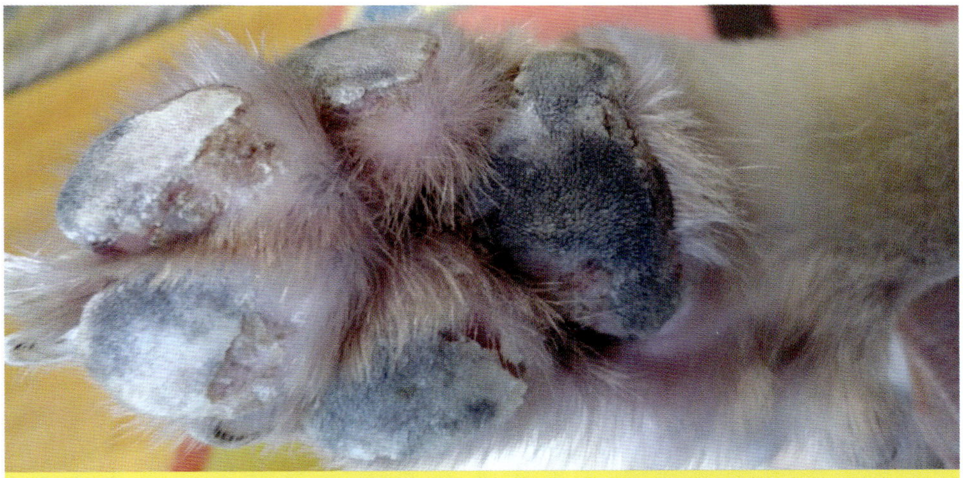

20 Paw pads in a dog with leishmaniasis.

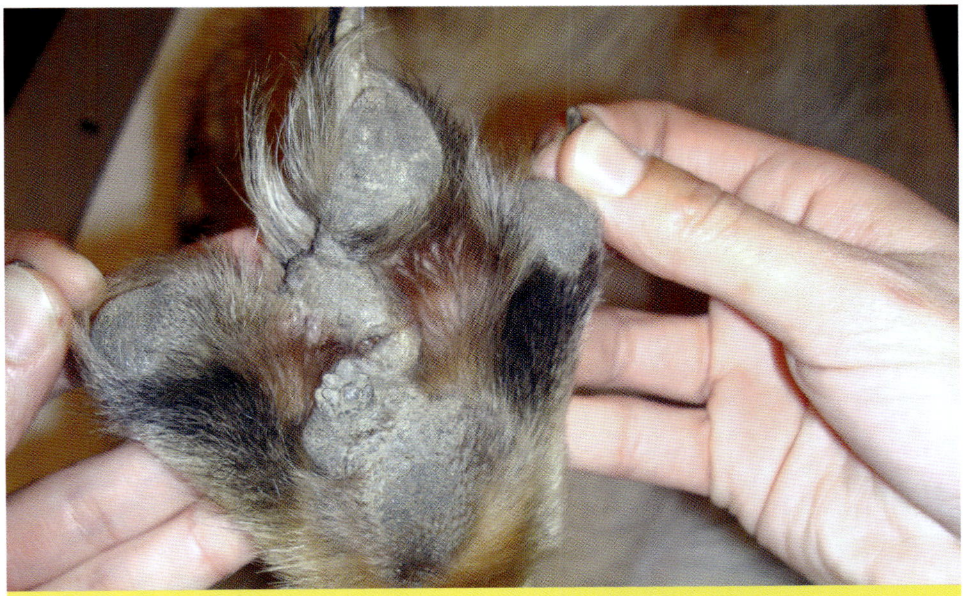

21 Hyperplastic and deformed paw pads in a dog with chronic allergy.

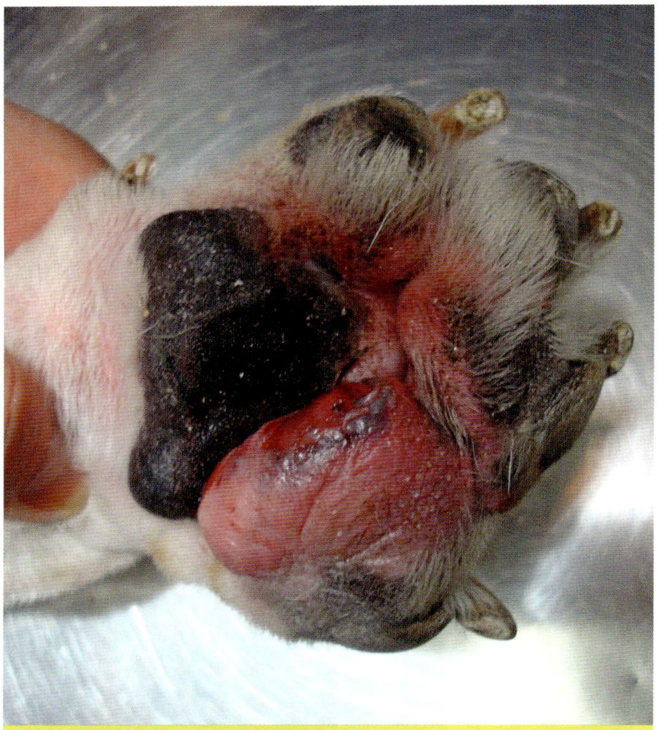
22 Paw pads of a dog with chronic *Malassezia* infection.

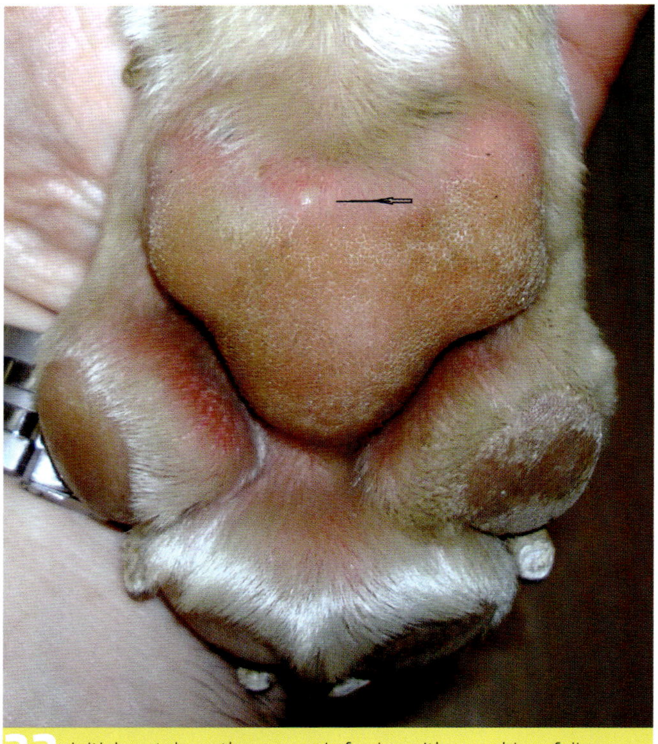
23 Initial pustule on the paw pad of a dog with pemphigus foliaceus.

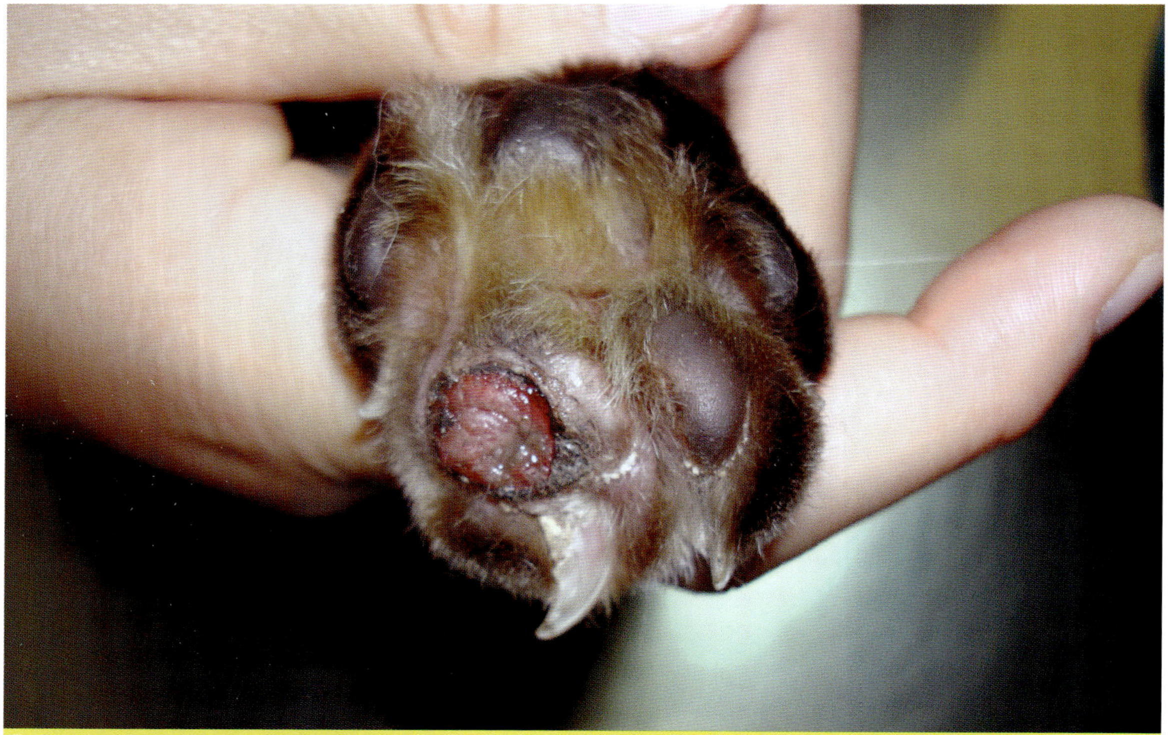
24 Cat with an ulcer of the paw pad due to vasculitis.

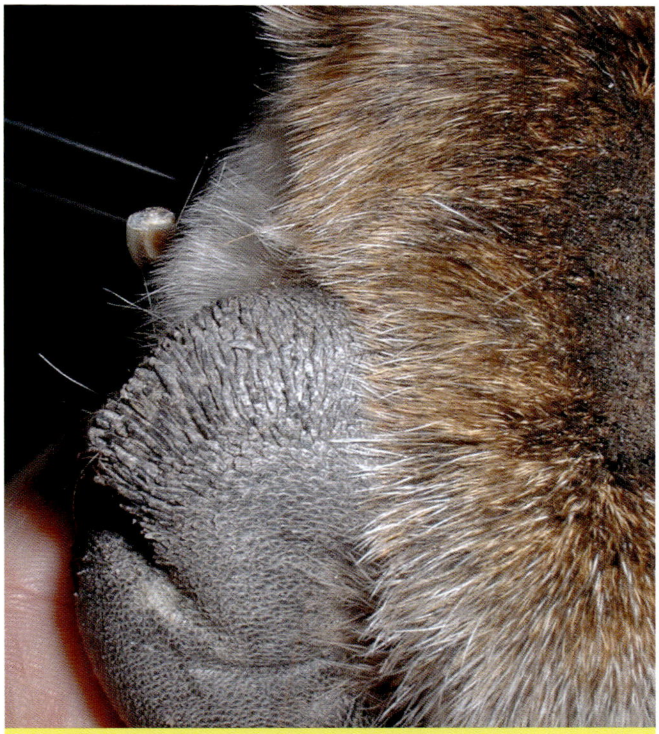

25 Dog with hyperkeratosis of the paw pad due to poor stance.

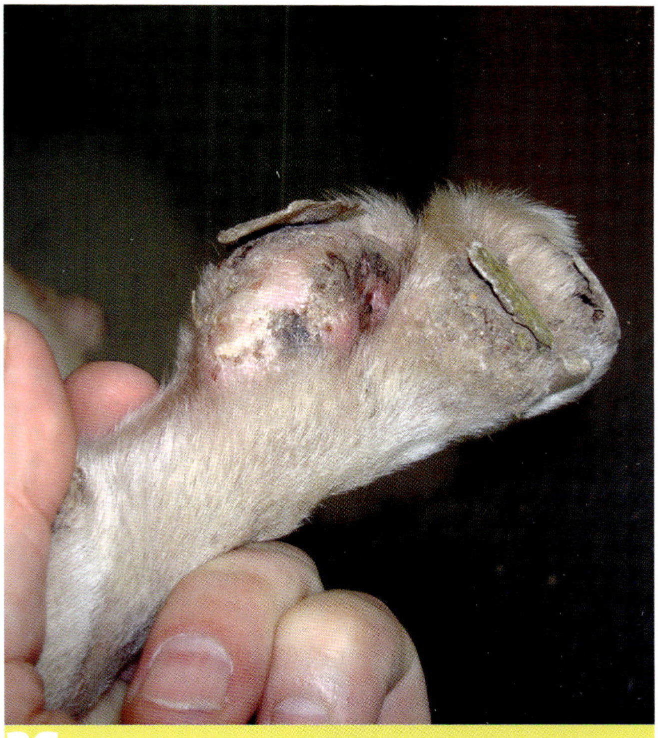

26 Paw pad detachment in a dog with an autoimmune disease.

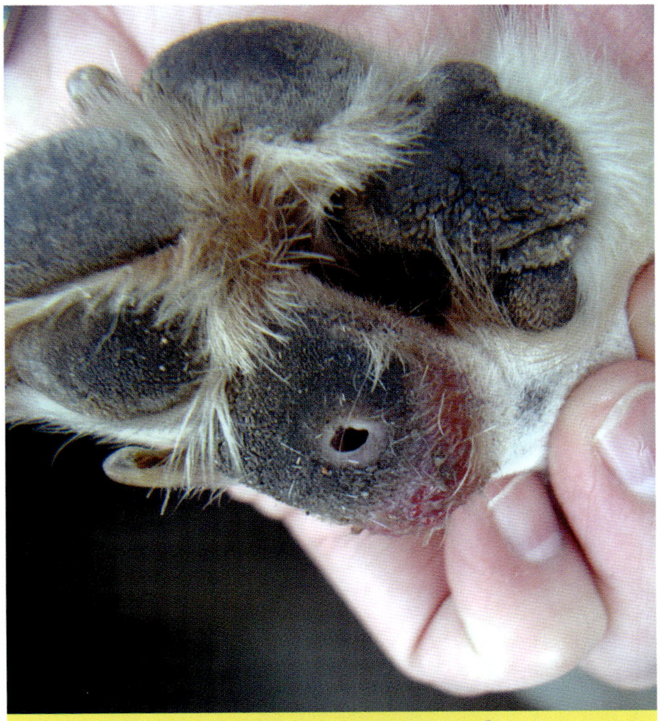

27 Perforation of the paw pad to drain a trichogranuloma on the posterior aspect of the pad.

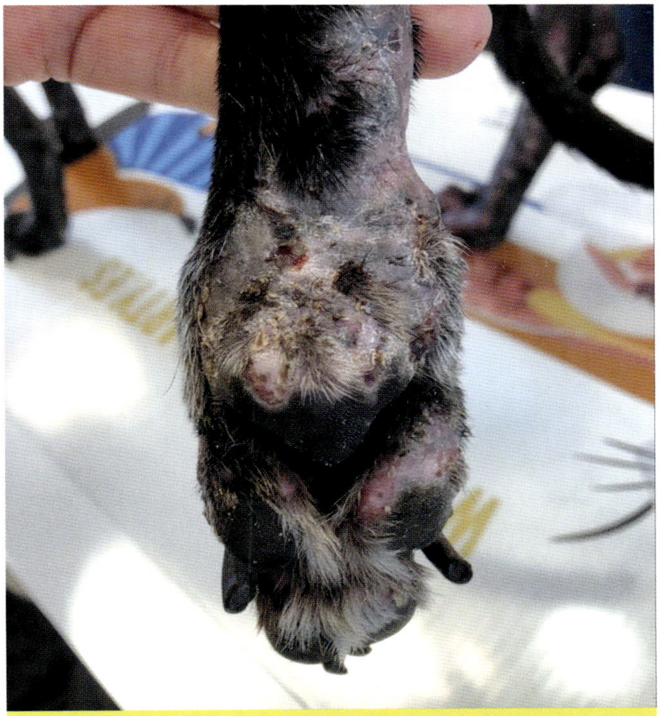

28 Drug reaction: paw pad involvement.

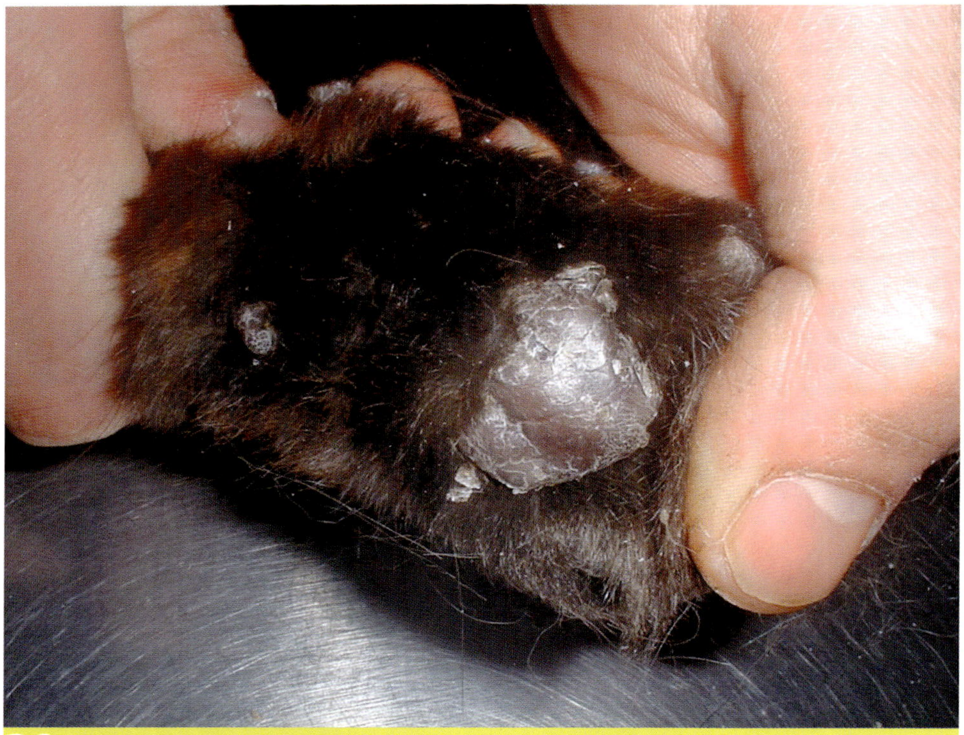

**29** Paw pad of cat with pemphigus foliaceus.

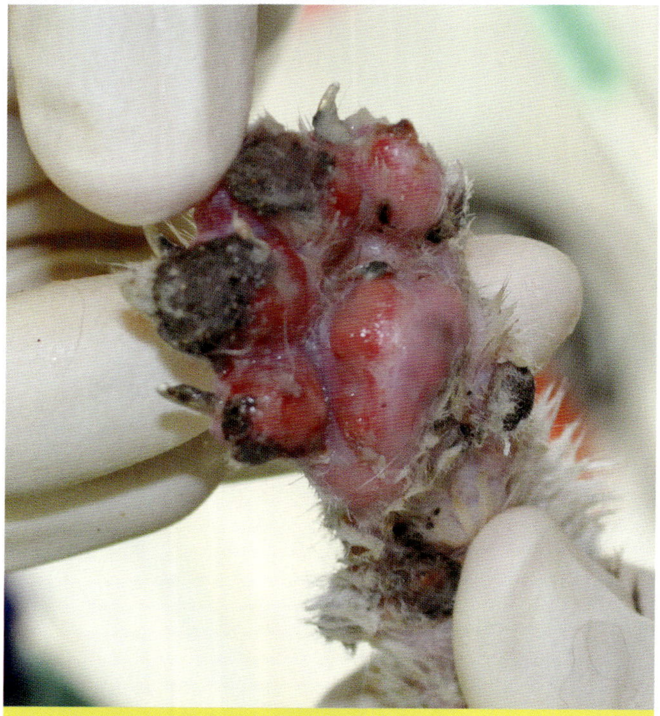

**30** Splitting of the paw pad in a cat with ischaemic dermatitis caused by Herpesvirus.

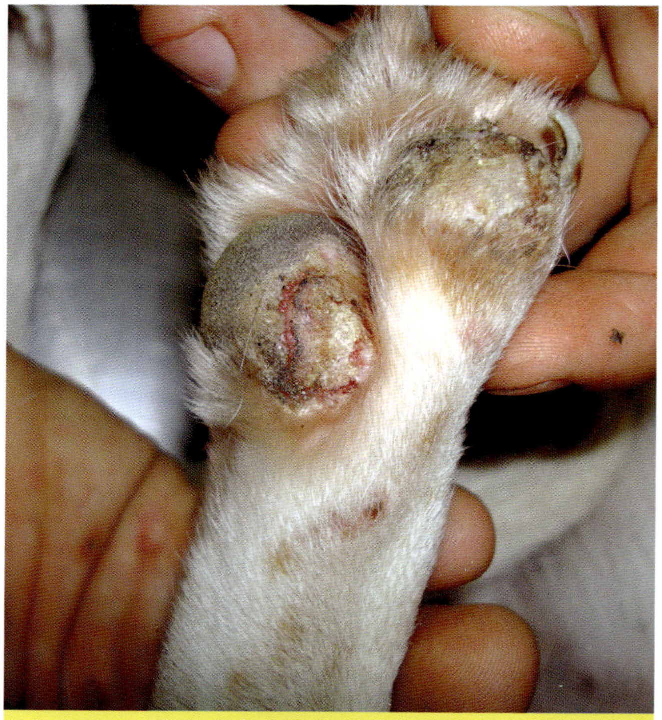

**31** Dermatophytosis: paw pad and peripheral tissue involvement.

# Canine facial dermatoses

The skin of the face can be affected by different primary or secondary skin diseases, as well as systemic diseases.

It is useful to have a series of images depicting the diseases that most frequently affect this region of the body in dogs and cats.

Sometimes the image is so characteristic that it can be practically diagnostic.

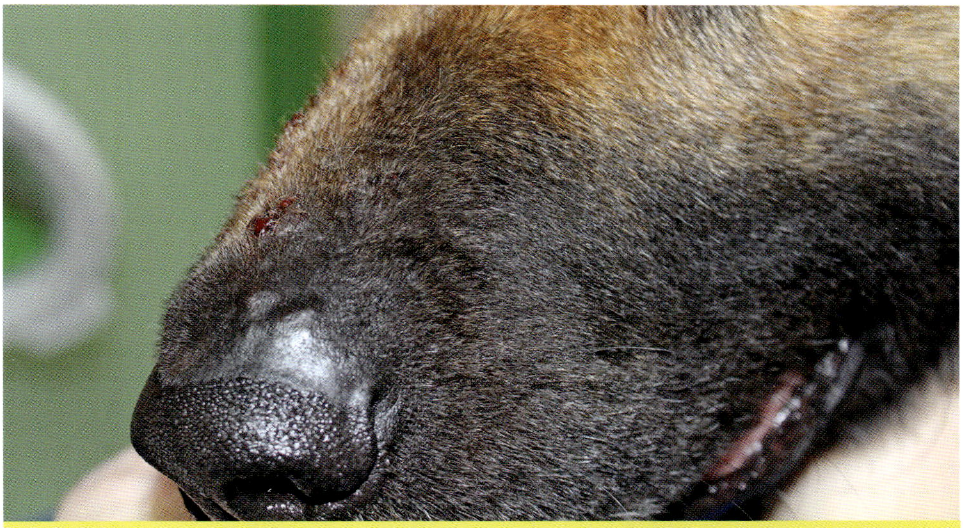

32 Onset of facial eosinophilic furunculosis with involvement of the nasal bridge caused by insect (usually *Hymenoptera*) bites and/or stings.

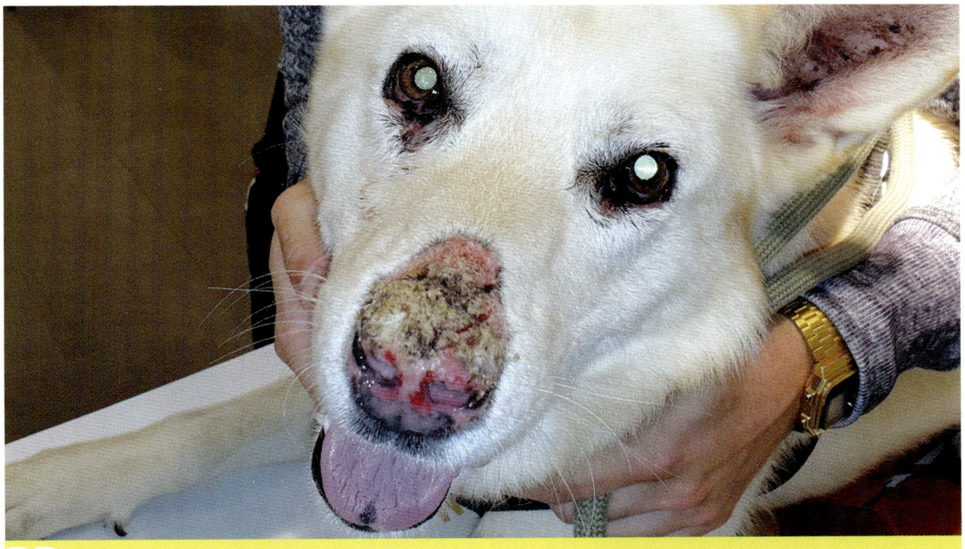

33 Cutaneous lupus affecting the face, specifically the nasal bridge, pinnae, and eyelids.

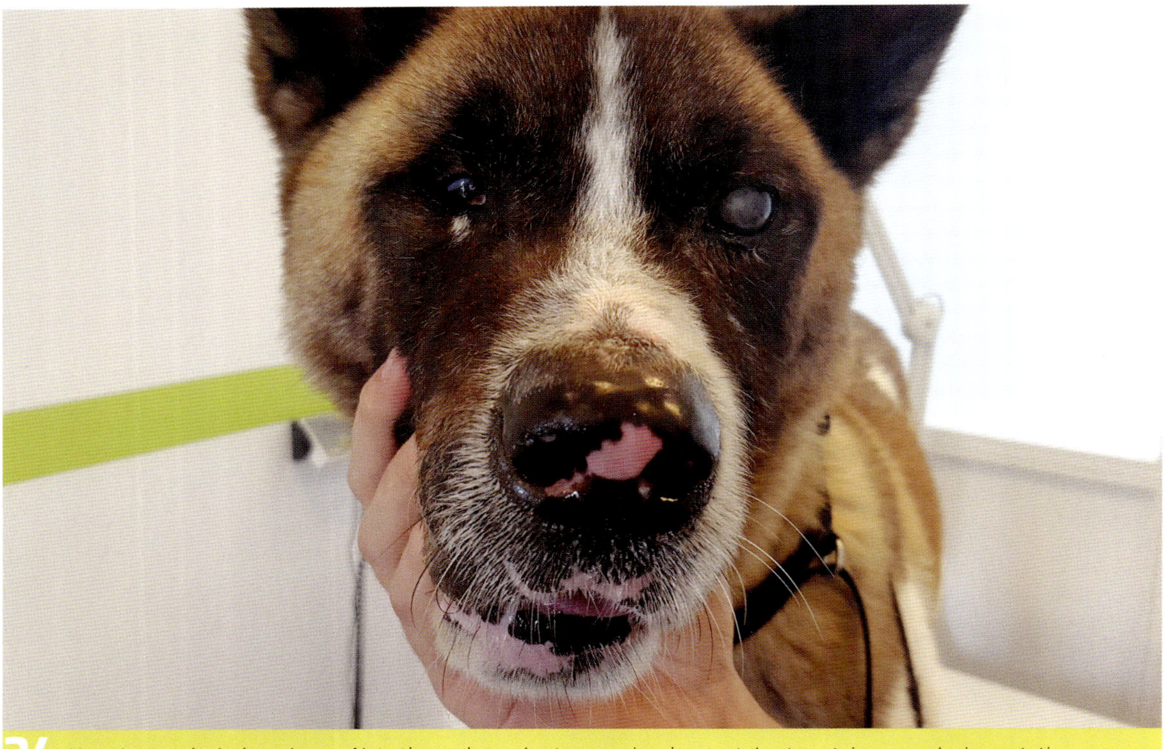

**34** Uveodermatological syndrome. Note the ocular and cutaneous involvement due to autoimmune depigmentation.

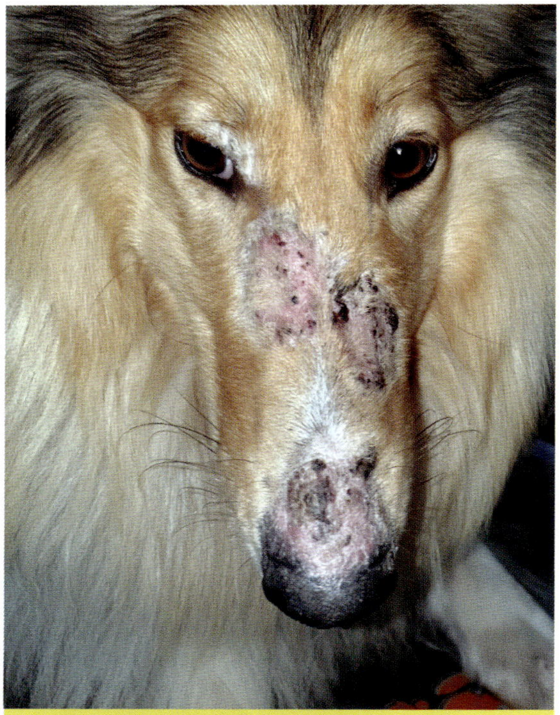

**35** Dermatomyositis in a Collie. Note the vasculitis lesions.

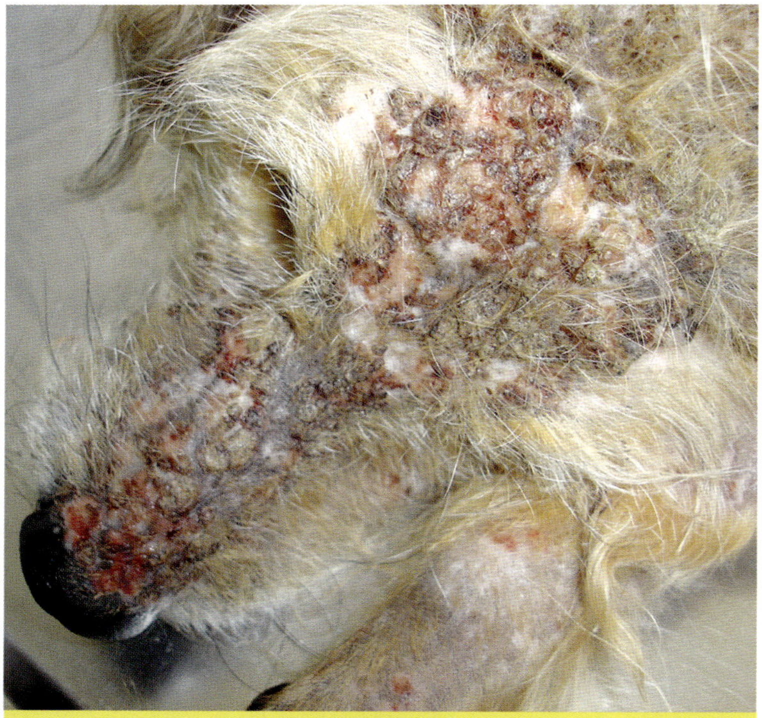

**36** Facial dermatosis due to pemphigus foliaceus. Formation of pustules and crusts.

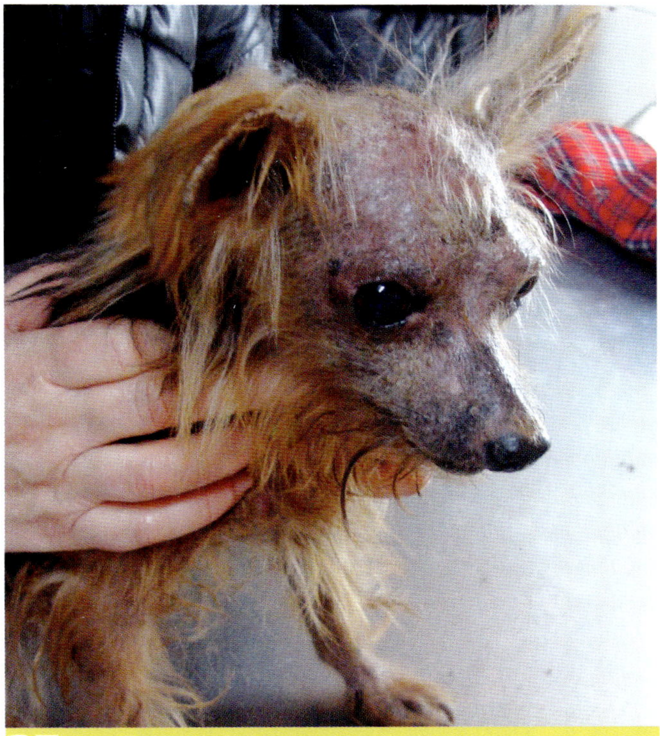

37 Disseminated facial dermatophytosis in a Yorkshire Terrier.

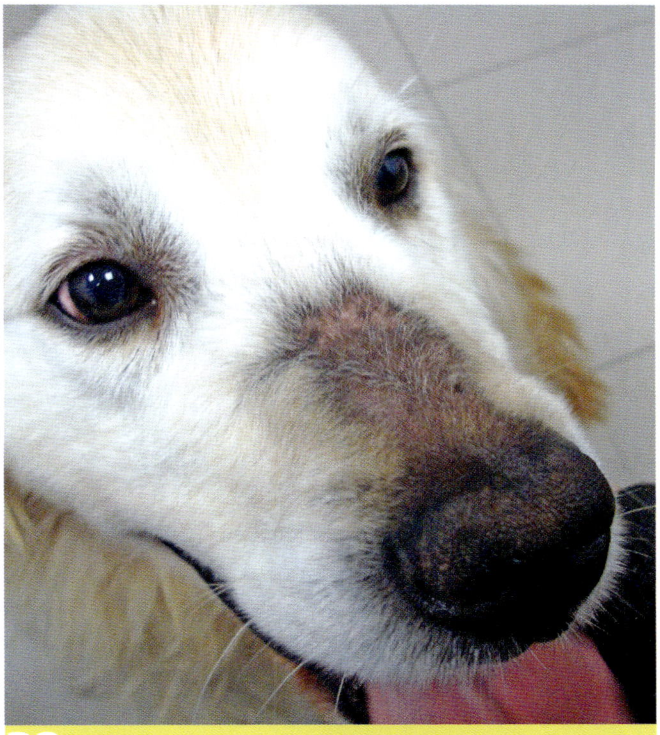

38 Recurrent alopecia on the nasal bridge of a dog.

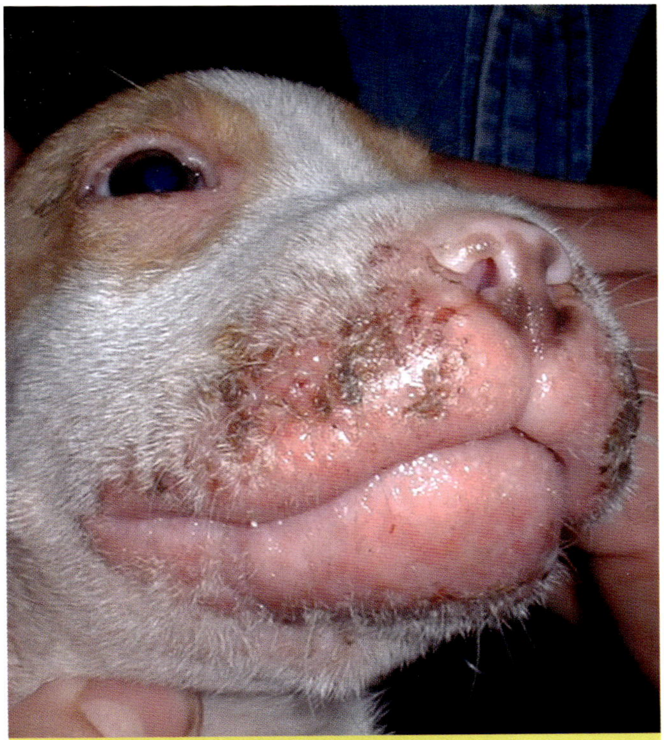

39 Classic facial presentation in a puppy with juvenile cellulitis.

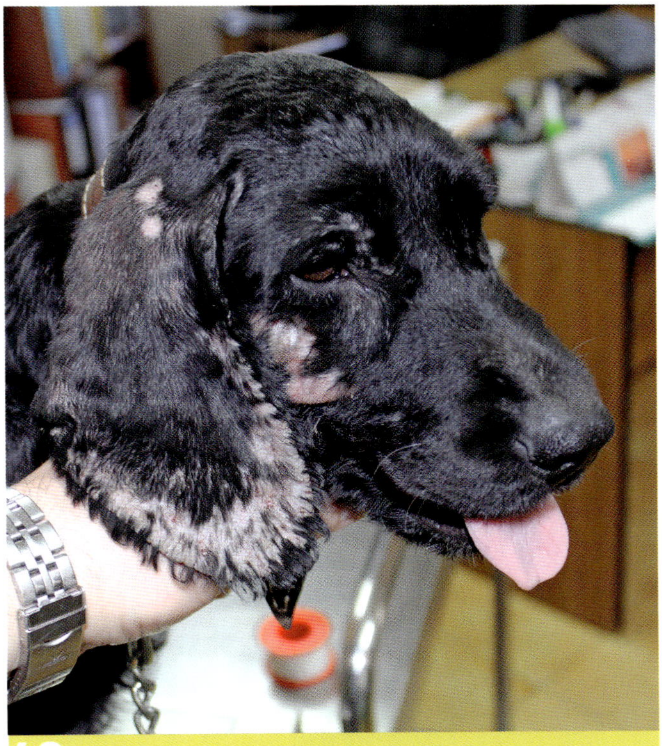

40 Scabies with involvement of the face and pinnae.

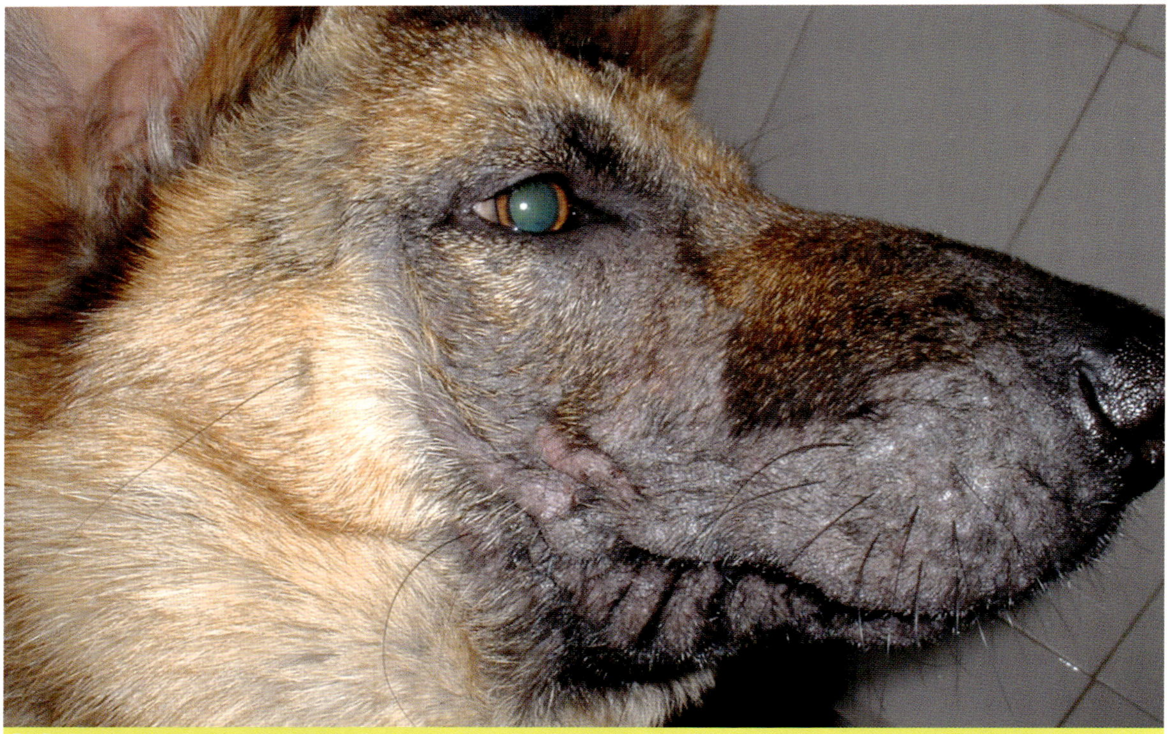

41 Alopecia and papules on the face of a dog with demodicosis.

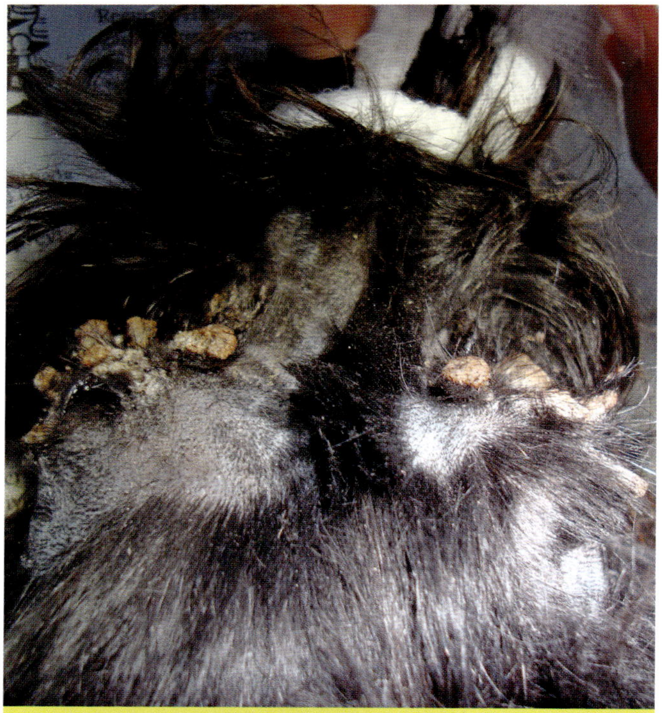

42 Lichenoid keratotic dermatosis on the eyelids caused by a chronic infection.

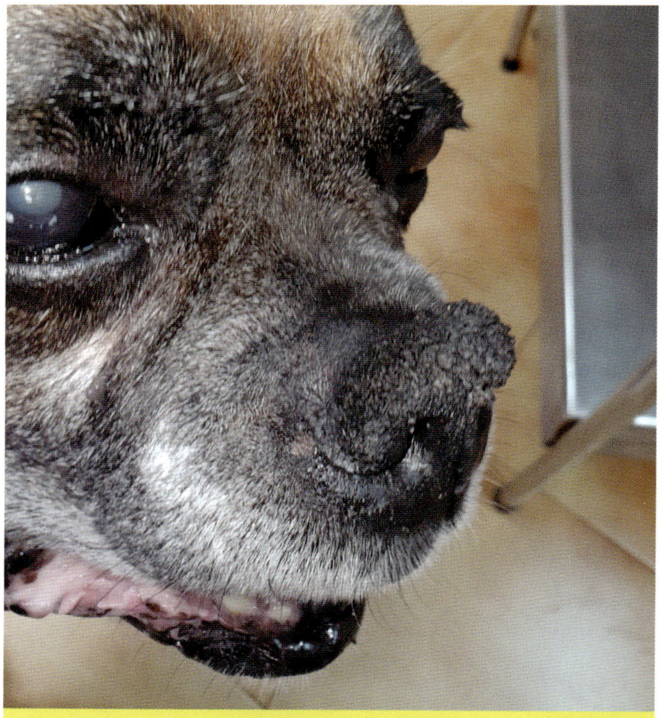

43 Hyperkeratosis on the nose of a senior dog.

# Acral mutilation syndrome

## Lesion aetiology/pathogenesis and clinical picture

Acral mutilation syndrome (AMS) is a rare hereditary, autosomal recessive disease characterised by sensory neuropathy that causes analgesia or sensory alterations in the distal limbs, with consequent self-mutilation.

It has been described in the Miniature Pinscher, English Springer Spaniel, English Pointer, and German Shorthaired Pointer. This acropathy usually occurs in puppies from 3 months of age, resulting in biting and licking of the digits and nails. This behaviour leads to self-mutilation of the digits all the way to the paw pads. The animal walks on the stumps, showing no signs of pain.

## Diagnostic method

Diagnosis is usually based on the clinical picture. A genetic DNA test can be performed to rule out carriers as breeders.

## Main differential diagnoses

- Other syndromes characterised by neuropathy due to lack of sensitivity
- Allergies with severe clinical signs

## Treatment

Gabapentin is a possible therapeutic option, although its efficacy is limited. Bandages may be the only treatment.

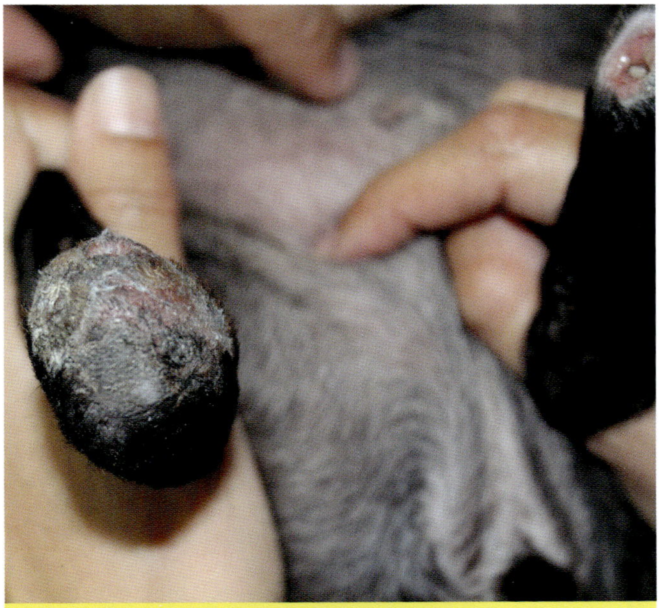

44 Self-mutilated limb of a Miniature Pinscher. In the other limb the exposed bone is visible.

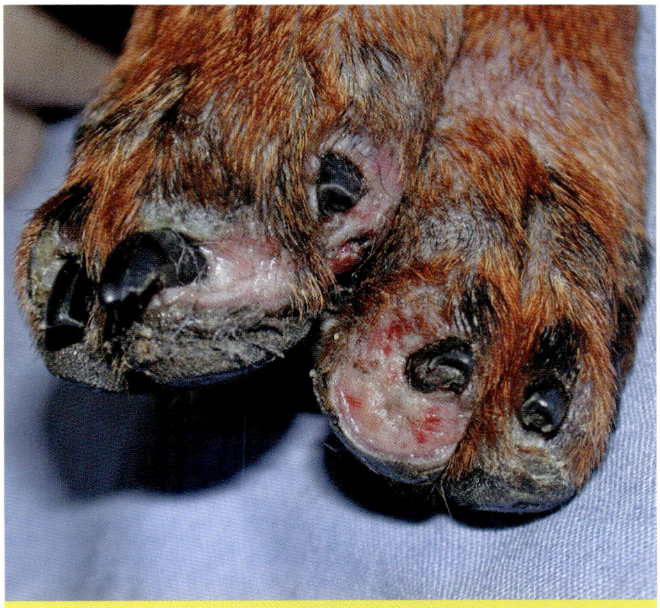

45 Onset of self-mutilation affecting both limbs. Image courtesy of Francesco Albanese.

# Collagen diseases

## Cutaneous asthenia

### Lesion aetiology/pathogenesis and clinical picture

These are likely congenital disorders and are characterised by alterations in collagen fibres. They usually manifest with abnormally fragile skin that is easily stretched and can even tear.

The underlying aetiology in veterinary medicine is poorly understood, although certain specific breeds are thought to be predisposed.

Cutaneous asthenia or dermatosparaxis is the most recognised disease within this group.

### Diagnostic method

Diagnosis is usually based on the patient's clinical presentation. Elasticity and fragility of the skin are characteristic.

Histopathology shows marked dermal abnormalities.

### Main differential diagnoses

- Wounds of other causes
- Scarring

### Treatment

Supplementation with vitamin C can be very helpful. These animals should not be used for breeding and should be protected for life against possible lacerations.

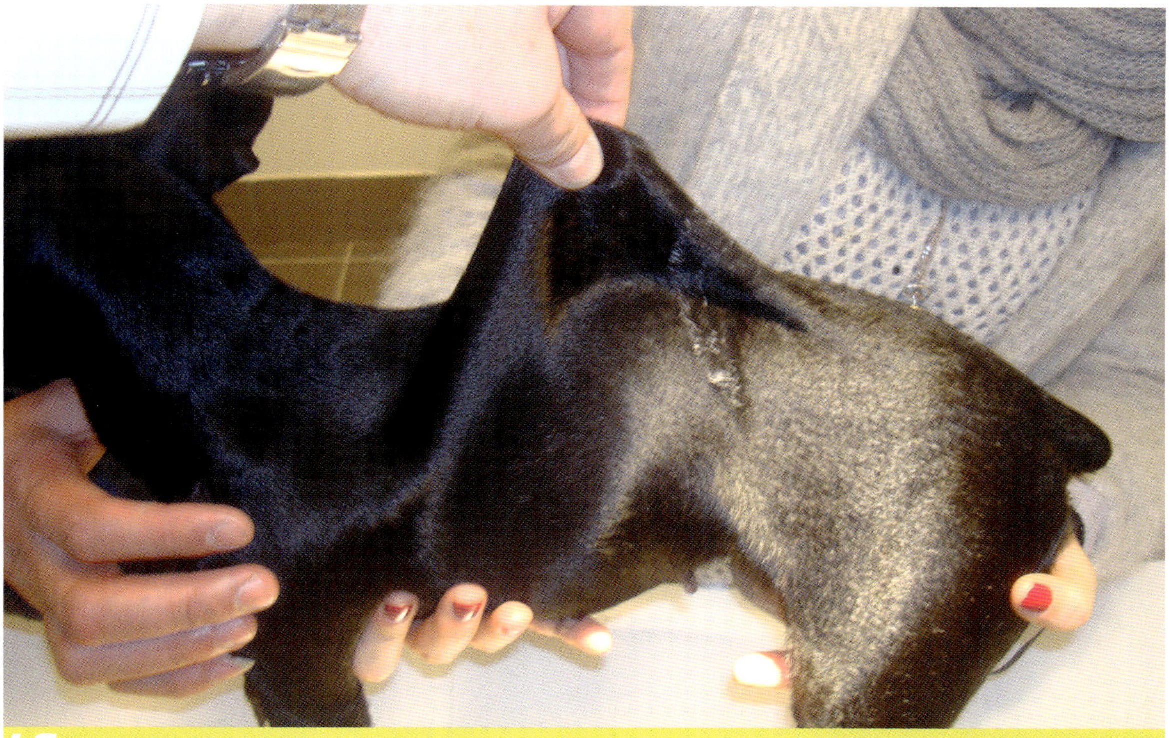

46 Marked cutaneous laxity in a dog with cutaneous asthenia.

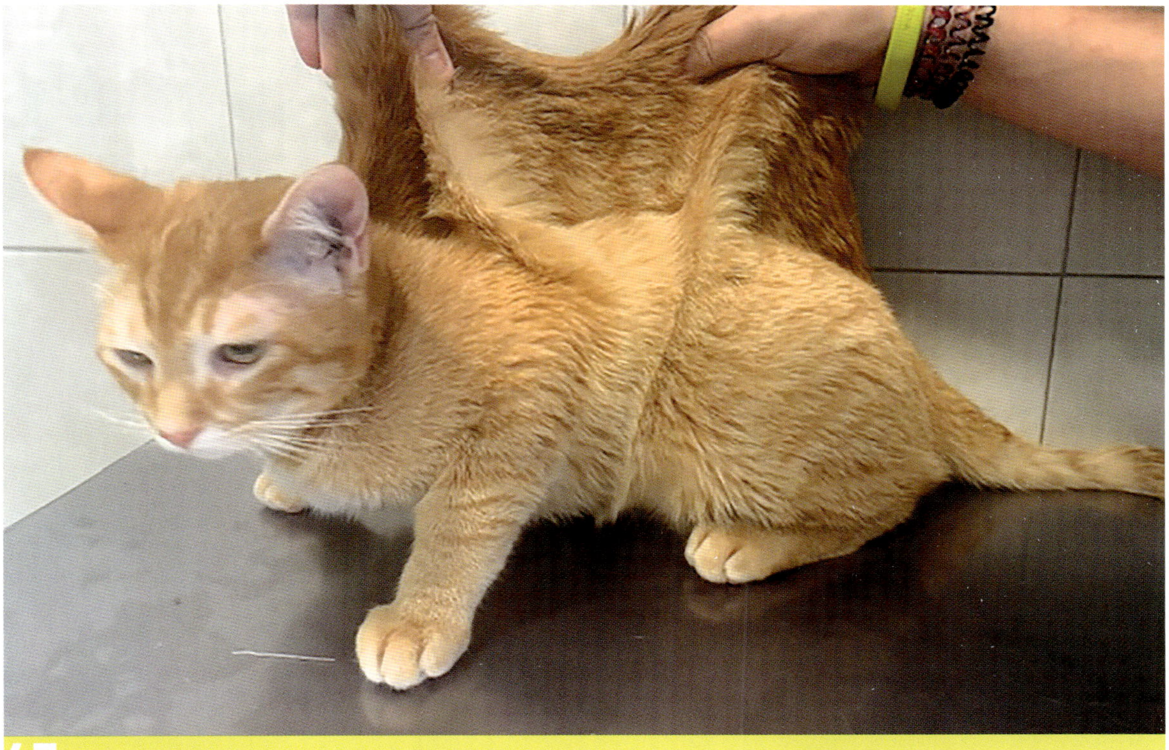

47 Cutaneous asthenia in a mixed-breed cat. Image courtesy of the Ronda Sur Veterinary Clinic.

## Feline auricular chondritis

### Lesion aetiology/pathogenesis and clinical picture

Feline auricular chondritis can be considered a form of relapsing polychondritis that causes inflammation and even necrosis of certain cartilaginous structures in the body, in this case the ears, mainly in cats. The aetiology is thought to involve an immune-mediated reaction targeting the collagen in cartilage. Some authors associate this process with prior trauma to the pinna.

Painful, swollen pinnae are quite characteristic.

### Diagnostic method

While the clinical picture is quite distinctive, biopsy is the only method that can confirm lymphoplasmacytic inflammation with necrosis.

### Main differential diagnoses

- Trauma
- Otohaematoma and subsequent retraction

### Treatment

Glucocorticosteroids have not shown great efficacy. Cyclosporine and dapsone are potential treatment options.

Surgical amputation provides a definitive solution to prevent pain.

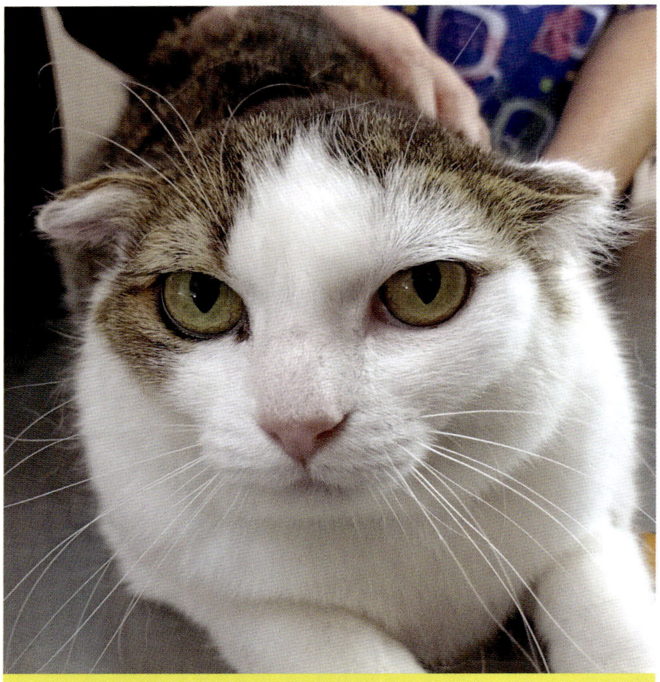

48 Folded pinnae in a cat with bilateral chondritis.

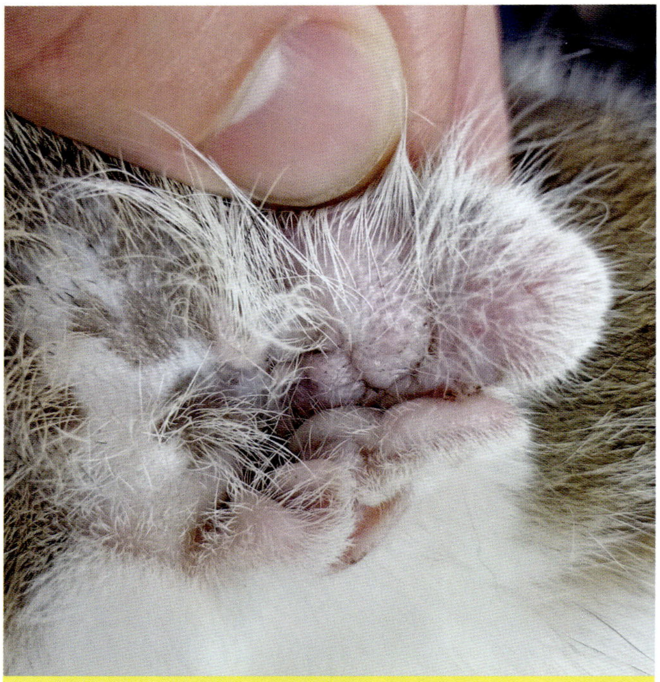

49 Pinna exhibiting inflammation and the onset of necrosis in a cat with chondritis.